Review of
Plastic
Surgery

D1428689

WITHDRAWN FROM
LIBRARY

BRITISH MEDICAL ASSOCIATION

0834805

Content Strategist: *Belinda Kuhn*
Content Development Specialist: *Poppy Garraway, Alexandra Mortimer*
Content Coordinator: *Trinity Hutton*
Project Manager: *Louisa Talbott*
Design: *Christian Bilbow*
Illustration Manager: *Emily Costantino*
Marketing Manager: *Melissa Fogarty*

Review of

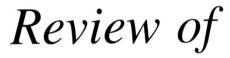

Plastic Surgery

Donald W. Buck II, MD

Assistant Professor

Plastic and Reconstructive Surgery
Washington University School of Medicine
St. Louis, MO, USA

Foreword by

Peter C. Neligan, MB, FRCS(I), FRCSC, FACS

Professor of Surgery, Division of Plastic Surgery
University of Washington
Seattle, WA, USA

Elsevier | ExpertConsult.com

For additional online content visit http://expertconsult.inkling.com

BMA LIBRARY
BRITISH MEDICAL ASSOCIATION

ELSEVIER   Edinburgh   London   New York   Oxford   Philadelphia   St. Louis   Sydney   Toronto   2016

ELSEVIER

© 2016, Elsevier Inc. All rights reserved.

No part of this publication may be reproduced or transmitted in any form or by any means, electronic or mechanical, including photocopying, recording, or any information storage and retrieval system, without permission in writing from the publisher. Details on how to seek permission, further information about the Publisher's permissions policies and our arrangements with organizations such as the Copyright Clearance Center and the Copyright Licensing Agency, can be found at our website: www.elsevier.com/permissions.

This book and the individual contributions contained in it are protected under copyright by the Publisher (other than as may be noted herein).

Notices

Knowledge and best practice in this field are constantly changing. As new research and experience broaden our understanding, changes in research methods, professional practices, or medical treatment may become necessary.

Practitioners and researchers must always rely on their own experience and knowledge in evaluating and using any information, methods, compounds, or experiments described herein. In using such information or methods, they should be mindful of their own safety and the safety of others, including parties for whom they have a professional responsibility.

With respect to any drug or pharmaceutical products identified, readers are advised to check the most current information provided (i) on procedures featured or (ii) by the manufacturer of each product to be administered to verify the recommended dose or formula, the method and duration of administration, and contraindications. It is the responsibility of practitioners, relying on their own experience and knowledge of their patients, to make diagnoses, to determine dosages and the best treatment for each individual patient, and to take all appropriate safety precautions.

To the fullest extent of the law, neither the Publisher nor the authors, contributors, or editors, assume any liability for any injury and/or damage to persons or property as a matter of products liability, negligence or otherwise or from any use or operation of any methods, products, instructions, or ideas contained in the material herein.

ISBN: 978-0-323-35491-2

your source for books,
journals and multimedia
in the health sciences

www.elsevierhealth.com

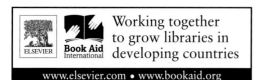

Working together
to grow libraries in
developing countries

www.elsevier.com • www.bookaid.org

The
publisher's
policy is to use
**paper manufactured
from sustainable forests**

Printed in China

Last digit is the print number: 9 8 7 6 5 4 3 2 1

Contents

Foreword

This book by Donald Buck is unique in several ways. It fills a niche segment of the plastic surgery literature, as it is aimed at residents and fellows training in plastic surgery. However, it is also of use to the full spectrum of those interested in plastic surgery, from medical students to attending physicians. This is not an encyclopedic textbook nor is it meant to be. It is meant as a review and that is exactly what it achieves. Each topic is presented in point format, excluding the fluff and including only what has to be known. Condensing material like this requires a lot of skill and knowledge, and Dr. Buck has achieved this with flying colors. The format and layout make it easy to read yet it is small enough to fit in a backpack or satchel. It is easy to find one's way round this book and it is ideal for quickly revisiting a topic before rounds or the operating room. It is extremely useful as a review for exams and for testing one's knowledge. This is really the genius of this book. Dr. Buck has invited renowned and recognized experts not specifically to write chapters, as most textbook editors do, but rather to write self-assessment questions that are fashioned as board-type questions. These individuals are not only household names in the specialty, but they are obviously experienced in the topic, as well as in educating residents and, more importantly, in examining them. This makes this book unique and incredibly useful.

Dr. Buck is to be congratulated not only in compiling this book but in having the wit to use his experts in an ingenious way. In doing so he has contributed invaluably to the education of the next generation of plastic surgeons. I think this book will become a standard resource for medical students, residents, and fellows.

by Peter C. Neligan

Preface

Plastic surgery is a vast specialty, encompassing the management of diseases and conditions from head to toe, in patients who are both young and old. With such a diverse and overarching surgical discipline, it comes as no surprise that our textbooks read like encyclopedias with seemingly limitless pages of detail and descriptions. An entire bookcase can easily be filled with textbook after textbook attempting to cover the topics that we encounter as plastic surgeons. As a student, resident, or young attending, the vastness of plastic surgery can become overwhelming, and it is easy to get lost in the details. One quick look at the six volumes required to cover our specialty in *Plastic Surgery 3rd Edition* alone can generate a tremendous amount of heartburn. This is particularly true during examination time, be it the in-service examination for trainees or the written examination for plastic surgery certification.

I vividly remember the anxiety surrounding the exam preparation process and my disbelief at the lack of a "go-to" plastic surgery review book highlighting frequently tested, high-yield facts for the in-service exam and written boards. It seemed that all other specialties had one: a handy companion book with tattered pages of fruitful facts, figures, and illustrations that covered the broad topics and themes of the specialty, perfect for focused studying and examination review. The purpose of this book is to fill that void and serve as a trustworthy companion to students, residents, and young plastic surgeons alike.

This book is not intended to be a replacement for your favorite plastic surgery textbooks or "encyclopedias," nor is it meant to cover the minutiae of our specialty. Instead, it is intended to provide a foundation of plastic surgery fundamentals and themes upon which further details can be added. It is also intended to serve as an added resource for treating the anxiety and heartburn of examination preparation by providing a useful, relevant, and easily accessible collection of high-yield topics and facts covering plastic surgery.

The book consists of 30 chapters, conveniently designed to align with the defined topics that are frequently covered in plastic surgery examinations. Within each chapter are numerous pearls of wisdom and abundant facts in bulleted format that cover some of the most frequently tested topics. These pearls are complemented by beautiful figures and illustrations that further drive home important concepts and themes. In addition, each chapter has dedicated exam-style multiple-choice questions written by topic experts from around the world, to test your knowledge and enhance your preparation through creation of a practice exam.

It is my sincere hope that you find this book useful and comforting and that it will help to alleviate some of the anxiety associated with rotations, examinations, and review of our awesome specialty. Best of luck!

Donald W. Buck II

List of Question Contributors

Sonya Agnew, MD
Assistant Professor
Division of Plastic Surgery, Department of
Surgery
Department of Orthopaedic Surgery and
Rehabilitation
Loyola University Medical Center
Maywood, IL, USA
*Chapter 15. Hand Masses, Vascular
Disorders, and Dupuytren's Contracture,
Questions 1–5*

Jamil Ahmad, MD, FRCSC
Lecturer, Division of Plastic and
Reconstructive Surgery
Department of Surgery
University of Toronto
Toronto, Ontario, Canada
*Chapter 27. Rhinoplasty and Nasal
Reconstruction, Questions 1–5*

C. Bob Basu, MD, MPH, FACS
Director, Basu Center for Aesthetics &
Plastic Surgery
Chief of Plastic Surgery
North Cypress Medical Center
Houston, TX, USA
*Chapter 1. Anesthesia, Practice Management,
Patient Safety, and Coding, Questions 1–5*

Phillip Blondeel, MD, PhD
Professor of Plastic Surgery
Department of Plastic and Reconstructive
Surgery
University Hospital Ghent
Ghent, Belgium
*Chapter 9. Breast Cancer and Breast
Reconstruction, Questions 1–5*

Lucas Boehm, PharmD
Medical College of Wisconsin
Milwaukee, WI, USA
*Chapter 8. Breast Anatomy, Embryology,
and Congenital Defects, Questions 1–15*

Donald W. Buck II, MD
Assistant Professor
Plastic & Reconstructive Surgery
Washington University School of Medicine
St. Louis, MO, USA
*Chapter 2. Head and Neck Anatomy and
Facial Palsy, Questions 1–5*
*Chapter 4. Craniofacial Trauma, Questions
1–5*
Chapter 7. Ear Reconstruction, Questions 1–5
*Chapter 19. Tendon Injuries and
Reconstruction. Questions 1–5*
*Chapter 20. Wound Healing and Tissue
Expansion, Questions 1–5*
*Chapter 22. Burns and Burn Reconstruction,
Questions 1–10*
*Chapter 25. Flaps and Microsurgery,
Questions 1–5*

Ming-Huei Cheng, MD, MBA, FACS
Professor and Vice President
Department of Plastic and Reconstructive
Surgery
Chang Gung Memorial Hospital
Taoyuan, Taiwan
*Chapter 13. Lower Extremity Reconstruction
and Lymphedema, Questions 1–5*

Brian M. Derby, MD
Private Practice
Sarasota Plastic Surgery Center
Sarasota, FL, USA
*Chapter 26. Eyelid Anatomy, Reconstruction,
and Blepharoplasty, Questions 1–5*

Brent Egeland, MD
Attending Surgeon
Institute of Reconstructive Plastic Surgery
University Medical Center Brackenridge
Austin, TX, USA
*Chapter 19. Tendon Injuries and
Reconstruction, Questions 6–10*

Marco Ellis, MD
Director of Craniofacial Surgery
Northwestern Specialists in Plastic Surgery
Northwestern University
University of Illinois Chicago
Chicago, IL, USA
*Chapter 26. Eyelid Anatomy, Reconstruction,
and Blepharoplasty, Questions 6–10*

Neil A. Fine, MD
President NSPS
Clinical Associate Professor
Division of Plastic Surgery
Northwestern University, Feinberg School
of Medicine
Chicago, IL, USA
*Chapter 9. Breast Cancer and Breast
Reconstruction, Questions 6–13*

Ida Fox, MD
Assistant Professor of Plastic Surgery
Department of Surgery
Washington University School of Medicine
St. Louis, MO, USA
*Chapter 12. Peripheral Nerve Injuries,
Brachial Plexus, and Compression
Neuropathies, Questions 1–5*

Robert D. Galiano, MD, FACS
Associate Professor
Director of Research
Division of Plastic Surgery
Northwestern University, Feinberg School
of Medicine
Chicago, IL, USA
*Chapter 20. Wound Healing and Tissue
Expansion, Questions 6–10*

Catharine B. Garland, MD
Chief Resident, Plastic Surgery
Department of Surgery
University of California San Francisco
San Francisco, CA, USA
*Chapter 27. Rhinoplasty and Nasal
Reconstruction, Questions 6–10*

Patrick B. Garvey, MD, FACS
Associate Professor of Plastic Surgery
Department of Plastic Surgery
The University of Texas MD Anderson
Cancer Center
Houston, Texas, USA
*Chapter 11. Trunk Reconstruction and
Pressure Sores, Questions 1–5*

Amanda Gosman, MD
Associate Professor
Division of Plastic Surgery
University of California San Diego
San Diego, CA, USA
*Chapter 4. Craniofacial Trauma, Questions
6–10*

Ronald P. Gruber, MD
Clinical Associate Professor
Divisions of Plastic and Reconstructive
Surgery
University of California
San Francisco, CA, USA
Adjunct Clinical Associate Professor
Stanford University Medical Center
Stanford, CA, USA
*Chapter 27. Rhinoplasty and Nasal
Reconstruction, Questions 6–10*

Anandev Gurjala, MD, MS
Attending Surgeon
Department of Plastic and Reconstructive
Surgery
Kaiser Permanente San Francisco
San Francisco, CA, USA
*Chapter 24. Malignant Skin Conditions,
Questions 1–5*

Jeffrey A. Gusenoff, MD
Associate Professor of Plastic Surgery
Co-Director, Life After Weight Loss
Program
Department of Plastic Surgery
University of Pittsburgh
Pittsburgh, PA, USA
*Chapter 29. Body Contouring and Suction-
Assisted Lipectomy, Questions 1–5*

Kristy L. Hamilton, MD
Plastic Surgery Resident
Division of Plastic Surgery
Baylor College of Medicine
Houston, TX, USA
*Chapter 11. Trunk Reconstruction and
Pressure Sores, Questions 1–5*

James P. Higgins, MD
Chief, Curtis National Hand Center
Union Memorial Hospital
Baltimore, MD, USA
*Chapter 18. Carpal Injuries and Hand
Arthritis, Questions 1–5*

John B. Hijjawi, MD, FACS
Program Director
Reconstructive Microsurgery Fellowship
Associate Professor
Department of Plastic Surgery
Medical College of Wisconsin
Milwaukee, WI, USA
*Chapter 8. Breast Anatomy, Embryology,
and Congenital Defects, Questions 1–15*

Elliot M. Hirsch, MD
Division of Plastic and Reconstructive
Surgery
Feinberg School of Medicine
Northwestern University
Chicago, IL, USA
*Chapter 23. Benign Skin Conditions and
Skin Disorders, Questions 1–5*

Peter S. Kim, MD
Clinical Instructor of Surgery
Department of Surgery
Beth Israel Deaconess Medical Center
Harvard Medical School
Boston, MA, USA
*Chapter 16. Hand Fractures and
Dislocations, Questions 1–10*

Grant M. Kleiber, MD
Assistant Professor of Surgery
Division of Plastic and Reconstructive
Surgery
Washington University School of Medicine
St. Louis, MO, USA
*Chapter 15. Hand Masses, Vascular
Disorders, and Dupuytren's Contracture,
Questions 6–10*

Jason H. Ko, MD
Assistant Professor of Surgery
Division of Plastic Surgery and Department
of Orthopaedics and Sports Medicine
University of Washington School of
Medicine
Seattle, WA, USA
*Chapter 17. Nail-Bed Injuries, Soft-Tissue
Amputations, and Replantation, Questions
1–10*

Jeffrey H. Kozlow, MD, MS
Assistant Professor
Section of Plastic Surgery
University of Michigan Health System
Ann Arbor, MI, USA
*Chapter 21. Soft-Tissue and Hand Infections,
Questions 1–5*

Brian I. Labow, MD, FACS, FAAP
Associate Professor of Surgery
Boston Children's Hospital, Harvard
Medical School
Boston, MA, USA
*Chapter 14. Congenital Hand Disorders,
Questions 1–5*

Victor L. Lewis, Jr., MD
Professor of Clinical Surgery
Division of Plastic Surgery
Feinberg School of Medicine
Northwestern University
Chicago, IL, USA
*Chapter 23. Benign Skin Conditions and
Skin Disorders, Questions 6–11*

Frank Lista, MD, FRCSC
Assistant Professor
Division of Plastic and Reconstructive
Surgery
Department of Surgery
University of Toronto
Toronto, Ontario, Canada
Chapter 10. Noncancer Breast Surgery,
Questions 1–5

Samir Mardini, MD
Professor of Surgery
Program Director
Division of Plastic Surgery
Department of Surgery
Mayo Clinic College of Medicine
Rochester, MN, USA
Chapter 3. Head and Neck Cancer,
Odontogenic Tumors, and Vascular
Anomalies, Questions 1–5

Derek L. Masden, MD
Plastic Surgery/Hand Surgery, Washington
Hospital Center
Assistant Clinical Professor
Department of Plastic Surgery, Georgetown
University Hospital
Washington, DC, USA
Chapter 18. Carpal Injuries and Hand
Arthritis, Questions 6–14

Martha S. Matthews, MD, FACS
Professor of Surgery
Department of Surgery
Division of Plastic Surgery, Cooper
Medical School of Rowan University
Camden, NJ, USA
Chapter 1. Anesthesia, Practice Management,
Patient Safety, and Coding, Questions 6–10

Mary H. McGrath, MD, MPH, FACS
Professor of Surgery and Associate Chair
Department of Surgery
Division of Plastic Surgery
University of California San Francisco
San Francisco, CA, USA
Chapter 24. Malignant Skin Conditions,
Questions 6–10

Amy M. Moore, MD
Assistant Professor of Surgery
Division of Plastic and Reconstructive
Surgery
Department of Surgery
Washington University School of Medicine
St. Louis, MO, USA
Chapter 14. Congenital Hand Disorders,
Questions 6–10

Gerhard S. Mundinger, MD
Craniofacial Surgery Fellow/Acting
Instructor
Division of Craniofacial and Plastic Surgery
Seattle Children's Hospital
Harborview Medical Center
University of Washington Medical Center
Seattle, WA, USA
Chapter 3. Head and Neck Cancer,
Odontogenic Tumors, and Vascular
Anomalies, Questions 6–10

Terence Myckatyn, MD
Associate Professor
Division of Plastic and Reconstructive
Surgery
Washington University School of Medicine
St. Louis, MO, USA
Chapter 10. Noncancer Breast Surgery,
Questions 6–10

Maurice Y. Nahabedian, MD
Professor and Vice Chairman
Department of Plastic Surgery
Georgetown University
Washington, DC, USA
Chapter 8. Breast Anatomy, Embryology,
and Congenital Defects, Questions 16–20

Peter C. Neligan, MB, FRCS(I), FRCSC,
FACS
Professor of Surgery
Division of Plastic Surgery
University of Washington
Seattle, WA, USA
Chapter 25. Flaps and Microsurgery,
Questions 6–10

Ashit Patel, MBChB, FACS
Associate Professor
Division of Plastic Surgery
Albany Medical Center
Albany, NY, USA
Chapter 21. Soft-Tissue and Hand Infections,
Questions 6–10

Kamlesh B. Patel, MD
Assistant Professor of Plastic Surgery
Department of Surgery
Washington University St. Louis
St. Louis, MO, USA
Chapter 5. Craniosynostosis and Craniofacial
Syndromes, Questions 1–5

Pravin K. Patel, MD, FACS
Professor of Surgery and Chief of
Craniofacial Surgery
Division of Plastic, Reconstructive, and
Cosmetic Surgery
The University of Illinois at Chicago
Chicago, IL, USA
Chapter 6. Clefts and Orthognathic Surgery,
Questions 1–5

Jason Roostaeian, MD
Assistant Clinical Professor
Division of Plastic Surgery
David Geffen School of Medicine
University of California Los Angeles
Los Angeles, CA, USA
Chapter 28. Rhytidectomy and Neck
Rejuvenation, Questions 1–10

Michel Saint-Cyr, MD, FRCS(C)
Director, Division of Plastic Surgery
Wigley Professorship in Plastic Surgery
Baylor, Scott & White Health
Scott & White Memorial Hospital
Temple, TX, USA
Chapter 11. Trunk Reconstruction and
Pressure Sores, Questions 6–10

Clark Schierle, MD, PhD, FACS
Director of Aesthetic Surgery
Northwestern Specialists in Plastic Surgery,
S.C.
Adjunct Assistant Professor, University of
Illinois at Chicago
Chicago, IL, USA
*Chapter 30. Injectables, Skin Resurfacing,
Lasers, and Hair Restoration, Questions 1–10*

Basel Sharaf, MD, DDS
Mayo Clinic
Rochester, MN, USA
*Chapter 3. Head and Neck Cancer,
Odontogenic Tumors, and Vascular
Anomalies, Questions 1–5*

John W. Shuck, MD
Resident Physician
Department of Plastic Surgery
Georgetown University Hospital
Washington, DC, USA
*Chapter 18. Carpal Injuries and Hand
Arthritis, Questions 1–5*

Alison Snyder-Warwick, MD
Assistant Professor of Surgery
Department of Surgery, Division of Plastic
and Reconstructive Surgery
Washington University School of Medicine
St. Louis, MO, USA
*Chapter 2. Head and Neck Anatomy and
Facial Palsy, Questions 6–10*

Jason M. Souza, MD
Lieutenant Commander
Medical Corps, US Navy
Division of Plastic and Reconstructive
Surgery
Walter Reed National Military Medical
Center
Bethesda, MD, USA
*Chapter 12. Peripheral Nerve Injuries,
Brachial Plexus, and Compression
Neuropathies, Questions 6–10*

Jordan P. Steinberg, MD, PhD
Pediatric Craniofacial Surgery Fellow
Children's Healthcare of Atlanta
Atlanta, GA, USA
*Chapter 5. Craniosynostosis and Craniofacial
Syndromes, Questions 6–10*

Jon Ver Halen, MD, FACS
Associate Professor of Surgery
Division of Plastic Surgery
Texas A&M University, Baylor Scott &
White Health
Temple, TX, USA
*Chapter 29. Body Contouring and Suction-
Assisted Lipectomy, Questions 6–10*

Aparna Vijayasekaran, MBBS, MDS
Plastic Surgery Resident
Department of Plastic and Reconstructive
Surgery
The Mayo Clinic
Rochester, MN, USA
*Chapter 11. Trunk Reconstruction and
Pressure Sores, Questions 6–10*

Albert S. Woo, MD
Chief, Pediatric Plastic Surgery
Director, Cleft Palate–Craniofacial Institute
St. Louis Children's Hospital
Associate Professor of Plastic Surgery
Department of Surgery
Washington University School of Medicine
St. Louis, MO, USA
*Chapter 6. Clefts and Orthognathic Surgery,
Questions 6–10*

Akira Yamada, MD, PhD
Department of Plastic Surgery
Northwestern University, Feinberg School
of Medicine
Ann & Robert Lurie Children's Hospital of
Chicago
Chicago, IL, USA
*Chapter 7. Ear Reconstruction, Questions
6–10*

Shuji Yamashita, MD, PhD
Assistant Professor
Department of Plastic and Reconstructive
Surgery
The University of Tokyo
Tokyo, Japan
*Chapter 13. Lower Extremity Reconstruction
and Lymphedema, Questions 6–10*

Acknowledgments

I must first thank the wonderful team at Elsevier for the incredible opportunity to create this book. It has been a true privilege working alongside Belinda Kuhn, Poppy Garraway, Alex Mortimer, and Trinity Hutton. I am indebted to their support, encouragement, expertise, and patience along the way. I would also like to thank all of the contributors to the book who have graciously added their expertise to this work—I am truly grateful!

Finally, and most important, I would like to thank my beautiful wife, Jennifer, and my children, Benjamin and Brooke, for their unwavering love and support. They inspire me to be better every day, and without them, none of this would have been possible.

DWB

Dedication

This book is dedicated to my family, teachers, mentors, and colleagues and to all plastic surgeons—past, present, and future—who carry the legacy of our specialty forward.

Anesthesia, Practice Management, Patient Safety, and Coding

Chapter

1

General Anesthesia

1. Intravenous agents: Primarily used for induction of anesthesia or sedation anesthesia, such as monitored anesthesia care (MAC) sedation.
   - Propofol is commonly used because it is short acting, associated with smooth emergence, and reduction of nausea and vomiting. Limitations of propofol include hypotension and pain on injection
   - Ketamine causes a dissociative state and is the only induction agent that increases blood pressure and heart rate.

   - Frequently used for conscious sedation in children
   - Intravenous ketamine has more rapid onset, shorter duration of action, and a lower risk of laryngospasm than intramuscular ketamine (see Table 1.1).

2. Inhalational agents: Often used today for maintenance of anesthesia after intravenous induction.
   - Supplemented by intravenous opioids for pain and muscle relaxants or paralytics
   - Most commonly used today are isoflurane, sevoflurane, and desflurane (see Table 1.2)

Table 1.1 Clinical Characteristics of Intravenous Induction Agents

IV INDUCTION AGENT	DOSE (MG/KG)	COMMENTS	SIDE EFFECTS	SITUATIONS REQUIRING CAUTION	RELATIVE INDICATIONS
Thiopental	2-5	Inexpensive; slow emergence after high doses	Hypotension	Hypovolemia; compromised cardiac function	Suitable for induction in many patients
Ketamine	1-2	Psychotropic side effects controllable with benzodiazepines; good bronchodilator; potent analgesic at subinduction doses	Hypertension; tachycardia	Coronary disease; severe hypovolemia	Rapid-sequence induction of asthmatics, patients in shock (reduced doses)
Propofol	1-2	Burns on injection; good bronchodilator; associated with low incidence of postoperative nausea and vomiting	Hypotension	Coronary artery disease; hypovolemia	Induction of outpatients; induction of asthmatics
Etomidate	0.1-0.3	Cardiovascularly stable; burns on injection; spontaneous movement during induction	Adrenal suppression (with continuous infusion)	Hypovolemia	Induction of patients with cardiac contractile dysfunction; induction of patients in shock (reduced doses)
Midazolam	0.15-0.3	Relatively stable hemodynamics; potent amnesia	Synergistic ventilatory depression with opioids	Hypovolemia	Induction of patients with cardiac contractile dysfunction (usually in combination with opioids)

Reprinted from Townsend, C.M., Beauchamp, R.D., Evers, B.M., et al. (Eds.), 2012. Sabiston Textbook of Surgery, 19th ed. Saunders.

Table 1.2 Important Characteristics of Inhalational Agents

ANESTHETIC	POTENCY	SPEED OF INDUCTION AND EMERGENCE	SUITABILITY FOR INHALATIONAL INDUCTION	SENSITIZATION TO CATECHOLAMINES	METABOLIZED (%)
Nitrous oxide	Weak	Fast	Insufficient alone	None	Minimal
Diethyl ether	Potent	Very slow	Suitable	None	10
Halothane	Potent	Medium	Suitable	High	20+
Enflurane	Potent	Medium	Not suitable	Medium	<10
Isoflurane	Potent	Medium	Not suitable	Minimal	<2
Sevoflurane	Potent	Rapid	Suitable	Minimal	<5
Desflurane	Potent	Rapid	Not suitable	Minimal	0.02

Reprinted from Townsend, C.M., Beauchamp, R.D., Evers, B.M., et al. (Eds.), 2012. Sabiston Textbook of Surgery, 19th ed. Saunders.

3. Neuromuscular blocking agents: Useful for muscle paralysis as well as rapid induction
   - Two categories of agents: Depolarizing and nondepolarizing
   - Succinylcholine
     - The only depolarizing agent still in use
     - Typically used only for rapid sequence intubation (produces rapid onset and short duration of action)
     - Disadvantages: Associated with malignant hyperthermia and hyperkalemia (especially with burns, paralyzed patients, and massive trauma patients)
   - Nondepolarizing agents
     - Most commonly used today
     - Longer duration of action
4. Opioids: Used as adjuncts to anesthesia for analgesia
   - Most common agents: Fentanyl- and synthetic fentanyl–based agents (e.g., sulfentanil, remifentanil, and alfentanil), morphine, hydromorphone, and meperidine
     - Fentanyl, and its synthetic derivatives, is frequently used because it is 100-150 times more potent than morphine and has a rapid onset and short duration of action.
   - Disadvantages of opioids: Respiratory depression

5. Benzodiazepines: Frequently used for anxiolysis before induction, amnesia, as well as in some conscious sedation protocols
   - Common agents include diazepam and midazolam
   - Useful for the treatment of local anesthetic toxicity

Local Anesthesia

1. Delivery of anesthetic to local tissues to provide focused anesthesia to the surgical site/field
2. Local anesthetic agents are frequently used with regional blocks, conscious sedation, and deep sedation techniques; may also be used with general anesthesia to provide postoperative anesthesia or assist with hemostasis (e.g., epinephrine effects).
3. Two classes: Esthers and amides
   - Esther compounds are more rapidly hydrolyzed by plasma pseudocholinesterases and have shorter durations of action.
     - Allergic reactions to local anesthetics are much more common with ester compounds.
   - Amide compounds are degraded by the liver.
4. Commonly used local anesthetic agents (see Table 1.3)

Table 1.3 Commonly Used Local Anesthetic Agents

AGENT	CLASS	DURATION OF ACTION (MIN)	RECOMMENDED DOSAGE GUIDELINES (MG/KG)	MAXIMUM TOTAL DAMAGE (MG)
Procaine (Novocain)	Ester	15-60	7	35-600
Chloroprocaine (Novocain)	Ester	15-30	Without epinephrine: 11 With epinephrine: 14	800 1000
Lidocaine (Xylocaine)	Amide	30-60	Without epinephrine: 4.5	300
		120-360	With epinephrine: 7	
Mepivacaine (Carbocaine)	Amide	45-90	7	400
Bupivacaine (Marcaine)	Amide	120-240 180-420	Without epinephrine: 2.5 With epinephrine: 2.5-4	175 225-400
Prilocaine (Citanest)	Amide	30-90	8	500-600

Reprinted from Mustoe, T.A., Buck, D.W., Lalonde, D.H., 2010. Plast. Reconstr. Surg. 126 (4), 165–176. Adapted from multiple sources.

5. 4% topical cocaine
   - Was commonly used for nasal surgery (e.g., rhinoplasty, septoplasty) because of rapid mucosal absorption and subsequent onset of action.
   - Maximum dosage: 1.5 mg/kg
   - Infrequently used today because of the potential for coronary vasoconstriction
6. Epinephrine
   - Frequently added to local anesthetics to provide
     - A slight increase in the maximum dosage of anesthetic allowed
     - Local vasoconstriction
       - Reduces the amount of anesthetic required for effect due to reduction in diffusion of the compound
       - Assists with hemostasis
   - Epinephrine-containing lidocaine compounds have been safely used in the digits
     - Treatment of ischemia related to epinephrine (e.g., a pale finger) injection includes conservative measures (e.g., elevation; consider warm/cold compresses) and phentolamine injection.
7. Toxicity
   - Although rare, systemic toxicity can be observed with excess local anesthetic administration.
   - Signs of toxicity
     - Headache, tinnitus, perioral and tongue paresthesias (early findings)
     - Restlessness
     - Seizures
     - Respiratory arrest and cardiac collapse (late finding)
   - Treatment
     - Respiratory and circulatory support (e.g., airway control, 100% oxygen administration, intravenous fluids)
     - Benzodiazepines (useful for early neurologic signs)
     - Intravenous lipid administration
   - Intra-arterial injection of bupivacaine can cause irreversible heart block and cardiac collapse.
8. Tumescent solution (also known as "wetting solution")
   - Prepared by combining lidocaine and epinephrine to saline to create a dilute solution of local anesthetic that can be safely infiltrated into the soft tissues.
   - Allows for much larger dosages of lidocaine use (up to 35 mg/kg).

- Systemic levels of lidocaine peak at 12 to 14 hours below the clavicles and 6 to 12 hours above the clavicles.
  - This is important when performing both trunk and head and neck procedures to prevent overlap of peaks and potential for toxicity
9. Topical anesthetics
   - Topical combination anesthetic formulations that are useful in children to provide anesthesia without the trauma of injection
   - Common agents
     - LET (lidocaine, epinephrine, and tetracaine)
     - Eutectic mixture of local anesthetics (EMLA), lidocaine, and prilocaine; small risk of methemoglobinemia because of the prilocaine
     - ELA-Max (liposomal lidocaine): More rapid onset of action
   - Disadvantages: Requires prolonged contact with site for anesthetic effect (e.g., 30-60 minutes)
10. Regional nerve block
    - Involves infiltration of local anesthetic in the vicinity of a sensory nerve distant from the surgical site to provide local anesthesia.
    - Advantages: Avoid tissue distortion from anesthetic infiltration; reduce the amount of anesthetic required for effect.
    - Bier block: Use of a double tourniquet and intravenous administration of lidocaine to provide upper extremity anesthesia
      - Lidocaine toxicity can occur with a nonfunctioning tourniquet, inappropriate early release of the tourniquet, and a poorly functioning tourniquet (e.g., a tourniquet that is too small or too large for the given extremity).
11. Conscious sedation
    - Uses a combination of anesthetics and opioids to provide an altered level of consciousness to a relaxed state while maintaining airway protection.
    - Titration of medications is tailored to the patient's vital signs and state of alertness.
    - Most recommend small, incremental dosing of sedation agents to maintain a stable level of anesthesia and reduce the risk for overmedication and oversedation.
    - Advantages: Reduced risk of deep venous thrombosis, postoperative nausea and vomiting, faster recovery, and fewer unplanned admissions.
    - Common agents for conscious sedation (see Table 1.4)

Table 1.4 Commonly Used Agents for Conscious Sedation

AGENT	CLASS	COMMON DOSAGE GUIDELINES	SIDE EFFECTS
Midazolam	Benzodiazepine	0.5-1 mg every 5-10 min per patient alertness	Respiratory depression, somnolence, amnesia
Diazepam	Benzodiazepine	10-50 mg preoperatively	Respiratory depression, somnolence
Lorazepam	Benzodiazepine	0.5-2 mg per os 0.25-1 mg intravenously	Respiratory depression, somnolence
Ketamine	Dissociative anesthetic	200-750 mcg/kg bolus, followed by 5- to 20-mcg/kg/min infusion	Hallucinogens, delirium, intracranial hypertension, increased respiratory secretions, cardiac simulation
Clonidine	Alpha-2 agonist	0.1-0.2 mg preoperatively	Hypotension, rebound tachycardia, flushing
Fentanyl	Opioid receptor agonist	25-50 mcg every 5-10 min per patient alertness	Respiratory depression, somnolence, nausea, vomiting
Reversal agents			
Flumazenil	Benzodiazepine receptor antagonist	0.2-mg incremental doses to maximum of 1 mg	Dizziness, blurred vision, headache, nausea, flushing, injection-site pain, agitation
Naloxone	Opioid antagonist	0.1- to 0.2-mg incremental doses every 2-3 min to desired degree of reversal	Hypotension, hypertension, arrhythmias, dyspnea, pulmonary edema, agitation, flushing, nausea

Reprinted from Mustoe, T.A., Buck, D.W., Lalonde, D.H., 2010. Plast. Reconstr. Surg. 126 (4), 165–176. Adapted from multiple sources.

Complications of Anesthesia

1. Allergy
2. Cardiovascular toxicity
3. Postoperative nausea and vomiting (PONV)
   - Affects approximately one-third of all surgical patients
   - Multifactorial etiology and includes the chemoreceptor trigger zone within the brain stem
     - The chemoreceptor trigger zone has receptors for dopamine, acetylcholine, histamine, and serotonin.
   - Risk factors: Female gender, nonsmoking status, history of PONV, history of opioid-induced nausea and vomiting, inhalational anesthetics, long operative duration
   - Treatment is pharmacologic, with a focus on prophylaxis in high-risk patients (see Table 1.5)
4. Malignant hyperthermia
   - Life-threatening hypermetabolic event that occurs after exposure to inhalational anesthetics (e.g., halothane, enflurane, isoflurane, sevoflurane) and depolarizing muscle relaxants (e.g., succinylcholine)
   - Autosomal dominant inheritance with variable penetrance
   - Clinical manifestations
     - Fever
     - Tachycardia
     - Arrhythmia
     - Acidosis
     - Muscle rigidity
     - Tachypnea
     - Skin flushing
     - Hypotension

Table 1.5 Commonly Used Antiemetic Agents

DRUG CLASS	COMMON SIDE EFFECTS
Dopamine Receptor Antagonists (DA-2)	

Phenothiazines
  Fluphenazine
  Chlorpromazine
  Prochlorperazine
Butyrophenones
  Droperidol
  Haloperidol
Substituted benzamide
Metoclopramide
	Sedation
	Dissociation
	Extrapyramidal effects

Antihistamines (H)	
Diphenhydramine Promethazine	Sedation Dry mouth
Anticholinergics	
Scopolamine Atropine	Sedation Dry mouth Tachycardia
Serotonin Receptor Antagonists	
Ondansetron Dolasetron	Headache
Corticosteroids	
Dexamethasone Methylprednisolone Hydrocortisone	Glucose intolerance Altered wound healing Immunosuppression Renal effects

Reprinted from Townsend, C.M. (Eds.), 2012. Sabiston Textbook of Surgery, 19th ed. Saunders.

- ■ Rhabdomyolysis
- ■ Increased end-tidal CO_2
  - • Treatment: Hyperventilation with 100% oxygen, dantrolene administration, termination of surgery, supportive care
5. Methemoglobinemia
   - • Rare, life-threatening complication associated with topical and local anesthetics (e.g., prilocaine, benzocaine, and lidocaine)
   - • The anesthetic oxidizes the iron component of hemoglobin such that it cannot bind and transport oxygen.
   - • Characterized by progressive signs including graying of skin, headache, weakness, cyanosis with brown discoloration of blood, arrhythmias, seizures, and finally anoxic brain injury and death.
   - • Treatment: Administration of 100% oxygen, intravenous methylene blue

Pain Control

1. Effective postoperative pain control is important for patient comfort, as well as surgical outcome, because untreated pain is associated with prolonged hospital stay, deep venous thrombosis, pulmonary embolus, pneumonia, bowel dysmotility, insomnia, and impaired wound healing.

2. Many analgesics today can be administered orally, intravenously, intramuscularly, or locally through indwelling pain "pumps" and patient-controlled systems.
3. For severe pain, multimodality and/or multidrug treatment is often necessary.
4. Commonly used analgesic agents (see Table 1.6)

Practice Management

1. HIPAA: Health Insurance Portability and Accountability Act
   - • Created to protect patient privacy. Covers medical records and photography.
   - • Patients must be notified of their rights with respect to their personal medical information.
     - ■ Right to restrict use/disclosure
     - ■ Right to inspect/copy records
     - ■ Right to amend records
     - ■ Right to audit the disclosure of records
   - • Personal medical information must be recorded in a de-identified manner for research purposes. This information includes
     - ■ Patient name
     - ■ Contact information
       - ○ Address
       - ○ Telephone/fax numbers
       - ○ Email address

Table 1.6 Commonly Used Analgesics

AGENT	CLASS	ROUTE	DOSAGE GUIDELINES	MAXIMUM DAILY DOSAGE	SIDE EFFECTS/ADVERSE REACTIONS
Acetaminophen	NSAID	PO, PR	325-650 mg every 6-8 hr	4000 mg	Hepatic dysfunction in overdose; reduce dose in alcoholics
Ibuprofen	NSAID	PO	200-800 mg	2400 mg	Bleeding, gastrointestinal discomfort, renal failure
Ketorolac	NSAID	IV	30 mg every 8 hr	90 mg	Bleeding, gastrointestinal discomfort, renal failure
Diclofenac	COX-2 inhibitor	PO	75 mg BID	150 mg	Bleeding, gastrointestinal discomfort, renal failure
Celecoxib	COX-2 inhibitor	PO	100-200 mg BID	200-400 mg	Gastrointestinal discomfort, CV risk
Rofecoxib	GABA analog	PO	12.5 mg daily	25 mg	Gastrointestinal discomfort, CV risk
Gabapentin	GABA analog	PO	300-600 mg TID	3600 mg (limit dose in renal failure patients)	Dizziness, somnolence, peripheral edema
Pregabalin	Weak opioid	PO	75-150 mg BID	300-450 mg	Dizziness, somnolence, confusion, dry mouth, blurred vision
Tramadol	Weak opioid	PO, IV, IM	50-100 mg QID		Sedation
Codeine	Weak opioid	PO	15-60 mg every 4 hr	3 mg/kg/day	Sedation
Morphine	Strong opioid	IV	1-2 mg every 2-4 hr		Respiratory depression, nausea, vomiting
Hydromorphone	Strong opioid	PO	2-10 mg every 6 hr		Respiratory depression, constipation, nausea, hypotension
		IV	0.25-1 mg every 2-4 hr		
Acetominophen/ hydrocodone	Mixed	PO	500 mg/5 mg every 4-6 hr	4000 mg acetaminophen	Lightheadedness, dizziness, nausea, vomiting

Reprinted from Mustoe, T.A., Buck, D.W., Lalonde, D.H., 2010. Plast. Reconstr. Surg. 126 (4), 165–176. Adapted from multiple sources.
BID, Twice daily; COX-2, cyclooxygenase-2; CV, cardiovascular; GABA, gamma-amniobutyric acid; IM, intramuscularly; IV, intravenously; NSAID, nonsteroidal anti-inflammatory drug; PO, per os (by mouth); PR, per rectum; QID, four times daily; TID, three times daily.

- Identification numbers
  - Social security number
  - Medical record number
  - Insurance numbers
  - Other account numbers
  - Driver's license number
  - Medical device serial numbers
- Photographs involving the full face or other identifiable body markers (e.g., tattoos)
- Date of birth
- Age and gender are not considered identifiers.
- Medical information cannot be discussed with anyone other than the patient unless prior consent and permission has been obtained from the patient or the patient is a minor (i.e., <18 years old).

2. Informed consent
- Elements of discussion and documentation that are required for adequate consent
  - Diagnosis requiring treatment
  - Procedural risks, potential complications, and potential side effects
  - Probability of success based on the patient's medical condition
  - Available alternative methods of treatment
  - Risks associated with noncompliance with postprocedure recommendations and/or restrictions

3. Employment policies/practices
- It is illegal to discriminate against an applicant, or employee, because of
  - Age
  - Religion
  - Nation of origin
  - Race
  - Sex
  - Child care responsibilities
  - Health-related disabilities
  - Arrest history
- As such, inquiries into any of the above aspects during the application or interview process are unethical and considered illegal.
- It is legal to ask questions about an applicant's or employee's background or to require a background check.

Patient Safety

1. American Society of Anesthesiologists (ASA) classification (see Table 1.7)
- Correlates with overall health of the patient and surgical outcome (i.e., higher ASA is associated with a patient in poorer health and with a greater risk for morbidity and/or mortality from surgery/anesthesia).

Table 1.7 ASA Classification

ASA I	Normal healthy patient without active disease
ASA II	Patient with mild systemic disease (e.g., hypertension under medical control)
ASA III	Patient with severe systemic disease
ASA IV	Patient with severe systemic disease that is a constant threat to life
ASA V	Patient who is moribund and not expected to survive without surgery
ASA VI	Patient who has been declared brain dead for organ donation

Reprinted from Halperin, B., 2013. In: Neligan, P.C. (Ed.), Plastic Surgery, 3rd ed. Elsevier, China.
ASA, *American Society of Anesthesiologists.*

2. Deep venous thrombosis
- Risk factors
  - History of prior venous disease
  - Obesity (body mass index [BMI] >30)
  - Immobility
  - Diabetes
  - Smoking
  - History of cancer
  - Increased age
  - Long duration of surgery
  - General anesthesia
  - Abdominoplasty and/or suction-assisted lipectomy
  - Prolonged hospital stay >4 days
  - Caprini score >8
- Prophylaxis
  - Compression stockings
  - Intermittent pneumatic compressive devices
    - Must be placed before induction of anesthesia
  - Preoperative and/or postoperative anticoagulation (e.g., low-molecular-weight heparin, subcutaneous heparin) is generally recommended for high-risk patients.
- Characterized by localized swelling and pain of the affected extremity, exacerbation in the dependent position
  - Often asymptomatic
  - Occasionally present with pulmonary embolus, tachycardia, hypotension, and respiratory distress.
- Diagnosis: High index of suspicion, duplex ultrasound
  - Ventilation-perfusion (VQ) scan, spiral chest CT for pulmonary embolus
- Treatment
  - Supportive care (e.g., supplemental oxygen, airway protection)
  - Anticoagulation (e.g., heparin, low-molecular-weight heparin, coumadin, fondaparinux in patients with heparin-induced thrombocytopenia)

Billing and Coding

1. Billing is performed based on current procedural terminology (CPT) codes used to describe the operation being performed, and/or the evaluation being conducted.
   - Evaluation and management (E/M) codes: Used to report evaluation and management services that are provided in the office, outpatient facility, ambulatory facility, hospital, and in consultation.
     - Level of service is dependent on evaluation of six of seven components (in order of importance): History, examination, medical decision making, counseling, coordination of care, nature of the presenting problem, time
   - Procedural Codes: Used to report the procedures/operations that were performed.
     - Surgical codes include preoperative visits, if the decision for surgery was made at a prior visit; local anesthesia; immediate postoperative care; writing orders; evaluation of the patient in the postanesthesia care unit; typical postoperative follow-up care (as defined by the global period)
2. Global period: Period following a procedure in which any associated aftercare, including office visits, is considered to be "included" in the CPT code billed.
   - The global period varies according to operation and is often based on complexity (e.g., most operations have a global period of 90 days, whereas skin excisions often have a global period of 10 days).
3. Many bundled or global CPT codes include most steps or components of an operation or procedure, such that each individual step cannot be coded separately. Common examples relevant to plastic surgery:
   - Excision of lesion codes (both benign and malignant) include simple closure (single layer); however, intermediate and/or complex closure codes can be listed separately.
   - Debridement codes cannot be used with wound closure codes because they are only used for wounds, which are allowed to heal secondarily.
     - Debridement codes are reported by the depth of tissue removed and surface area.
     - If debridement is performed in the operating room before wound closure, the "surgical preparation of wound bed" codes should be used.
   - Free-flap CPT codes include exposure of recipient vessels, microvascular anastomosis and use of the surgical microscope, flap harvest and elevation, and primary closure of the donor site.
     - If closure of the donor site requires additional procedures (e.g., split thickness skin graft, adjacent tissue transfer, etc.), these procedures can be coded as well.
   - Adjacent tissue transfer codes include the excision of a skin lesion, and thus, the excision cannot be separately coded.
   - Nerve decompression codes generally include external neurolysis but do not include internal neurolysis (e.g., carpal tunnel release).
   - Use of the surgical microscope is included in all microsurgery/free-flap codes, except for codes involving nerve repair.
4. Billing for combined reconstructive cosmetic and reconstructive procedures (e.g., abdominoplasty and umbilical hernia repair)
   - The patient must be billed separately for the cosmetic portion of the operation, including the associated hospital and anesthesia fees.
   - This separation is based on time during the operation.
     - The surgeon informs the operating room staff when the cosmetic surgery portion is being performed and the time is documented.

Common CPT Code Definitions

1. Lesion excisions are coded according to the longest diameter of lesion plus the margin.
2. Skin closure methods are coded according to the length of the closure.
   - If multiple closure procedures are performed on a patient, the closure method is coded according to the sum of the lengths closed using that particular method (e.g., all simple closure lengths are added, intermediate closure lengths are added, etc.).
3. Skin closure definitions
   - Simple repair includes all simple one-layered closures.
     - Simple repair is included in all excision codes.
   - Intermediate repair includes all multilayer closures or single-layer closure of heavily contaminated wounds.
   - Complex repair includes wounds requiring more than a one-layered closure (e.g., scar revision, debridement, extensive undermining, stents or retention sutures, etc.).
   - Adjacent tissue transfer includes all types of local tissue rearrangement (e.g., local flaps, Z plasty, rotation-advancement flaps, bilobed flaps, rhomboid flaps, Ryan flaps, etc.) that is not based on a defined pedicle or axial blood supply.
     - Coded according to the area of the defect plus the donor site
     - Coded per defect, not per flap
     - Excision of a lesion is included in all adjacent tissue transfer codes
4. Code modifiers: Used to further define or describe the procedure
   - 22 modifier identifies increased complexity or procedural services required for that particular code.
   - 52 modifier identifies decreased complexity or procedural services required for that particular code.
   - 50 modifier identifies bilateral cases (e.g., breast reduction, brachioplasty, etc.).
   - 51 modifier identifies multiple combined procedures performed.
   - 59 modifier identifies procedures that were distinct and should be considered independent (e.g., resection of multiple malignant lesions from the same anatomic area).

- 62 modifier identifies procedure that was performed with a cosurgeon, where each surgeon is performing a separately documented part of the operation.

Suggested Reading

American Medical Association, 2014. CPT 2015 Standard Codebook, Standard Ed. American Medical Association, pp. 1–770.

Buck, D.W., Mustoe, T.A., Kim, J.Y.S., 2006. Postoperative nausea and vomiting in plastic surgery. Semin. Plast. Surg. 20 (4), 249–255.

Haeck, P.C., 2013. Chapter 4: The role of ethics in plastic surgery. In: Neligan, P.C. (Ed.), Plastic Surgery, 3rd ed. Elsevier, China, pp. 55–63.

Halperin, B., 2013. Chapter 8: Patient safety in plastic surgery. In: Neligan, P.C. (Ed.), Plastic Surgery, 3rd ed. Elsevier, China, pp. 124–136.

Hill, J., Singh, V.M., Sen, S.K., 2013. Chapter 4: Anesthesia for upper extremity surgery. In: Neligan, P.C. (Ed.), Plastic Surgery, 3rd ed. Elsevier, China, pp. 92–105.

Hultman, C.S., 2013. Chapter 5: Business principles for plastic surgeons. In: Neligan, P.C. (Ed.), Plastic Surgery, 3rd ed. Elsevier, China, pp. 64–91.

Krizek, T.J., 2010. Chapter 11: Ethics in plastic surgery. In: Weinzweig, J. (Ed.), Plastic Surgery Secrets Plus, 2nd ed. Mosby Elsevier, Philadelphia, pp. 61–71.

Kulaylat, M.N., Dayton, M.T., 2012. Chapter 13: Surgical complications. In: Townsend, C.M., Beauchamp, R.D., Evers, B.M., et al. (Eds.), Sabiston Textbook of Surgery, 19th ed. Elsevier Saunders, Philadelphia, pp. 281–327.

McDaniel, W.L., Jarris, R.F., 2011. Chapter 5: Local and topical anesthetic complications. In: Pfenninger, J.L., Fowler, G.D. (Eds.), Pfenninger and Fowler's Procedures for Primary Care, 3rd ed. Elsevier Mosby, pp. 25–27.

Mottura, A.A., 2013. Chapter 9: Local anesthetics in plastic surgery. In: Neligan, P.C. (Ed.), Plastic Surgery, 3rd ed. Elsevier, China, pp. 137–149.

Murphy-Lavoie, H., LeGros, T.L., 2013. Chapter 188: Local and regional anesthesia. In: Adams, J.G. (Ed.), Emergency Medicine, 2nd ed. Saunders, pp. 1578–1586.

Mustoe, T.A., Buck, D.W., Lalonde, D.H., 2010. The safe management of anesthesia, sedation, and pain in plastic surgery. Plast. Reconstr. Surg. 126 (4), 165–176.

Pannucci, C.J., Dreszer, G., Wachtman, C.F., et al., 2011. Postoperative enoxaparin prevents symptomatic venous thromboembolism in high-risk plastic surgery patients. Plast. Reconstr. Surg. 128 (5), 1093–1103.

Prohibited Employment Policies/Practices. U.S. Equal Employment Opportunity Commission. Found at: <http://www.eeoc.gov/laws/practices/.> Accessed on: November 30, 2014.

Reisman, N.R., 2013. Chapter 6: Medico-legal issues in plastic surgery. In: Neligan, P.C. (Ed.), Plastic Surgery, 3rd ed. Elsevier, China, pp. 92–103.

Sherwood, E.R., Williams, C.G., Prough, D.S., 2012. Chapter 16: Anesthesiology principles, pain management, and conscious sedation. In: Townsend, C.M., Beauchamp, R.D., Evers, B.M., et al. (Eds.), Sabiston Textbook of Surgery, 19th ed. Saunders, pp. 389–417.

Summary of the HIPAA Privacy Rule. United States Department of Health & Human Services. Found at: <http://www.hhs.gov/ocr/privacy/hipaa/understanding/summary/privacysummary.pdf.> Accessed on: November 30, 2014.

Chapter

Head and Neck Anatomy and Facial Palsy

2

1. Facial nerve (cranial nerve VII)
   - Facial nerve anatomy
     - Course
       - Brain stem → pontomedullary junction → traverses internal auditory meatus → geniculate ganglion → stylomastoid foramen → parotid → muscles of facial expression
     - Intratemporal branches
       - Chorda tympani: Parasympathetic, taste to anterior two-thirds of tongue
       - Stapedius nerve: Motor to stapedius muscle
       - Greater petrosal nerve: Parasympathetic
     - Stylomastoid foramen branches
       - Posterior auricular nerve
       - Posterior belly of digastric nerve
       - Stylohyoid nerve
     - Parotid branches
       - Temporal/frontal branch: Found within the superficial temporal or temporoparietal fascia
       - Zygomatic branch: Overlap with buccal branch; near parotid duct, superficial to masseter muscle
       - Buccal branch: Overlap with zygomatic branch; near parotid duct, superficial to masseter muscle
       - Marginal mandibular nerve: Motor to lower lip depressors and mentalis muscles, located up to 1 cm below mandibular border, crosses facial vessels.
       - Cervical nerve: Lowest division, motor to platysma (see Figure 2.1)
   - Temporal anatomy
     - Layers from superficial to deep in this region include (1) skin, (2) subcutaneous tissue, (3) superficial temporal fascia, also known as the temporoparietal fascia, (4) superficial layer of the deep temporal fascia, (5) superficial temporal fat pad, (6) deep layer of the deep temporal fascia, and (7) temporalis muscle.
       - When the coronal flap is raised, as soon as the yellow superficial temporal fat pad is seen beneath the superficial layer of the deep temporal fascia, the superficial layer of the deep temporal fascia must be incised and included with the coronal flap to protect the frontal branch, which is in the superficial temporal fascia (temporoparietal fascia), one layer superficial to this (see Figure 2.2).

2. Facial palsy
   - Etiology
     - Most common cause in children is idiopathic (Bell's palsy), followed by infectious (and traumatic, neoplastic, and congenital) etiologies
     - Bell's palsy: Most common, suddenly acquired, unilateral facial palsy
       - Associated with diabetes mellitus (DM), pregnancy, upper respiratory infections; must exclude stroke, tumor
       - Other symptoms include pain, epiphora, oral incompetence, hyperacusis, taste impairment.
       - Treatment: Observation; 85% will show improvement in neurologic function within 3 weeks.
       - No evidence for facial nerve decompression
     - Pontine lesions (tumor, motor neuron disease, Mobius, infarction)
       - Millard-Gruber and Raymond-Foville syndromes: Pontine stroke
         - Facial and abducens palsy, contralateral hemiplegia
       - Mobius: Most common, bilateral, congenital facial palsy
         - Often associated with abducens palsy as well
     - Infranuclear lesions (Guillain-Barré, Bell's), muscle diseases (myasthenia gravis, myotonic dystrophy, facioscapulohumeral dystrophy)
       - Ramsay Hunt syndrome: Herpes zoster virus involvement of facial nerve leading to extreme ear pain, with shingles/vesicles along the facial nerve course, accompanying facial palsy
     - Trauma
       - Location is important
         - Penetrating injury anterior to a vertical line drawn down from the lateral canthus often not explored (ends too difficult to find due to small

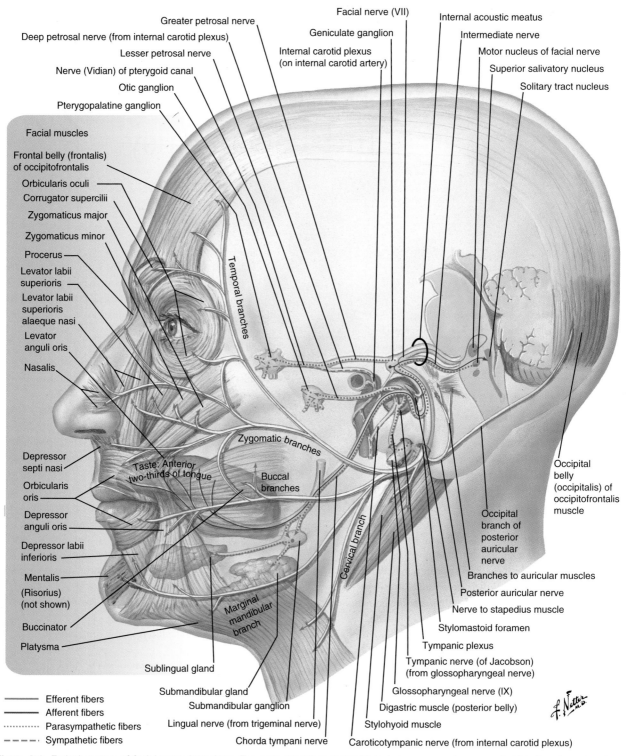

Figure 2.1. Typical pattern of facial nerve branching. The main branch is divided into two components, each of which then branches in a random manner to all parts of the face. Extensive distal arborization and interconnections are apparent. *(Reprinted with permission from www.netterimages.com ©Elsevier Inc. All rights reserved.)*

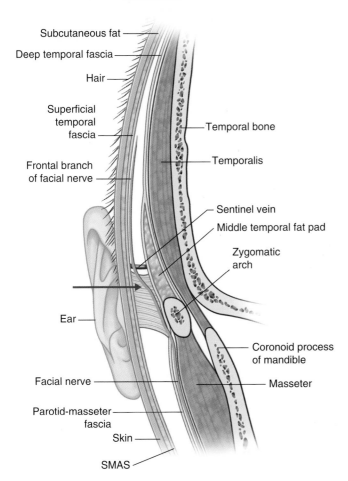

Subcutaneous fat
Deep temporal fascia
Hair
Superficial temporal fascia
Frontal branch of facial nerve
Temporal bone
Temporalis
Sentinel vein
Middle temporal fat pad
Zygomatic arch
Ear
Coronoid process of mandible
Facial nerve
Masseter
Parotid-masseter fascia
Skin
SMAS

Figure 2.2. Facial layers of the temporal region. The fat/fascia in the subaponeurotic plane *(red arrow;* between the temporal fascia and deep temporal fascia) is intimately related to the facial nerve. Some investigators believe that there is a separate fascial layer in this space, referred to as the parotidomasseteric fascia. *(Reprinted from Neligan, P.C., 2013. Plastic Surgery, 3rd ed. pp. 3–22.)*

diameter); in addition, with buccal branch injury, extensive overlap may allow reinnervation.
→ Some would argue that even these anterior injuries should be explored operatively, even if repair is unlikely.
○ Major buccal branch of facial nerve travels with parotid duct; suspect injuries to duct for any lacerations that violate a line from tragus to upper lip or when upper lip dysfunction is noted.
◆ For parotid duct injuries: Cannulate Stensen duct intraorally, inject saline or methylene blue to diagnose duct injury, and repair over stent or feeding tube if disrupted.
○ Distal nerve end can be stimulated up to 72 hours after injury, after which time it undergoes Wallerian degeneration (important implications for direct repair)
■ Tumors

3. Facial nerve repair/reconstruction
• Primary direct repair
■ Gives best results when end-to-end coaptation can be performed without significant tension (otherwise, nerve graft is advised).
■ Performed in a clean wound, ideally within 72 hours of injury because during this time, the distal nerve end can still be stimulated to ensure proper target identification.
• Nerve grafting
■ Success depends on relative number of axons, potential for regeneration through the graft, and status of facial muscles (motor end plate loss occurs from 12 to 24 months postinjury).
■ Common donor nerves for facial palsy include great auricular, branches of cervical plexus, and sural.
• Nerve transfer
■ Useful when distal stumps are present and facial musculature motor end plates are still intact.
■ Cranial nerve donors include trigeminal and hypoglossal.
■ Ipsilateral motor nerve to masseter also now used.
■ Cross-face nerve grafting is most favorable option in terms of restoring spontaneous facial movement.
○ Note that temporal and marginal mandibular branches have less overlap with other branches in terms of function, so degree of donor morbidity may be higher for cross-face nerve grafting.
○ Often better to graft from larger branch over to affected side and leave smaller branch behind on normal side, such that function is slightly weakened on the normal side; will give better symmetry.
○ Cross-face nerve grafts are passed through the upper buccal sulcus region to the opposite side and coapted to the distal stumps on the affected side.
• Free neurotized muscle transfer (e.g., for reanimation)
■ More likely to get spontaneous smile development compared to that with regional muscle transfer (e.g., temporalis transfer, where biting motion must initiate the smile); regional muscles also have suboptimal vector of pull.
■ Use of gracilis popularized by Zuker and Manktelow
○ Can be harvested in segmental fashion (1/2 to 1/3 of muscle) to reduce bulk in face; harvested with obturator nerve.
■ Inset to deep temporal fascia and oral commissure (modiolus) with appropriate tensioning; vector parallels course of zygomaticus major m (see Table 2.1).
■ Cross-face nerve grafting can be used to innervate versus ipsilateral motor nerve to masseter.
○ Cross-face nerve graft is not as powerful but allows total spontaneity of smile.
◆ Must wait for Tinel's sign with cross-face nerve graft (or nerve biopsy) to establish that axons have reached the distal end before free muscle transfer.

Table 2.1 Dimensions of the Levators of the Upper Lip

MUSCLE	LENGTH (MM)	WIDTH (MM)	THICKNESS (MM)
Zygomaticus major	70	8	2
Levator labii superioris	34	25	1.8
Levator anguli oris	38	14	1.7

Reprinted from Freilinger, G., Gruber, H., Happak, W., et al., 1987. Surgical anatomy of the mimic muscle system and the facial nerve: Importance for reconstructive and aesthetic surgery. Plast. Reconstr. Surg. 80, 686.

> ○ Cross-face nerve graft with free gracilis is a two-stage procedure, whereas coaptation to ipsilateral masseteric nerve is done in one stage.
> - Brow asymmetry
>   - For recent occurrence of facial paralysis in which extent of recovery is unclear, asymmetry can be addressed with botulinum toxin injection into the unaffected side to weaken it.
>   - Once it is clear that recovery is unlikely and denervation probable, can consider static procedures to correct asymmetry (e.g., forehead lift, brow lift, blepharoplasty, canthoplasty).
> - Facial dyskinesis
>   - Hyperkinesis after facial reanimation surgery can be addressed with injection of botulinum toxin into facial muscles that are most hyperkinetic.
>   - Synkinesis may also be addressed with injection of botulinum toxin (e.g., eyelid closure with chewing in patient who has recovered from Bell's palsy) (see Box 2.1)

4. Trigeminal nerve (cranial nerve V)
   - Trigeminal nerve anatomy
     - The ophthalmic division of the trigeminal nerve (V1)
       - ○ Sensation to the forehead and anterior scalp
       - ○ Exits the skull through the supraorbital foramen.
         - ◆ Three sensory branches: Lacrimal, frontal, and nasociliary nerves
         - ◆ Nasociliary nerve courses above the optic nerve and below the superior rectus muscle.
           - → First branch is the posterior ethmoidal nerve, which provides sensation to the posterior ethmoid sinuses.
           - → The terminal branches are the anterior ethmoidal nerve and the infratrochlear nerves, which supply the septum and lateral walls.
           - → The dorsal nasal nerve, which supplies innervation to the tip.
     - The maxillary division of the trigeminal nerve (V2)
       - ○ Sensation to the cheek and upper lip and to the upper teeth via the superior alveolar nerve
       - ○ Transmitted through the infraorbital foramen

BOX 2.1 MOST COMMON SURGICAL OPTIONS FOR EACH REGION OF THE FACE

Brow (Brow Ptosis)
Direct brow lift (direct excision)
Coronal brow lift with static suspension
Endoscopic brow lift
Upper Eyelid (Lagophthalmos)
Gold weight
Temporalis transfer
Spring
Tarsorrhaphy
Lower Eyelid (Ectropion)
Tendon sling
Lateral canthoplasty
Horizontal lid shortening
Temporalis transfer
Cartilage graft
Nasal Airway
Static sling
Alar base elevation
Septoplasty
Commissure and Upper Lip
Nerve transfer either directly or via nerve graft to reinnervate recently paralyzed muscles
Microneurovascular muscle transplantation with the use of ipsilateral seventh nerve, cross-facial nerve graft, or other cranial nerve for motor innervation
Temporalis transposition with or without masseter transposition
Static slings
Soft-tissue balancing procedures (rhytidectomy, mucosal excision, or advancement)
Lower Lip
Depressor labii inferioris resection (on normal side)
Muscle transfer (digastric, platysma)
Wedge excision

Reprinted from Zuker, R.M., Gur, E., Hussain, G., et al., 2013. In: Neligan, P.C. (Ed.), Plastic Surgery, 3rd ed. Elsevier, China.

- Mandibular division (V3): Inferior alveolar, buccal, mandibular nerves
  - ○ Inferior alveolar nerve
    - ◆ Enters the mandible on the medial side of the ramus ~10 mm below the sigmoid notch.
    - ◆ Courses through the canal closest to the buccal cortical plate in the region of the ramus, angle, and down to the third molar with an average distance of 1.8 mm ± 1 mm.
    - ◆ The nerve then swerves away at a position of 4.1 mm + 1 mm from the buccal cortex as it passes the region of the first and second molars.
    - ◆ As it traverses the mandibular body, it is lowest and closest to the inferior cortex (7.5 mm + 1.5 mm) near its exit site at the level of the first molar and second premolar via the mental foramen on the anterior surface of the mandible.
    - ◆ The mental nerve supplies the skin of the lower lip and chin, right up to the midline.

5. Essential sensory innervation of head and neck structures (see Figures 2.3 and 2.4)
   - Sensory innervation of the ear
     - Great auricular nerve: Sensory to earlobe and lower half of ear
     - Auricular branch of vagus nerve (Arnold's nerve): Concha
     - Auriculotemporal nerve: Anterior and superior helix/external auditory canal
     - Lesser occipital nerve: Posterior superior ear
   - Sensory innervation of the nose
     - See above
   - Sensory innervation of the lips
     - Infraorbital nerve
       ○ The maxillary canine may be used as a landmark for needle insertion toward the infraorbital foramen during infiltration of the infraorbital nerve.
       ○ Bilateral blockade of the infraorbital nerve in the midline provides complete anesthesia to all central components of the upper lip, including the vermillion, Cupid's bow, and philtrum.
     - Mental nerve
       ○ Bilateral mental nerve blocks effectively anesthetize the central section of the lower lip.
     - Buccal nerve: Branch of cranial nerve (CN) V3; supplies sensory to the commissure
       ○ For lacerations near the commissure, you must inject anesthetic locally
   - Sensory innervation of the cheek
     - Buccal nerve: Central cheek
     - Landmark: Retromolar fossa, posterior to the mandibular third molar

   - Sensory innervation of the forehead
     - Supraorbital nerve (SON): Superficial division—paramedian forehead and anterior scalp; deep division—frontoparietal scalp
       ○ The deep division travels initially along the temporal periosteum and then more cephalad pierces the deep galea plane and enters the galea fat pat. This information is key to avoiding injury when performing a forehead lift.
       ○ Superficial branch travels superficial to frontalis.
     - Supratrochlear nerve: Medial skin of the forehead. The supratrochlear nerve also runs superficial to the frontalis muscle.
   - Innervation to tongue
     - Sensory
       ○ Anterior two-thirds: Lingual nerve (branch of CN V3)
       ○ Posterior third: Glossopharyngeal (CN IX)
     - Motor
       ○ Hypoglossa nerve: If injured, results in ipsilateral tongue paralysis
     - Sense of taste
       ○ Anterior 2/3rds: Chorda tympany from CN VII (join linguinal nerve)
       ○ CN V (lingual): Sensations of salt, bitter, sweet, and sour
         ◆ A 7-9% decrease in taste of these sensations after septoplasty/rhinoplasty
       ○ Post 1/3rd: Glossopharyngeal (CN IX)

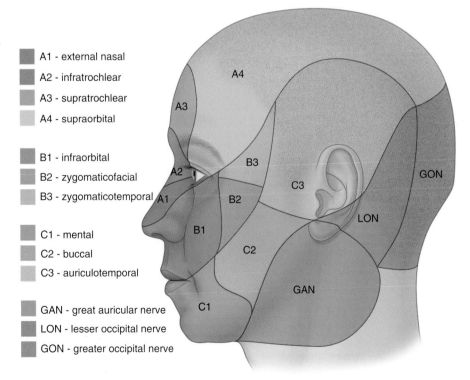

A1 - external nasal
A2 - infratrochlear
A3 - supratrochlear
A4 - supraorbital

B1 - infraorbital
B2 - zygomaticofacial
B3 - zygomaticotemporal

C1 - mental
C2 - buccal
C3 - auriculotemporal

GAN - great auricular nerve
LON - lesser occipital nerve
GON - greater occipital nerve

Figure 2.3. Sensory supply of the face. *(Reprinted from Neligan, P.C., 2013. Plastic Surgery, 3rd ed. pp. 3–22.)*

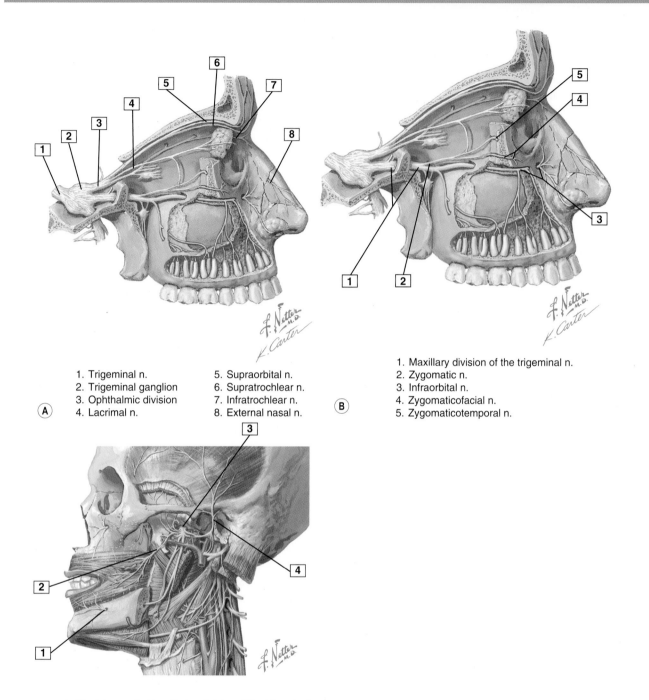

1. Trigeminal n. 5. Supraorbital n.
2. Trigeminal ganglion 6. Supratrochlear n.
3. Ophthalmic division 7. Infratrochlear n.
4. Lacrimal n. 8. External nasal n.

(A)

1. Maxillary division of the trigeminal n.
2. Zygomatic n.
3. Infraorbital n.
4. Zygomaticofacial n.
5. Zygomaticotemporal n.

(B)

1. Mental n. 3. Mandibular division of the trigeminal n.
2. Buccal n. 4. Auriculotemporal n.

(C)

Figure 2.4. A-C, Sensory nerves of the face. *(Reprinted with permission from www.netterimages.com ©Elsevier Inc. All rights reserved.) n, nerve.*

6. Essential anatomical foramen/structures
   - Foramen
     - Foramen lacerum: Internal carotid artery
     - Foramen ovale: Mandibular division trigeminal nerve (V3)
     - Foramen rotundum: Maxillary division trigeminal nerve (V2)
     - Stylomastoid foramen: Facial nerve
     - Jugular foramen: Glossopharyngeal nerve (CN IX), vagus (CN X), spinal accessory (CN XI) (see Figures 2.5 and 2.6)
   - Stensen duct
     - The maxillary second molar is a landmark typically used to locate the opening of the Stensen duct.
     - The parotid (Stensen) duct opens into the mouth at the level of the upper second molar. It is ~4 to 7 cm long,

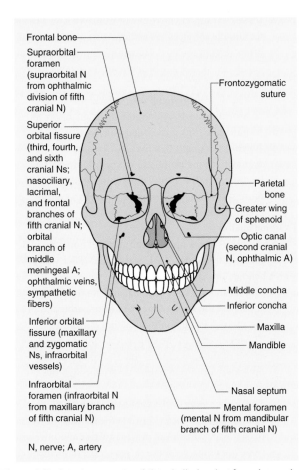

Figure 2.5. Anterior aspects of the skull showing foramina and their contents. *(Reprinted from Craven, J., 2014. Anatomy of the skull learning objectives. Anaesth. Intensive Care Med. 15 (4), 146–148.)*

extends from the anterior border of the superficial lobe of the parotid gland, and is frequently accompanied by accessory parotid tissue. The duct runs anteriorly over the masseter muscle about halfway between the zygomatic arch and the angle of the mouth. It turns medially beyond the anterior border of the masseter muscle, pierces the buccinator muscle, and opens into the mouth through the parotid papilla at about the level of the upper second molar.

○ Zygomatic and buccal branches of the facial (VII) nerve may cross superficially over the parotid duct.

■ Location of the parotid duct has implications for placement of surgical incisions.

○ Vertical incisions at the anterior border of the parotid gland may cause injury to the parotid duct or to branches of the facial (VII) nerve. Horizontal incisions are less likely to damage these structures.

✦ Because of the parotid septae, parotid abscesses tend to be compartmentalized and may not be fluctant.

✦ Pitting edema over the parotid gland usually indicates an abscess.

✦ Abscesses may need to be drained via multiple horizontal incisions.

• The buccinator muscle is the only muscle of facial expression that compresses the cheeks, an essential function for playing air-based instruments such as the trumpet.

■ Ordinarily contributes to the function of forming a food bolus during mastication.

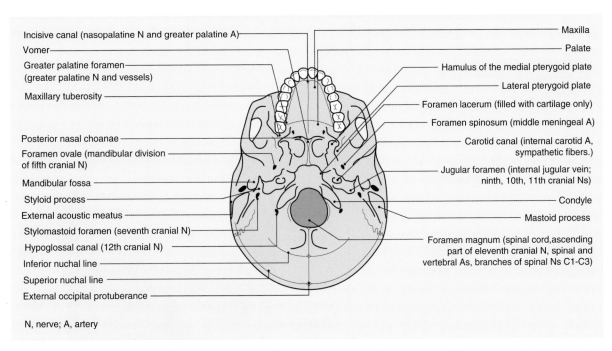

Figure 2.6. Inferior aspect of the skull showing foramina and their contents. *(Reprinted from Craven, J., 2014. Anatomy of the skull learning objectives. Anaesth. Intensive Care Med. 15 (4), 146–148.)*

- Both the buccinator and the orbicularis oris compress the lips, also necessary for playing trumpets.
- The levator labii superioris, risorius, and zygomaticus major muscles all have a function that contributes to separating the lips, which releases pressure from inside the mouth.
  - These muscles arise from bone and fascia and attach to the lips.
- Only two muscles would be in the area of a high bifurcation of the carotid that may need to be cut for better exposure during microsurgical cases: Posterior belly of the digastric and the stylohyoid, which span across the skull base to the hyoid.
- The supraorbital and supratrochlear arteries are branches of the internal carotid artery via the ophthalmic artery, and therefore, receive their blood supply from the internal carotid.
- The branches of the external carotid artery, from proximal to distal, are as follows:
  - Superior thyroid
  - Ascending pharyngeal
  - Lingual, occipital, facial
  - Posterior auricular
  - Maxillary arteries
- The arteries of the scalp travel through the subcutaneous fat from the periphery toward the vertex, then anastomose in the midline with branches of the ophthalmic artery. They are branches of the external carotid directly (occipital, posterior auricular) or from the superficial temporal.

7. Layers of the face: The skin, subcutaneous tissue, superficial muscular aponeurotic system (SMAS), fascia, and facial (VII) nerve
   - Dissection within the subcutaneous plane is safe because this plane does not contain the facial (VII) nerve.
   - The SMAS is a heterogenous structure, consisting of facial muscles and fibrous and adipose tissue.
     - Cephalad: The SMAS continues as the temporoparietal fascia.
   - Dissection superficial to the SMAS layer is safe because the muscles of facial animation are innervated from below, except for the buccinator, mentalis, and levator anguli oris muscles, which are innervated via their superficial surfaces.
     - The depressor anguli oris, orbicularis oculi, orbicularis oris, and zygomaticus major are all innervated from their deep surfaces.
   - When dissecting below the SMAS plane, the zygomaticus major muscle serves as an important landmark. In this plane, dissection should proceed more superficially to preserve innervation of the zygomaticus major muscle.

8. Orbital anatomy
   - Seven bones make up the orbit: Frontal bone, maxilla, zygoma, ethmoid, lacrimal, greater and lesser wings of the sphenoid, and palatine
     - The frontal, maxilla, zygoma, and ethmoid bones constitute the strong outer rim of the orbit and protect the more delicate bones in the interior orbit.
     - The lesser wing of the sphenoid forms the posterior aspect of the roof of the orbit and transmits the optic nerve and ophthalmic artery through the optic canal.
     - The greater wing of the sphenoid contains the superior orbital fissure, which transmits the lacrimal nerve, frontal nerve, trochlear nerve, superior and inferior branches of the oculomotor nerve, the nasociliary nerve, and the abducens nerve (see Figure 2.7).

9. Tooth eruption
   - First molar is the first permanent tooth to erupt; this typically occurs between ages 6 and 7 years.
     - Age of mixed dentition, in which both deciduous (primary) and permanent (secondary) teeth erupt in the oral cavity simultaneously, begins with eruption of the first molars.
   - Central incisors erupt between ages 6 and 8 years, lateral incisors between ages 7 and 9, canine teeth between ages 9 and 12, and first premolars between ages 10 and 12.

Figure 2.7. Surgical anatomy of the orbits. *(Reprinted from Guyuron, B., Eriksson, E., Persing, J.A., et al. [Eds.], 2009. Plastic Surgery: Indications and Practice, Elsevier, pp. 619–644.)*

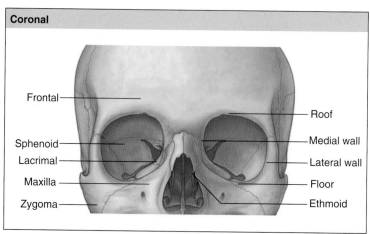
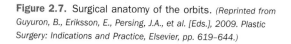

10. Commonly tested congenital disorders
- Choanal atresia
  - Cyanosis that is relieved by crying (paradoxical cyanosis): Classic symptoms
    - Inability to pass catheter through the nose to nasopharynx. Computed tomography (CT) scan shows narrow posterior nasal cavity secondary to medial displacement of lateral nasal wall and pterygoid plates
- Thyroglossal duct cyst
  - May form anywhere along the thyroglossal duct, which extends from the foramen cecum of the tongue to the final position of the thyroid gland in the neck, below the laryngeal cartilage.
  - Normally, the thyroglossal duct atrophies and disappears.
    - However, a remnant of it may persist and form a cyst in the tongue or anterior midline of the neck, most commonly inferior to the hyoid bone.
  - Often asymptomatic unless it becomes infected
- Reactive lymph nodes
  - Most common neck mass in children.
  - Usually found laterally in the submandibular and jugulodigastric areas
- Branchial cleft remnants (sinuses and cysts)
  - Arise from a remnant cleft between the 2nd and 3rd branchial arches. They are located laterally, along the anterior border of the sternocleidomastoid muscle, usually just inferior to the angle of the mandible.
  - Can be bilateral in 30% of cases.
  - Histo: Lined with squamous epithelium, contains keratin, hair follicles, sweat glands, and sebaceous glands.
  - Must be completely excised to prevent recurrence.
- Lingual thyroid glands
  - A type of ectopic thyroid located within the tongue, along the course of the thyroglossal duct, resulting from failure of thyroid to descend.
  - Unlike thyroglossal duct cysts, they represent the only thyroid tissue present in the patient.
- Ranula
  - A mucocele or mucous extravasation phenomenon in the floor of the mouth, arising from the ducts of the sublingual or submandibular glands, often as a sequela of obstruction of the sublingual gland
  - Usually presents as a unilateral swelling of the floor of the mouth that is fluctuant and tinted blue or glossy white
  - Treatment includes marsupialization or surgical excision including the sublingual gland.
  - The ranula may herniate through the muscles of the floor of the mouth and present as a cervical mass.
- Failed closure of the fonticulus frontalis, an embryonic fontanel between the inferior frontal bone and nasal bone, may result in three main types of midline anterior anomalies: Nasal dermal sinus, anterior cephalocele, and nasal glioma.
  - Although closure may be affected by various factors such as gender and race, the anterior fontanel closes by 24 months of age in 96% of children.
  - Nasal gliomas: Thought to originate as encephaloceles but fail to maintain their intracranial connections
    - May be external, internal, or a combination of both
    - External gliomas typically appear at or just lateral to the nasal root.
      - They are reddish, firm, noncompressible, lobular lesions that exhibit telangiectasias of the overlying skin but do not transilluminate or pulsate.
      - Bony defects, intracranial connections, and cerebrospinal fluid leakage occur only rarely.
      - Histologic evaluation shows astrocytic neuroglial cells and fibrous and vascular connective tissue that is covered with skin or nasal mucosa.
  - Nasal dermoid cyst arises from a dermoid sinus, the cutaneous inward passage lined with stratified squamous epithelium.
    - May also be external or internal
    - External nasal dermoid: Firm, noncompressible, nonpulsatile lesion that does not transilluminate and may be lobulated
    - Although bony defects are infrequent, cerebrospinal fluid leakage and meningitis may occur.
    - Derived from ectoderm and mesoderm and thus contains adnexal structures including hair follicles, pilosebaceous glands, and smooth muscles.
  - Encephaloceles involve herniation of cranial tissue through a skull defect.
    - Classified as meningoceles (containing meninges only), meningoencephaloceles (containing meninges and brain), or meningoencephalocystoceles (containing meninges, brain, and part of the ventricular system)
    - External, or sincipital, encephaloceles are soft, bluish, compressible, pulsatile masses located at the nasal root and transilluminate.
      - They typically enlarge with crying and Valsalva maneuver.

Suggested Readings

Adour, K.K., Hilsinger, R.L., Callan, E.J., 1985. Facial paralysis and Bell's palsy: A protocol for differential diagnosis. Am. J. Otol. (Suppl.), 68–73.

Afifi, A.M., Djohan, R., 2013. Chapter 1: Anatomy of the head and neck. In: Neligan, P.C. (Ed.), Plastic Surgery, 3rd ed. Elsevier, pp. 3–22.

Berkovitz, B.K.B., Moxham, B.J., 2002. The face. In: Berkovitz, B.K.B., Moxham, B.J. (Eds.), Head and Neck Anatomy: A clinical reference. Informa Healthcare, London, pp. 108–113.

Burggasser, G., Happak, W., Gruber, H., et al., 2002. The temporalis: Blood supply and innervation. Plast. Reconstr. Surg. 109, 1862–1869.

Clemente, C.D., 1997. Neck and head. In: Clemente, C.D. (Ed.), Anatomy: A Regional Atlas of the Human Body, 4th ed. Williams & Wilkins, Baltimore, pp. 435–576.

Coker, N.J., Vrabec, J.T., 2001. Acute paralysis of the facial nerve. In: Bailey, B.J. (Ed.), Head and Neck Surgery/Otolaryngology, 3rd ed. Lippincott Williams & Wilkins, Philadelphia, pp. 1843–1858.

Goldenberg, D.V., Alonso, N., Ferreira, M.C., 2009. Chapter 48: Facial trauma. In: Guyuron, B., Eriksson, E., Persing, J.A., et al. (Eds.), Plastic Surgery: Indications and Practice, Elsevier, pp. 619–644.

Hedlund, G., 2006. Congenital frontonasal masses: Developmental anatomy, malformations, and MR imaging. Pediatr. Radiol. 36, 647–662 quiz 726–727.

Janfaza, P., Cheney, M.L., 2001. Superficial structures of the face, head, and parotid region. In: Janfaza, P., Nadol, J.B., Galla, R., et al. (Eds.), Surgical Anatomy of the Head and Neck, Lippincott Williams & Wilkins, Philadelphia, pp. 2–48.

Janfaza, P., Rubin, P., Azar, N., 2001. Orbit. In: Janfaza, P., Nadol, J.B., Galla, R.J., (Eds.), Surgical Anatomy of the Head and Neck, Lippincott Williams & Wilkins, Philadelphia, pp. 149–222.

Kendell, B.D., Frost, D.E., 2005. Applied surgical anatomy of the head and neck. In: Fonseca, R.J., Walker, R.V., Betts, N.J., et al. (Eds.), Oral and Maxillofacial Trauma, 3rd ed. Elsevier Saunders, St. Louis, pp. 281–328.

Knize, D.M., 1995. A study of the supraorbital nerve. Plast. Reconstr. Surg. 96, 564–569.

Moore, K., 1985. The tongue. In: Moore, K. (Ed.), Clinically Oriented Anatomy, vol. 2. Williams & Wilkins, Baltimore, p. 935.

Moore, K.L., Dalley, A.F. II, 1999. Head. In: Moore, K.L., Dalley, A.F., II (Eds.), Clinically Oriented Anatomy, 4th ed. Lippincott Williams & Wilkins, Philadelphia, pp. 870–871.

Moore, K.L., Dalley, A.F., II., 1999. Summary of cranial nerves. In: Moore, K.L., Dalley, I.I.A.F. (Eds.), Clinically Oriented Anatomy, 4th ed. Lippincott Williams & Wilkins, Philadelphia, pp. 1082–1096.

Moore, K.L., Persaud, T.V.N., 2008. The Developing Human: Clinically Oriented Embryology, 8th ed. WB Saunders, Philadelphia, pp. 159–196.

Netter, F., 1989. Head and neck. In: Netter, F.H. (Ed.), Atlas of Human Anatomy, Ciba-Geigy Corporation, Tarrytown, New York, p. 56.

Roth, J.J., Granick, M.S., Solomon, M.P., 1997. Pediatric neck masses. In: Bentz, M. (Ed.), Pediatric Plastic Surgery, Appleton & Lange, Stamford, pp. 494–498.

Snell, R.S., 2006. Skeletal muscles. In: Snell, R.S. (Ed.), Clinical Anatomy by Systems, Lippincott Williams & Wilkins, Philadelphia, pp. 441–445.

Snell, R.S., 2006. The upper and lower airway and associated structures. In: Snell, R.S. (Ed.), Clinical Anatomy by Systems, Lippincott Williams & Wilkins, Philadelphia, pp. 55–56.

Wexler, A., 1997. Anatomy of the head and neck. In: Ferraro, J.W. (Ed.), Fundamentals of Maxillofacial Surgery, Springer-Verlag, New York, pp. 53–114.

Ziccardi, V.B., Zuniga, J.R., 2005. Traumatic injuries of the trigeminal nerve. In: Fonseca, R.J., Walker, R.V., Betts, N.J., et al. (Eds.), Oral and Maxillofacial Trauma, 3rd ed. Elsevier Saunders, Philadelphia, pp. 877–914.

Zide, B.M., Swift, R., 1998. How to block and tackle the face. Plast. Reconstr. Surg. 101, 840–851.

Zuker, R.M., Gur, E., Hussain, G., et al., 2013. Chapter 11: Facial paralysis. In: Neligan, P.C. (Ed.), Plastic Surgery, 3rd ed. Elsevier, pp. 278–306.

Head and Neck Cancer, Odontogenic Tumors, and Vascular Anomalies

Salivary Gland Tumors

1. Salivary glands include the parotid, submandibular, and sublingual glands.
2. The majority (80%) of salivary gland tumors occur in the parotid gland and are benign pleomorphic adenomas (80%). Tumors that arise in the submandibular and/or sublingual glands are more likely to be malignant (see Table 3.1).

Table 3.1 Tumors of the Salivary Glands

	BENIGN (%)	MALIGNANT (%)
Parotid	80	20
Submaxillary	60	40
Sublingual	40	60
Minor salivary glands	20	80

Reprinted from Neligan, P.C., Rodrigueze, E.D. (Eds.), 2013. Plastic Surgery, vol. 3, 3rd ed. Elsevier, China, 360–379.

3. Diagnosis of neck masses often includes fine-needle aspiration and imaging (ultrasound, computed tomography [CT], and/or magnetic resonance imaging [MRI])
4. Benign salivary gland tumors
   - Pleomorphic adenoma ("benign mixed tumor")
     - Most common tumor of the salivary glands (parotid)
     - Characterized by a painless, firm mass that does not cause facial nerve dysfunction.
     - Treatment: Superficial parotidectomy with protection of the facial nerve
   - Papillary cystadenoma lymphomatosum ("Warthin's tumor")
     - 2nd most common tumor of the parotid glands
     - Male predilection, between 50 and 60 years old
     - Characterized by a smooth, painless mass that can be bilateral in ~10% of patients.
     - Treatment: Surgical excision with narrow margins
   - Hemangioma
     - Most common parotid mass in children
     - Characterized by typical growth pattern of hemangiomas: Rapid growth after birth, followed by involution
     - Treatment: Oral prednisone for enlarging lesions
       ○ If lesion regresses with prednisone, treatment continues
       ○ If lesion continues to grow despite treatment, surgical excision may be indicated.
5. Malignant salivary gland tumors
   - Mucoepidermoid carcinoma
     - Most common malignant salivary gland tumor
     - Characterized by slow-growing, firm mass that can cause facial nerve dysfunction
     - Treatment is based on tumor grade (low vs. high)
       ○ Low-grade tumors can be treated with superficial parotidectomy +/− radiation therapy, depending on surgical margins.
       ○ High-grade tumors are more aggressive and have a higher rate of lymph node and facial nerve involvement. These tumors require total parotidectomy, resection of involved nerve branches, neck dissection, and adjuvant radiation therapy.
   - Adenoid cystic carcinoma
     - 2nd most common malignant tumor of the parotid gland; most common malignancy of the submandibular and sublingual glands
     - Characterized by a painful, firm, fixed lesion with an affinity for nerve invasion resulting in facial nerve and/or trigeminal nerve dysfunction
     - Treatment: Total parotidectomy and resection of all involved nerves in the path of the tumor
   - Acinic cell carcinoma
     - Characterized by solid or cystic multifocal masses in the parotid gland
     - Can be bilateral in ~3% of patients
     - Treatment: Total parotidectomy, resection of the facial nerve, and repair with nerve grafts, neck dissection

- Adenocarcinoma
  - Characterized by slow-growing, firm, fixed masses
  - Often involve the facial nerve, with metastases to cervical nodes or systemically
  - Treatment: Total parotidectomy, resection of the facial nerve, cervical node dissection, and adjuvant radiation
6. Frey's syndrome
  - Gustatory sweating that can occur after parotidectomy, secondary to interconnection of the parasympathetic nerve fibers from the parotid gland and the sympathetic nerve fibers of the sweat glands in the overlying skin
  - Diagnosis: Clinical history, starch-iodine test
  - Treatment options
    - Reelevation of the cheek flap with insertion of fascia or acellular dermal matrix to separate the nerve endings
    - Botox chemodenervation

Oral Cavity and Pharyngeal Cancer

1. Cancer of the oral cavity and pharynx in the United States is commonly caused by chronic substance abuse, including tobacco and alcohol, and in South Asia by tobacco and betel nut use. In addition, these cancers are secondary to viral infections (e.g., Epstein-Barr virus, human papilloma virus).
   - There is also an association with some occupational exposure, including nickel and radium.
2. Most cancers of the oral cavity and pharynx present as squamous cell carcinoma (SCC), with advanced disease, including nodal metastases (see Figure 3.1).

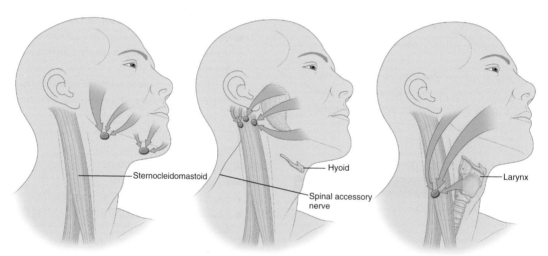

Level IA
- Floor of mouth, anterior oral tongue, anterior mandibular alveolar ridge, lower lip

Level IB
- Oral cavity, anterior nasal cavity, soft tissue of midface, submandibular gland

Level IIA & IIB
- Oral cavity, nasal cavity, nasopharynx, oropharynx, hypopharynx, larynx, parotid gland (Greater risk of metastases from oral and larynx tumors to level IIA. Greater risk of metastases from oropharynx tumors to level IB)

Level III
- Oral cavity, nasopharynx, oropharynx, hypopharynx, larynx

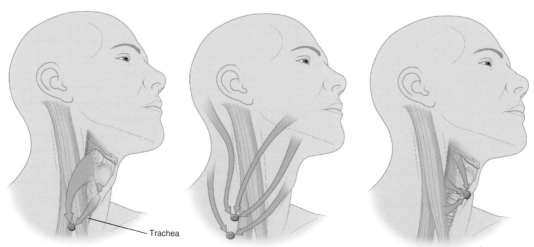

Level IV
- Hypopharynx, thyroid, cervical esophagus, larynx

Level VA & VB
- Nasopharynx, oropharynx, posterior scalp/neck skin

Level VI
- Thyroid gland and subglottic larynx, apex of piriform sinus, cervical esophagus

Figure 3.1. Drainage pattern of head and neck lymph nodes. *(Reprinted from Neligan, P.C., Rodrigueze, E.D. [Eds.], 2013. Plastic Surgery, vol. 3, 3rd ed. Elsevier, China, 420–439).*

3. Staging of lip, oral cavity, and pharyngeal cancer follows the tumor/node/metastasis (TNM) classification (see Table 3.2).

Table 3.2 TNM Clinical Staging System for Lip and Oral Cavity

Tx	Primary tumor cannot be assessed	Nx	Nodes cannot be assessed
T0	No evidence of primary tumor	N0	No evidence of nodal metastasis
Tis	Carcinoma in situ		
T1	≤2 cm in greatest dimension	N1	Single ipsilateral node <3 cm
T2	2-4 cm	N2a	Single ipsilateral node 3-6 cm
		N2b	Multiple ipsilateral nodes 3-6 cm
		N2c	Bilateral or contralateral nodes <6 cm
		N3	Any lymph node >6 cm
T3	>4 cm		
T4a	Lip: Invasion of mandible, skin, floor of mouth, nerve OC: Invasion of mandible, extrinsic tongue, maxilla, skin		
T4b	Invasion of masticator space, skull base, or carotid sheath		
Stage			
0	TisN0M0		IVA T4aN012M0
I	T1N0M0		T123N2M0
II	T2N0M0		IVB T4B any NM0
III	T3N0M0		T1-4A N3
	T123N1M0		IVC any T any NM1

Modified from Patel, S.G., Shah, J.P., 2005. TNM staging of cancers of the head and neck: Striving for uniformity among diversity. CA Cancer J. Clin. 55, 242–258.
OC, Occult; TNM, tumor, node, metastasis.

4. Treatment often depends on stage. In general,
   - For stage-I or -II disease (no nodal metastases), complete surgical resection +/– neck dissection versus radiation therapy to the primary site
     - Radiation therapy is frequently used for stage-I or -II lesions of the larynx, hypopharynx, and nasopharynx.
     - Surgery is frequently recommended for lesions of the oropharynx, oral cavity, and paranasal sinuses (e.g., maxillary sinus).
   - For stage-III or -IV disease, complete surgical resection, neck dissection, adjuvant radiation therapy
5. Complications of head and neck cancer resection and reconstruction
   - Recurrence
   - Wound Infection
     - Treated with antibiotics, debridement of nonviable tissue, and local wound care

- Stable bony hardware may be left in place and mobile hardware must be removed.
- Suture dehiscence and salivary fistula
- Osteoradionecrosis
  - Devitalization and necrosis of bone secondary to radiation therapy
  - Mandible is most commonly affected.
  - Risk factors: Infection, higher levels of radiation, trauma, dental caries
  - Treatment: Hyperbaric oxygen and limited sequestrectomy may be an option for early-stage disease, with radical debridement and free vascularized bone graft (e.g., free fibula flap) for advanced disease.

6. Lip Cancer
   - Greater than 90% of cases are SCC.
   - Most common site of head and neck cancer, excluding skin malignancies
   - Characterized by an ulcerated or exophytic lesion (especially of the lower lip)
   - Lesions >2 cm should have a CT scan to evaluate for cervical nodal metastases.
     - Commonly metastasize to level-I nodes (submandibular or submental area)
   - Treatment: Surgical excision is the primary management. Radiation therapy is limited to patients who cannot tolerate surgery.
   - Reconstructive options depend on defect location and size. The primary goal is oral competence. Layered closure of the defect, including the orbicularis oris, is critical (see Figures 3.2 and 3.3).

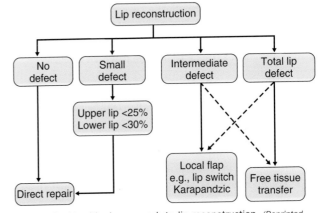

Figure 3.2. Algorithmic approach to lip reconstruction. *(Reprinted from Neligan, P.C., Rodrigueze, E.D. [Eds.], 2013. Plastic Surgery, vol. 3, 3rd ed. Elsevier, China, 254–277.)*

   - In general, primary closure can be performed for lesions <1/3rd of the lower lip and <1/4th of the upper lip.
   - Lesions involving commissure typically require an Estlander flap.
   - Large central lesions can be reconstructed with Karapandzic, Gillies, or Webster-Bernard flaps.
   - Central upper lip defects can often be reconstructed with an Abbe or lip-switch flap.

■ Total lower lip reconstruction can be performed with a free radial forearm flap, commonly using the palmaris tendon as a fascial sling for oral competence.

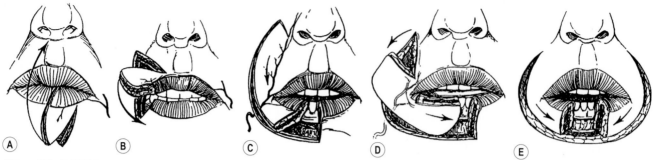

Figure 3.3. Full-thickness musculocutaneous flaps for lip reconstruction. These flaps can be based on the right or left superior or inferior labial arteries and are useful for lip and oral sphincter reconstruction. **A,** Abbe flap arc to central upper lip. **B,** Estlander flap arc to oral commissure and lower lip. **C,** Gillies fan flap to central upper lip. **D,** McGregor flap arc to central lower lip. **E,** Karapandzic flap arc to central lower lip. *(Reprinted from Weinzweig, J. [Ed.], 2010. Plastic Surgery Secrets Plus, 2nd ed. Mosby, 401–408.)*

7. Floor of mouth (FOM) cancer
   • Difficult to evaluate because of proximity to mandible and dentition
   • Approximately 30% will present with nodal metastasis.
   • Treatment: Surgical excision plus adjuvant radiation therapy in patients with >1 positive lymph node, extranodal invasion, perineural invasion, close margins
     ■ May require a mandibulotomy for exposure
     ■ A marginal mandibular resection is required for tumors that abut the lingual mandibular cortex. Involves surgical excision of the alveolus only
     ■ A segmental mandibular resection is required for tumors that invade the mandible.
   • Reconstructive options depend on defect size.
     ■ For large FOM resections without segmental mandibular resection, a free radial forearm flap is an excellent option.
     ■ For large composite defects, including bone, a vascularized osteocutaneous flap may be necessary (e.g., fibula flap, scapular flap).

8. Tongue cancer
   • Most commonly, SCC that arises from areas of preexisting leukoplakia or erythroplasia
   • Tongue cancer has the highest rate of regional metastases of all oral cavity cancers.
   • Base of tongue tumors are often more infiltrative and have a higher incidence of nodal metastases, including the possibility of bilateral nodal metastases.
   • Treatment: Most recommend surgical excision with wide margins, neck dissection, and adjuvant radiation therapy.
   • Reconstructive options depend on defect size.
     ■ Lesions <4 cm of the anterior and middle 1/3rd of the tongue can often be closed primarily.
     ■ Larger, more posterior lesions can be reconstructed with a skin graft or fasciocutaneous free flaps (e.g., radial forearm free flap, anterolateral thigh [ALT] free flap)

■ Subtotal tongue reconstruction is often performed with a free ALT flap.

9. Hypopharyngeal and laryngeal cancer
   • The hypopharynx is the area inferior to the oropharynx and base of tongue, behind the larynx, and superior to the cervical esophagus.
     ■ Most patients with cancer of the hypopharynx present with dysphagia, whereas most patients with laryngeal cancer present with hoarseness.
     ■ Majority develop in the piriform sinus and invade surrounding structures (e.g., larynx, thyroid, thyroid cartilage, esophagus).
     ■ Treatment often requires total laryngopharyngectomy with adjuvant radiation therapy in advanced disease. Small, localized lesions can be treated with radiation therapy alone or partial laryngopharyngectomy.
   • Larynx consists of the epiglottis, glottis (vocal cords), and subglottis (1 cm below the vocal cords to the inferior edge of the cricoid cartilage).
     ■ Most patients with laryngeal cancer present with hoarseness.
     ■ Treatment
       ○ Small supraglottic cancers are often treated with radiation therapy, whereas other small lesions can be removed via transoral laser resection or partial laryngectomy.
       ○ Advanced disease and/or larger lesions often require total laryngectomy with or without adjuvant radiation.
   • Reconstructive options often depend on defect size and typically rely on free-flap reconstruction including jejunum flaps, tubed ALT flaps, or tubed radial forearm flaps (see Table 3.3).

Table 3.3 Advantages and Disadvantages of Commonly Used Flaps for Pharyngoesophageal Reconstruction

	ALT	JEJUNUM	RADIAL FOREARM	PECTORALIS
Flap elevation	Moderately difficult	Moderately difficult	Easy	Easy
Flap reliability	Good	Good	Good	Variable
Flap thickness	Can be too thick	Good	Good	Too thick
Primary healing	Good	Best	Good	Can be poor
Donor site morbidity rates	Low	High	Moderate	Moderate
Recovery time	Quick	Can be slow	Quick	Quick
Fistula rates	Low	Low	Moderate	High
Stricture rates	Low	High	Moderate	Moderate
TEP voice	Good	Poor	Good	Unknown
Swallowing	Good	Good	Good	Fair
Use for circumferential defects	Yes	Yes	Second choice	No
Use for partial defects	Yes	No	Yes	Yes
Contraindications	Obesity, with a very thick thigh	High-risk disease, severe COPD, prior abdominal surgery	Thin patient with a small arm, radial dominance	Female gender, obesity, smoking, circumferential defects

Reprinted from Yu, P., 2009. Intraoral, pharynx, and esophagus. In: Butler, C.E. (Ed.), Head and Neck Reconstruction, Elsevier, 167–196.
ALT, Anterolateral thigh (flap); COPD, chronic obstructive pulmonary disease; TEP, tracheoesophageal puncture.

Mandibular Tumors

1. Odontogenic keratocyst (OKC)
   - OKCs are benign cystic lesions, lined by keratinized epithelium, that occur over a large age range and typically begin after odontogenesis of the first permanent tooth.
   - Peak incidence is in the 2nd to 3rd decade of life, with a predilection for the mandible (especially in the mandibular third molar area).
   - Characterized by a radiolucent, well-demarcated, cystic mass within the mandible that can cause scalloping of the mandibular border.
   - Treatment often centers on enucleation, with removal of the entire cyst lining for small lesions and resection for larger lesions.
   - Recurrence rate is relatively high, and patients should be followed regularly.
   - Multiple OKCs is suggestive of nevoid basal cell carcinoma syndrome or Gorlin syndrome.
     - Autosomal dominant disease with multiple manifestations
       - Basal carcinomas
       - OKCs
       - Palmar and plantar pits
       - Calcification of the falx cerebri
       - Bifid ribs
       - Skeletal abnormalities
       - Cardiac and ovarian fibromas
       - Brain tumors
     - Treatment involves close observation and individual treatment of manifestations.

2. Ameloblastoma
   - Benign, odontogenic tumor that can arise from the lining of an odontogenic cyst (intraosseous ameloblastoma) or the gingiva or alveolar mucosa (peripheral ameloblastoma).
   - Intraosseous ameloblastomas occur in the mandible in 80% of cases.
   - Classically described as a radiolucent, well-demarcated cystic lesion with a "soap bubble" or "honeycomb" appearance on X ray
   - Pathologic features include columnar basilar cells in a palisading pattern.
   - Most aggressive of the benign odontogenic tumors and can spread locally through cortical bone and periosteum into adjacent vital structures
   - Treatment: Recommended is segmental mandibular resection with 1-cm margins. If tumor is contained within the mandibular cortex or periosteum, soft tissue need not be excised.
     - Although successful results with enucleation and curettage have been reported, recurrence can occur.
   - Reconstructive options depend on defect location and size and can include nonvascularized or vascularized bone grafts.

3. Bisphosphonate-related osteonecrosis (BRON)
   - Necrosis of the mandible after therapeutic dosages of bisphosphonates
   - Risk factors: Patients taking bisphosphonates with a history of cancer, dentoalveolar surgery, periodontal, and/or dental abscess; age older than 65; chemotherapy
   - Characterized by swelling, pain, infection, exposed bone, halitosis

- Treatment: Chlorhexidine mouth rinse, antibiotics. Superficial debridement or resection is recommended only in advanced disease with exposed necrotic bone that extends beyond the alveolus, concomitant pathologic fracture, or extraoral fistula.

Vascular Anomalies

1. Hemangioma
   - Vascular tumors that frequently appear within the first 4 weeks of life
     - Affects females more commonly than males.
   - Characterized by a red, spongy lesion with a rapid growth phase, followed by involution.
     - In general, 70% of hemangiomas will involute by 7 years of age.
     - Two types of congenital hemangiomas are possible. Compared to infantile hemangioma, congenital hemangiomas are negative for glucose transporter-1 (GLUT-1).
       - Rapidly involuting congenital hemangioma (typically involutes by 12 months of age)
       - Noninvoluting congenital hemangioma (will not involute)
   - Diagnosis: Often made through history, physical examination, and growth patterns
     - MRI and CT scan are useful for evaluation and demonstrate a well-defined vascular tumor.
   - Treatment options
     - Initial observation
     - Involution may be induced by steroid administration or propranolol treatment.
       - Cardiac monitoring is necessary for propranolol treatment
     - Surgical excision is indicated for persistent bleeding, when tumor location or growth impairs function or cosmesis (e.g., obstruction of globe, ear), or if the patient develops a platelet consumptive coagulopathy (Kassabach-Merritt syndrome).
     - Laser ablation is also a possibility.
   - Syndromic hemangioma disorders
     - von Hippel-Lindau syndrome
       - Characterized by retinal hemangiomas and hemangioblastomas of the cerebellum and viscera.
       - Associated with seizures and mental retardation.
     - PHACE Syndrome
       - Characterized by **p**osterior fossa cerebrovascular anomalies, large facial **h**emangiomas, **a**rterial anomalies, **c**ardiovascular abnormalities, and **e**ye abnormalities.
       - Diagnosis can be made by the presence of a hemangioma of the face plus one of the above extracutaneous manifestations discovered by MRI/magnetic resonance angiogram (MRA) of the brain, echocardiogram, and ophthalmologic exam.

2. Vascular malformations (VMs)
   - Arise from disorders in the embryologic development of the vascular system
   - Characterized by a lesion that is present at birth, grows proportionally with the child, and never involutes
   - Categorized based on vascular flow: Low or high
     - High-flow VMs
       - Contain an arterial component (e.g., arterial malformation, arteriovenous malformation [AVM])
         - Painless mass that is not compressible
         - May lead to distal ischemia or high-output cardiac failure.
       - Treatment: Selective embolization with subsequent resection
     - Low-flow VMs
       - Venous malformation
         - Most common low-flow VM
         - Bluish discoloration, compressible, painful secondary to thrombus formation or dependent position
         - Treatment: Sclerotherapy for symptomatic lesions, followed by surgical excision when amenable
       - Lymphatic malformation
         - Enlarge as a result of fluid accumulation, cellulitis, or inadequate drainage
         - Propensity for infection
         - May cause bone hypertrophy.
         - Treatment: First-line treatment is sclerotherapy for symptomatic lesions, and this can be followed by surgical resection when amenable.
       - Capillary malformation
         - "Port-wine stain"
         - Red or pink macular stains that can follow dermatomal distribution
         - Treatment: Pulse dye laser
         - Sturge-Weber syndrome
           - Characterized by capillary malformation in the distribution of the 1st and 2nd divisions of the trigeminal nerve (V1, V2), ocular abnormalities (e.g., glaucoma), and leptomeningeal VM.
           - Can be associated with soft-tissue or bony overgrowth
           - Requires close ophthalmology follow-up and MRI

3. Syndromic vascular anomalies
   - Sturge-Weber syndrome (see above)
   - Klippel-Trenaunay syndrome
     - Characterized by presence of a slow-flow capillary-lymphatic-venous malformation of an extremity with underlying soft-tissue or bony overgrowth.
     - Most commonly affects the lower extremities.
     - MRI will assist in diagnosis.
     - Treatment: Epiphysiodesis for limb-length discrepancies, sclerotherapy and compression of lymphatic and venous malformation components, staged contour resection for circumferential overgrowth

- Parkes Weber syndrome
  - Characterized by a fast-flow VM (typically an AVM), with associated soft-tissue and/or bony overgrowth and an overlying capillary malformation.
  - Most commonly affects the lower extremities.
  - Angiography will demonstrate the AVM.
  - Treatment depends on symptoms. Development of high-output cardiac failure because of shunting requires embolization.

Suggested Readings

Ariyan, S., Narayan, D., Ariyan, C.E., 2013. Chapter 14: Salivary gland tumors. In: Neligan, P.C., Rodrigueze, E.D. (Eds.), Plastic Surgery, vol. 3, 3rd ed. Elsevier, pp. 360–379.

Basal Cell Carcinoma Nevus Syndrome Life Support Network. Found at: <http://www.gorlinsyndrome.org/default.aspx.> Accessed on: October 23, 2014.

Boutros, S., 2007. Chapter 36: Reconstruction of the lips. In: Thorne, C.H., Beasley, R.W., Aston, S.J., et al. (Eds.), Grabb and Smith's Plastic Surgery, 6th ed. Wolters Kluwer, pp. 367–374.

Cheng, M.H., Huang, J.J., 2013. Chapter 12: Oral cavity, tongue, and mandibular reconstructions. In: Neligan, P.C., Rodrigueze, E.D. (Eds.), Plastic Surgery, vol. 3, 3rd ed. Elsevier, pp. 307–335.

Coleman, J.J., Tufaro, A.P., 2013. Chapter 16: Tumors of the lips, oral cavity, oropharynx, and mandible. In: Neligan, P.C., Rodrigueze, E.D. (Eds.), Plastic Surgery, vol. 3, 3rd ed. Elsevier, pp. 398–419.

Greene, A.K., Mulliken, J.B., 2013. Chapter 29: Vascular anomalies. In: Neligan, P.C., Gurtner, G. (Eds.), Plastic Surgery, vol. 1, 3rd ed. Elsevier, China, pp. 676–706.

Gulani, A.C., Hampton, R. von Hippel-Lindau Disease, emedicine.com. Found at: <http://emedicine.medscape.com/article/1219430-overview.> Accessed on: October 24, 2014.

Hellstein, J.W., 2010. Chapter 93: Odontogenesis, odontogenic cysts, and odontogenic tumors. In: Flint, P.W., Haughey, B.H., Lund, V.J., et al. (Eds.), Cummings Otolaryngology Head & Neck Surgery, 5th ed. Mosby, pp. 1259–1278.

Jackson, I.T., 2013. Chapter 18: Local flaps for facial coverage. In: Neligan, P.C., Rodrigueze, E.D. (Eds.), Plastic Surgery, vol. 3, 3rd ed. Elsevier, China, pp. 440–460.

Kupferman, M.E., Sacks, J.M., Chang, E.I., 2013. Chapter 17: Carcinoma of the upper aerodigestive tract. In: Neligan, P.C., Rodrigueze, E.D. (Eds.), Plastic Surgery, vol. 3, 3rd ed. Elsevier, pp. 420–439.

Metry, D., Heyer, G., Hess, C., et al., 2009. Consensus statement on diagnostic criteria for PHACE syndrome. Pediatrics 124 (5), 1447–1456.

Mulliken, J.B., 2007. Chapter 22: Vascular anomalies. In: Thorne, C.H., Beasley, R.W., Aston, S.J., et al. (Eds.), Grabb and Smith's Plastic Surgery, 6th ed. Wolters Kluwer, pp. 191–200.

Neligan, P.C., 2013. Chapter 10: Cheek and lip reconstruction. In: Neligan, P.C., Rodrigueze, E.D. (Eds.), Plastic Surgery, vol. 3, 3rd ed. Elsevier, China, pp. 254–277.

Saadeh, P.B., Delacure, M.D., 2007. Chapter 32: Head and neck cancer and salivary gland tumors. In: Thorne, C.H., Beasley, R.W., Aston, S.J., et al. (Eds.), Grabb and Smith's Plastic Surgery, 6th ed. Wolters Kluwer, pp. 333–346.

Seki, J.T., 2010. Chapter 60: Lip reconstruction. In: Weinzweig, J. (Ed.), Plastic Surgery Secrets Plus, 2nd ed. Mosby, pp. 401–408.

Yu, P., 2009. Chapter 8: Intraoral, pharynx, and esophagus. In: Butler, C.E. (Ed.), Head and Neck Reconstruction, Elsevier, pp. 167–196.

Yu, P., 2013. Chapter 13: Hypopharyngeal, esophageal, and neck reconstruction. In: Neligan, P.C., Rodrigueze, E.D. (Eds.), Plastic Surgery, vol. 3, 3rd ed. Elsevier, pp. 336–359.

Craniofacial Trauma

Chapter

4

General Anatomy

1. Facial buttresses: Provide structural support to the facial skeleton. Stability of buttresses is critical for maintenance of skeletal integrity, facial width and height, and balance of forces (see Figure 4.1).
   - Vertical buttresses (four)
     - Nasomaxillary
     - Zygomaticomaxillary
     - Pterygomaxillary
     - Mandibular ramus and condyle
   - Horizontal buttresses (four)
     - Supraorbital rim
     - Infraorbital rim (upper transverse maxillary)
     - Nasal floor and maxillary alveolus
     - Mandibular arch

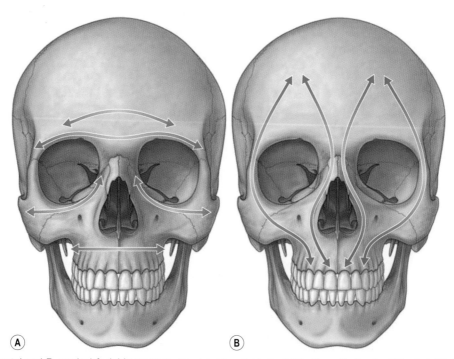

Figure 4.1. A, Horizontal and **B,** vertical facial buttresses. *(Reprinted from Goldenberg, D.C., Alonso, N., Ferreira, M.C., et al. (Eds.), 2009. Plastic Surgery: Indications and Practice, 1st ed. Elsevier, 619–644.)*

2. Scalp layers
   - Skin
   - Subcutaneous fat
   - Galea aponeurosis
   - Loose areolar tissue
     - Layer at which traumatic avulsion injury occurs
   - Pericranium

Preoperative Considerations

1. Airway, breathing, circulation (ABC), and trauma resuscitation
2. In high-energy injuries (e.g., motor vehicle collisions, "whiplash" injuries, facial injury from relatively fixed object), must rule out concomitant cervical spine injury.
   - Reported incidence of 5% to 15%
3. Operating room airway control is important when planning fixation of fractures.
   - In the setting of nasal, midface, and mandibular fractures, tracheostomy should be considered.
   - For mandible fractures, nasotracheal intubation is preferred.
4. Presence of facial laceration warrants thorough facial nerve examination.
   - Ask the patient to elevate brow, close eyes, smile, evert lower lip, and purse lips.
   - Intact facial nerve motor function on exam obviates the need for facial nerve exploration.
5. Presence of cheek laceration warrants evaluation for concomitant parotid duct (Stenson duct) injury.
   - The course of the parotid duct (~5 cm in length) loosely follows a line drawn from the lower margin of the concha to midway between the red margin of the upper lip and the ala of the nose.
   - The papilla of the duct can be found within the mucosa of the cheek at the level of the 2nd maxillary molar.
   - Diagnosis of parotid duct injury
     - Cannulation of the intraoral papilla and subsequent saline (or methylene blue) flush: Presence of fluid rush or methylene blue within the laceration during the flush is consistent with injury.
   - Treatment of parotid duct injuries
     - Distal duct injuries can be treated with silastic stenting or intraoral drainage.
     - Proximal duct injuries can be treated with direct repair over a stent or ligation (if repair is impossible).
       - Ligation often leads to atrophy of the parotid gland but can also result in sialocele formation.

Frontal Sinus and Frontal Bone Fractures

1. Frontal sinus development
   - Absent at birth
   - Begins to develop at age 2
   - Appears on radiographs near age 7
   - Fully developed at age 15

2. Frontal sinus anatomy
   - Anterior "table"
     - Forms part of the forehead, brow, and glabella
     - Most resistant facial bone to fracture
     - Thickness or width can range from 4 to 12 mm.
   - Posterior "table"
     - Adjacent to the dura and cranial fossa
     - Thickness or width can range from 0.1 to 4.8 mm.
   - Nasofrontal duct (also known as frontonasal duct or nasofrontal outflow tract [NFOT])
3. Injury pattern, nasofrontal duct (or NFOT) function, and presence or absence of cerebrospinal fluid leak dictates general management algorithms (see Figure 4.2).
4. Isolated anterior table fractures
   - Nondisplaced (patent nasofrontal duct): No operative treatment warranted unless cosmetic concerns; consider antibiotic prophylaxis.
   - Displaced: Open reduction and internal fixation (ORIF) for improved contour
   - Fracture with involvement of nasofrontal duct: Obliteration of nasofrontal duct and sinus
5. Posterior table fractures
   - Nondisplaced posterior table fractures: No operative fixation warranted; antibiotic prophylaxis, observation for cerebrospinal fluid (CSF) leak
   - Displacement of fractures by 1 table width or greater: Many advocate for cranialization of the sinus with obliteration of the nasofrontal duct.
   - Significant displacement of both the anterior and posterior tables: Cranialization of the sinus with obliteration of the nasofrontal duct
   - Fracture with involvement of nasofrontal duct: Obliteration of the nasofrontal duct and cranialization depending on the degree of comminution and/or displacement
6. Nasofrontal duct injury
   - Warrants operative treatment with removal of sinus mucosa and duct obliteration. If posterior table is also involved, see recommendations above for general cranialization indications.
   - Obliteration can be accomplished with vascularized soft-tissue (e.g., pericranium) flaps, cancellous bone, muscle, fat, and/or synthetic bone cements.
     - Pericranium and cancellous bone are preferred.
     - Free fat and muscle grafts are associated with high rates of necrosis and resorption.
   - Mucocele
     - Sterile fluid-filled cyst
       - Can become infected (mucopyocele)
     - Typically occurs in patients with untreated frontal sinus fractures with missed nasofrontal duct injury
     - Can also develop after treatment/obliteration of the sinus secondary to retained sinus mucosa
7. CSF leak
   - Greater risk leak with posterior table fractures displaced >1 table width because of higher risk for associated dural tear

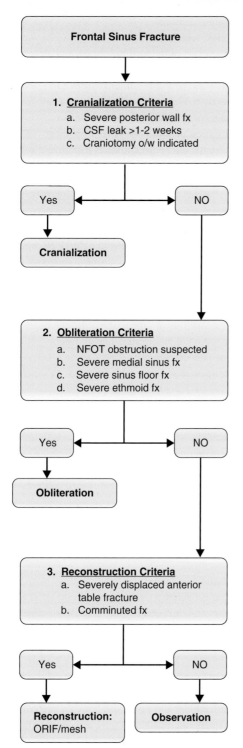

Figure 4.2. Frontal sinus fracture treatment algorithm. *CSF,* cerebrospinal fluid; *fx,* fracture; *NFOT,* nasofrontal outflow tract; *ORIF,* open reduction and internal fixation; *o/w,* otherwise. *(Reprinted from Echo, A., Troy, J.S., Hollier, L.H., 2010. Frontal sinus fractures. Semin. Plast. Surg. 24 (4), 375–382.)*

- Diagnosis
  - Clear appearing fluid
  - Positive beta-2 transferrin test ("send out test"); most reliable
  - "Halo" sign
    - Place drop of fluid on filter paper. CSF fluid will diffuse faster than blood and give the appearance of a "halo" around a center stain.
  - Elevated glucose on fluid chemistry
- CSF rhinorrhea is caused by a fracture of the cribriform plate with underlying dural injury.
- Treatment options
  - Observation with head elevation >30 degrees, bed rest, and antibiotics
  - If CSF leak lasts >4 days, can place a lumbar drain.
  - If CSF leak lasts >7-10 days, despite lumbar drainage, can proceed to craniotomy, dural repair, and treatment of frontal sinus injury (obliteration vs. cranialization).

Orbital Fractures

1. Commonly occur after assault, falls, or motor vehicle collisions.
2. A direct blow to the orbit typically results in force transmission and dissipation of the acute increase in intraorbital pressure through the weak points within the orbital framework (e.g., lamina papyracea, medial orbital wall, orbital floor; see Figure 4.3).

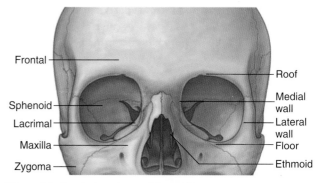

Figure 4.3. Surgical anatomy of the orbits. *(Reprinted from Goldenberg, D.C., Alonso, N., Ferreira, M.C., et al. (Eds.), 2009. Plastic Surgery: Indications and Practice, 1st ed. Elsevier, 619–644.)*

3. In the trauma setting, orbital fractures are often associated with concomitant zygoma and midface and nasal fractures.
4. Fractures of the orbit require careful examination to rule out entrapment of extraocular muscles, direct trauma to the globe, and/or optic nerve injury.
   - An ophthalmology exam is generally warranted for all orbit fractures.
   - Entrapment of the inferior rectus requires emergent operative treatment, especially in the pediatric population.
     - Delayed repair of entrapment in the pediatric population (typically >72 hours) can result in permanent visual deficit.

Craniosynostosis and Craniofacial Syndromes

General Craniosynostosis Nomenclature and Information

1. Craniosynostosis: Abnormal fusion of cranial sutures leading to abnormal head shape
   - May lead to increased intracranial pressure (ICP) and developmental delay
     - Increased ICP can be diagnosed by papilledema and "thumb printing" on radiographic studies.
   - Prevalence: ~1:2500 live births
   - Most common synostosis: Sagittal, followed by unilateral coronal, bilateral coronal, metopic, and lambdoid
   - Most infants with single-suture synostosis are nonsyndromic, whereas most with multisuture synostosis do have a syndrome.
   - Most syndromic craniosynostoses are related to fibroblast growth factor receptor (FGFR) genes and present with bilateral coronal craniosynostosis in isolation or in association with other suture synostoses.
   - Syndromic craniosynostoses and their related gene mutations
     - Apert syndrome: FGFR-2
     - Crouzon syndrome: FGFR-2
     - Pfeiffer syndrome: FGFR-2
     - Saethre-Chotzen syndrome: TWIST 1

2. Cranial sutures (see Figure 5.1)
   - Act as growth centers for the cranium and allow skull deformation for passage through the birth canal
   - With an open suture, the bone grows perpendicular to the suture line.
   - When the suture is fused, compensatory bone growth occurs parallel to the suture line (see Table 5.2).

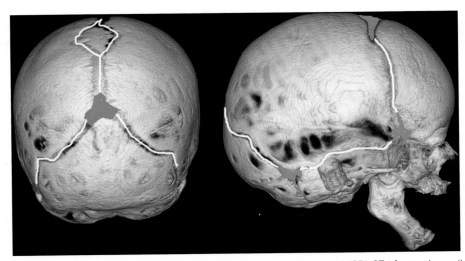

Figure 5.1. Normal sutures and fontanels. Posterior and lateral views of a three-dimensional (3D) CT of a newborn. *(Left)* Posterior view of the skull, demonstrating the posterior fontanel *(blue)*, the sagittal and the paired lambdoid sutures *(white lines)*. The sagittal suture contains an incidental wormian bone. *(Right)* Right lateral view demonstrating the mastoidal fontanel posteriorly, the sphenoidal fontanel anteriorly, and at the vertex the anterior fontanel *(blue)*, which is only partially seen. The right coronal, squamosal, and right lambdoid sutures are patent *(white lines)*. *(Reprinted from Kirmi, O., Lo, S.J., Johnson, D., et al., 2009. Craniosynostosis: a radiological and surgical perspective. Sem. Ultrasound CT MRI 30 (6), 492–512.)*

3. Suture closure (see Figure 5.2)
   - Order of closure: Metopic suture (8-9 months), sagittal suture (22 years of age), coronal suture (24 years), lambdoid suture (26 years), and squamosal suture (>60 years)

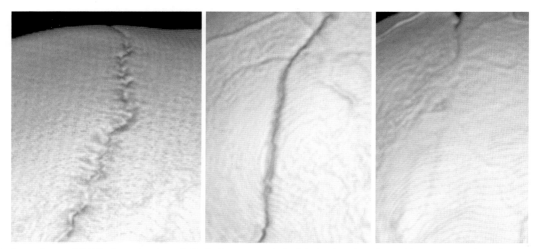

Figure 5.2. Fusing sutures. 3D CT: Normal suture *(left)*, fusing suture *(middle)* that has lost its architecture, and bone bridging of a fused suture *(right)*. *(Reprinted from Kirmi, O., Lo, S.J., Johnson, D., et al., 2009. Craniosynostosis: a radiological and surgical perspective. Sem. Ultrasound CT MRI 30 (6), 492–512.)*

4. Common craniofacial terms
   - Hypertelorism: Abnormal increase in the distance between the bony orbits
   - Hypotelorism: Decreased distance between the bony orbits
   - Telecanthus: Increased distance between the medial canthi
   - Exorbitism: Protrusion of the globe due to decreased volume of orbit

Craniosynostoses

See Figure 5.3.
1. Metopic craniosynostosis
   - Also known as trigonocephaly ("triangular-shaped" head)
   - Characterized by
     - Keel-shaped forehead
     - Metopic ridge (in mild cases)
     - Bitemporal narrowing
     - Parietal expansion
     - Hypotelorism
   - Most likely to be associated with midline brain abnormalities
2. Sagittal craniosynostosis
   - Also known as scaphocephaly ("boat-shaped head") or dolichocephaly
   - Characterized by
     - Bilateral frontal and occipital bossing
     - Elongated head in the anteroposterior direction
     - Decreased biparietal width

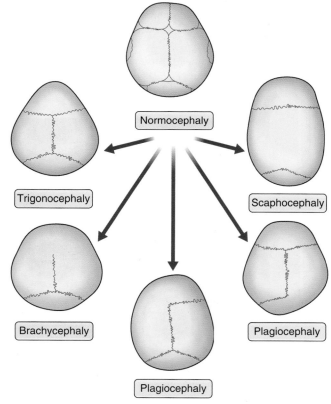

Figure 5.3. Characteristic skull shape depending on sutural involvement in craniosynostosis. *(Reprinted from Neligan, P.C., Losee, J. [Eds.], 2013. Plastic Surgery, 3rd ed. Elsevier, 726–748.)*

- Treatment: Endoscopic resection of the sagittal suture with postoperative helmet molding can often safely be performed on patients at 3 months of age.

3. Coronal craniosynostosis
   - Unilateral coronal craniosynostosis is also known as anterior plagiocephaly; bicoronal craniosynostosis is known as brachycephaly ("short, flat head").
   - Unilateral coronal synostosis is characterized by
     - Flattening of the ipsilateral forehead and supraorbital rim
     - Contralateral forehead bossing
     - "Harlequin" eye deformity: Flattened supraorbital rim, raised eyebrow, widened palpebral opening, deficient lateral orbital rim, steep superior orbital fissure, and sphenoid wing
     - Anterior displacement of the ipsilateral ear
     - Deviation of the nasal root toward the affected side
   - Bilateral coronal synostosis is characterized by
     - Symmetric, flat forehead
     - Increased biparietal width
     - Decreased anteroposterior length
     - Turricephaly or turribrachycephaly; can occur in certain patients in which there is a compensatory increase in parietal height leading to a "tall, flat head"

4. Lambdoid craniosynostosis
   - Also known as posterior plagiocephaly; very rare
   - Distinguished from deformational plagiocephaly by a "trapezoid"-shaped head
   - Characterized by
     - Flattening of the ipsilateral occiput
     - Inferior displaced mastoid bulge on affected side
     - Contralateral forehead bossing
     - Inferior displacement of the ipsilateral ear

5. Multisuture craniosynostosis
   - Involves premature fusion of multiple sutures
   - In the most severe form (pansutural synostosis), patients can develop a "cloverleaf" skull deformity (also known as the kleeblattschädel skull deformity)
     - Characterized by a "moth-eaten" appearance of bone on computed tomography (CT) imaging
     - May lead to severe increases in ICP and airway anomalies

6. Treatment of craniosynostosis depends on severity, appearance, and functional concerns.
   - Goals of surgery: Suture release to allow brain growth and development; normalization of head shape; reduction of functional deficits (e.g., increased intracranial pressure, developmental delay, etc.)
   - Timing of surgery is often dependent on the severity of the abnormality, with the more severe or symptomatic (e.g., increased ICP) patient often requiring surgery between 6 and 12 months of age.

7. Surgical treatment options (see Table 5.1)
   - Cranial vault remodeling: Multiple techniques have been described.
     - Surgery is often performed between 6 and 12 months of age.
   - Distraction osteogenesis
     - Useful for advancements >1 cm
     - Latency phase
       ○ The phase following osteotomy and application of the distractor device in which there is no bony movement
       ○ A typical latency phase lasts between 1 and 7 days.
     - Activation phase
       ○ The phase following the latency period in which the distractor is moved at a set rate (e.g., 1 mm/day)
       ○ Encourages bone formation
     - Consolidation phase
       ○ The distraction is completed, the device is left in place, and the new bone is allowed to consolidate and calcify.
       ○ A typical consolidation period is twice the duration of the active distraction.
   - Midface advancement
     - Often, LeFort I or III advancements
   - Rhinoplasty

Table 5.1 Skull Deformity in Craniosynostosis and Operative Techniques Used for Correction

FUSED SUTURE	SKULL SHAPE	HYPOPLASTIC ELEMENTS	COMPENSATORY GROWTH	OPERATIVE TECHNIQUES
Sagittal	Scaphocephaly	Biparietal, bitemporal	AP lengthening, frontal bossing, occipital protrusion	Strip craniectomy, cranial vault remodeling, spring-assisted cranioplasty
Unicoronal	Plagiocephaly	Ipsilateral frontal flattening, orbital rim recession	Contralateral frontal and temporal bulging, ipsilateral facial sutures (facial scoliosis)	FOA
Bicoronal	Brachycephaly	Occipital flattening, AP shortening	Elevation in skull height	FOA
Lambdoid	Plagiocephaly	Ipsilateral parieto-occipital flattening	Bulging of contralateral parieto-occipital bone	Lambdoid strip craniectomy, biparietal occipital remodeling
Metopic	Trigonocephaly	Hypotelorism, superior orbital rim recession, bitemporal narrowing	Parietal flaring	FOA

Reprinted from Kirmi, O., Lo, S.J., Johnson, D., et al. 2009. Sem. Ultrasound CT MRI 30 (6), 492–512.
AP, Anterior-posterior; FOA, fronto-orbital advancement.

Deformational Plagiocephaly

1. Not a true synostosis; abnormal head shape related to external forces and positioning
   - Increase in prevalence correlates with the "Back to Sleep" Campaign, instituted by the American Academy of Pediatrics
   - Other associated factors: Male gender, multiparity, torticollis
2. Distinguished from true synostosis (e.g., lambdoid or coronal craniosynostosis) by "parallelogram"-shaped head (see Figure 5.4)

Table 5.2 Cephalic Index, Based on Maximal Cranial Length and Maximal Cranial Width

CI	SUGGESTED DIAGNOSIS
<71	Hyperdolichocephalic
71-76	Dolichocephalic/scaphocephalic (as with sagittal)
76-81	Mesocephalic
81-81.5	Brachycephalic (as with bicoronal)
>85.5	Hyperbrachycephalic

Reprinted from Bennaceur, S., Petavy-Blanc, A.S., Chauve, J., et al. 2005. Human cephalic morphology. Anthropometry. In: Laffont, A., Durieuz, F. (Eds.), Encyclopédie Médicochirurgicale, Elsevier, 85–103.
CI, Cephalic index; CI = Wd/L × 100, where Wd is the maximal cranial width and L the maximal cranial length.

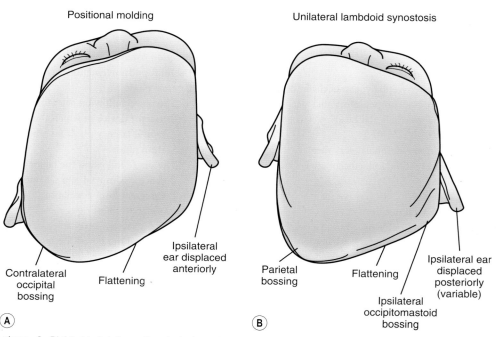

Positional molding — Contralateral occipital bossing, Flattening, Ipsilateral ear displaced anteriorly **(A)**

Unilateral lambdoid synostosis — Parietal bossing, Flattening, Ipsilateral occipitomastoid bossing, Ipsilateral ear displaced posteriorly (variable) **(B)**

Figure 5.4. Vertex views. **A,** Right-sided deformational plagiocephaly exhibiting a parallelogram head shape. **B,** Right-sided lambdoid craniosynostosis exhibiting a trapezoid-like head shape. *(Reprinted from Zitelli, B.J., McIntire, S.C., Nowalk, A.J. [Eds.], 2012. Atlas of Pediatric Physical Diagnosis, 6th ed. Elsevier, 889–912.)*

3. Characterized by
   - Flattening of the ipsilateral occiput
   - Ipsilateral forehead bossing
   - Anterior displacement of the ipsilateral ear
4. Treatment: Conservative
   - Helmet molding
   - Positioning (e.g., increase "tummy time")
   - Observation
   - Treatment of torticollis if contributing to positioning issues

Syndromic Craniosynostosis

1. Apert syndrome (acrocephalosyndactyly; see Figure 5.5)
   - Autosomal dominant
   - *FGFR-2* gene mutation
   - Characterized by turribrachycephaly, midface hypoplasia, *complex syndactylies of the hands and feet,* exorbitism, and often intellectual disability

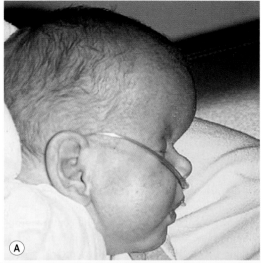

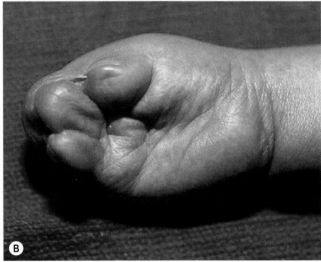

Figure 5.5. Apert syndrome. **A,** Lateral view of a child with Apert syndrome. **B,** Syndactyly of the hand. *(Reprinted from Zitelli, B.J., McIntire, S.C., Nowalk, A.J. [Eds.], 2012. Atlas of Pediatric Physical Diagnosis, 6th ed. Elsevier, 889–912.)*

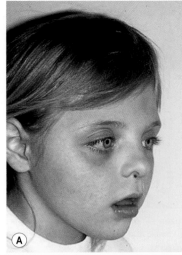

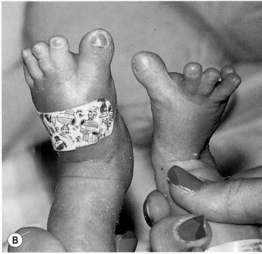

Figure 5.6. Pfeiffer syndrome. **A,** Lateral view. **B,** Great toe anomalies. *(Reprinted from Zitelli, B.J., McIntire, S.C., Nowalk, A.J. [Eds.], 2012. Atlas of Pediatric Physical Diagnosis, 6th ed. Elsevier, 889–912.)*

2. Saethre-Chotzen syndrome (acrocephalosyndactyly)
   - Autosomal dominant
   - *TWIST-1* gene mutation
   - Characterized by bicoronal craniosynostosis, *eyelid ptosis,* low hairline, proptosis, antimongoloid slanting of palpebral fissures, and syndactyly of the hands and/or feet
3. Pfeiffer syndrome (acrocephalosyndactyly; see Figure 5.6)
   - Autosomal dominant
   - *FGFR-1* or *FGFR-2* gene mutation
   - Characterized by bicoronal craniosynostosis, *enlarged thumbs and halluces,* and mild partial syndactyly of the hands and feet

4. Crouzon syndrome (craniofacial dysostosis; see Figure 5.7)
   - Autosomal dominant
   - *FGFR-2* and/or *FGFR-3* gene mutation
   - Characterized by bicoronal craniosynostosis (occasionally turribrachycephaly), midface hypoplasia, exorbitism, and *normal hands and feet*
   - Increased chance of ocular herniation due to hypolastia of the greater wing of the sphenoid

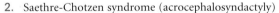

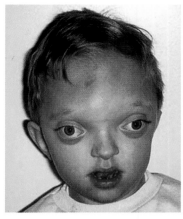

Figure 5.7. Crouzon syndrome. Frontal view. *(Reprinted from Zitelli, B.J., McIntire, S.C., Nowalk, A.J. [Eds.], 2012. Atlas of Pediatric Physical Diagnosis, 6th ed. Elsevier, 889–912.)*

5. Carpenter syndrome
   - Autosomal recessive
   - Characterized by mutlisutural craniosynostosis (e.g., sagittal, lambdoid, coronal), *preaxial polydactyly of the feet, symbrachydactyly (shortness) of the hands,* developmental delay, and *ocular findings*
6. Muenke syndrome
   - Autosomal dominant
   - *FGFR-3* gene mutation
   - Characterized by unicoronal or bicoronal craniosynostosis, midface hypoplasia, *carpal or tarsal fusions,* sensorineural hearing loss
7. Waardenburg Syndrome
   - Autosomal dominant with variable penetrance
   - *PAX3* or *MITF* gene mutations
   - Characterized by
     - Sensorineural hearing loss
     - *Telecanthus*
     - *White forelock of hair*
     - Craniosynostosis
     - Broad nasal bridge and high-arched cleft palate
     - Congenital heart disease, neural tube defects

Nonsynostotic Syndromes

1. Craniofacial microsomia (oculoauriculovertebral [OAV] spectrum disorder)
   - Second most common craniofacial anomaly after cleft lip and palate
   - Exact etiology is unknown, although some postulate that it may be related to a defect of the stapedial artery.
   - Highly variable presentation affecting structures of the first and second branchial arches; more commonly unilateral
   - Three main features
     - Auricular hypoplasia: May include small ears, auricular skin tags, and/or microtia
     - Mandibular hypoplasia: Typical presentation includes hypoplasia or absence of the mandibular ramus and/or

condyle, chin deviation to the affected side, and an occlusal cant upward on the affected side (see Figure 5.8).
     - Maxillary hypoplasia: Hypoplasia of the ipsilateral maxillary dentoalveolar process (contributes to the occlusal cant)
   - Cranial nerve abnormalities are also common and most frequently involve the facial nerve.
     - The most common finding is dysfunction of the marginal mandibular nerve on the affected side (see Table 5.3).
   - Treatment
     - Commissuroplasty for macrostomia repair: Reconstruction of the orbicularis oris and layered closure is paramount for successful commissuroplasty.
     - Mandibular distraction: Useful for patients with Type-IIA or -IIB mandibular deformity
     - Rib or iliac crest bone grafts are useful in the absence of the ramus and condyle (Type-III mandibular defects as above); the cartilaginous portion should be removed on rib grafts to reduce the risk for overgrowth.
     - Microtia/ear reconstruction: Typically performed when a child is 6 to 7 years of age or 10 years of age (if using the Nagata technique)
     - Orthognathic surgery: Reserved for skeletally mature patients when indicated
2. Goldenhar syndrome (OAV dysplasia/sequence)
   - A variant of craniofacial microsomia
   - Characterized by
     - *Epibulbar dermoids*
     - Preauricular skin tags
     - Spinal anomalies
     - Hypoplasia of the ear, mandible, and maxilla
   - Occasionally associated with cleft lip and palate
3. Treacher Collins syndrome ("mandibulofacial dysostosis")
   - Autosomal dominant; always bilateral and almost always symmetric
   - *TCOF1* gene mutation
   - Characterized by
     - Normal intelligence
     - *Lower lid colobomas* with absence of cilia
     - Downward slanting of the palpebral fissures
     - *Hypoplasia of the maxilla and zygoma,* with absence of the zygomatic arch
     - Tessier 6, 7, or 8 orofacial cleft
     - Conductive hearing loss
     - Mandibular hypoplasia and retrognathia
   - Other associated anomalies: Cleft palate and velopharyngeal insufficiency (in 33% of cases) (see Figure 5.9)
   - Treatment: Staged reconstruction. Example:
     - Within first year, macrostomia repair, tracheostomy
     - At 12 months, cleft palate repair
     - At 2 to 3 years, staged eyelid reconstruction (e.g., wedge resection of coloboma vs. tripier flap vs. graft), mandibular distraction

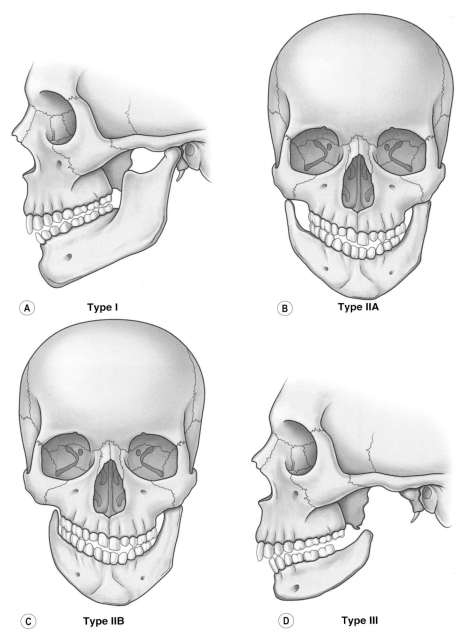

Figure 5.8. Pruzansky classification of the mandibular deformity, as modified by Kaban et al. **A,** Type I: Mandibular deficiency is only mild. **B,** Type IIA: Condyle and ramus are small, but condyle and glenoid fossa are anatomically oriented. Note that a flattened condyle can be hinged on a flat, often hypoplastic, infratemporal surface, and the coronoid process may be absent. **C,** Type IIB: Similar to type IIA except that the vertical or superoinferior plane of the condyle ramus is medially displaced. There is no functioning glenoid fossa. **D,** Type III: Absence of the ramus, condyle, and coronoid process. *(Reprinted from Neligan, P.C., Losee, J. [Eds.], 2013. Plastic Surgery, 3rd ed. Elsevier, 761–791.)*

- At 7 to 10 years, bone grafting for zygoma reconstruction, ear reconstruction
- Skeletal maturity: Orthognathic surgery, genioplasty, rhinoplasty
4. Nager syndrome (acrofacial dysostosis)
   - Autosomal recessive; extremely rare
   - Craniofacial features similar to Treacher Collins syndrome
- Characterized by
   - Hypoplasia of the zygoma, maxilla, and mandible
   - Pierre Robin sequence with cleft palate and velopharyngeal insufficiency (VPI)
   - *Radial hand deformities:* Thumb and/or radial hypoplasia, camptodactyly, syndactyly, clinodactyly

Table 5.3 Spectrum and Incidence of Associated Extracranial Malformations in Craniofacial Microsomia

PRINCIPAL ANOMALIES		ASSOCIATED ANOMALIES	
Mandibular	Mandibular hypoplasia (89-100%), malformed glenoid fossa (24-27%)	Craniofacial	VPI (35-55%), palatal deviation (39-50%), orbital dystopia (15-43%), ocular motility disorders (19-22%), epibulbar dermoids (4-35%), cranial base anomalies (9-30%), cleft lip and/or palate (15-22%), eyelid defects (12-25%), hypodontia/dental hypoplasia (8-25%), lacrimal drainage abnormalities (11-14%), frontal plagiocephaly (10-12%), sensorineural hearing loss (6-16%), preauricular sinus (6-9%), parotid gland hypoplasia, other cranial nerve defects (e.g., V, IX, XII)
Ear	Microtia (66-99%), preauricular tags (34-61%), conductive hearing loss (50-66%), middle-ear (ossicle) defects	General	Vertebral/rib defects (16-60%), cervical spine anomalies (24-42%), scoliosis (11-26%), cardiac anomalies (4-33%), pigmentation changes (13-14%), extremity defects (3-21%), central nervous system defects (5-18%), genitourinary defects (4-15%), pulmonary anomalies (1-15%), gastrointestinal defects (2-12%)
Midfacial	Maxillary and zygomatic hypoplasia, occlusal canting		
Soft-Tissue	Masticatory muscles hypoplasia (85-95%), macrostomia (17-62%), seventh-nerve palsy (10-45%)		

The prevalence rates were summarized from 19 reports that appeared in the literature from 1983 to 1996. Studies based on selected samples were omitted to minimize selection bias. The authors recognized that the prevalence rate may be falsely elevated because the reporting tertiary centers may have a referral bias of more severely affected patients.
VPI, Velopharyngeal insufficiency.
Adapted from Cousley, R.R., Calvert, M.L. 1997. Current concepts in the understanding and management of hemifacial microsomia. Br. J. Plast. Surg. 50, 536–551.

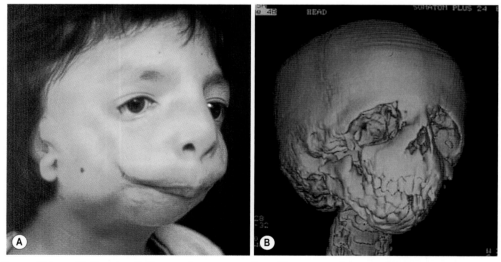

Figure 5.9. A, A 7-year-old boy with Treacher Collins syndrome presenting with severe coloboma of the lower eyelids, hypoplastic maxilla, and underprojected and narrow maxilla. There is bilateral microtia and macrostomia. The mandible shows severe hypoplasia, including at the menton. **B,** 3D-CT scan showing absence of the zygoma and malar bone and lack of inferolateral orbital floor. The mandible has a very short ascending ramus and the posterior aspect of the maxilla is also very short vertically. *(Reprinted from Neligan, P.C., Losee, J. [Eds.], 2013. Plastic Surgery, 3rd ed. Elsevier, 828.)*

5. Binder syndrome (nasomaxillary dysplasia)
   - Autosomal recessive, with incomplete penetrance
   - Exact etiology unknown, although some postulate that this is related to an underdevelopment of the nasomaxillary spine.
   - Characterized by
     - *Absent or reduced anterior nasal spine,* leading to a short nose, short columella, and flat nasal bridge
     - Acute nasolabial angle
     - Class-III malocclusion
     - Concave facial profile ("dish face")
   - Treatment: Orthognathic surgery (LeFort I or II osteotomy advancement) followed by dorsal nose augmentation
6. Mobius syndrome
   - Often sporadic, but autosomal dominant and recessive familial patterns have been reported.
   - Characterized by
     - *Bilateral congenital abducens and facial nerve palsies*
     - Other cranial nerve involvement (e.g., hypoglossal, vagus)
     - Musculoskeletal abnormalities (e.g., clubfoot)
     - Congenital heart defects

- Occasionally associated with cleft palate, retrogenia, and microstomia
- Treatment: Eye protection, facial reanimation with free functioning muscle transfer after the age of 5
  - For bilateral cases, operations are often spaced 3 to 6 months apart.

7. Parry-Romberg syndrome/disease (progressive hemifacial atrophy)
   - Etiology unknown, although some postulate that it may be related to an autoimmune disorder or a variant of scleroderma.
   - Characterized by *progressive hemifacial atrophy* beginning between 5 and 15 years of age and involves skin, soft tissue, muscle, and bone within the *trigeminal nerve dermatomes*
     - Classic sign: Linear indentation along the forehead ("coup de sabre")
   - Patients have normal facial appearance until the disease occurs.
   - Can be associated with seizures or other neurologic symptoms
   - Treatment: Fat grafting or microvascular fasciocutaneous flaps (e.g., parascapular or scapular flaps) to restore facial contour; immunosuppression in combination with methotrexate has been shown to stop progression of disease
     - Should be delayed until disease progression has stopped

8. Stickler syndrome (hereditary arthro-ophthalmopathy)
   - Autosomal dominant
   - Collagen production gene mutations (e.g., *COL2A1*, *COL11A1*, *COL11A2*)
   - Characterized by deficits of the eyes, craniofacial skeleton, ears, and joints, including
     - Cataract
     - Retinal detachment

- Myopia
- *Micrognathia and Pierre Robin sequence*
- Midface hypoplasia and malar bridge depression
- *Bifid uvula and submucous cleft palate*
- Early-onset degenerative joint disease

Suggested Readings

Buchanan, E.P., Xue, A.S., Hollier, L.H., 2014. Craniofacial syndromes. Plast. Reconstr. Surg. 134 (1), 128e–153e.

Campbell, C.A., Yu, J.C., Lin, K.Y., 2010. Chapter 38: Craniofacial microsomia. In: Weinzweig, J. (Ed.), Plastic Surgery Secrets Plus, 2nd ed. Mosby, pp. 253–256.

Fearon, J., 2013. Chapter 35: Syndromic craniosynostosis. In: Neligan, P.C., Losee, J. (Eds.), Plastic Surgery, 3rd ed. Elsevier, pp. 749–760.

Forrest, C.R., Hopper, R.A., 2013. Craniofacial syndromes and surgery. Plast. Reconstr. Surg. 131 (1), 86e–109e.

Jones, K.L., Jones, M.C., Casanelles Del Campo, M., 2013. Craniosynostosis syndromes. In: Smith's Recognizable Patterns of Human Malformation, 7th ed. Saunders Elsevier, Philadelphia, pp. 530–559.

Kirmi, O., Lo, S.J., Johnson, D., et al., 2009. Craniosynostosis: a radiological and surgical perspective. Sem. Ultrasound CT MRI 30 (6), 492–512.

Kirschner, R.E., Nah, H.D., 2009. Chapter 28: Craniofacial growth: Genetic and morphological processes in craniosynostosis. In: Guyuron, B., Eriksson, E., Persing, J.A., et al. (Eds.), Plastic Surgery: Indications and Practice, 1st ed. Elsevier, pp. 317–330.

Lin, A.Y., Losee, J.E., 2012. Chapter 22: Pediatric plastic surgery. In: Zitelli, B.J., McIntire, S.C., Nowalk, A.J. (Eds.), Atlas of Pediatric Physical Diagnosis, 6th ed. Elsevier, pp. 889–912.

McCarthy, J.G., Grayson, B.H., Hopper, R.A., et al., 2013. Chapter 36: Craniofacial microsomia. In: Neligan, P.C., Losee, J. (Eds.), Plastic Surgery, 3rd ed. Elsevier, pp. 761–791.

Molina, F., 2013. Chapter 39: Treacher-Collins syndrome. In: Neligan, P.C., Losee, J. (Eds.), Plastic Surgery, 3rd ed. Elsevier, p. 828.

Persing, J.A., Knoll, B., Duncan, C.C., 2009. Chapter 33: Non-syndromic craniosynostosis. In: Guyuron, B., Eriksson, E., Persing, J.A., et al. (Eds.), Plastic Surgery: Indications and Practice, 1st ed. Elsevier, pp. 389–404.

Steinbacher, D.M., Bartlett, S.P., 2013. Chapter 34: Nonsyndromic craniosynostosis. In: Neligan, P.C., Losee, J. (Eds.), Plastic Surgery, 3rd ed. Elsevier, pp. 726–748.

Taub, P.J., Silver, L., Torok, K.S., 2013. Chapter 37: Hemifacial atrophy. In: Neligan, P.C., Losee, J. (Eds.), Plastic Surgery, 3rd ed. Elsevier, pp. 792–802.

Tewfik, T.L. Manifestations of Craniofacial Syndromes. Meyers, A.D., Ed. Emedicine.com. Available at: <http://emedicine.medscape.com/article/844209-overview.> Accessed on: November 20, 2014.

Weinzweig, J., Whitaker, L.A., 2010. Chapter 30: Craniosynostosis. In: Weinzweig, J. (Ed.), Plastic Surgery Secrets Plus, 2nd ed. Mosby, pp. 196–211.

Clefts and Orthognathic Surgery

Chapter

6

Embryology

1. The formation of the face occurs between the 4th and 10th weeks of human development, secondary to fusion of the midline frontonasal prominence and the paired maxillary, lateral nasal, and mandibular prominences (see Figure 6.1).

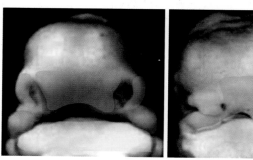

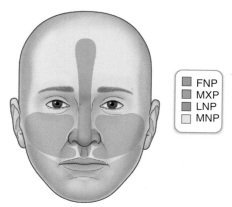

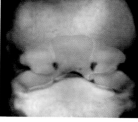

Figure 6.1. Prominences of vertebrate face. Frontonasal prominence *(FNP),* which contributes to forehead, middle of the nose, philtrum, and primary palate; maxillary prominence *(MXP),* which contributes to sides of face, lip, and secondary palate; lateral nasal prominence *(LNP),* which forms sides of nose; and mandibular prominence *(MNP),* which produces lower jaw. *(Reprinted from Neligan, P.C., Losee, J. [Eds.], 2013. Plastic Surgery, vol. 3, 3rd ed. Elsevier, 503–516.)*

- Frontonasal prominence
  - Forms the forehead, midline of the nose, philtrum, middle portion of the upper lip, and the primary palate
  - Gives rise to the lateral and medial nasal processes
- Lateral nasal prominence/process
  - Forms the nasal alae
- Maxillary prominence
  - Forms the upper jaw, sides of the face, sides of the upper lip, and the secondary palate
- Mandibular prominence
  - Forms the lower jaw and lip

2. Cleft lip deformities
   - From disruptions occurring during the 3rd to 7th weeks of gestation
   - Unilateral cleft lip: Failure of fusion of the medial nasal process and the maxillary prominence on one side
   - Bilateral cleft lip: Failure of fusion of the merged medial nasal processes with the maxillary prominences bilaterally

3. Cleft palate deformities
   - From disruptions occurring during the 5th to 12th weeks of gestation
   - Cleft of the primary palate (anterior to the incisive foramen): Failure of fusion of the frontonasal prominence (median palatine process) and maxillary prominences (lateral palatine process)
   - Cleft of the secondary palate (posterior to the incisive foramen): Failure of fusion of the maxillary prominences (lateral palatine processes)
   - Fusion of the palate proceeds from anterior to posterior as the tongue drops and the lateral palatal shelves rotate from a vertical to horizontal orientation (~7 to 8 weeks gestation).

Epidemiology

1. Isolated cleft palate and cleft lip with or without cleft palate are thought to be two genetically distinct deformities (see Table 6.1).
   - The incidence of cleft lip/palate differs among ethnicities and is approximately 1:1000 in those of Caucasian descent, 1:2000 of African, and 1:500 of Asian.
   - The incidence of isolated cleft palate is approximately 1:2000 in Caucasians.

Table 6.1 Incidence of Cleft Lip/Palate in Differing Ethnic Groups

ETHNICITY	INCIDENCE PER 1000 BIRTHS
Amerindian	3.6
Japanese	2.1
Chinese	1.7
White	1.0
African-American	0.3

Data from Wyszynski, D.F., Beaty, T.H., Maestri, N.E., 1996. Genetics of nonsyndromic oral clefts revisited. Cleft Palate Craniofac. J. 33, 406–417; Vieira, A.R., Orioli, I.M., 2001. Candidate genes for nonsyndromic cleft lip and palate. ASDC J. Dent. Child. 68 (229), 272–279.

- Cleft lip/palate is more common in boys.
- Isolated cleft palate is more common in girls.
- Cleft lip/palate affects the left side more often.

2. Isolated cleft palate is associated with a craniofacial syndrome in as many as 50% of patients, whereas only 30% of cleft lip/palate patients have an associated syndrome.
   - Van der Woude syndrome
     - One of the most common syndromes associated with clefts
     - Autosomal dominant
     - Characterized by lower lip sinus tracts ("pits"), cleft lip/palate, or cleft palate
   - 22q chromosomal deletion ("velocardiofacial syndrome")
     - Common syndrome associated with clefts (particularly, cleft palate)
     - Characterized by "bird-like" facial appearance, soft-palate dysfunction, developmental delay, congenital heart disease, B-cell immune dysfunction, and medialization of the carotid arteries
   - Pierre Robin sequence
     - Characterized by the triad of micrognathia, glossoptosis, and respiratory distress
     - 60-90% have associated cleft palate, which is typically of the soft palate and is U shaped or wide
     - Associated with Stickler syndrome (autosomal dominant inheritance, myopia, and joint problems), craniofacial microsomia, and Treacher Collins syndrome
     - Initial treatment is conservative and focused on airway protection including prone positioning and/or tongue-lip adhesion. In cases that have failed conservative measures, mandibular distraction or tracheostomy should be considered.
3. Inheritance of clefts
   - Cleft lip/palate
     - Unaffected parents with one affected child: Recurrence risk of 4%
     - Unaffected parents with two affected children: Recurrence risk of 9%
     - One affected parent and no affected children: Recurrence risk of 4%

- One affected parent and one affected child: Recurrence risk of 17%
- Cleft palate
  - Unaffected parents with one affected child: Recurrence risk of 2%
  - Unaffected parents with two affected children: Recurrence risk of 1%
  - One affected parent and no affected children: Recurrence risk of 6%
  - One affected parent and one affected child: Recurrence risk of 15%

General Anatomy

1. Unilateral cleft lip
   - Orbicularis abnormally inserts onto the columella on the noncleft side and the ala on the cleft side
   - Complete: Cleft includes the nasal sill.
   - Incomplete: Nasal sill contains some soft-tissue elements ("Simonart's band").
2. Bilateral cleft lip (see Figure 6.2)
   - Orbicularis oris abnormally inserts onto the ala bilaterally.
   - Prolabium is void of any orbicularis muscle and is often protruded forward.
   - Severe deficiency of columellar height
   - Wide alar bases

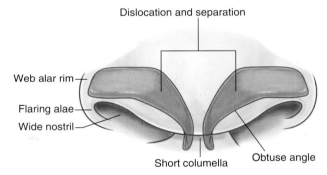

Figure 6.2. Bilateral cleft nose deformity involves bilateral displacement and distortion of osseocartilaginous skeleton of nose. Shortened columella plays prominent role in bilateral deformity and must be lengthened in subsequent procedures. *(Reprinted from Neligan, P.C., Losee, J. [Eds.], 2013. Plastic Surgery, vol. 3, 3rd ed. Elsevier, 631–654.)*

3. Cleft palate
   - Levator palatini abnormally inserts onto the hard palate instead of decussating in the midline.
     - Affects speech
     - Leads to severe Eustachian tube dysfunction; chronic otitis media found in 96% to 100% of patients (see Figure 6.3)
   - Classification
     - Kernahan Y classification (see Figure 6.4)
     - Veau classification (see Figure 6.5)

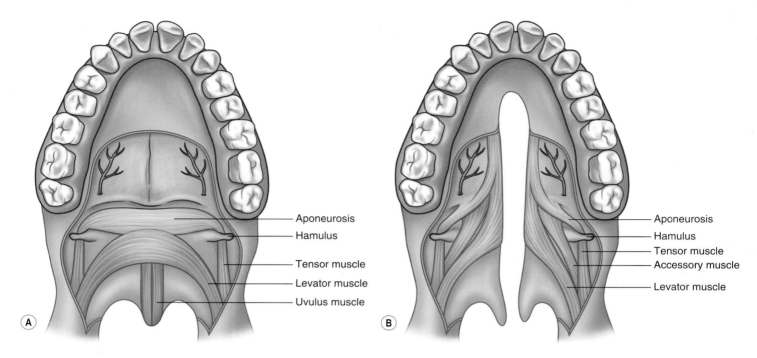

Figure 6.3. A, Normal anatomy: Levator veli palatini muscle can be seen forming a sling across soft palate; tensor veli palatini is shown coming around hamulus to fuse with levator. **B,** Cleft palate: Muscles are seen running more or less parallel with cleft margin. *(Reprinted from Neligan, P.C., Losee, J. [Eds.], 2013. Plastic Surgery, vol. 3, 3rd ed. Elsevier, 569–583.)*

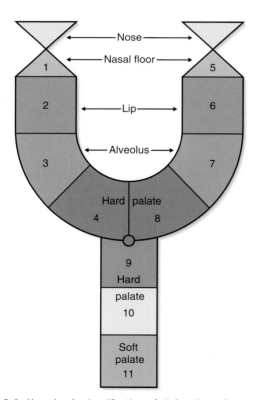

Figure 6.4. Kernahan's classification of clefts allows for standardized reporting of severity of both cleft lip and palate. *(Reprinted from Neligan, P.C., Losee, J. [Eds.], 2013. Plastic Surgery, vol. 3, 3rd ed. Elsevier, 569–583.)*

- Submucous cleft palate
  - Occurs when the palate has mucosal continuity but levator palatini muscle is discontinuous and abnormally oriented.
  - Characterized by Calnan's triad: Midline clear zone ("zona pellucida"), bifid uvula, palpable notch of the posterior hard palate
  - Requires speech evaluation to determine symptomatology.
  - If asymptomatic, submucous cleft palate requires no treatment. In symptomatic patients (~33% of cases), palatoplasty is required. A common technique includes the Furlow double-opposing Z plasty.
4. Unilateral cleft nasal deformity
   - Septum is deviated toward the cleft side.
   - Anterior nasal spine and nasal tip are deviated toward the noncleft side.
   - Piriform and alveolus on the cleft side are displaced posteriorly.
   - Ala on the cleft side is flattened and displaced inferior, posterior, and lateral
   - Columella is deficient (see Figure 6.6).

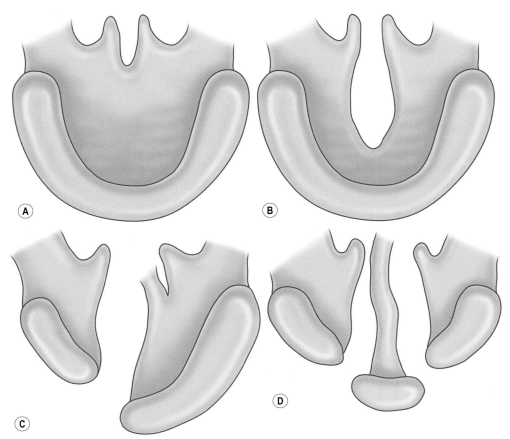

Figure 6.5. Veau classification system. **A,** Veau I cleft of soft palate. **B,** Veau II cleft of soft and hard palates. **C,** Veau III unilateral cleft. **D,** Veau IV bilateral cleft. *(Reprinted from Butler, C.E. [Ed.], 2009. Head and Neck Reconstruction, Elsevier, 271–294.)*

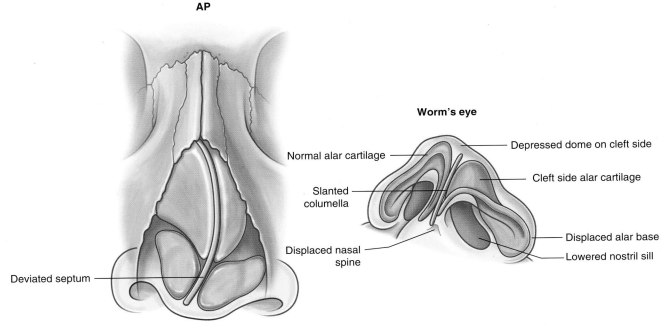

Figure 6.6. Key aspects of cleft nose deformity involve abnormalities of osseocartilaginous skeleton. *AP,* Anteroposterior. *(Reprinted from Neligan, P.C., Losee, J. [Eds.], 2013. Plastic Surgery, vol. 3, 3rd ed. Elsevier, 631–654.)*

Cleft Care

1. Requires multidisciplinary team care.
2. Initial treatment should focus on parental reassurance and counseling, feeding, and infant growth.
3. General sequence and timing of repair (see Table 6.2).

Table 6.2 Surgical Protocol

3 months	Primary cleft lip and nose
8 months	Two-flap palatoplasty
5 years (35%)	Secondary minor lip–nose
7-9 years (100%)	Cancellous iliac bone graft to alveolar cleft
7 years (full growth)	Distraction osteogenesis >12 mm, occlusal class III
Full growth (25-30%)	Orthognathic surgery
12-18 years	Rhinoplasty; other secondary soft tissue

Reprinted from Guyuron, B., Eriksson, E., Persing, J.A., et al. (Eds.), 2009. Plastic Surgery: Indications and Practice, 1st ed. Elsevier, 473–492.

4. Presurgical orthopedics
   - Useful in wide clefts to align lip/alveolar segments, reduce overall cleft width, and improve cleft nasal deformity (e.g., lengthen columella in bilateral cases).
   - Several techniques available, including passive devices (nasoalveolar molding [NAM]), active devices (Latham appliance), lip adhesion, and taping.
5. Unilateral cleft lip repair (see Figures 6.7 and 6.8)
   - Often performed at 3 months of age, following the "rule of 10s": 10 weeks, 10 g hemoglobin, 10 kg.
   - Several techniques have been described and all are variations of the Millard rotation-advancement technique.
   - Many current techniques involve some component of early cleft nasal repair via release of abnormal alar cartilage and suture techniques.
   - Noncleft side is the rotational component and the cleft side/lateral lip element is the advancement component of the repair.
   - Full release of the abnormally inserted orbicularis oris muscle with meticulous layered closure is critical to a successful repair.
   - L flap is taken from the residual mucosa of the lateral lip element and used when necessary to assist with nasal lining.
   - C flap is created on noncleft side and used to lengthen the columella.

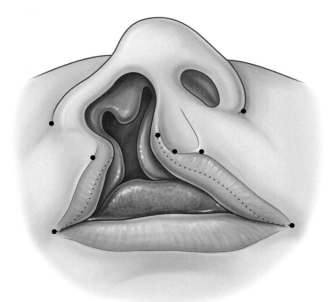

Figure 6.7. Preoperative markings. *(Reprinted from Guyuron, B., Eriksson, E., Persing, J.A., et al., [Eds.], 2009. Plastic Surgery: Indications and Practice, 1st ed. Elsevier, 473–492.)*

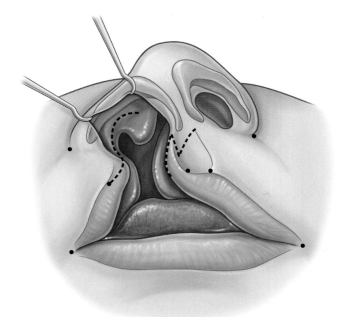

Figure 6.8. Preoperative incisions (dotted lines). *(Reprinted from Guyuron, B., Eriksson, E., Persing, J.A., et al., [Eds.], 2009. Plastic Surgery: Indications and Practice, 1st ed. Elsevier, 473–492.)*

- Complications of unilateral cleft lip repair include
  - Dehiscence: If early, perform re-repair with adequate soft-tissue release to allow tension-free closure.
  - Poor scarring: Treat early scar contracture conservatively because most will settle.
  - Whistle deformity: May require surgical correction with dermal fat grafts, vermillion lip-switch flaps, or re-repair.
  - Inadequate rotation: May perform re-repair with rotation-advancement flap technique.
6. Bilateral cleft lip repair (see Figures 6.9 and 6.10)
  - Prolabial skin is used to create a philtrum.
  - Prolabial mucosa is discarded or used to provide lining to the upper labial sulcus.
  - Lateral lip vermillion is used to create the median tubercle.
  - Orbicularis oris must be reapproximated at the midline beneath the prolabial skin flap.
  - Length of philtral flap is typically set at 6 to 7 mm, with a width of 2 mm at columellar-labial junction, and 3.5 to 4 mm between Cupid's bow peaks.

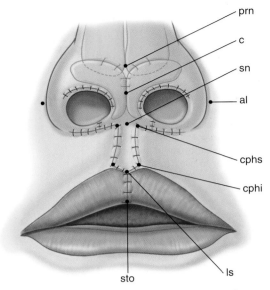

Figure 6.10. Using cautery Colorado needle dissection in preperiosteal plane for additional exposure. (Reprinted from Neligan, P.C., Losee, J. [Eds.], 2013. Plastic Surgery, vol. 3, 3rd ed. Elsevier, 550–568.)

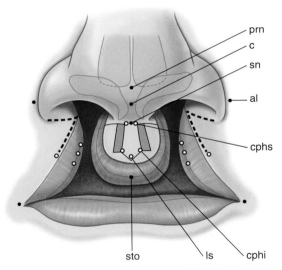

Figure 6.9. Markings for synchronous repair of bilateral cleft lip and nasal deformity. (White circles) Tattooed dots. Anthropometric points: Pronasale (prn); highest point of columella nasi (c); subnasale (sn); ala nasi (al); crista philtri superior (cphs); crista philtri inferior (cphi); labiale superius (ls); stomion (sto). (Reprinted from Neligan, P.C., Losee, J. [Eds.], 2013. Plastic Surgery, vol. 3, 3rd ed. Elsevier, 550–568.)

- Complications of bilateral cleft lip repair
  - Dehiscence: As above for unilateral cleft lip repair
  - Poor scarring
  - Tight lip: May require scar release and Abbe flap for correction.
7. Cleft palate repair
  - Often performed at 9 to 12 months of age
  - Palate repair surgery is often a balance between obtaining a closed functioning velum and limiting future maxillary growth disturbances.
  - Several techniques are available for primary cleft palate repair
    - Furlow double-opposing Z plasty (see Figure 6.11)
    - Two-flap palatoplasty (see Figure 6.12)
    - Von Langenbeck repair (see Figure 6.13)
    - Veau-Wardill-Kilner (VWK) repair (see Figure 6.14)
  - Complications after cleft palate repair
    - Dehiscence: If early, re-repair can be performed.
    - Fistula: See below
    - Velopharyngeal dysfunction (VPD): See below
8. Palatal fistula repair
  - Symptomatic fistulas require repair.
  - First option in fistula repair is often local random-pattern tissue flaps or reelevation of tissues and layered closure.
  - If local random pattern flaps are not possible or reelevation fails, then more advanced techniques include
    - Acellular dermis interposition with mucosal reelevation and layered closure
    - Facial artery myomucosal (FAMM) flap: Based off buccal branch of the facial artery; includes buccinator muscle (see Figure 6.15).

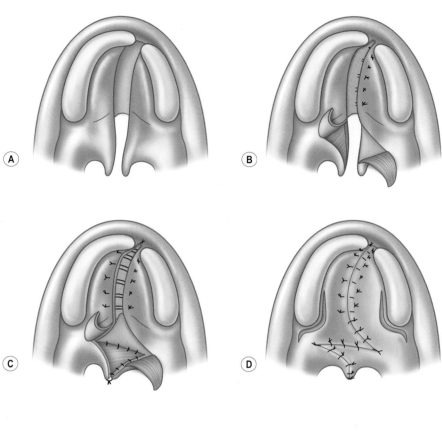

Figure 6.11. Furlow double-opposing Z plasty. **A,** Oral flap design shown with posteriorly based flap on left side. If necessary, relaxing incisions can be continued up to cleft margin behind alveolus, similar to two-flap palatoplasty for hard palate closure. **B,** Left-sided oral flap is raised with levator muscle, the right-sided flap above muscle. Reverse pattern is planned for oral side. Vomer flap is shown closing nasal mucosa anteriorly. **C,** Nasal flaps transposed and anterior oral mucosa closed. **D,** Final appearance after transposition of oral flaps. (*Reprinted from Neligan, P.C., Buck, D.W. [Eds.], 2013. Core Procedures in Plastic Surgery, Elsevier, 156–165.*)

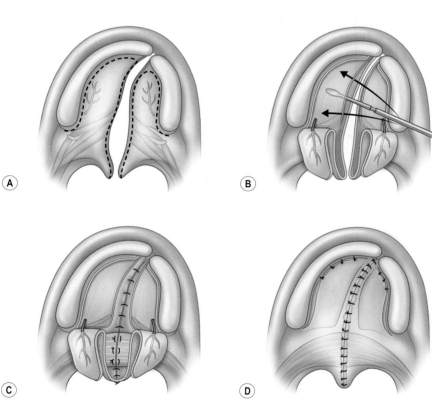

Figure 6.12. Two-flap palatoplasty. **A,** Incisions similar to von Langenbeck repair but they meet cleft margin just behind alveolar ridge. **B,** Mucoperiosteal flaps developed on both sides with preservation of greater palatine vessels. **C,** Levator veli palatini muscle is freed from posterior border of hard palate and sutured across midline. **D,** Final closure. It is often possible to close much of lateral incision and minimize raw areas. (*Reprinted from Neligan, P.C., Buck, D.W. [Eds.], 2013. Core Procedures in Plastic Surgery, Elsevier, 156–165.*)

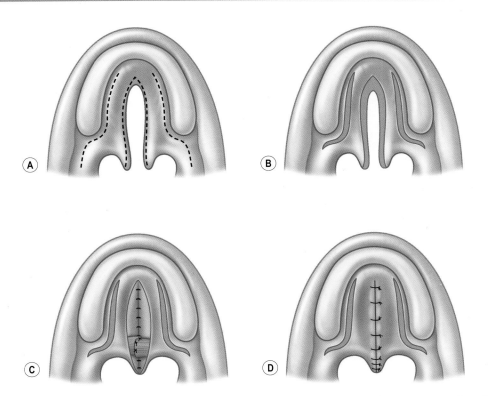

Figure 6.13. von Langenbeck repair. **A,** Relaxing incisions made behind alveolar ridge, creating bilateral bipedicle flaps for midline closure. Greater palatine vessels must be preserved. **B,** Cleft margins incised in a manner to leave adequate nasal mucosa for complete closure. **C,** Closure of nasal mucosa and muscle repair. **D,** Final appearance. *(Reprinted from Neligan, P.C., Buck, D.W. [Eds.], 2013. Core Procedures in Plastic Surgery, Elsevier, 156–165.)*

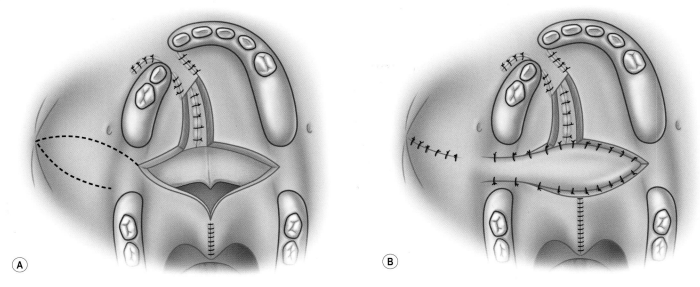

Figure 6.14. A, Buccal mucosal flap. Kaplan advocated use of this flap to elongate nasal mucosa. **B,** Flap transposed into nasal surface. In some situations, bilateral flaps can be used with second flap lining oral surface. *(Reprinted from Neligan PC, Buck, D.W. [Eds.], 2013. Core Procedures in Plastic Surgery, Elsevier, 156–165.)*

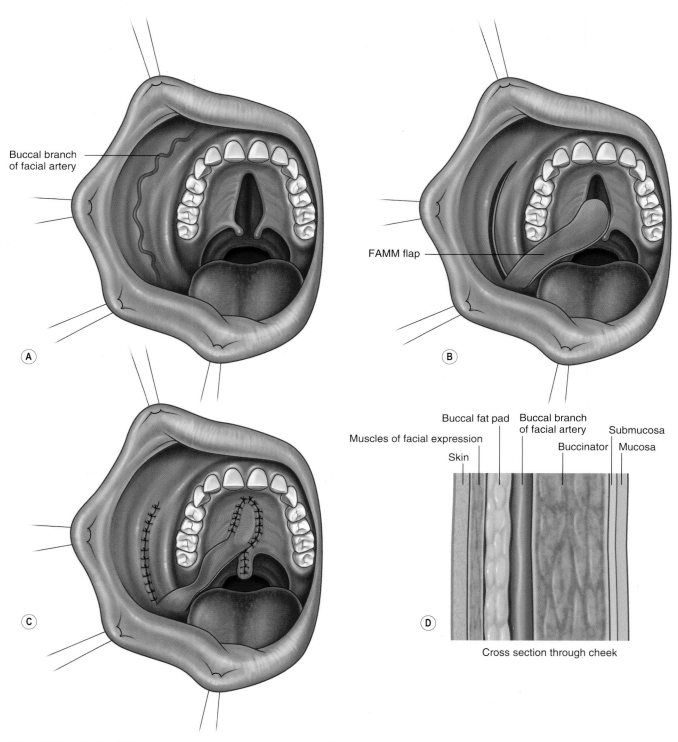

Buccal branch
of facial artery

A

FAMM flap

B

C

Buccal fat pad   Buccal branch
of facial artery   Submucosa

Muscles of facial expression   Mucosa

Skin   Buccinator

D

Cross section through cheek

Figure 6.15. A-D, Buccal tissue can be harvested via axial pattern flap based off facial artery. *FAMM,* Facial artery myomucosal. *(Reprinted from Neligan, P.C., Losee, J. [Eds.], 2013. Plastic Surgery, vol. 3, 3rd ed. Elsevier, 631–654.)*

- Tongue flap: Based off lingual artery; often used as last resort because tongue must be tethered for 2 to 3 weeks (see Figure 6.16).

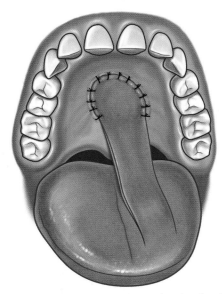

Figure 6.16. The tongue offers another regional option for palatal fistula repair. *(Reprinted from Neligan, P.C., Losee, J. [Eds.], 2013. Plastic Surgery, vol. 3, 3rd ed. Elsevier, 631–654.)*

Velopharyngeal Dysfunction

1. Borders of the velopharyngeal port
   - Soft palate (anterior)
   - Lateral pharyngeal walls
   - Posterior pharyngeal wall
2. Muscles involved in velopharyngeal port function
   - Levator veli palatini
   - Palatoglossus (anterior tonsillar pillar)
   - Palatopharyngeus (posterior tonsillar pillar)
   - Musculus uvulae
   - Superior pharyngeal constrictor
3. All muscles of the velopharynx are innervated by the pharyngeal plexus (cranial nerves IX, X, and XI) except the tensor veli palatini, which is innervated by the mandibular branch of the trigeminal nerve (cranial nerve V3).
4. Levator veli palatini is primary muscle responsible for velopharyngeal closure.
5. Velopharyngeal insufficiency: Inadequate closure of velopharyngeal port secondary to anatomic or structural defects (e.g., clefts, postsurgical cicatrix, etc.)
6. Velopharyngeal incompetence: Inability to close velopharyngeal port secondary to neuromuscular or neurologic deficits
7. Diagnosis of VPD
   - Speech assessment (see Box 6.1)

BOX 6.1 COMMON SPEECH PATHOLOGY TERMINOLOGY

Intelligibility: Perceived amount of speech (i.e., number of words) understood

Resonance: Perceptual balance of oral and nasal sound energy in speech. Speakers with VPD have an abnormal escape of excessive nasal sound energy through velopharyngeal port and into nasal cavity, referred to as hypernasality.

Hypernasality: Perception of excessive nasal sound energy in speech, typically on vowels, glides (W, Y), and liquid sounds (L, R).

Hyponasality: Perception of decreased nasal sound energy in speech, typically on nasal sounds M and N, and usually due to structural obstruction (e.g., enlarged adenoid pad, nasal congestion).

Mixed resonance: Combination of hypernasality and hyponasality perceived by listener. Cul-de-sac resonance is sometimes considered a form of mixed resonance, in which sound energy escapes to anterior nasal cavity and becomes trapped by some form of nasal obstruction or constriction, such as a deviated septum.

Nasal emission: Abnormal escape of airflow through nose during consonant production (audible or inaudible). When audible, may also be referred to as nasal turbulence.

Compensatory articulation errors: Category of articulation errors typically observed in populations with cleft palate or VPD, believed to result from an active strategy to regulate pressure and airflow for speech. Typically includes a pattern of producing sounds in a posterior place of vocal tract, such as pharynx or larynx, where pressure and airflow can be "valved" before their escape to level of velopharynx or oral cavity.

Glottal stop substitutions: Most common type of compensatory articulation errors seen in children with cleft palate or history of VPD, produced by adducting vocal folds together and abruptly releasing pressure beneath to create sound of an oral pressure consonant. Often used as a replacement (substitution) for pressure consonants such as P, B, T, D, K, and G.

Nasal substitutions: Active replacement of oral sounds P, B, T, and D with nasal sounds M and N.

Active nasal fricative: Learned articulatory behavior in which oral sound (usually S, SH, CH) is replaced with voiceless nasal sound (i.e., all airflow is emitted through the nose); sometimes accompanied by nasal grimace.

Weak pressure consonants: Perception of decreased pressure in oral consonants such as P, B, T, D, and F, resulting from fistula or velopharyngeal gap, causing these sounds to take on nasalization (e.g., B sound is perceived as an M; D perceived as an N), even though speaker is accurately attempting to produce correct sound. Often co-occurs with nasal emission.

Sibilant distortions: Incorrect tongue placement resulting from faulty learning or malocclusion, resulting in imprecise production of sounds S and Z.

Reprinted from Neligan, P.C., Losee, J. (Eds.), 2013. Plastic Surgery, vol. 3, 3rd ed. Elsevier, 614–630.

- Videofluoroscopy
- Nasopharyngoscopy

8. Surgical treatments: Treatment is often directed by the motion or lack thereof detected on videofluoroscopy and nasopharyngoscopy.
    - Furlow palatoplasty
        - Useful to lengthen a velum that is too short to contact the posterior pharyngeal wall.
    - Posterior pharyngeal flap (see Figure 6.17)

- Useful when there is good lateral wall motion and poor posterior wall motion.
- Flap is often superiorly based, and donor site closed primarily.
- Take care when dissecting the flap in patients with velocardiofacial syndrome because of risk for medialization of carotid vessels.
- A flap that is too wide can cause severe airway obstruction and/or obstructive sleep apnea.

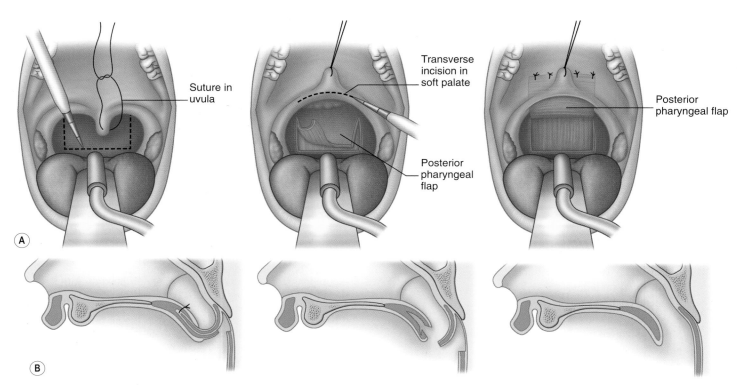

Figure 6.17. A,B, Posterior pharyngeal flap. *(Reprinted from Neligan, P.C., Losee, J. [Eds.], 2013. Plastic Surgery, vol. 3, 3rd ed. Elsevier, 614–630.)*

- Sphincter pharyngoplasty
    - Useful when there is good posterior wall motion, and poor lateral wall motion
    - The palatopharyngeus muscles/posterior tonsillar pillars are elevated bilaterally and interdigitated to create a sphincter.
    - Similar risks to pharyngeal flaps (see Figure 6.18).
- Posterior pharyngeal wall augmentation
    - Useful in patients who have good overall velar motion with a small gap, in which augmentation may reduce the overall port size.
    - Typically used as a secondary option for VPD
    - Possible materials used for augmentation can include autologous fat, calcium hydroxyapatite, or other soft-tissue fillers.

9. Nonsurgical treatments: Often used if surgery is not possible or desired.
    - Prostheses: Palatal lift and speech bulb
    - Behavioral speech therapy

Orthognathic Surgery

1. Orthognathic surgery: Surgical movement of the maxilla and mandible to optimize facial harmony and occlusion
2. Orthognathic surgery should not be performed until skeletal maturity is reached.
3. Patient selection and planning rely on history, physical exam, and cephalometric analysis (see Figure 6.19).
    - Sella-nasion-subspinale (SNA) angle
        - Provides information regarding position of maxilla in the anteroposterior plane.

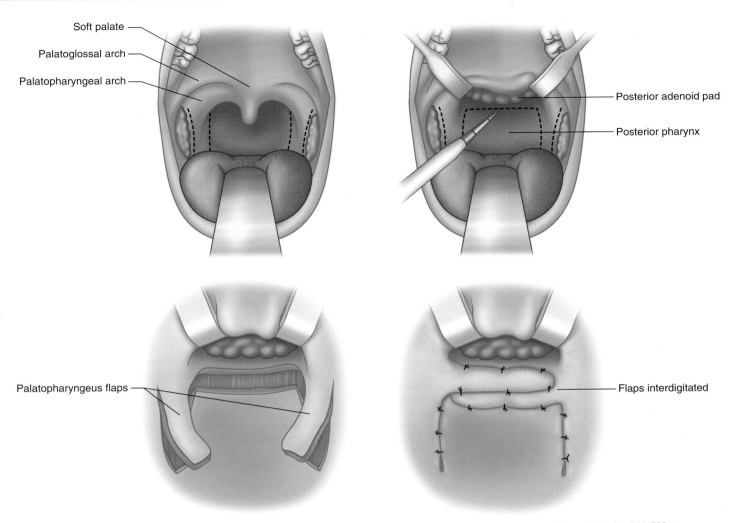

Figure 6.18. Sphincter pharyngoplasty. *(Reprinted from Neligan, P.C., Losee, J. [Eds.], 2013. Plastic Surgery, vol. 3, 3rd ed. Elsevier, 614–630.)*

Labels (clockwise): Soft palate, Palatoglossal arch, Palatopharyngeal arch, Posterior adenoid pad, Posterior pharynx, Flaps interdigitated, Palatopharyngeus flaps

- Normal SNA is 82 degrees (Caucasian) and 85 degrees (African-American).
- If less than normal, maxilla is in abnormal posterior position with respect to cranial base and vice versa.
- Sella-nasion-supramentale (SNB) angle
  - Provides information regarding position of mandible in the anteroposterior plane.
  - Normal SNB is 80 degrees (Caucasian) and 81 degrees (African-American).
  - If less than normal, mandible is in abnormal posterior position with respect to cranial base and vice versa.
- Subspinale-nasion-supramentale (ANB) angle
  - Provides information on relationship of maxilla to mandible in the anteroposterior plane.
  - Normal ANB is 2 degrees (i.e., maxilla protrudes 2 degrees more anterior than mandible with respect to cranial base.).
- Frankfurt horizontal plane: Line from porion (midpoint of upper contour of external auditory canal) to orbitale (lowest point on inferior margin of bony orbit)

- Ricketts' esthetic plane
  - In a patient with normal proportions, a line extending from nasal tip toward soft tissues of chin should touch lower lip, with upper lip 2 mm behind it.
  - If chin is retruded, it will be behind this line.
4. Occlusion
  - Often described according to the Angle classification
    - Class-II malocclusion: ANB less than normal; retrognathic mandible, increased overjet
    - Class-III malocclusion: SNA less than normal or ANB greater than normal; retruded maxilla or prognathic mandible, negative overjet (see Figure 6.20).
  - Overbite: Vertical overlap between upper and lower incisal edges with the teeth in occlusion
  - Overjet: Horizontal between labial surface of upper incisor and lower incisor with the teeth in occlusion
5. LeFort I osteotomy
  - Developed to provide segmental movements of maxilla
  - Maxilla can be advanced, impacted, set back, or moved in multiple planes with multipiece osteotomies (see Figure 6.21).

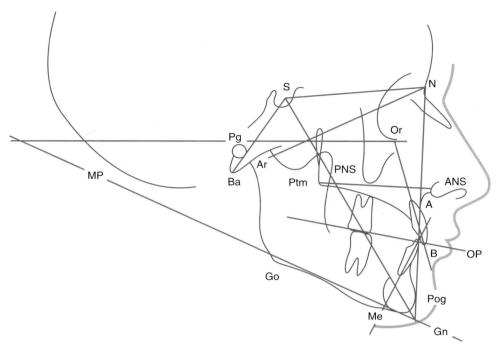

Figure 6.19. Cephalometric radiograph identifies skeletal landmarks used in determining lines and angles that reflect facial development. These measurements aid in determining extent to which each jaw contributes to dentofacial deformity. *S,* Sella turcica, midpoint of sella turcica; *N,* nasion, anterior point of intersection between nasal and frontal bones; *A,* "A point," innermost point in depth of concavity of maxillary alveolar process; *Ar,* articulare; *B,* "B point," innermost point on contour of mandible between incisor tooth and bony chin; *Ba,* basale, most inferior point of skull base; *Pog,* pogonion, most anterior point on contour of chin; *Go,* gonion, most inferior and posterior point at angle formed by ramus and body of mandible; *Po,* porion, uppermost lateral point on roof of external auditory meatus; *Or,* orbitale, lowest point on inferior margin of orbit; *PNS,* posterior nasal spine, most posterior point on maxilla; *Ptm,* pterygomaxillary fissure; *ANS,* anterior nasal spine, most anterior point on maxilla; *Gn,* gnathion, center of inferior contour of chin; *Me,* menton, most inferior point on mandibular symphysis; *MP,* mandibular plane, line connecting Go and Gn; *OP,* occlusal plane. *(Reprinted from Neligan, P.C., Losee, J. [Eds.], 2013. Plastic Surgery, vol. 3, 3rd ed. Elsevier, 655–670.)*

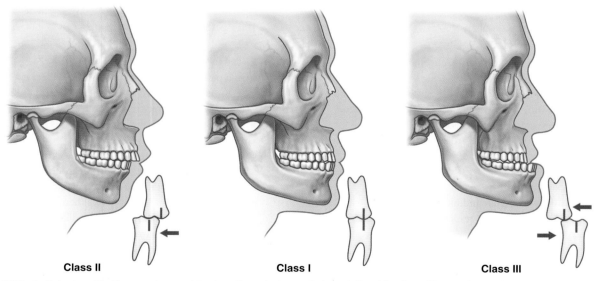

| Class II | Class I | Class III |

Figure 6.20. Angle's classification may be used to describe anterior-posterior relationship of maxillary and mandibular dental arches. In class-I relationship, mesial buccal cusp of upper first molar articulates in buccal groove of mandibular molar. In class-II relationship, mesial buccal cusp of upper first molar articulates between mandibular first molar and second premolar. In class-III relationship, mesial buccal cusp of upper first molar articulates between first and second mandibular molar teeth; mandible is said to be prognathic (more anterior) when compared with maxilla. *(Reprinted from Neligan, P.C. [Ed.], 2013. Plastic Surgery, 3rd ed. Elsevier, 354–372.)*

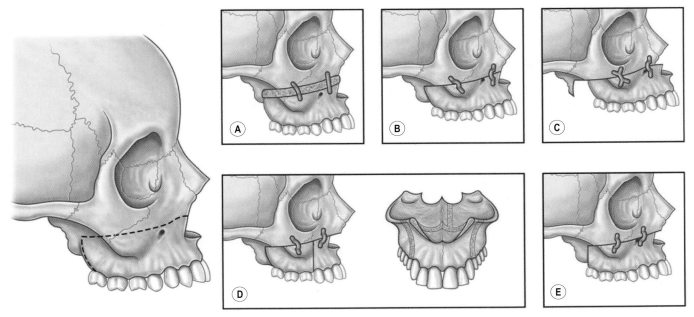

Figure 6.21. A-E, LeFort I osteotomies demonstrating maxillary advancement, impaction, setback, and multipiece LeFort. *(Reprinted from Neligan, P.C., Losee, J. [Eds.], 2013. Plastic Surgery, vol. 3, 3rd ed. Elsevier, 655–670.)*

- In patients with history of cleft lip/palate, there is a concern that VPD will develop after advancement.
- Many advocate limiting movements to less than 1 cm to reduce risk of relapse, nonunion, and/or instability.
  - In situations requiring movements greater than 1 cm, distraction should be considered.
- In patients with narrow alveolar arches, perform palatal expansion before LeFort I osteotomies.
- LeFort I osteotomy with impaction is the most common method for treating patients with "long face syndrome."
  - Long face syndrome is characterized by increased vertical maxillary height, increased gingival show, and lip incompetence.
  - Impaction of maxilla can lead to decreased nasolabial angle, widened alar base, and anterior positioning of the chin.
- Take care to cauterize or clip descending palatine arteries during downfracture of maxilla to prevent significant postoperative bleeding.

6. Bilateral sagittal split osteotomy
   - Developed to provide segmental movements of mandible
   - Mandible can be advanced, impacted, and/or rotated.
   - Take care to avoid injury to the inferior alveolar nerve.
   - Lower lip paresthesias extremely common postoperatively, with most resolving over time (see Figure 6.22).

7. "Double jaw" surgery
   - Movement of maxilla and mandible in one procedure may be necessary in select patients.
   - In general, maxillary osteotomies are completed first; maxilla is placed into its new position and plated; and then the mandibular osteotomies are completed.

8. Genioplasty
   - Chin position can be evaluated by measuring the sella-nasion-pogonion (SNPg) angle or using Ricketts' esthetic line.
   - When manipulating mandible or maxilla, may be necessary to adjust chin position to account for unnecessary changes.
   - Chin segment can be advanced, impacted, reduced, or angled inferiorly and fixed into place.
   - Make transverse osteotomy at least 3 mm below mental foramen (located between first and second premolar) to avoid injury to mental nerve.
   - Resuspend mentalis muscle during closure to prevent lower lip ptosis and/or "witch's chin" deformity.

Craniofacial Clefts

9. Rare deformities of face and cranium that occur in many patterns and degrees of severity
10. Classification system of cleft patterns established by Tessier (see Figure 6.23).
11. Tessier 3 cleft involves alar base and medial canthus.
12. The Tessier 4 cleft spares the nose and is often referred to as "oro-ocular."
13. Tessier 7 cleft is the most common craniofacial cleft and is frequently associated with craniofacial microsomia first and second branchial arch syndrome, Goldenhar syndrome, and Treacher Collins syndrome.
    - Treatment of Tessier 7 cleft involves a full-thickness incision with meticulous layered closure involving reorientation and restoration of orbicular oris muscle at commissure.

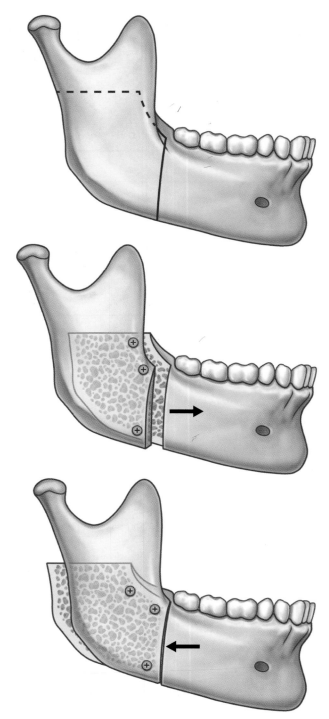

Figure 6.22. Mandibular sagittal split osteotomies demonstrating mandibular advancement *(middle)* and setback *(bottom)*. *(Reprinted from Neligan, P.C., Losee, J. [Eds.], 2013. Plastic Surgery, vol. 3, 3rd ed. Elsevier, 655–670.)*

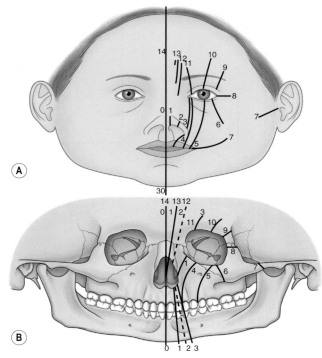

Figure 6.23. Tessier classification of craniofacial clefts. **A,B,** Illustrations of Tessier clefts: Skeletal locations of numeric clefts are depicted on right side of face *(left half of drawings)*. Soft-tissue landmarks are outlined on left side of face *(right half of drawings)*. Facial clefts are numbered 0 through 7 and cranial clefts 8 through 14. Mandibular midline facial cleft is number 30. *(Reprinted from Neligan, P.C., Losee, J. [Eds.], 2013. Plastic Surgery, vol. 3, 3rd ed. Elsevier, 701–725.)*

14. Tessier 8 cleft is located at lateral canthus and is called the "equator of the Tessier craniofacial time zones." It divides facial clefts from cranial clefts.
15. Treacher Collins syndrome has a combination of Tessier 6, 7, and 8 clefts.
16. Tessier 0-14 clefts occur in midline forehead and cranium and may represent encephaloceles.

Suggested Readings

Afshar, M., Brugmann, S.A., Helms, J.A., 2013. Chapter 22: Embryology of the craniofacial complex. In: Neligan, P.C., Losee, J. (Eds.), Plastic Surgery, vol. 3, 3rd ed. Elsevier, pp. 503–516.

Bradley, J.P., Kawamoto, H.K., 2013. Chapter 33: Craniofacial clefts. In: Neligan, P.C., Losee, J. (Eds.), Plastic Surgery, vol. 3, 3rd ed. Elsevier, pp. 701–725.

Chen, K.-T.C., Noordhoff, S.M., Fisher, D.M., et al., 2013. Chapter 8: Cleft lip repair. In: Neligan, P.C., Buck, D.W. (Eds.), Core Procedures in Plastic Surgery, Elsevier, pp. 134–155.

Chen, P.K.T., Noordhoff, M.S., Kane, A., 2013. Chapter 23: Repair of the unilateral cleft lip. In: Neligan, P.C., Losee, J. (Eds.), Plastic Surgery, vol. 3, 3rd ed. Elsevier, pp. 517–549.

Cole, P.D., Stal, S., 2009. Chapter 13: Cleft lip repair: Evaluation, planning, and surgical approach to single and bilateral defects. In: Butler, C.E. (Ed.), Head and Neck Reconstruction, Elsevier, pp. 295–307.

Feldman, E.M., Koshy, J.C., Hollier, L.H., et al., 2013. Chapter 29: Secondary deformities of the cleft lip, nose, and palate. In: Neligan, P.C., Losee, J. (Eds.), Plastic Surgery, vol. 3, 3rd ed. Elsevier, pp. 631–654.

Goldstein, J.A., Bakter, S.B., 2013. Chapter 30: Cleft and craniofacial orthognathic surgery. In: Neligan, P.C., Losee, J. (Eds.), Plastic Surgery, vol. 3, 3rd ed. Elsevier, pp. 655–670.

Gosman, A.A., 2007. Chapter 19: Cleft lip. In: Janis, J.E. (Ed.), Essentials of Plastic Surgery, 1st ed. QMP, pp. 176–182.

Gosman, A.A., 2007. Chapter 20: Cleft palate. In: Janis, J.E. (Ed.), Essentials of Plastic Surgery, 1st ed. QMP, pp. 183–196.

Hoffman, W.Y., 2013. Chapter 25: Cleft palate. In: Neligan, P.C., Losee, J. (Eds.), Plastic Surgery, vol. 3, 3rd ed. Elsevier, pp. 569–583.

Kirschner, R.E., Baylis, A.L., 2013. Chapter 28: Velopharyngeal dysfunction. In: Neligan, P.C., Losee, J. (Eds.), Plastic Surgery, vol. 3, 3rd ed. Elsevier, pp. 614–630.

Lam, A., Koudela, C.L., 2010. Chapter 25: Dental basics. In: Weinzweig, J. (Ed.), Plastic Surgery Secrets Plus, 2nd ed. Mosby, pp. 165–170.

Losee, J.E., Smith, D., 2009. Chapter 12: Cleft palate repair. In: Butler, C.E. (Ed.), Head and Neck Reconstruction, Elsevier, pp. 271–294.

Marchac, A.C., Cheng, M.S., Michienzi, J.W., et al., 2009. Chapter 38: Unilateral cleft lip repair. In: Guyuron, B., Eriksson, E., Persing, J.A., et al. (Eds.), Plastic Surgery: Indications and Practice, 1st ed. Elsevier, pp. 473–492.

Mulliken, J.B., 2013. Chapter 24: Repair of bilateral cleft lip. In: Neligan, P.C., Losee, J. (Eds.), Plastic Surgery, vol. 3, 3rd ed. Elsevier, pp. 550–568.

Neligan, P.C., Buck, D.W. 2013. Chapter 9: Cleft palate repair. In: Neligan, P.C., Buck, D.W. (Eds.), Core Procedures in Plastic Surgery, Elsevier, pp. 156–165.

Parker, T.H., 2007. Chapter 21: Velopharyngeal incompetence. In: Janis, J.E. (Ed.), Essentials of Plastic Surgery, 1st ed. QMP, pp. 197–203.

Shivapuja, P.K., Spolyar, J.L., 2010. Chapter 27: Cephalometrics. In: Weinzweig, J. (Ed.), Plastic Surgery Secrets Plus, 2nd ed. Mosby, pp. 179–186.

Sommerlad, B.C. 2009. Chapter 40: Cleft palate. In: Guyuron, B., Eriksson, E., Persing, J.A., et al. (Eds.), Plastic Surgery: Indications and Practice, 1st ed. Elsevier, pp. 505–520.

Taub, D.I., Jacobs, J.M.S., Jacobs, J.S., 2013. Chapter 16: Anthropometry, cephalometry, and orthognathic surgery. In: Neligan, P.C. (Ed.), Plastic Surgery, 3rd ed. Elsevier, pp. 354–372.

Ear Reconstruction

1. Embryology (see Figure 7.1)
   - The 6 branchial arches: At the 4th week of gestation, develop within the walls of the anterior foregut with subsequent branchial clefts/grooves (externally) and pharyngeal pouches (internally)
   - The ear arises from the 1st (mandibular) and 2nd (hyoid) branchial arches, which are further defined by the development of six hillocks, appearing during 6th week.
     - 1st arch: Anterior hillocks (1 to 3) form tragus, root of the helix, and superior helix; Meckel's cartilage ossifies to become malleus and incus.
     - 2nd arch: Posterior hillocks (4 to 6) form posterior helix, antihelix, antitragus, and lobule; Reichert's cartilage ossifies to form stapes.
   - The external acoustic meatus develops from the first branchial groove.
   - The middle ear and eustachian tube are formed from the first pharyngeal pouch.
   - The second, third, and fourth branchial grooves are obliterated within the cervical sinus during the later stages of development.
   - The lymphatic drainage of the ear follows embryologic development.
     - 1st arch structures drain to the parotid lymph nodes.
     - 2nd arch structures drain to cervical lymph nodes.

2. Anatomy
   - The external ear: A three-tiered cartilaginous framework with skin on its anterior surface
     - The complete ear includes the scapha, concha, helix, antihelix, tragus, and lobule as shown in Figure 7.2.

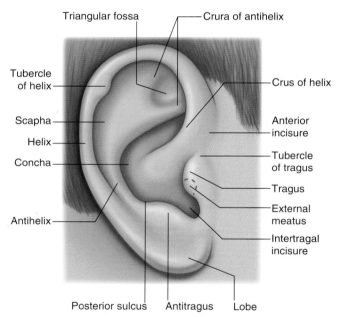

Figure 7.2. Anatomical structure of the ear. *(Reprinted with permission from Janis, J.E., Rohrich, R.J., Gutowski, K.A., 2005. Otoplasty. Plast. Reconstr. Surg. 115 [4], 60e–72e.)*

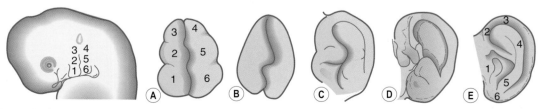

Figure 7.1. Stages in the development of the external ear. *(From Carlson, B.M., 2009. Human Embryology and Developmental Biology, 4th ed. Mosby, Philadelphia.)*

- Blood supply: Primary supply to ear is via posterior auricular artery; multiple perforators pierce cartilage to supply anterior ear (see Figures 7.3 and 7.4).
  - The superficial temporal artery supplies only a small portion of the auricle and the triangular fossa.
  - The occipital artery supplies minor contribution to posterior ear.

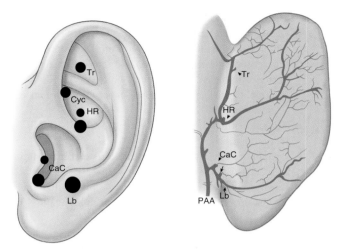

Figure 7.4. Perforating sites of the posterior auricular artery. *Left,* Anterior surface; *right,* posterior surface. *CaC,* cavum conchae; *Cyc,* cymba conchae; *HR,* helical root; *Lb,* earlobe; *PAA,* posterior auricular artery; *Tr,* Triangular fossa. *(Adapted from Park, C., Lineaweaver, W.C., Rumly, T.O., et al., 1992. Plast. Reconstr. Surg. 90, 38–44.)*

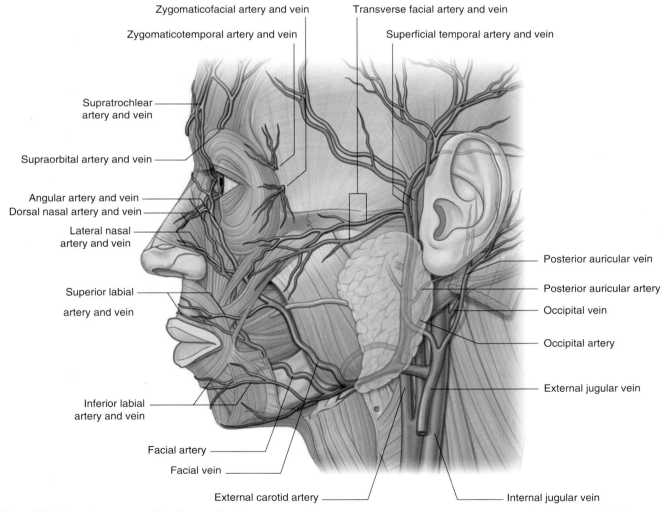

Figure 7.3. Vascular anatomy of the face and neck. *(Reprinted from Drake, R.L., Vogl, A.W., Mitchell, A.V.M. [Eds.], 2015. Gray's Anatomy for Students. Elsevier, 835–1135.)*

- Sensory innervation of the external ear
  - Great auricular nerve (C2, C3) ascends from Erb's point, 6.5 cm below the level of the tragus on the midpoint of the sternocleidomastoid (SCM) and travels just slightly posterior to the external jugular vein (EJV)
    - Supplies sensory to lower half of ear (anterior and posterior)
  - Auriculotemporal nerve (V3) ascends with superficial temporal vessels.
    - Supplies the tragus and the anterior/superior portions of auricle and external auditory canal
  - Lesser occipital nerve (C2, C3) emerges higher than the greater auricular nerve (GAN) and travels along the posterior border of SCM
    - Supplies the posterosuperior aspect of auricle
  - Arnold's nerve (auricular branch of vagus; cranial nerve 10 [CN X]) travels along the ear canal.
    - Supplies the concha and posterior auditory canal
  - External ear block: Place a ring of local anesthetic around the ear.
    - Exception: The concha and posterior auditory canal are innervated by Arnold's nerve (the auricular branch of the vagus nerve (X), which travels along the ear canal).
3. The normal ear (see Figures 7.5 and 7.6)
   - 85% to 90% of normal ear development is largely complete by 5 to 6 years of age, although the width of the ear and its distance from the scalp will increase until 10 years of age. The superior level of the ear is at the same height as the lateral brow, whereas the inferior aspect of the ear is at the same height as the nasal base.
   - On frontal view, the helical rim should be seen more lateral than the antihelical rim.
   - The vertical axis of the ear is tilted posteriorly (when relating the apex of the helix to the lobule) ~15 to 20 degrees, which roughly correlates with the angle of the nasal dorsum.
   - The vertical height of the ear is roughly equal to the distance from the lateral orbital rim to the helical root at the level of the brow.
   - Ideal ear size
     - Male: 63 mm × 35 mm
     - Female: 59 mm × 32 mm
     - Width of ear is 55% of height.
   - Normal helical rim-to-head measurements for each third of the ear are 10 to 12 mm at the helical apex, 16 to 18 mm at the midpoint, and 20 to 22 mm at the lobule.
   - Projection of the helical rim is 1 to 2.5 cm from the mastoid skin, with a normal scapha-conchal angle of 90 degrees and a normal auriculocephalic (AC) angle of 20 to 30 degrees.
     - Projection >20 mm or 45 degrees corresponds to a prominent ear.

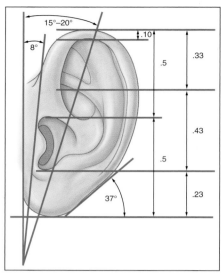

Figure 7.5. Anatomical relationships of the normal ear. *(Reprinted with permission from Bauer, B.S., 1998. Congenital anomalies of the ear. In: Bentz, M.L. [Ed.], Pediatric Plastic Surgery. Appleton & Lange, Stamford, 359–392.)*

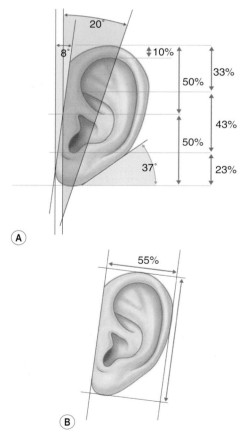

Figure 7.6. Proportional analyses of an ideal auricle, as described by Tolleth. *(Reprinted from Guyuron, B., Eriksson, E., Persing, J.A., et al. [Eds.], 2009. Plastic Surgery: Indications and Practice, 1st ed. Elsevier, 671–699.)*

4. Prominent ear
   - Increased conchoscaphal angle, deepened conchal bowl, and prominent lobule
   - The superior and middle thirds of the ear are most likely to be affected.
     - The most likely cause of a prominent superior third: Absence or effacement of the superior crus of the antihelix.
       - The conchoscaphal angle is >90 degrees and the helix is positioned >12 to 15 mm from the temporal region.
       - The cephaloauricular angle is also increased and typically measures >25 degrees.
     - Prominence of the middle third of the ear is most likely caused by hypertrophy of the concha cavum.
       - The concha cavum has a depth of >1.5 cm.
       - The middle third of the ear is located >16 to 18 mm from the mastoid region.
   - Various corrective methods have been described, including rasping of the anterior surface of the antihelix (Stenstrom), placement of retention sutures to recreate the antihelical fold (Mustarde), conchal bowl resection, and suturing of the conchal bowl to the mastoid fascia (Furnas).
   - At birth, the neonate's ears are soft and pliable, which makes molding therapy of ear deformities more successful.
     - Due to maternal estrogen, which increases cartilage content of hyaluronic acid
     - After 6 weeks, infant's estrogen levels begin to fall and ears become less malleable. Breastfed babies have higher levels of estrogen for a longer time; thus, their ears may be moldable for a longer period.
     - Molding is most effective in infants <3 months.
     - Custom-made mold can be fashioned out of soft putty and affixed into the ear with surgical tape or Steri-Strips.
       - Depending on severity, molding can be continued for several weeks to a few months.
   - The top two causes of prominent ears are (1) inadequate formation of the antihelical fold and (2) conchal hypertrophy.
     - An antihelical fold can be created by a posterior approach and suturing techniques.
     - Conchal reduction can be performed via an anterior approach (reduction of skin and cartilage) or a posterior approach (reduction of cartilage only).
   - Surgical repair of deformational or prominent ears are reserved for older children with residual deformities.
5. Ear deformations/congenital malformations
   - Lop ear/cup ear/constricted ear (see Figure 7.7)
     - Deformity that involves a constricted helical rim with the superior portion of the helix often folding over the scapha
     - Acquired in utero and related to softened cartilage of the upper helix from circulating maternal estrogens. This cartilage lacks sufficient stiffness to support the upper helix.
       - Infants: Respond to shaping with a molding splint formed to match the normal helix

   - Recurrent or older child: Cartilage rasping or surgical options work, including detaching the helix from the scapha and resuturing it to the scapha at a proper angle (see Figure 7.8).

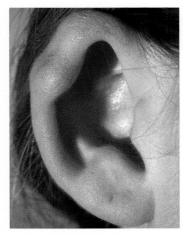

Figure 7.7. Moderately constricted ear. *(Reprinted from Brent, B., 1980. The correction of microtia with autogenous cartilage grafts. II. Atypical and complex deformities. Plast. Reconstr. Surg. 66, 13.)*

   - Cryptotia
     - An adherence of the superior portion of the helix to the temporal skin with varying degrees of severity.
     - In some cases, the helix can be "pulled" out to normal position.
       - Surgical correction involves release of this abnormal connection and frequently requires skin grafting, or posterior auricular flaps, depending on the severity of the deformity (see Figure 7.9).
   - Stahl's ear
     - A hereditary auricular deformity caused by an abnormal cartilaginous pleat that extends from the crus antihelix to the edge of the helix, deforming the regular curvature of the ear
     - Primarily includes a "third antihelical crus"
       - One method of treatment is wedge excision of the third crus (see Figure 7.10).
   - Microtia (see Figure 7.11)
     - Congenital malformation with abnormal/rudimentary development and/or absence of ear structures
       - Occurs in 1 in 7000 births; more males than females; more in right ear than left; highest incidence in Asian/Hispanics; 15% family history (hx)
         50% associated with other craniofacial (CF) syndromes/disorders involving 1st or 2nd branchial arch
         - Orbital auricular vertebral syndrome (Goldenhar)
         - CF microsomia
         - Tessier 7 cleft
         - Treacher Collins syndrome (more common)
       - Inner ear not typically involved (not derived from 1st/2nd branchial arch)

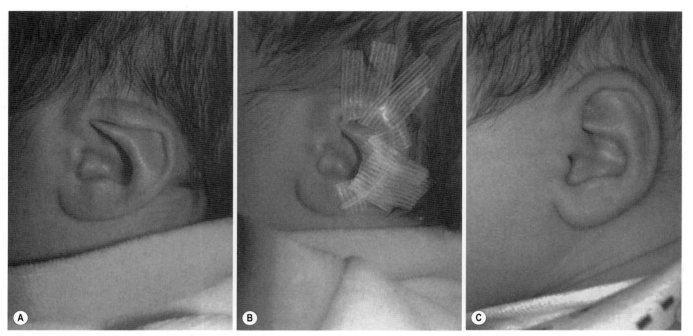

Figure 7.8. Neonate with lop ear. *(Reprinted from Tan, S.T., Abramson, D.L., MacDonald, D.M., et al., 1997. Molding therapy for infants with deformational auricular anomalies. Ann. Plast. Surg. 38, 263.)*

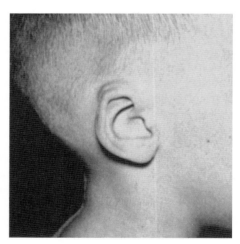

Figure 7.9. Cryptotia. *(Reprinted from Neligan, P.C., 2013. Plastic Surgery. Elsevier, 187–225.)*

- In children, treatment is frequently performed with autologous cartilage grafts when the patient is 6 to 7 years of age (sufficient cartilage present for adequate reconstruction; Nagata technique waits until 10 years of age or chest circumference of 60 cm).
- Reconstruction is not an option for infants or younger children, although surgery to place bone-conduction hearing aids will improve hearing on the affected side and can be placed at 6 to 12 months of age.
- In patients with unilateral microtia, creation of an ear canal or insertion of bone-anchored hearing aids (BAHAs) should be delayed until *after* ear reconstruction

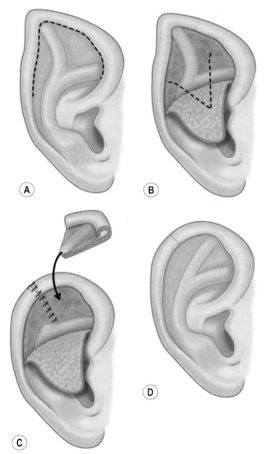

Figure 7.10. Correction of Stahl's ear. *(Redrawn from Kaplan, H.M., Hudson, D.A., 1999. A novel surgical method of repair for Stahl's ear: a case report and review of current treatment modalities. Plast. Reconstr. Surg. 103, 566–569.)*

(13 to 19 years of age) to minimize scarring and avoid interference with reconstruction.

- Alloplastic frameworks, such as porous polyethylene, can be placed in younger patients. However, they have a greater incidence of extrusion and infection.

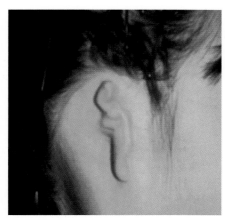

Figure 7.11. Lobule-type microtia. *(Reprinted from Guyuron, B., Eriksson, E., Persing, J.A., et al. [Eds.], 2009. Plastic Surgery: Indications and Practice, 1st ed. Elsevier, 671–699.)*

- Postoperative management is imperative in total auricular reconstruction.
  - Skin coaptation to the carved cartilage construct is best provided by continuous closed suction drainage for the first 5 postoperative days. The reported complication rate is <1%.
  - The quantity and quality of drainage can be monitored, and any potential hematoma should be removed before it obscures the framework details.
  - Pressure dressings risk skin necrosis over the new cartilage framework and are not preferred over closed suction drainage.
  - If early cellulitis/infection is suspected, aggressive incision and drainage, placement of irrigating drains, and antibiotics are first-line therapies made in an attempt to preserve the cartilage construct.
    - If fever and cellulitis do not improve quickly, the construct must be removed.

6. Total auricular reconstruction
   - Goal: Restore the cosmesis of the auricle and the function of the superior helical rim to provide support for eyeglasses
     - The most difficult problem in elderly patients: Fabrication of cartilage framework from calcified and extremely brittle costal cartilage; therefore, prosthetics or osseointegration (OI) is probably best.
     - In younger patients, the major difficulty is attainment of sufficient skin surface area to cover the fabricated cartilage frame without resorting to skin grafts.
   - Autogenous reconstruction most often requires 2 to 4 stages. If perichondrium is kept intact, construct should grow with child.
     - Stage 1: Creation of a cartilage framework and placement under vascularized tissue (usually temporoparietal fascia [TPF] if lack posterior auricular skin)
     - Stage 2: Elevation of the framework
     - Stage 3: Lobule transposition
     - Stage 4: Conchal excavation (see Figures 7.12 and 7.13)
   - Medpor (porous polyethylene)/prosthetic reconstruction
     - Rate of extrusion can be reduced with TPF flap coverage.
     - Can have some soft-tissue incorporation/ingrowth.
       - Small areas of exposure/extrusion can be treated initially with dressing changes and topicals.
       - Contraindicated in infected wound beds or areas without adequate soft-tissue coverage
   - Autogenous versus prosthetic techniques
     - Pediatric microtia patients: Autogenous reconstruction
     - Traumatic or ablative defects in adults: Prosthetic reconstruction
     - Patients with severe soft-tissue hypoplasia, low or unfavorable hairline, and failed autogenous reconstruction: Prosthetic reconstruction
   - Indications for osseointegrated implants: Major cancer extirpation, poor local tissue, absence of the lower half of the ear, salvage following unsuccessful surgery, and poor-operative-risk patients (see Figure 7.14)
7. Traumatic reconstruction
   - Upper third: Defects of helix/antihelix
     - In an older patient, a partial middle ear defect can be treated by wedge resection and direct closure.
       - In a younger patient, the cupping of the ear resulting from this approach would be esthetically unacceptable; therefore, a more complete reconstruction is required.
     - Partial-thickness injuries involving the upper third of the ear with exposed perichondrium are best approached with conservative debridement and topical treatment to prevent dessication until devitalized tissues demarcate.

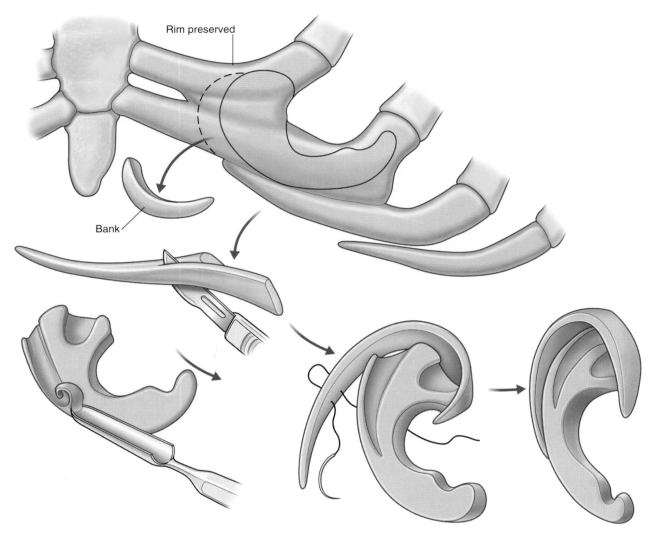

Figure 7.12. Rib cartilage harvest for ear framework fabrication. Note that the upper border of the sixth cartilage is preserved; this will help prevent subsequent chest deformity as the child grows. The entire "floating cartilage" will be used to create the helix. To produce the acute flexion necessary to form the helix, the cartilage is deliberately warped in a favorable direction by thinning it on its outer, convex surface. The thinned helix is affixed to the main sculptural block with horizontal mattress sutures of 4-0 clear nylon; the knots are placed on the framework's undersurface. *(Reprinted from Neligan, P.C. [Ed.], 2013. Plastic Surgery, 3rd ed. Elsevier, 187–225.)*

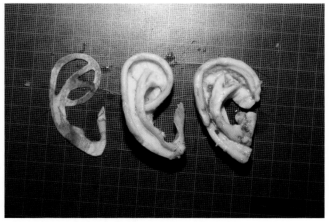

Figure 7.13. Nagata three-dimensional framework for microtia reconstruction. *(Reprinted from Guyuron, B., Erikkson, E., Persing, J., et al. [Eds.], 2009. Plastic Surgery: Indications and Practice. Elsevier, 671–699.)*

- A full-thickness loss of rim, antihelical fold, and/or variable amount of concha can be reconstructed only with a flap.
  - The postauricular transposition skin flap is the best solution for large defects (>2 to 2.5 cm).
    - The flap is based at the edge of the hairline, and the width of the flap is equal to that of the defect.
      - After 10 days, the base of the flap is divided and the remainder of the flap is used to resurface the posterior part of the ear.
      - The donor area, if small, will heal spontaneously or a skin graft may be used.

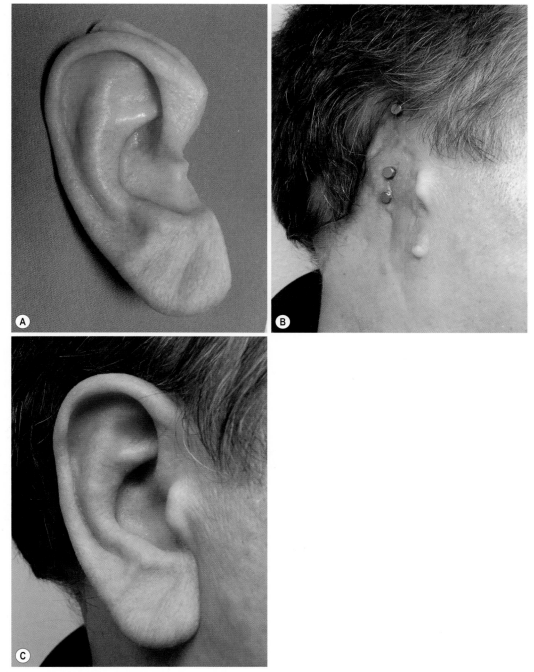

Figure 7.14. Osseointegrated implants with ear prosthesis. *(Courtesy Gregory G. Gion, M.M.S, C.C.A.)*

○ A rim-only defect <1.5 cm can be treated with a small triangular kite flap or a rim advancement flap (Antia-Buch; see Figure 7.15).

  ◆ Antia-Buch flap: A local chondrocutaneous flap that uses tissue from the helical rim based on the postauricular skin to reconstruct the helical margin

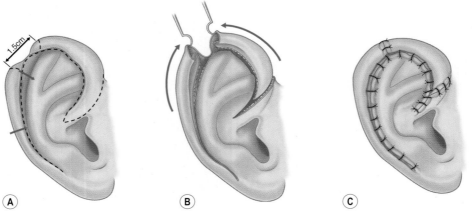

Figure 7.15. Antia-Buch advancement flap. **A,** A 1.5-cm defect and proposed incisions. **B,** The two segments of the helical rim are advanced. **C,** Final result with an overall reduction in size of the ear. *(Modified from Thorne, C.H., 2006. The external ear. In: McCarthy, J.G., Galiano, R.D., Boutros, S.G. [Eds.], Current Therapy in Plastic Surgery. Elsevier, Philadelphia, 103.)*

- ○ The postauricular revolving door island flap is ideal for defects of the conchal area.
  - ◆ Design: Partially on posterior ear and partially on the mastoid area
    - → A skin incision is made around the island and the flap is raised posteriorly and anteriorly.
    - → The skin is incised through the anterior surface of the ear, and the posterior skin elevation stops at the ear/mastoid groove.

- → This vertical attachment becomes the pedicle or hinge of the flap.
- → The posterior skin island can be rotated like a revolving door into the interior conchal defect, the conchal defect is reconstructed, and the posterior defect is closed primarily.
- ○ For larger/more complex lesions
  - ◆ Geometric wedge resection (see Figure 7.16)

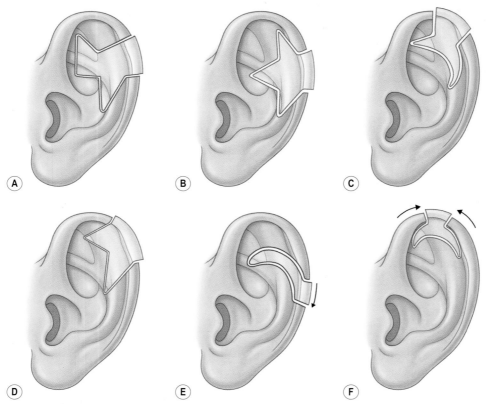

Figure 7.16. Techniques for reducing the auricular circumference and decreasing tension at the suture line in primary closure of helical defects of the upper or middle thirds. **A-F,** Various patterns of excision. *(Modified from Converse, J.M. [Ed.], 1977. Reconstructive Plastic Surgery, 2nd ed. WB Saunders, 1671–1719.)*

- Cartilage graft with posterior auricular tunnel procedure of Converse (see Figure 7.17).
- Orticochea chondrocutaneous flap: A full-thickness incision is made outlining the entire concha. The flap is pedicled off of the helical rim, which must be at least 1 cm wide. The flap is rotated to fill the defect and the donor site is closed primarily (see Figure 7.18).

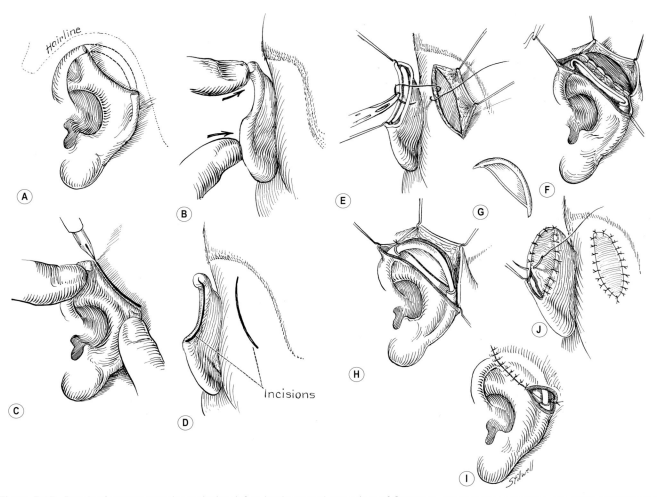

Figure 7.17. Repair of posterosuperior auricular defect by the tunnel procedure of Converse. *(Reprinted from Converse, J.M., 1958. Reconstruction of the auricle. Plast. Reconstr. Surg. 22, 150–230.)*

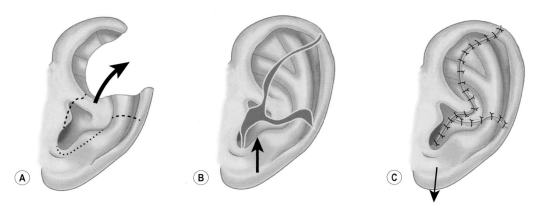

Figure 7.18. Orticochea procedure of conchal rotation for the repair of upper- and middle-third auricular defects. *(Adapted from Ha, R.Y., Trovato, M.J. Plastic Surgery of the Ear, Selected Readings in Plastic Surgery, 11 [R3], 2013.)*

- Middle-third defects
  - Many of the same techniques described above, including wedge excision and Antia-Buch flaps, can be used for small defects.
- For larger composite defects involving variable portions of the antihelix and concha, a conchal cartilage or rib graft with retroauricular skin flap coverage is useful (see Figures 7.19 and 7.20).

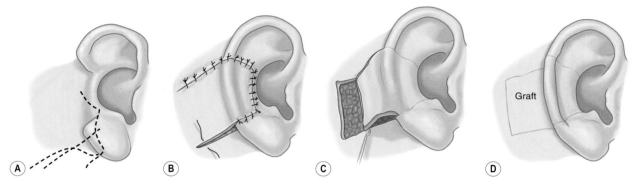

Figure 7.19. Dieffenbach's technique for reconstruction of the middle third of the auricle, drawn from his description (1829-1834). **(A)** The defect and outline of the flap. **(B)** The flap advanced over the defect. **(C,D)** In a second stage, the base of the flap is divided and the flap is folded around the posteromedial aspect of the auricle. A skin graft covers the scalp donor site. *(Reprinted from Neligan, P.C., 2013. Plastic Surgery, 3rd ed. Elsevier, 187–225.)*

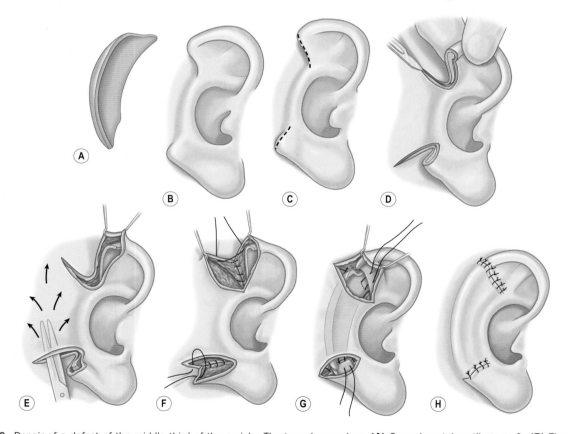

Figure 7.20. Repair of a defect of the middle third of the auricle: The tunnel procedure. **(A)** Carved costal cartilage graft. **(B)** The defect. **(C)** Incisions through the margins of the defect. **(D)** Incisions through the edge of the defect are extended backward through the skin of the mastoid area. **(E)** The skin of the mastoid area is undermined between the two incisions. **(F)** The medial edge of the incision at the border of the auricular defect is sutured to the edge of the postauricular incision. A similar type of suture is placed at the lower edge of the defect. **(G)** The cartilage graft is placed under the skin of the mastoid area and anchored to the auricular cartilage with sutures. **(H)** Suture of the skin incision. *(Reprinted from Converse, J.M., 1958. Reconstruction of the auricle. Plast. Reconstr. Surg. 22, 150–230. Copyright © 1958, The Williams & Wilkins Company, Baltimore.)*

- Lower-third defects
  - Involve the lobule only, which is a skin-only reconstruction (see Figure 7.21)
    - Reconstructive plan depends on size of defect
    - Wedge excision and closure
    - Staged reconstruction with septal cartilage
    - Multiflap techniques

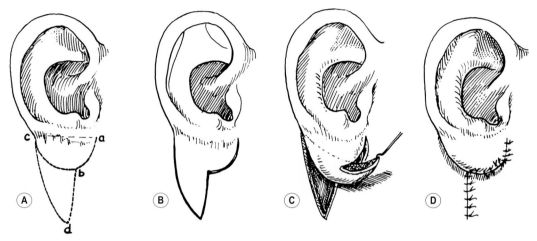

Figure 7.21. Reconstruction of the earlobe. **A,** The curved line *abc* outlines the proposed earlobe as measured on the unaffected contralateral auricle. A vertical flap is outlined; line *bd* is equal in length to line *ab*, and *cd* is equal to *ca*. **B,** Incisions are made through the outlined skin and subcutaneous tissue. **C,** The vertical flap is raised from the underlying tissue as far upward as the horizontal line *ac*, and the apex of the flap is sutured to point *a*. **D,** The operation completed. *(Modified from Alanis, S.Z., 1970. A new method for earlobe reconstruction. Plast. Reconstr. Surg. 45, 254.)*

8. Ear replantation
   - Microsurgical ear replantation provides best esthetic result in select cases of ear amputation.
     - Venous congestion occurs to some extent in nearly every case and is the most common cause of postreplantation complications.
     - There have been several case reports of successful ear replantation without a venous anastomosis, although venous anastomosis is recommended whenever possible.
       - Postoperative congestion can be managed with leech therapy for vascular compromise.
       - Arterial compromise demands reexploration, whereas venous compromise can be managed nonoperatively.
   - Because the large arteries to the ear enter on the posterior aspect, anastomosis is most appropriate on the posterior surface (recipient vessels include branches of the external carotid artery, the anterior auricular branch of the superficial temporal artery, and a branch of the occipital artery).
   - Despite reports of banking amputated cartilage pieces in abdomen and/or forearm, later retrieval often yields warped cartilage that has lost its strength.
     - Because of these disadvantages, microvascular replantation should be used, when possible, to give the best chance for preserving the native auricular architecture.

9. Complications of otoplasty/ear reconstruction/trauma
   - The most common complication is recurrence
   - Persistent prominence of the lobule after otoplasty results from inadequate cavum concham reduction before Furnas suture placement in cases with significant conchal hypertophy.
   - Pinned-back appearance results from overtightening of scapha-mastoid sutures.
   - Auricular chondritis and perichondritis: A serious surgical infection requiring immediate surgical intervention as the primary course of treatment in traumatic cases
     - Culture swabs will guide antibiotic therapy.
     - Chondritis complicating elective otoplasty: Intravenous antibiotics, removing a few sutures to allow drainage/insertion of irrigating drains
       - If no response, open incision and drainage (I&D), remove all sutures, and plan for a delayed otoplasty.
   - Hematoma can cause cauliflower ear deformity (fibrosis of cartilage; see Figures 7.22 and 7.23).
     - Presents as severe, acute ear pain
     - Most appropriate management is complete evacuation via a small incision, with application of a bolster dressing to prevent reaccumulation of the fluid or blood.
     - Resection of the posterior cartilage and sculpting of the anterior cartilage is the treatment option for chronic calcification or cauliflower ear deformity.

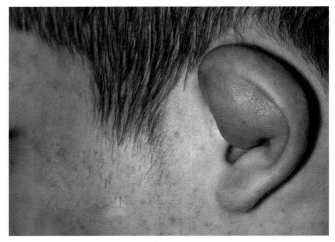

Figure 7.22. An auricular hematoma. *(Reprinted from Neligan, P.C., Plastic Surgery, 3rd ed., 23–48.)*

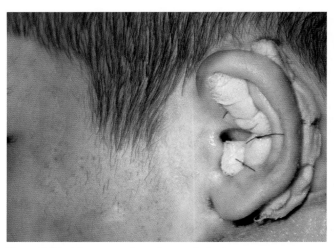

Figure 7.23. After evacuation of an auricular hematoma. *(Reprinted from Neligan, P.C., Plastic Surgery, 3rd ed. 23–48.)*

10. Burned ear reconstruction
    • Conchal transposition flap (orticochea) has minimal donor site morbidity, low complication rate, and can allow eyeglass wear.
       ▪ Auricular osteointegrated prostheses have a high complication rate in burn patients.
       ▪ Silastic prostheses with temporoparietal flap coverage have very high exposure and infection rates.
11. Chondrodermatitis nodularis helicis (see Figure 7.24)
    • A benign condition commonly found in older men often associated with trauma from sleeping. It begins as an area of cartilage inflammation and then ulcerates through the skin. On exam, patient presents with a painful, scabby area with a central crater.
       ▪ Treatment is excision of the cartilage and closure of the skin.
       ▪ Can mimic a skin cancer on physical examination
       ▪ Recurrence rate is high.
          ○ Preventive measures to decrease the recurrence rate include avoidance of sleeping on the affected ear.

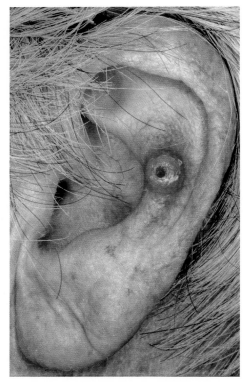

Figure 7.24. This firm nodule with a central crater is seen on the antihelix of an elderly woman with chondrodermatitis nodularis helicis; antihelical lesions are more common in women. *(Reprinted from Thompson, L.D.R., Goldblum, J.R. [Eds.], 2013. Head and Neck Pathology, 2nd ed. Elsevier, 399–420. Courtesy Dr. S.A. Norton.)*

12. Auricular composite grafts
    • Unlike skin grafts, composite grafts only interface with the recipient bed along their perimeter; therefore, graft size should be no larger than 1.5 cm in diameter, so the center of the graft is never more than 5 to 8 mm from a blood supply.
    • The clinical appearance of a healing composite graft follows a reproducible pattern.
       ▪ 6 to 8 hours: Very white
       ▪ 8 to 24 hours: Slight pink tinge signaling revascularization
       ▪ 24 hours to 1 week: Cyanosis 2/2 venous congestion
       ▪ After 1 week: Graft ultimately becomes pink and then redder as revascularization intensifies.
       ▪ 6 months to 1 year: Redness will fade, and the tissue acquires its final tone.
          ○ A lingering whitish area in the center of a cyanotic graft most likely represents impending necrosis.
             ◆ However, even if eschar develops, it should not be debrided.
                → Removing the eschar may dislodge the surviving portion of the graft and also places it at increased risk for infection.
                → Observation is the most prudent initial step in management.

- Postoperative cooling is recommended to decrease the metabolic rate of the grafted tissue until secondary revascularization has taken place.

13. Otoplasty
   - Commonly calls for a combination of procedures
     - Create an antihelical fold.
       - Stenstrom cartilage abrasion
         - Partial-thickness scoring, scratching, or abraiding of anterior surface of antihelix causing cartilage to bend *away* from the scoring (relieves internal stress)
       - Mustarde sutures
         - Mattress sutures on posterior aspect of ear cartilage to create an antihelical fold (see Figure 7.25)
     - To reduce conchal hypertrophy: Cartilage reduction
     - To reduce conchal bowl projection: Furnas sutures (see Figure 7.26)
       - Only method known for placement of conchomastoid sutures
       - Designed to correct ears with deep conchae (>2.5 cm)
       - Mattress sutures from conchal cartilage to mastoid periosteum

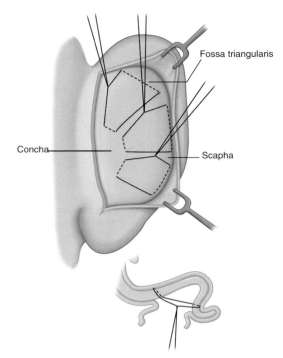

Figure 7.25. Placement of Mustarde sutures. *(Reprinted with permission from Janis, J.E., Rohrich, R.J., Gutowski, K.A., 2005. Otoplasty. Plast. Reconstr. Surg. 115 [4], 60e–72e.)*

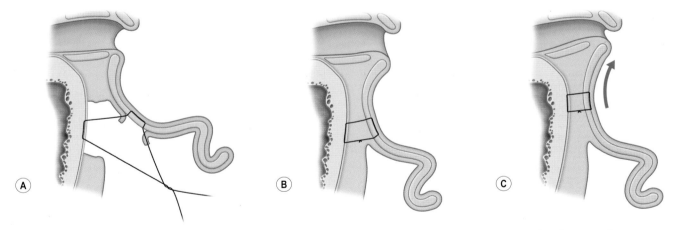

Figure 7.26. Placement of Furnas conchomastoid sutures. Note that suture placement too close to the external auditory canal can constrict the canal *(far right)*. *(Reprinted with permission from Janis, J.E., Rohrich, R.J., Gutowski, K.A., 2005. Otoplasty. Plast. Reconstr. Surg. 115 [4], 60e–72e.)*

14. Cleft lobe repair (see Figure 7.27)
   - Extremely common, usually a traumatic etiology (pulling) or slow stretch over time (may be caused by heavy earrings)
   - Many techniques including straight line wedge excision and layered closure versus incorporation of Z plasty

   - Refrain from repiercing until 6 weeks (if remote from scar line) or 12 weeks (if within scar line)
     - Alternatively, techniques have been described for repair and preservation of a perforation for an earring.
   - Key is approximation of lower lobule skin to prevent notching (most common complaint)

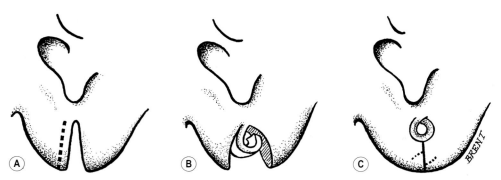

Figure 7.27. Repair of an earlobe cleft with preservation of the perforation for an earring. **A,** A flap is prepared by a parallel incision on one side of the cleft; the other side is "freshened" by excision of the margin. **B,** The flap is rolled in to provide a lining for preservation of the earring track. **C,** Closure is completed; a small Z plasty may be incorporated. *(Modified from Pardue, A.M., 1973. Repair of torn earlobe with preservation of the perforation for an earring. Plast. Reconstr. Surg. 51, 472.)*

Suggested Readings

Aguilar, E.F., 2004. Ear reconstruction. Clin. Plast. Surg. 31, 87–91.

Bauer, B.S., Patel, P.K., 1998. Congenital deformities of the ear. In: Bentz, M.L. (Ed.), Pediatric Plastic Surgery. Appleton & Lange, Stamford, CT, pp. 359–392.

Beahm, E.K., Walton, R.L., 2002. Auricular reconstruction for microtia: part I. Anatomy, embryology, and clinical evaluation. Plast. Reconstr. Surg. 109, 2473–2482.

Brent, B., 2002. Microtia repair with rib cartilage grafts: a review of personal experience with 1000 cases. Clin. Plast. Surg. 29 (2), 257–271, vii.

Brent, B., 1999. Technical advances in ear reconstruction with autogenous rib cartilage grafts: personal experience with 1200 cases. Plast. Reconstr. Surg. 104, 319–334.

Brent, B.D., 2013. Reconstruction of the ear. In: Neligan, P.C. (Ed.), Plastic Surgery, 3rd ed. Elsevier, pp. 187–225.

Byrd, H.S., Langevin, C.J., Ghidoni, L.A., 2010. Ear molding in newborn infants with auricular deformities. Plast. Reconstr. Surg. 126 (4), 1191–1200.

Cho, B.H., Ahn, H.B., 1999. Microsurgical replantation of an ear, with leech therapy. Ann. Plast. Surg. 43, 427–429.

Dancey, A., Jeynes, P., Nishikawa, H., 2005. Acrylic ear splints for treatment of cryptotia. Plast. Reconstr. Surg. 115 (7), 2150–2152.

Donelan, M.B., 1989. Conchal transposition flap for postburn ear deformities. Plast. Reconstr. Surg. 83, 641–654.

Elsahy, N.I., 2002. Acquired ear defects. Clin. Plast. Surg. 29, 175–186.

Elsahy, N.I., 2002. Reconstruction of the ear after skin and cartilage loss. Clin. Plast. Surg. 29, 201–212.

Eppley, B.L., 1999. Alloplastic implantation. Plast. Reconstr. Surg. 104, 1761.

Furnas, D.W., 2002. Otoplasty for prominent ears. Clin. Plast. Surg. 29 (2), 273–288, viii.

Furnas, D.W., 2000. Otoplasty for protruding ears, cryptotia, or Stahl's ear. In: Evans, G.R.D. (Ed.), Operative Plastic Surgery. McGraw-Hill, New York, pp. 417–448.

Ha, R.Y., Trovato, M.J., 2013. Plastic surgery of the ear. In: Selected Readings in Plastic Surgery, vol. 11. (R3), pp. 1–52.

Hackney, F.L., 2001. Plastic surgery of the ear. In: Selected Readings in Plastic Surgery, vol. 9. pp. 1–26.

Jackson, I.T., 2002. Ear reconstruction. In: Jackson, I.T. (Ed.), Local Flaps in Head and Neck Reconstruction. Quality Medical Publishing, St. Louis, pp. 251–271.

Janis, J.E., Rohrich, R.J., Gutowski, K.A., 2005. Otoplasty. Plast. Reconstr. Surg. 115 (4), 60e–72e.

Janz, B.A., Cole, P., Hollier, L.H. Jr., et al., 2009. Treatment of prominent and constricted ear anomalies. Plast. Reconstr. Surg. 124 (1 Suppl.), 27e–37e.

Kind, G.M., 2002. Microvascular ear replantation. Clin. Plast. Surg. 29, 233–248.

Nagata, S., 2000. Microtia: auricular reconstruction. In: Achauer, B.M., Eriksson, E., Guyuron, B., et al. (Eds.), Plastic Surgery: Indications, Operations and Outcomes. Mosby, St. Louis, pp. 1023–1056.

Nagata, S., 1994. Modification of the stages in total reconstruction of the auricle: parts I-IV. Plast. Reconstr. Surg. 93 (2), 221–266.

Park, C., Lew, D.H., Yoo, W.M., 1999. An analysis of 123 temporoparietal fascial flaps: anatomic and clinical considerations in total auricular reconstruction. Plast. Reconstr. Surg. 104, 1295–1306.

Park, C., Lineaweaver, W.C., Rumly, T.O., et al., 1992. Arterial supply of the anterior ear. Plast. Reconstr. Surg. 90 (1), 38–44.

Snik, A., Leijendeckers, J., Hol, M., et al., 2008. The bone-anchored hearing aid for children: recent developments. Int. J. Audiol. 47, 559.

Stal, S., Klebuc, M., Spira, M., 2001. Otoplasty. In: Goldwyn, R.M., Cohen, M.N. (Eds.), The Unfavorable Result in Plastic Surgery, Avoidance and Treatment. Lippincott Williams & Wilkins, Philadelphia, pp. 437–450.

Stelnicki, E.J., 2004. Infections of the face. In: Greer, S.E., Benhaim, P., Lorenz, H.P., et al. (Eds.), Handbook of Plastic Surgery. Marcel Dekker, New York, pp. 141–143.

Thorne, C., Brecht, L.E., Bradly, J.P., et al., 2001. Auricular reconstruction: indications for autogenous and prosthetic technique. Plast. Reconstr. Surg. 107, 1241–1251.

Thorne, C.H., 2006. Otoplasty and ear reconstruction. In: Thorne, C.H., Beasley, R.W., Aston, S.J., et al. (Eds.), Grabb and Smith's Plastic Surgery, 6th ed. Lippincott Williams & Wilkins, Philadelphia, pp. 304–310.

Van Wijk, M.P., Breugem, C.C., Kon, M., 2009. Non-surgical correction of congenital deformities of the auricle: a systematic review of the literature. J. Plast. Reconstr. Aesthet. Surg. 62 (6), 727–736.

Walton, R.L., Beahm, E.K., 2002. Auricular reconstruction for microtia. Part II: surgical techniques. Plast. Reconstr. Surg. 110, 234–249.

Zaren, H.A., Lowe, N.J., 1997. Benign growth and generalized skin disorders. In: Aston, S.J., Beasley, R.W. Thorne, C.H.M. (Eds.), Grabb and Smith's Plastic Surgery, 5th ed. Lippincott & Raven, Philadelphia, pp. 141–148.

Breast Anatomy, Embryology, and Congenital Defects

Chapter

8

1. Breast embryology/development
   - Embryologic development
     - Ectodermal breast bud develops during the 5th to 6th week of gestation.
     - Ectodermal thickening from the axilla to the pelvis forms the milk line or "milk streak" (see Figure 8.1)
       - Most of this atrophies by the 9th week except in the pectoral region, which forms the mammary ridge.

   - Basal cells within the mammary ridge proliferate to form the nipple bud during the 9th week of gestation.
   - Mammary ducts and lobular buds are formed by the 12th week of gestation.
   - The lactiferous ducts form by 16 to 24 weeks.
2. Breast anatomy (see Figures 8.2 and 8.3)
   - General
     - Coopers suspensory ligaments support the breast parenchyma.
       - Attenuation of these ligaments leads to breast ptosis.
     - Breast lobule
     - Up to 50% of the breast is fat.
     - Lymphatic drainage occurs via the axillary and parasternal nodes.

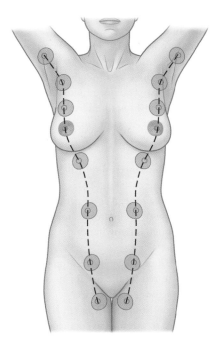

Figure 8.1. The milk lines. *(Reprinted with permission from Standring, S. [Ed.], 2008. Gray's Anatomy, 40th ed. Churchill Livingstone, London, 1712.)*

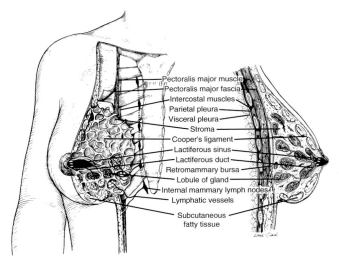

Figure 8.2. Tangential and sagittal view of the breast. The breast lies in the superficial fascia just deep to the dermis, attached to the skin by the suspensory ligaments of Cooper. The retromammary bursa separates it from the investing fascia of the pectoralis major muscle. Cooper's ligaments form fibrosepta in the stroma that provide support for the breast parenchyma. From 15 to 20 lactiferous ducts extend from lobules comprised of glandular epithelium to openings located on the nipple. Subcutaneous fat and tissue are distributed around the lobules of the gland and account for much of its mass. *(Reprinted from Copeland, E.M. III, Bland, K.I., 2004. The Breast, 4th ed. WB Saunders, Philadelphia, 21–38.)*

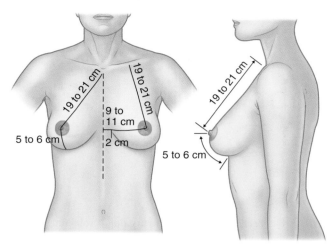

Figure 8.3. Statistical standards for the dimensions of the breast. *(Reprinted from Neligan, P.C. [Ed.], 2013. Plastic Surgery, 3rd ed. Elsevier, 1–12.)*

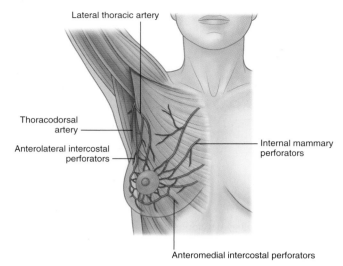

Figure 8.5. Blood supply to the breast; cross-sectional view. *(Reprinted from Neligan, P.C. [Ed.], 2013. Plastic Surgery, 3rd ed. Elsevier, 1–12.)*

- Arterial supply of the breast (see Figures 8.4-8.6)
  - Dominant supply via the 2nd and 3rd internal mammary artery (IMA) perforators
    - Nipple-areolar complex (NAC): Perforators from the two IMA vessels
    - Superior/superomedial pedicle: 2nd and 3rd intercostal IMA perforators
    - Medial pedicle: 3rd intercostal IMA perforators
    - Inferior pedicle: Intercostal a. perforators
    - Central mound pedicle
  - Other sources: Perforators from intercostal arteries, lateral thoracic a., thoracodorsal a., and thoracoacromial a.

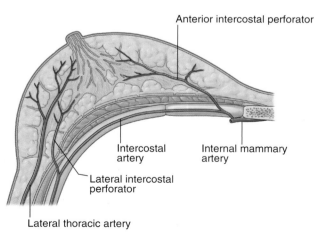

Figure 8.4. Blood supply to the breast. *(Reprinted from Neligan, P.C. [Ed.], 2013. Plastic Surgery, 3rd ed. Elsevier, 1–12.)*

- Sensory innervation
  - Multiple contributions from cutaneous nerves
  - Sensitivity decreased with increased age, breast size/volume, and breast ptosis
    - Superior pole: Supraclavicular branches of the cervical plexus
      - Most sensitive area to light pressure
    - Lateral breast: Anterior rami of lateral cutaneous branches of 3rd to 6th intercostal n.
    - Medial breast: Anterior cutaneous branches of 2nd to 6th intercostal n.
    - NAC
      - Dominant innervation: Lateral cutaneous branch of 4th intercostal n. (T4)
        - Danger zone: Nerves perforate the fascia just lateral to the pectoralis major m. border through interdigitation of the serratus anterior muscle.
          - Blunt dissection recommended in this region to reduce the risk for nerve injury and NAC sensory disturbance.
      - Also contributions from 5th lateral cutaneous n. and 3rd to 4th medial cutaneous n.
        - Dominant innervation with medially based pedicles is T3-T4 intercostal n.
      - NAC most sensitive to vibration (areola) and least sensitive to light pressure (nipple).

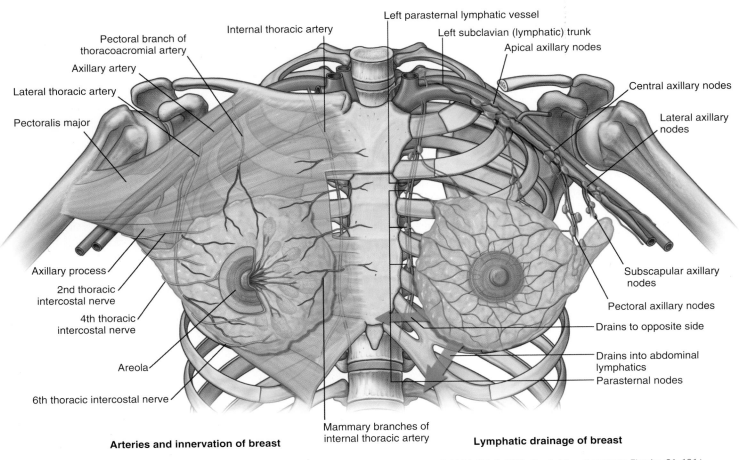

Figure 8.6. Comprehensive breast anatomy. *(Reprinted from Drake, R.L., Vogl, A.W., Mitchell, A.V.M. [Eds.], 2015. Gray's Atlas of Anatomy. Elsevier, 61–131.)*

- Innervation of the pectoralis m.
  - Medial pectoral nerve
    - From medial cord of brachial plexus and innervates lateral and inferior portion of pectoralis major (after passing up through pectoralis minor)
  - Lateral pectoral nerve: From lateral cord of brachial plexus and innervates the medial and superior portions of pectoralis major
- Pubertal development (see Figure 8.7)
  - Tanner stages
    - Stage I: No breast development or pubic hair
    - Stage II: Onset of breast development (thelarche); pubic hair appears.
      - Darkening and widening of the areola
      - Areola forms a mound that is elevated from the underlying palpable breast bud.
    - Stage III: Breast bud enlarges beyond areola; darker, coarser, and wider distribution of pubic hair
    - Stage IV: Areola/nipple for a secondary mound projecting above the underlying breast mound; adult-like pubic hair sparing the medial thighs
    - Stage V: Recession of secondary mound to create a mature adult breast with projection of the nipple; adult-like pubic hair
  - Menarche can begin at Tanner stages II-V
  - Benign premature thelarche: Breast development before pubic hair development or menarche

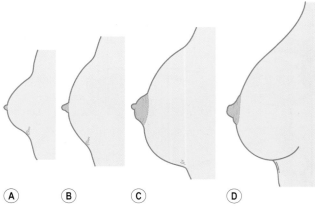

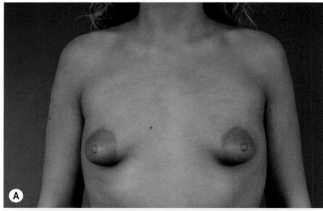

Figure 8.7. Stages of breast development at puberty. **A,** Breast bud elevation; **B,** growth and protrusion of the nipple; **C,** elevation of the secondary areolar mound; **D,** regression of the areolar mound to the level of the general breast contour. *(Reprinted from Mansel, R.E., Webster, D.J.T., Sweetland, H.M., et al. [Eds.], 2009. Hughes, Mansel, & Webster's Benign Disorders and Diseases of the Breast, 3rd ed. Elsevier, 25–40.)*

3. Congenital breast/chest wall abnormalities
   - Amastia
     - Absence of glandular tissue and the nipple
   - Amazia
     - Absence of the glandular tissue only
     - Can result from surgical removal of the breast bud, radiation, or congenital absence (e.g., Jeune syndrome)
   - Athelia
     - Absence of the nipple only
   - Ectopic breast tissue
     - Breast tissue found outside of the milk line
       - For example, scalp, ear, back, shoulder, epigastrium, and posterior thigh
   - Accessory breast tissue (polymastia)
     - Extra breast tissue found along the milk line (polymastia)
       - Most localized to the chest region, although may also involve the axilla, groin, vulva, and medial thigh
       - Can cause pain, restrict arm movement, affect cosmesis, and develop malignancy
     - Treatment recommendation is for surgical removal.
   - Polythelia
     - Extra nipple tissue due to failure of complete regression of the milk line
   - Tuberous breast deformity (see Figure 8.8)
     - Classic signs: Narrowed breast base, high and constricted inframammary fold (IMF), hypertrophy, and herniation of the NAC
     - Treatment recommendation is augmentation with radial gland scoring and areola reduction.

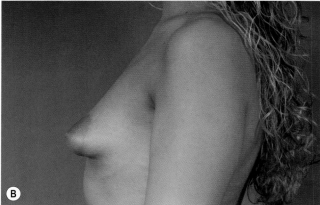

Figure 8.8. Preoperative appearance of a 19-year-old woman with a fully developed "classic" tuberous breast deformity. The breast is hypoplastic in general and whatever parenchyma is present is located mainly under the NAC. There does not appear to be normal peripheral expansion of the breast mound. As a result, growth of the constricted breast bud projects through the elastic areolar skin, creating an areolar "pseudoherniation." Along with this is seen a concomitant enlargement of the areolar diameter. As a result of the failure of the breast bud to expand peripherally, the surrounding breast skin remains tight and the IMF that does form is malpositioned superiorly. *(Reprinted from Hammond, D.C. [Ed.], 2009. Atlas of Aesthetic Breast Surgery. Elsevier, 183–194.)*

- Juvenile breast hypertrophy
  - Severe diffuse breast enlargement (unilateral or bilateral) without mass or nodularity
  - Occurs early in puberty and rarely regresses spontaneously
    - Etiology: Abnormal end-organ responsiveness to estrogen, with normal levels of hormone and hormone receptors
  - Treatment recommendation is observation until size has stabilized (1 year or more), followed by reduction mammaplasty
    - Reduction mammaplasty can be performed even if patient is younger than 18 years of age.
- Fibroadenoma (see Figure 8.9)
  - Most common breast neoplasm in adolescent females
  - Differentiated from juvenile hypertrophy by presence of palpable mass

- Classic signs of giant fibroadenoma: Rapid asymmetric breast enlargement just after onset of puberty, with prominent overlying veins, a palpable mass >5 cm in size, and occasional pressure-induced skin ulceration
- Treatment recommendation is enucleation using reduction mammoplasty techniques to obtain symmetry with contralateral breast.

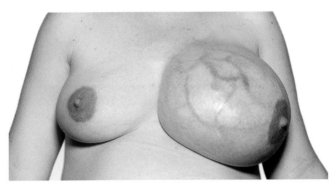

Figure 8.9 Benign giant fibroadenoma of adolescence. Rapid growth, vascularity, and pressure skin necrosis raised the question of malignancy. *(Reprinted from Mansel, R.E., Webster, D.J.T., Sweetland, H.M., et al., 2009. Hughes, Mansel, & Webster's Benighn Disorders and Diseases of the Breast, 3rd ed. Elsevier, 81–106.)*

- Anterior thoracic hypoplasia
  - Anterior chest wall depression from posteriorly displaced ribs
  - Hypoplasia of ipsilateral breast with a superiorly displaced NAC and a normal sternum and pectoralis major muscle
- Pectus excavatum
  - Most common congenital chest wall abnormality
  - A concave anterior chest wall defect from abnormal formation of the ribs and sternum
  - Most commonly involves the lower third of the sternum
- Pectus carinatum
  - A convex or anteriorly projecting sternum and ribs
  - Often creates the appearance of a "pigeon's chest"
- Poland syndrome (see Figure 8.10)
  - Often unilateral
  - Classic signs: Absence of the sternal head of the pectoralis major, hypoplasia or aplasia of the breast or nipple, deficiency of subcutaneous fat and axillary hair, abnormalities of the rib cage, and upper extremity anomalies
  - Complex presentations include hypoplasia or aplasia of the chest wall musculature or total absence of the anterolateral ribs with herniation of the lung.

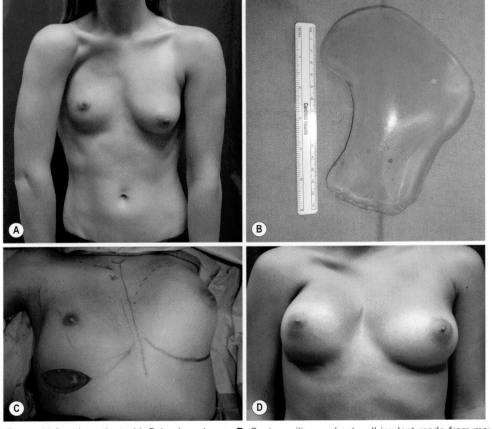

Figure 8.10. A, A 17-year-old female patient with Poland syndrome. **B,** Custom silicone chest wall implant made from moulage. **C,** Chest wall implant placed through inframammary incision. **D,** Breast implant placed in front of chest wall implant at separate stage. *(Reprinted from Neligan, P.C., 2013. Plastic Surgery, 3rd ed. Elsevier, 548–557.)*

- Reconstructive options include the insertion of subcutaneous tissue expanders in young patients, followed by latissimus flap reconstruction with permanent implants once breast development is completed.
- Sternal cleft
  - Failure of midline fusion of the sternum
  - Potential for the lack of protection to the heart and great vessels
  - Not associated with aplasia or hypoplasia of the breast

4. Gynecomastia
   - Abnormal benign enlargement of the male breast that correlates with hormonal changes
     - Infancy: Secondary to circulating maternal estrogens
     - Adolescence: Secondary to transient increase of estradiol at the onset of puberty
       - Reported to affect up to 65% of adolescent males
     - Increasing age: Results from decreased testosterone production with age and increased peripheral conversion of testosterone to estrogen
   - Conditions associated with gynecomastia (see Box 8.1)
   - Drugs associated with gynecomastia (see Box 8.2)

BOX 8.1 ETIOLOGY OF GYNECOMASTIA

Physiologic
  Neonatal period
  Puberty
  Advanced age
States of androgen deficiency
  Hypogonadism
    Primary
      Klinefelter syndrome
      Kallman syndrome
      Congenital anorchia
      Adrenocorticotropic hormone (ACTH) deficiency
      Defects in synthesis of androgens
    Secondary
      Trauma
      Orchitis
      Cryptorchidism
      Irradiation
      Hydrocele
      Spermatocele
      Varicocele
  Renal failure
  Androgen insensitivity syndrome
States of estrogen excess
  Testicular sources
    Germ cell tumor
      Choriocarcinoma
      Seminoma
      Teratoma

Non–germ cell tumor
  Leydig cell tumor
  Granulosa-theca tumor
  Sertoli cell tumor
True hemaphroditism
Liver disease
  Cirrhosis
Malnutrition
  Protein deficiency
  Fat deficiency
Infectious sources
  Sparganum or plerocercoid larva of the tapeworm
Neoplastic
  Breast carcinomas
  Adrenal cortical carcinomas
  Lung carcinomas
  Liver carcinomas
Systemic diseases with idiopathic mechanisms
  Non-neoplastic conditions of the lung
  Trauma
  Obesity
  AIDS
Familial

Reprinted from Guyuron, B., Eriksson, E., Persing, J.A., et al. (Eds.), 2009. Plastic Surgery: Indications and Practice, 1st ed. Elsevier, 727–736.

BOX 8.2 PHARMACOLOGIC SOURCES OF GYNECOMASTIA

Estrogen-like activity
  Estrogens
  Heroin
  Marijuana
  Digitalis
  Digoxin
  Digitoxin
  Anabolic steroids
Inhibit testosterone
  Cimetidine
  Ketoconazole
  Phenytoin
  Spironolactone
  Antineoplastic agents
  Diazepam

Cytoproterone
Flutamide
Gonadotropins
  Human chorionic gonadotropin
Central nervous system agents
  Phenothiazines
  Amphetamines
  Sympathetic modifiers
Idiopathic mechanisms
  Reserpine
  Theophylline
  Verapamil
  Tricyclic antidepressants
  Fuorosemide
  Methyldopa

Reprinted from Guyuron, B., Eriksson, E., Persing, J.A., et al. (Eds.), 2009. Plastic Surgery: Indications and Practice, 1st ed. Elsevier, 727–736.

- Diagnosis (see Figure 8.11)
  - Thorough history and physical examination
    - Testicular examination and/or ultrasound
      - Especially in adolescents
    - Persistence of symptoms
  - Labs
    - Estrogen/androgen ratio
      - Increased in testicular tumors, Klinefelter syndrome
    - Thyroid function tests
    - Luteinizing hormone (LH)/follicle-stimulating hormone (FSH)
  - Karyotyping
    - Klinefelter Syndrome
      - Rare, XXY chromosomal abnormality
      - Increased risk of breast cancer (elevated FSH, LH, estrogen receptor [ER], progesterone receptor [PR] and decreased testosterone)
      - 50% to 65% of patients will develop gynecomastia.
      - Bilateral mastectomy may be recommended in symptomatic patients.

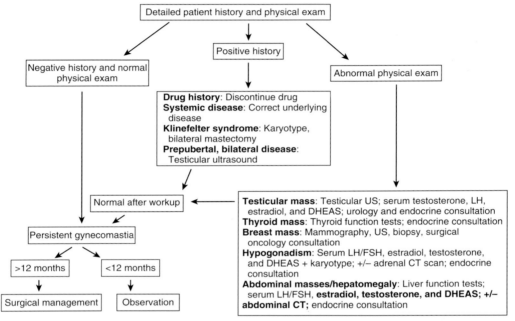

Figure 8.11. Rohrich algorithm. *CT,* Computed tomography; *DHEAS,* dehydroepiandrosterone; *FSH,* follicle-stimulating hormone; *LH,* luteinizing hormone; *US,* ultrasound. *(Adapted from Rohrich, R.J., Ha, R.Y., Kenkel, J.M., et al., 2003. Classification and management of gynecomastia: defining the role of ultrasound-assisted liposuction. Plast. Reconstr. Surg. 111, 909.)*

- Classification: Based on degree of skin excess and glandular excess
  - Simon's classification (see Table 8.1)

Table 8.1 Classification of Gynecomastia

GRADE	BREAST ENLARGEMENT	SKIN EXCESS
I	Small	Absent
IIA	Moderate	Absent
IIB	Moderate	Present
III	Large	Present

Reprinted from Guyuron, B., Eriksson, E., Persing, J.A., et al. (Eds.), 2009. Plastic Surgery: Indications and Practice, 1st ed. Elsevier, 727–736.

- Treatment options include ultrasound-assisted liposuction, traditional suction lipectomy, concentric circumareolar resection, periareolar resection with adjunctive suction lipectomy, and breast amputation with free nipple grafting.
  - Treatment reserved for symptoms present for >12 months.
  - For resection techniques, a Wise pattern reduction is not recommended because it will produce a conical, projecting breast.
  - The decision between liposuction and resection largely depends on the degree of skin excess.
    - Liposuction for gynecomastia requires disruption of the IMF for best results.
  - In severe gynecomastia with significant ptosis, skin excision is often necessary. In these cases, the ideal configuration and location of the male nipple is within the 4th or 5th intercostal space, 3 cm in diameter, and oval in shape.

5. Galactorrhea
   - Abnormal breast/nipple discharge
     - Rare in regularly menstruating women who have never been pregnant; however, reportedly can occur in 25% of women with prior pregnancies.
   - Etiology
     - History of pregnancy
     - Hypothyroidism
     - Pituitary tumor (prolactinoma)
     - Medications: Tricyclic antidepressants, fluoxetine
   - Diagnosis
     - Thorough history and physical examination
     - Labs
       ○ Prolactin
       ○ Thyroid function tests (hypothyroidism) and a history of all medications, including tricyclic antidepressants and fluoxetine
     - Imaging
       ○ Magnetic resonance imaging (MRI) of brain to rule out a pituitary tumor in women with elevated prolactin levels
   - Treatment recommendations: Bromocriptine to suppress prolactin secretion

Suggested Readings

Beer, G.M., Budi, S., Seifert, B., et al., 2001. Configuration and localization of the nipple-areola complex in men. Plast. Reconstr. Surg. 108 (7), 1947–1952.

Berrino, P., Berrino, V., 2013. Chapter 23: Poland syndrome. In: Neligan, P.C. (Ed.), Plastic Surgery, 3rd ed. Elsevier, pp. 548–557.

Cederna, P.S., 2009. Chapter 54: Gynecomastia. In: Guyuron, B., Eriksson, E., Persing, J.A., et al. (Eds.), Plastic Surgery: Indications and Practice, 1st ed. Elsevier, pp. 727–736.

De La Torre, J., Davis, M.R., 2013. Chapter 1: Anatomy for plastic surgery of the breast. In: Neligan, P.C. (Ed.), Plastic Surgery, 3rd ed. Elsevier, pp. 1–12.

Ferri, F.F., 2014. Gynecomastia. In: Ferri, F. (Ed.), Ferri's Clinical Advisor 2014. Mosby, pp. 511.

Mansel, R.E., 2009. Chapter 3. In: Mansel, R.E., Webster, D.J.T., Sweetland, H.M., et al. (Eds.), Hughes, Mansel, & Webster's Benign Disorders and Diseases of the Breast, 3rd ed. Elsevier, pp. 25–40.

Muti, E., 2013. Chapter 23: Congenital anomalies of the breast. In: Neligan, P.C. (Ed.), Plastic Surgery, 3rd ed. Elsevier, pp. 521–547.

Rohrich, R.J., Ha, R.Y., Kenkel, J.M., et al., 2003. Classification and management of gynecomastia: defining the role of ultrasound-assisted liposuction. Plast. Reconstr. Surg. 111, 909.

Sabel, M.S., 2009. Chapter 1: Anatomy and physiology of the breast. In: Sabel, M.S. (Ed.), Essentials of Breast Surgery: A Volume in the Surgical Foundations Series, 1st ed. Mosby, pp. 1–17.

Weinzweig, J., 2010. Chapter 90: Chest wall reconstruction. In: Weinzweig, J. (Ed.), Plastic Surgery Secrets Plus, 2nd ed. Mosby, pp. 587–593.

Breast Cancer and Breast Reconstruction

Chapter 9

1. Breast cancer epidemiology
   - Most common noncutaneous malignancy among women
     - Affects 1:8 women
   - Independent risk factors
     - Exposure to estrogen
       - Early age at menarche
       - Late menopause
       - First full-term pregnancy after 30 years of age (yo)
     - Personal history of breast cancer or benign proliferative breast disease
     - BRCA mutation (occurs in <1% of women; accounts for 5% of breast cancers; 60% to 80% lifetime risk)
       - BRCA1 mutation associated with the following malignancies: Breast (85%), ovarian (62%), male breast, pancreatic, testicular, and early-onset prostate cancers
       - BRCA2 associated with the following malignancies: Breast (85%), ovarian (25%), male breast (7%), pancreatic, and prostate cancers
     - Breast cancer in a first-degree relative
       - Age of affected <50 yo → Risk ratio (RR) 2.3
       - Age of affected >50 yo → RR 1.8
       - Bilateral breast cancer → RR 5.5
2. Breast cancer diagnosis
   - Clinical breast exam
   - Mammography
     - Radiographic imaging of the breast that is an excellent screening tool for abnormal masses or calcifications
       - Linear or branching calcifications may suggest malignancy.
       - Pleomorphic/granular calcifications may suggest malignancy.
       - Popcorn-like calcifications suggest fibroadenoma.
       - Large rod-like calcifications suggest secretory ducts.
       - Round eggshell calcifications suggest oil cysts.
       - Dystrophic/coarse calcifications suggest fat necrosis.
         - Calcifications can be found in ~25% of women who have had inferior pedicle breast reductions.
     - Patients with implants may get mammograms; however, they require a special view called the Eklund view, where the prosthesis is pushed against the chest wall and the breast parenchyma is pulled anteriorly around and away from the implant.
       - Implant position, capsular contracture, and small native breasts can compromise the reliability of mammography.
         - Implant size has not been shown to affect mammography.
   - Magnetic resonance imaging (MRI)
     - Newer tool for evaluating the breast for breast cancer
     - Especially useful for screening high-risk patients
     - May have high false-positive rate, resulting in increased secondary procedures such as biopsy and mastectomy
   - Ultrasound
     - Widely used as a diagnostic modality; often used as a secondary study to work up a mass
     - Useful in women with dense breasts (i.e., younger women)
     - Ultrasound findings can help differentiate between malignant and benign lesions.
       - The following ultrasound findings suggest malignancy: Spiculations, asymmetric mass, calcifications, angular margins, hypoechoic lesion with posterior shadowing, heterogenous
   - Histologic diagnostic modalities
     - Core biopsy
       - Image guided
     - Fine-needle aspiration
       - Disadvantages
         - Does not provide structural information to determine invasive from in situ
         - High false-negative rates from sampling error (2% to 22%)
     - Excisional biopsy
       - Indications: Disagreement between mammography and histology, atypical ductal hyperplasia on percutaneous biopsy, radial scar on mammography, or percutaneous biopsy
3. Breast cancer types
   - Ductal carcinoma in situ (DCIS)
   - Lobular carcinoma in situ (LCIS)
   - Invasive ductal carcinoma (IDC)
   - Invasive lobular carcinoma (ILC)

- Inflammatory breast carcinoma
    - Can often involve chest wall, requiring a modified radical mastectomy with wide skin defect
        - Treatment options include a rectus abdominal myocutaneous flap (preferred choice, especially if breast reconstruction desired), latissimus (lat) flap +/− split thickness skin graft, omental flap + split thickness skin graft.
4. Breast cancer staging (see Tables 9.1 and 9.2)

Table 9.1 Staging of Breast Cancer: TNM System

Tumor Size: T (Largest Diameter)	
TX	Primary tumor cannot be assessed
T0	No evidence of primary tumor
Tis	Carcinoma in situ
Tis (DCIS)	Ductal carcinoma in situ
Tis (LCIS)	Lobular carcinoma in situ
Tis (Paget's)	Paget's disease of the nipple *not* associated with invasive carcinoma and/or carcinoma in situ (DCIS and/or LCIS) in the underlying breast parenchyma. Carcinomas in the breast parenchyma associated with Paget's disease are categorized based on the size and characteristics of the parenchymal disease, although the presence of Paget's disease should still be noted.
T1	Tumor ≤20 mm in greatest dimension
T1mi	Tumor ≤1 mm in greatest dimension
T1a	Tumor >1 mm but ≤5 mm in greatest dimension
T1b	Tumor >5 mm but ≤10 mm in greatest dimension
T1c	Tumor >10 mm but ≤20 mm in greatest dimension
T2	Tumor >20 mm but not ≤50 mm in greatest dimension
T3	Tumor >50 mm in greatest dimension
T4	Tumor of any size with direct extension to chest wall or skin (includes inflammatory carcinoma)
Nodal Involvement: N (Nodal Status)	
NX	Regional lymph nodes cannot be assessed (e.g., previously removed, not removed).
N0	No regional lymph node metastases histologically
N1	Metastases to movable ipsilateral level-I, -II axillary lymph node(s)
N2	Metastases in ipsilateral level-I, -II axillary lymph nodes that are clinically fixed or matted or in clinically detected* ipsilateral internal mammary nodes in the *absence* of clinically evident axillary lymph node metastases
N3	Metastases in ipsilateral infraclavicular (level-III axillary) lymph node(s) with or without level-I, -II axillary lymph node involvement, clinically detected* ipsilateral internal mammary lymph node(s) with clinically evident level-I, -II axillary lymph node metastases, or ipsilateral supraclavicular lymph node(s) with or without axillary or internal mammary lymph node involvement
N3a	Metastases in ipsilateral infraclavicular lymph node(s)
N3b	Metastases in ipsilateral internal mammary lymph node(s) and axillary lymph node(s)
N3c	Metastases in ipsilateral supraclavicular lymph node(s)
Metastases: M	
M0	No clinical or radiographic evidence of distant metastases
cM0(i+)	No clinical or radiographic evidence of distant metastases, but deposits of molecularly or microscopically detected tumor cells that are no larger than 0.2 mm in circulating blood, bone marrow, or other nonregional nodal tissue in a patient without symptoms or signs of metastases
M1	Distant detectable metastases as determined by classic clinical and radiographic means and/or histologically proven larger than 0.2 mm

From 2010. AJCC Cancer Staging Manual and Handbook, 7th ed. Springer-Verlag, New York.
*Detected by imaging studies (excluding lymphoscintigraphy) or by clinical examination and having characteristics highly suspicious for malignancy or a presumed pathologic macrometastasis based on fine-needle biopsy with cytologic examination.
TNM, Tumor/node/metastasis.

Table 9.2 TNM Stage and Survival

STAGE	TNM CATEGORY*	RECURRENCE FREE AT 10 YEARS (NO SYSTEMIC ADJUVANT THERAPY)
0	TisN0M0	98%
I	T1N0M0 T <1 cm T >1-2 cm	80% (all stage-I patients) 90% 80-90%
IIA	T0N1M0 or T2N0M0 T1N1M0	60-80% 50-60%
IIB	T2 N1M0 T3N0M0	5-10% worse than IIA and based on node status 30-50%
IIIA	T0, T1, or T2N2M0; T3N1; or N2M0	10-40%
IIIB	T4N0, N1, or N2M0	5-30%
IIIC	Any T and N3M0	15-20%
IV	Any T, any N, and M1	<5%

See Table 9.1 for TNM definitions.
TNM, Tumor/node/metastasis.

5. Breast cancer treatment
   - Breast-conserving therapy
     - Lumpectomy and radiation
       ○ Equivalent to mastectomy in long-term survival
       ○ Requires adjunctive radiation to limit risk for local recurrence
       ○ General indications
         ◆ Women who have small, easily accessible cancer with relatively large breasts and desire to avoid mastectomy
       ○ Contraindications
         ◆ Large cancer with small breasts, such that tumor removal would result in significant distortion of the remaining breast
       ○ Complications
         ◆ Contracture and scarring
         ◆ Radiation-related complications
         ◆ Unfavorable esthetic outcomes (estimated to be 20% to 35%)
       ○ Reconstructive options (see Figures 9.1 and 9.2)
         ◆ Oncoplastic reduction or mastopexy
           → Balancing the resection with breast landmarks and shape to preserve aesthetics
         ◆ Lat flap

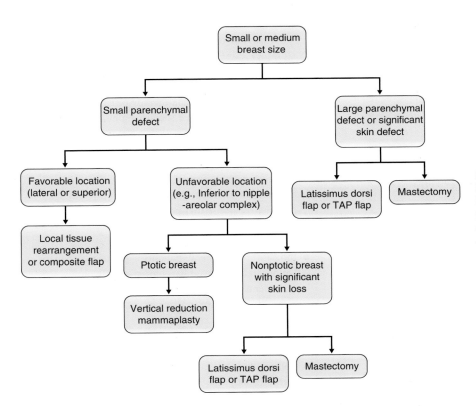

Figure 9.1. Proposed algorithm for partial breast reconstruction in small- or medium-breasted patients. *TAP,* thoracodorsal artery perforator. *(Reprinted from Beahm, E., 2013. In: Neligan, P.C. [Ed.], Plastic Surgery, 3rd ed. Elsevier, 266.)*

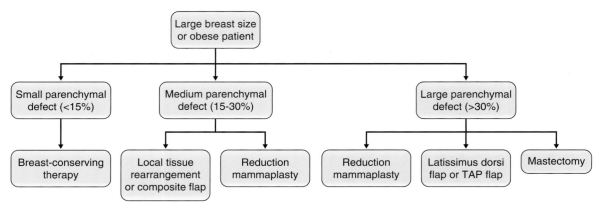

Figure 9.2. Proposed algorithm for partial breast reconstruction in obese or large-breasted patients. *TAP,* thoracodorsal artery perforator. *(Reprinted from Beahm, E., Lang, J.E., 2013. In: Neligan, P.C. [Ed.], Plastic Surgery, 3rd ed. Elsevier, 266.)*

- Mastectomy
  - Removal of all breast parenchyma
  - Mastectomy types
    - Radical: Wide excision of all breast tissue, overlying skin, pectoralis major muscle, and en bloc dissection of level-I, -II, and -III nodes
    - Modified radical: All of the above, except pectoralis muscle resection, with en bloc removal of the level-I and -II axillary lymph nodes
    - Skin sparing: Resection of all breast tissue through a circumareolar incision, including the nipple-areolar complex (NAC), but preserving as much of the skin envelope as possible to facilitate immediate reconstruction
      - Reported recurrence rate of 2% at 4 years
    - Nipple sparing: Excision of breast tissue with preservation of the NAC
      - Requires intraoperative retroareolar frozen section
      - Indications: Isolated single-tumor focus <3 cm, located >2 cm from the NAC; prophylactic mastectomy patients
      - Contraindications: Multifocal disease, tumor in close proximity to NAC (<2 cm), tumor >3 cm, clinical invasion of the NAC, positive retroareolar frozen section, positive nodal disease
      - Complications: NAC compromise
        - Risk factors: Large periareolar scar, thin mastectomy flaps
        - Preferred incisions for nipple-sparing mastectomy (NSM) include radial incisions +/− periareolar extension and inframammary fold incisions.
    - Prophylactic: Resection of a breast that does not have a diagnosis of cancer
      - Indications: Women with known genetic predisposition and those with unilateral breast cancer who desire contralateral mastectomy

- Sentinel lymph node biopsy
  - Indicated for all oncologic breast interventions to sample for possibility of lymphatic spread
  - Not indicated in prophylactic interventions
- Lymph node dissection
  - Indications: Positive sentinel lymph node biopsy or clinically positive nodes found to be positive for cancer preoperative or intraoperative
  - Complications
    - Lymphedema
    - Sensory disturbance of the upper, medial arm from injury to the intercostobrachial n. and the medial brachial cutaneous n.
- Neoadjuvant therapy
  - Indications: Use of chemotherapy or endocrine therapy to reduce tumor burden such that a lumpectomy may be feasible or to determine whether a patient responds to a given therapy that is useful to determine prognosis
  - Currently, there is no survival advantage for neoadjuvant therapy versus traditional or surgery + adjuvant approaches unless the patient develops a pathologic complete response that portends a favorable prognosis.
  - Complications: See below
- Chemotherapy
  - Indications: In general, patients with positive axillary lymph nodes are candidates for chemotherapy.
    - Patients with estrogen-receptor- or progesterone-receptor-positive invasive breast cancer should receive adjuvant endocrine therapy (i.e., tamoxifen for premenopausal women and aromatase inhibitors for postmenopausal women).
  - Complications: Wound healing derangements, nausea/vomiting, alopecia, immunosuppression

- Radiation
  - Indications: Women undergoing breast-conservation therapy, tumors >5 cm (T3), 4 or more positive lymph nodes (N2); strongly recommended for 1 to 3 axillary lymph node involvement
    - Radiation therapy is also considered for patients with lymphovascular invasion or close surgical margins.
  - Complications: Skin damage, fibrosis of soft tissue, poor wound healing, reduced cosmesis of reconstruction, increased postreconstruction complications (especially with implant-based reconstruction)
  - Radiation skin damage progression
    - Acute changes: Vessel thrombosis, erythema
    - Chronic changes: Impaired neutrophil activation and fibroblast function, leading to poor wound healing
      - Late radiation tissue injury (LRTI) occurs in approximately 5% to 15% of long-term survivors and can occur months to years after exposure.
        - → Characterized by progressive tissue deterioration followed by fibrotic replacement
        - → Development of late or new ulceration within radiation field is concerning for possible malignancy and biopsy should be considered.
          - ➡ Squamous cell carcinoma (Marjolin's ulcer)
          - ➡ Radiation-induced sarcoma
        - → Chronic radiation wound management requires autologous tissue.
          - ➡ Latissimus dorsi flap is preferred option
  - Safest option after immediate expander insertion with unexpected need for postoperative radiation therapy is explantation, followed by delayed autologous reconstruction.
6. Reconstructive options
   - Reconstruction timing
     - Immediate: At the time of the mastectomy
       - Advantages: Psychosocial benefits, take advantage of available skin, supple soft tissues that are relatively free of scar
       - Disadvantages: Formal pathologic evaluation not completed, risk of mastectomy flap necrosis that could compromise esthetic results
     - Delayed: Delayed for some time after the mastectomy incisions have healed
       - Advantages: Full pathologic evaluation completed along with any necessary adjunctive therapies
       - Disadvantages: Operating in a scarred field, greater skin requirement than immediate reconstructions, delayed psychosocial benefits of reconstruction
       - Delayed autologous reconstruction is the preferred reconstructive choice in the setting of adjuvant radiotherapy.

- Reconstruction types
  - Implant-based breast reconstruction
    - Tissue expanders, placed in the subpectoral space, used to stretch the skin envelope, followed by expander-implant exchange at a second stage
    - Preferred option in patients who do not need adjuvant radiation therapy and desire a quick recovery with minimal scarring
    - Advantages: Relatively short operative time, no second donor site, good symmetry achieved in bilateral reconstructions, patient participation in choosing size of reconstruction
    - Disadvantages: High risk of wound healing complications, infection, exposure in setting of radiation therapy; symmetry with contralateral native breast is difficult in unilateral reconstructions; requires two operative stages and multiple office visits; less natural in appearance and feel than autologous reconstruction, implant-related complications
    - Can include a lat flap or perforator flap to improve appearance or as salvage of an exposed or infected implant
    - Can be used with acellular dermal matrix
      - Advantages: Increased initial fill of the expander, potentially decreased capsular contracture
      - Disadvantages: Increased seroma and infection rate, cost
    - Newer expanders on the market use an osmotic gradient to allow self-filling
      - Advantages: Frequent postoperative office visits not required for expansion; no external expander access required, which reduces risk
      - Disadvantages: No external control of expansion process, expansion occurs at a set rate that cannot be adjusted, fill malfunction
  - Autologous tissue reconstruction
    - Use of second donor site to reconstruct breast with patient's own tissue
    - Transverse rectus abdominis myocutaneous (TRAM) flap (see Figure 9.3)
      - Based off epigastric a./venae comitantes
        - → Can be pedicled (superior epigastric a.) or "free" (inferior epigastric a.)
          - ➡ Pedicled TRAM: Shorter operative time, decreased risk of total flap loss, higher incidence of fat necrosis and partial flap loss, increased length of hospital stay
          - ➡ Free TRAM: More flexibility in flap shaping and insetting, decreased abdominal wall morbidity, recommended for patients who are diabetic, overweight, or cigarette smokers

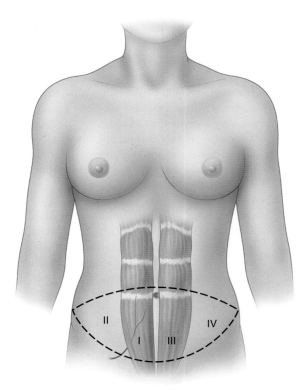

Figure 9.3. Zones of skin perfusion in the lower abdomen. Zone I overlies the rectus abdominis muscle ipsilateral to the pedicle, zone II lies lateral to this, zone III lies over the contralateral rectus abdominis muscle, and zone IV lies lateral to this. Zones I and II have the most reliable perfusion, with variable perfusion across the midline. *(Reprinted from Hall-Findlay, E.J., Evans, G.R.D. [Eds.], 2010. Esthetic and Reconstructive Surgery of the Breast. Elsevier, 117–146.)*

- ◆ Muscle-sparing (MS) free TRAM
  - → MS-0: Entire width of rectus m. harvested, partial length
  - → MS-1: Medial or lateral strip of rectus muscle spared during flap harvest
  - → MS-2: Medial and lateral strip of rectus muscle spared during flap harvest
  - → MS-3: Entire rectus m. spared during harvest. Flap perfusion based off of perforators through the rectus m. (deep inferior epigastric artery perforator [DIEP] flap)
- ◆ Advantages: Ability to create a natural-appearing breast, secondary benefit of improved abdominal contour, avoids risks associated with implants, better symmetry with contralateral native breast in unilateral reconstructions
- ◆ Disadvantages: Long surgery, donor site morbidity (bulge, hernia, scarring, seroma/hematoma, weakness), free-flap surgery requires expertise in microsurgery
  - ○ Superficial inferior epigastric artery (SIEA) flap
    - ◆ Free flap based off of the superficial epigastric vessels

- ◆ Advantages: Avoids incisions within rectus fascia and dissection of rectus muscle, leading to least abdominal morbidity when compared to TRAM and DIEP
- ◆ Disadvantages: Reliable SIEA vessel present in <33% of patients, unpredictable perfusion of tissue leading to higher frequency of total flap loss, fat necrosis
  - ○ Superior gluteal artery perforator (SGAP) flaps/ inferior gluteal artery perforator (IGAP) flaps
    - ◆ Based off of perforators from the gluteal arteries
    - ◆ Indicated when abdominal donor site is not available or desired and patient prefers to avoid implants.
    - ◆ Disadvantages: Requires positioning changes during operation, scar across buttock, relatively thick and firm adipose tissue that is difficult to mold and shape into breast, size limitations with reconstruction
  - ○ Transverse upper gracilis (TUG) myocutaneous flaps
    - ◆ Based off of cutaneous perforators from the underlying gracilis m. and descending branch of the medial circumflex femoral a. source vessel
    - ◆ Indicated when abdominal donor site is not available or desired by patient
    - ◆ Advantages: Reliable vascular anatomy
    - ◆ Disadvantages: Size limitations, donor site along medial thigh, reliability of skin paddle perfusion
  - ○ Lat dorsi myocutaneous flap
    - ◆ Based off of the thoracodorsal vessels
    - ◆ Transposed through subcutaneous tunnel within axilla
    - ◆ Most commonly used in combination with an expander implant (see below)
    - ◆ Extended lat dorsi flap includes subcutaneous adipose tissue in lumbar, scapular, and parascapular regions in an effort to eliminate the need for an implant.
    - ◆ Advantages: Local, pedicled option; provides skin and muscle coverage for salvage operations; enhances natural appearance and feel of implant reconstruction
    - ◆ Disadvantages: Requires second donor site; harvest of muscle can lead to loss of shoulder extension, adduction, and medial rotation (compensated for by teres major); seroma (most common complication); size limitations with skin paddle
- ■ Combination
  - ○ Use of expanders and implants + autologous tissue (typically, lat dorsi myocutaneous flap)
  - ○ Advantages: Allows use of implants in reconstructive efforts in setting of radiation therapy, enhances the natural/esthetic appearance and feel of implant-based reconstruction
  - ○ Disadvantages: Requires a second donor site, implant-related complications

7. Anaplastic large cell lymphoma (ALCL)
   - Women with breast implants may have a very small but increased risk of developing ALCL in the scar capsule adjacent to the prosthesis.
     - Generally more indolent, with a favorable prognosis when compared to patients with systemic ALCL
   - Diagnosis should be considered in patients who have late-onset persistent seroma.
   - Diagnosis made through histologic examination of the capsule for giant cells
   - The Food and Drug Administration (FDA) does not recommend removing implants in asymptomatic patients.
   - Currently developing a registry of these patients to better understand the disease and potential association

8. Phyllodes tumor (see Figure 9.4)
   - Most commonly occurring nonepithelial neoplasm of the breast
     - Accounts for 1% of all breast tumors
     - Approximately 85% of phyllodes tumors are benign.
   - Characterized by a large (~5 cm), smooth, mobile, and sharply demarcated mass
   - Suggested treatment options
     - Wide local excision with 1-cm margins
     - Mastectomy (if mass size precludes breast-conserving surgery)

9. Common preoperative considerations
   - Smoking
     - Increased risk of mastectomy flap necrosis as well as donor site skin necrosis and wound healing complications, umbilical necrosis, hernia in autologous reconstructions
   - Antibiotics
     - Preoperative and intraoperative redosing as necessary
     - No evidence to support postoperative antibiotics
     - Oral antibiotics recommended as initial treatment for early/minor infection of prosthetic reconstruction
   - Anticoagulation
     - Preoperative anticoagulation with subcutaneous heparin or low-molecular-weight heparin is effective in reducing the risk of deep venous thrombosis and pulmonary embolus

10. Common postoperative considerations
    - Severe pain with expansion
      - Initial treatment recommendation is to remove fluid from the expander because overfill can lead to ischemia.
    - Mastectomy skin flap necrosis in setting of implant-based reconstruction
      - Initial treatment recommendations depend on presence or absence of expander exposure.
        - If necrosis occurs over area with no muscle coverage, debridement and primary closure of skin, if possible, is preferred.
        - If necrosis occurs over area with muscle coverage, dressing changes and healing by secondary intent can be performed.
    - Secondary procedures
      - Reconstruction revision
        - Skin excision
        - Fat grafting for contour deformities (especially in the upper pole)
        - Capsulectomy/capsuloraphy
      - Contralateral procedures for symmetry
        - Reduction mammoplasty
        - Mastopexy
        - Augmentation
      - Donor site revision
        - Scar revision
        - Dog-ear excision
        - Abdominal bulge/hernia repair

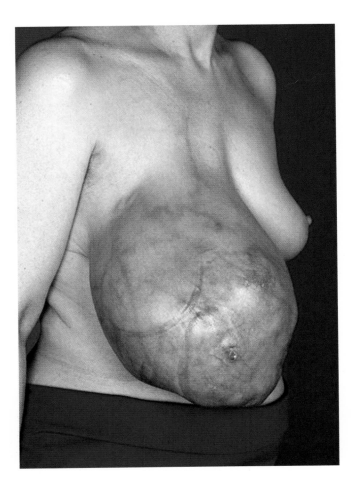

Figure 9.4. Benign phyllodes tumor of the breast with a diameter of 30 cm in a 55-year-old patient. The visible vessels and thinned skin are characteristics of large phyllodes tumors. *(Reprinted from Lenhard, M.S., Kahlert, S., Himsl, I., et al., 2008. Euro. J. Obstet. Gyn. Reprod. Biol. 138 [2], 217–221.)*

Suggested Readings

American Cancer Society, 2010. Breast Cancer Facts and Figures. Available at: <http://www.cancer.org/Research/CancerFactsFigures/CancerFactsFigures/cancer-facts-and-figures-2010/> Accessed on: January 8, 2015.

Beahm, E., Lang, J.E., 2013. Chapter 10: Breast cancer: Diagnosis, therapy, and oncoplastic techniques. In: Neligan, P.C. (Ed.), Plastic Surgery, 3rd ed. Elsevier, pp. 266.

Belz, J.M., Woo, A.S., Tung, T.H.H., 2014. Chapter 25: Breast cancer reconstruction. In: Woo, A.S., Shahzad, F., Snyder-Warwick, A.K. (Eds.), Plastic Surgery Case Review. Thieme, pp. 109–112.

Davidson, N., 2012. Chapter 204: Breast cancer and benign breast disorders. In: Goldman, L., Schafer, A.I. (Eds.), Goldman's Cecil Medicine, 24th ed. Elsevier, pp. 1309–1317.

Fosnot, J., Serletti, J.M., 2013. Chapter 17: Free TRAM breast reconstruction. In: Neligan, P.C. (Ed.), Plastic Surgery, 3rd ed. Elsevier, pp. 411–434.

Fosnot, J., Serletti, J.M., 2013. Chapter 18: Autologous breast reconstruction using abdominal flaps. In: Neligan, P.C., Buck, D.W. (Eds.), Core Procedures in Plastic Surgery. Elsevier, pp. 278–308.

Lenhard, M.S., Kahlert, S., Himsl, I., et al., 2008. Phyllodes tumor of the breast: clinical follow-up of 33 cases of this rare disease. Euro. J. Obstet. Gynecol. Reprod. Biol. 138 (2), 217–221.

Lipa, J.E., 2010. Chapter 9: DIEP flap breast reconstruction. In: Hall-Findlay, E.J., Evans, G.R.D. (Eds.), Aesthetic and Reconstructive Surgery of the Breast. Elsevier, pp. 117–146.

Losken, A., 2013. Chapter 11: The oncoplastic approach to partial breast reconstruction. In: Neligan, P.C. (Ed.), Plastic Surgery, 3rd ed. Elsevier, pp. 296–313.

LoTempio, M.M., Allen, R.J., Blondeel, P.N., 2013. Chapter 19: Alternative flaps for breast reconstruction. In: Neligan, P.C. (Ed.), Plastic Surgery, 3rd ed. Elsevier, pp. 457–471.

Nahabedian, M.Y., Momen, B., Galdino, G., et al., 2002. Breast reconstruction with the free TRAM or DIEP flap: patient selection, choice of flap, and outcome. Plast. Reconstr. Surg. 110 (2), 466–475.

Narod, S.A., 2010. BRCA mutations in the management of breast cancer: the state of the art. Nat. Rev. Clin. Oncol. 7 (12), 702–707.

Nava, M.B., Catanuto, G., Pennati, A., et al., 2013. Chapter 14: Expander-implants breast reconstructions. In: Neligan, P.C. (Ed.), Plastic Surgery, 3rd ed. Elsevier, pp. 336–369.

National Comprehensive Cancer Network, 2014. NCCN Guidelines for Invasive Breast Cancer. Available at: <http://www.nccn.org/professionals/physician_gls/f_guidelines.asp#breast/> Accessed on: August 6, 2014.

Neligan, P.C., Grotting, J.C., 2013. Chapter 17: Implant based breast reconstruction. In: Neligan, P.C., Buck, D.W. (Eds.), Core Procedures in Plastic Surgery. Elsevier, pp. 263–277.

Said, H.K., Javid, S.H., Colohan, S., et al., 2014. Chapter: Breast reconstruction following mastectomy: indications, techniques, and results. In: Cameron, J.L., Cameron, A.M. (Eds.), Current Surgical Therapy, 11th ed. Saunders, pp. 621–624.

Spear, S.L., Clemens, M.W., 2013. Chapter 15: Latissimus dorsi flap breast reconstruction. In: Neligan, P.C. (Ed.), Plastic Surgery, 3rd ed. Elsevier, pp. 370–392.

Noncancer Breast Surgery

Chapter

10

General Information

1. Noncancer breast surgery includes all of the techniques aimed at restoring an esthetic, more youthful appearance of the breasts in the setting of various benign conditions.
2. Indications
   - A motivated patient who desires improvement in the appearance of her breasts with the presence of macromastia, micromastia, and/or breast ptosis
3. Contraindications: Similar for all esthetic surgery
   - Patient is being pushed into surgery by others or desires to please others.
   - Patient seeking esthetic breast surgery because of marital problems or familial disapproval
   - Patient with unrealistic expectations or with minimal deformity and a distorted sense of their appearance (body dysmorphic disorder)
   - Patient who has been "doctor shopping" or has had multiple prior surgeries but is still dissatisfied

Reduction Mammaplasty

1. Macromastia signs and symptoms
   - Back pain, shoulder and neck pain, trapezius m. hypertrophy, shoulder strap grooving, and inframammary fold (IMF) intertrigo
2. Preoperative considerations
   - Degree of ptosis and hypertrophy and desired postoperative size will help determine the amount of parenchymal reduction required and assist with selection of skin incision pattern and pedicle location.
   - Postoperative nipple-areolar complex (NAC) perfusion and sensation
     - Most important determinant of postoperative sensation is location of glandular resection and pedicle selection (lateral pedicle, inferior pedicle, or medial pedicle are best), *not* reduction volume, preoperative breast volume, skin incision pattern, and/or sternal notch-to-nipple distance.

- Postoperative lactation
  - Rates of breast-feeding in women after breast reduction surgery are similar to those of child-bearing women who have not had breast reduction surgery.
    - Approximately 30% of women after inferior pedicle breast reduction breast-feed either exclusively or with formula supplementation.
  - Most important determinant of ability to breast-feed after breast reduction surgery is pedicle thickness
    - Pedicle type and reduction volume has no effect.
    - Impossible with free nipple grafting.
- Smoking cessation
- Breast measurements (see Figures 10.1 and 10.2)
  - Sternal notch-to-nipple distance
  - Nipple-to-IMF distance
  - Nipple-to-midline distance
  - Breast base width

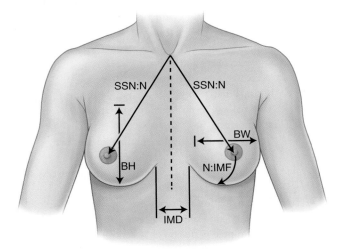

Figure 10.1. Preoperative measures (taken before breast augmentation) include *BH* (breast height), *BW* (breast width), *N:IMF* (nipple to inframammary fold), *IMD* (intermammary distance), and *SSN:N* (suprasternal notch to nipple). *(Reprinted from Neligan, P.C., Buck, D.W. [Eds.], 2013. Core Procedures in Plastic Surgery. Elsevier, 225.)*

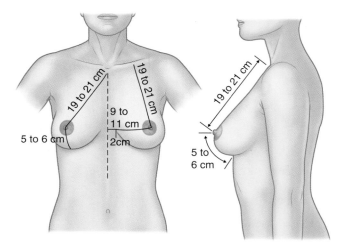

Figure 10.2. Statistical standards for the dimensions of the breast. *(Reprinted from Neligan, P.C., Buck, D.W. [Eds.], 2013. Core Procedures in Plastic Surgery. Elsevier, 235.)*

- Many advocate for preoperative mammography before surgery with any breast masses, breast complaints, or at-risk women (>35-40 years old [yo]) whose mammogram is over 1 year old.
  - Risk of occult breast cancer occurrence in reduction specimen is extremely rare (reportedly 0.2%).
  - When found, cancer is often early stage or in situ carcinoma.
3. Techniques
   - Suction lipectomy
     - Can be used alone in select patients
     - Contraindicated in patients with breast ptosis or who will likely require skin reduction
     - Advantages
       - Minimal scars
       - Rapid recovery and return to work
       - Decreased operative time
       - Minimal risk to nipple sensation/perfusion
       - Minimal risk to postoperative lactation
     - Disadvantages
       - Unable to pathologically examine lipoaspirate
       - High risk of inadequate reduction
       - Skin contraction unpredictable, leading to excess skin
       - Unable to correct breast ptosis
   - Traditional reduction mammaplasty
     - Combines a skin excision pattern with a pedicle to maintain nipple perfusion
       - Skin patterns include Wise pattern, keyhole, vertical, and no-vertical-scar techniques
       - Pedicle options include superior, medial, superomedial, inferior, lateral, and central pedicle
         - The inferior pedicle can achieve significant volume reduction and reduce the vertical dimension of the breast.
           - Can be used for all reductions, including moderate to severe reductions (>800 g)

- Vertical mammaplasty
  - Uses a vertical-only skin excision that reduces scar burden and narrows the breast, thereby increasing projection
  - The initial breast shape is poor with a characteristic flattened, lower pole and inferior dog ears; however, this improves after 3 to 6 months.
  - This technique is generally used for moderate reductions (<800 g) or smaller but is contraindicated with a long pedicle length >9 cm because of concerns with nipple perfusion.
4. Complications: Risk factors include obesity, reduction volume >1000 g, and smoking.
   - Infection
   - Scarring
     - Long-term complication most associated with patient dissatisfaction
   - Seroma, hematoma
     - Greatest risk factor for hematoma is hypotensive anesthesia
     - Drains have not reduced the incidence of hematoma.
   - Fat necrosis
     - Characteristic finding: Development of delayed, firm, and nontender masses
   - Asymmetry
   - Skin loss and wound development (especially at the inferior T junction in Wise pattern reductions)
     - Most common complication in obese patients with large reduction volume
   - Under-resection
     - May require reoperation
   - NAC complications
     - Incidence <5%
     - Risk factors: Smoking, elevated body mass index (BMI), and long pedicle
     - Etiology
       - Intrinsic physiologic risk (obesity, smoking)
       - Excessive nipple-to-IMF distance/pedicle length and excessive sternal notch-to-nipple distance
       - Torsion of the pedicle
       - Excessive tension on the closure
     - Management
       - If immediately after reduction, pedicle exploration with release of tension
       - If pedicle release does not result in improvement, convert to free nipple graft
         - Be sure to graft to well-vascularized tissue and not the compromised skin flap or pedicle.
       - If nipple compromise occurs after early postoperative period, observation and conservative wound care

Mastopexy

1. Many similarities with reduction mammoplasty; however, primary goal is to lift the breast and correct breast ptosis

2. Breast ptosis: Relationship of the NAC to the IMF and lower contour of the breast (see Figures 10.3 and 10.4)
   - Regnault classification
     - Grade I: NAC within 1 cm of the IMF and above the lower contour of the breast
     - Grade II: NAC is 1-3 cm below the IMF but above the lower contour of the breast
     - Grade III: NAC >3 cm below the IMF and at the lower contour of the breast
     - Grade IV (pseudoptosis): NAC at the level of the IMF, but the majority of the breast volume has descended below the IMF
       - Increased nipple-to-IMF distance in setting of stable sternal notch-to-nipple distance

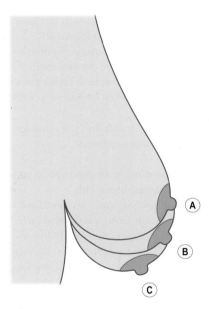

Figure 10.3. Breast ptosis classification as described by Regnault. **(A)** Minimal ptosis: Nipple is at the level of or just inferior to the inframammary crease. **(B)** Moderate ptosis: Nipple is 1-3 cm below the inframammary crease. **(C)** Severe ptosis: Nipple is >3 cm below the inframammary crease. *(Redrawn from Georgiade, G.S., Georgiade, N.G., Riefkohl, R., 1991. Esthetic breast surgery. In: McCarthy, J.G. [Ed.], Plastic Surgery. WB Saunders, Philadelphia, 38–39.)*

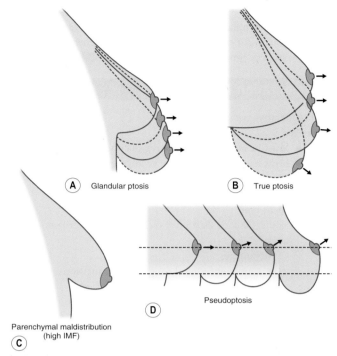

A Glandular ptosis **B** True ptosis

C Parenchymal maldistribution (high IMF) **D** Pseudoptosis

Figure 10.4. Different types of breast ptosis. *IMF*, inframammary fold. *(Redrawn after Brink, R.R., 1993. Management of true ptosis of the breast. Plast. Reconstr. Surg. 91, 657–662.)*

3. Preoperative considerations
   - Degree of ptosis often correlates with particular surgical plan.
     - Grade-I ptosis can often be treated with augmentation alone or may sometimes require a crescentric or periareolar mastopexy.
     - Grade-II ptosis often requires a vertical or infra-areolar mastopexy.
     - Grade-III ptosis often requires a Wise pattern mastopexy because of the amount of skin resection required.
   - Massive weight loss patients
     - Presentation: Grade-III ptosis, deflated superior breast pole, medicalization of the NAC with lateralization of the breast mound, extension of the skin excess, and ptosis to the lateral axilla and back
   - Mastopexy after removal of implants
     - Degree of preoperative breast ptosis will determine whether mastopexy is required after explantation.
     - If the amount of native breast parenchyma overlying the implant is inadequate (<4 cm), or there is severe ptosis requiring nipple elevation >4 cm, mastopexy should be delayed for at least 3 months following explantation to reduce the risk of NAC compromise.
4. Techniques
   - Techniques are similar to those used in reduction mammoplasty; however, the glandular resection is minimal with a goal to lift the gland through excess skin removal and parenchymal anchoring.

5. Complications
   - Similar complications to reduction mammoplasty
   - See below for complications specific to augmentation-mastopexy procedures.

Augmentation Mammaplasty

1. Preoperative consideration
   - Age
     - Must be at least 22 yo to have silicone prostheses
     - Must be at least 18 yo to have augmentation mammoplasty with saline implants (unless for reconstructive purposes)
   - Implant type
     - Saline: Silicone elastomer shell filled with sterile normal saline
       - Advantages
         - Can be inserted through smaller incisions
         - Volume/fill can be adjusted or varied
         - Less capsular contracture, particularly in the subglandular pocket
         - Ruptures are evident almost immediately
       - Disadvantages
         - Higher rate of rippling, visibility
         - Higher rate of deflation
         - Less natural to touch
     - Silicone
       - Advantages
         - Natural appearance and feel
         - Lower rate of rippling, deflation
       - Disadvantages
         - Requires larger incision for insertion
         - Higher rates of capsular contracture, particularly in the subglandular pocket
         - Ruptures are often silent.
           → The Food and Drug Administration (FDA) recommends a magnetic resonance imaging (MRI) scan at 3 years postoperatively, followed by every 2 years after that to screen for rupture.
         - Silicone can obscure some breast tissue on mammogram.
           → No increase in incidence or late diagnosis of cancer
       - Silicone prosthesis generations
         - 1st generation: Thick shell, viscous gel, and Dacron patches
         - Removed from market because of capsular contracture and hardness
         - 2nd generation (1973-1985): Thinner shell, lower viscosity gel that resulted in softer, and more natural-feeling prosthesis
           → Removed from market because of rates of rupture, bleed, and capsular contracture
         - 3rd generation: Thicker shell with inner barrier and increased cross linking of the silicone elastomer, more viscous (cohesive) gel
           → Designed to reduce silicone bleeding prostheses
         - 4th generation: Cohesive gel ("gummy bear") implant
       - Moratorium in 1990s on use of silicone breast prostheses because of fears over possible systemic effect of silicone; lifted in early 2000s
         - Multiple studies in Europe and North America have failed to determine a causative association between silicone breast prostheses and any traditional or atypical connective tissue diseases or autoimmune diseases.
   - Texture
     - Textured implants have lower rates of capsular contracture compared to smooth implants (particularly with subglandular pocket placement).
       - Texturing alters the capsule response by making the collagen pattern more disorganized.
     - Textured saline implants have higher rates of rippling and deflation rates when compared to smooth saline implants.
       - No difference in deflation rates between textured and smooth silicone prostheses
   - Implant size
     - Most important factor for determining prosthesis size is the patient's breast base width.
     - Large prostheses (>350 mL) are associated with
       - Long-term soft-tissue attenuation including thinning, stretching, atrophy, rippling, and ptosis
       - Greater effect on vascularity, which increases potential risk of NAC loss, skin flap loss, infection, exposure, malposition, and deformity
   - Implant position
     - Subglandular
       - Implant is placed in the subglandular/prepectoral space.
       - Contraindicated in patients who have a pinch test <2 cm, which signals inadequate soft-tissue coverage of the implant
       - Higher rates of capsular contracture compared to subpectoral placement
       - Preferred implant position for patients who are weight lifters, athletes, or active and want to minimize disruption of their pectoralis m.
     - Subpectoral
       - Implant is placed beneath the pectoralis major m.
       - Lower rates of capsular contracture
       - Lower rates of palpability/visibility
       - Contraction of pectoralis m. postoperative can lead to distortion/animation deformity

- **Dual plane**
  - Combination of subpectoral and subglandular placement
  - Inferior attachments of pectoralis m. are released.
    - Superior pole of implant covered by pectoralis m.
    - Inferior pole of implant covered by breast parenchyma
- Incision placement
  - Periareolar
  - IMF
  - Transaxillary
  - Umbilical

2. Special techniques
   - Transaxillary augmentation
     - Pocket dissection and implant inserted through incision along anterior axillary crease
     - Often used with endoscope for aid in visualization and implant positioning
     - Disadvantages
       - High rate of malposition
         - Minimized with endoscopic techniques
       - Potential injury to intercostobrachial n. and medical brachial cutaneous n. during dissection within axilla, leading to numbness and paresthesias of medial upper arm
         - Danger zone: Dissection deep into the axillary fat posterior to the lateral border of the pectoralis m.
           - → Reduce risk by staying in the subdermal plane until lateral border of pectoralis m. is reached.
   - Augmentation/mastopexy
     - Balance of volume increase with implant placement and excess skin reduction for ptosis correction
     - Implant should be inserted first, before the mastopexy is performed.
     - Compared to mastopexy alone, the length of incisions required to correct ptosis is reduced and the amount of excess skin removed is often less because of the volume by the implant.
     - Disadvantages
       - Higher rates of ptosis recurrence because of weight of prosthesis on the incision
       - Increased risk of nipple malposition because the nipple is moved at the same time as the implant

3. Complications
   - Reoperation
     - 10-year risk for reoperation for any implant-related indication: 25%
     - Often secondary to deflation of the implant, capsular contracture, hematoma, wound infection, and seroma
   - Malposition
     - Lateral displacement
       - Often a result of inadequate medial pocket dissection, aggressive lateral pocket dissection, or activity of pectoralis m.

- **Double bubble deformity**
  - Type A: Implant sits **a**bove the native breast parenchyma.
  - Type B: Implant has fallen **b**elow the IMF and sits **b**elow the native breast parenchyma.
- Infection
  - Frank infection denoted by gross purulence around the implant
    - Treatment: Removal of the implant, irrigation of the pocket, debridement of the capsule, and reinsertion of an implant 6 months later
  - Mild infection
    - Treatment: Removal of the implant, irrigation of the pocket, capsule debridement, and immediate insertion of new implants
  - Triple-antibiotic solutions for irrigation
    - Improved broad-spectrum activity against bacteria commonly cultured around breast implants
      - 10% povidone iodine, gentamicin, and cefazolin (for silicone implants)
      - Bacitracin, gentamicin, and cefazolin (for saline implants)
        - → Iodine contraindicated with saline implants
  - Nontuberculosis mycobacterium infection
    - Indolent infection that presents late
    - Symptoms: Erythema; swelling; turbid, odorless, and clear fluid
    - Treatment: Long-term course of ciprofloxacin and Bactrim
- Rupture
  - Mean age of implant rupture is 13.4 years.
  - MRI is most effective for assessing potential implant rupture.
    - Reportedly, at 7 to 10 years, 50% of implants show evidence of rupture on MRI.
    - "Linguine sign": Fraying of the elastomer shell, suggesting silicone rupture
  - Suggested management
    - Explantation and capsulectomy
    - Reinsertion of implants if desired. If not, follow guidelines above for mastopexy after explantation.
- Capsular contracture
  - Development of scar around the implant
    - Foreign body response to surface-bound protein fibrinogen
  - Baker classification of capsular contracture (see Table 10.1)

Table 10.1 Grades of Capsular Contracture Divided into the Following Four Types

GRADE	DESCRIPTION
I	Capsular contracture of the augmented breast feels as soft as an unoperated breast.
II	Capsular contracture is minimal, breast is less soft than an unoperated breast, implant can be palpated but is not visible
III	Capsular contracture is moderate, breast is firmer, implant can be palpated easily and may be distorted or visible
IV	Capsular contracture is severe and breast is hard, tender, and painful, with significant distortion present. The capsule thickness is not directly proportional to palpable firmness, although some relationship may exist.

Reproduced with permission from Spear, S.L., Baker, J.L., Jr., 1995. Classification of capsular contracture after prosthetic breast reconstruction. Plast. Reconstr. Surg. 96 (5), 1119–1124.

- If contracture persists after multiple revisions (capsulectomies with implant replacement), next step is latissimus flap.
- Suggested management
  - Capsulectomy with implant replacement
  - Change of implant position (if original position is subglandular)
  - Some have advocated for the use of acellular dermal matrix.
  - If contracture recurs after multiple revisions, can consider latissimus flap.
- Patient dissatisfaction with size
  - Risks of increasing implant size
    - Soft-tissue thinning
    - Atrophy of native breast parenchyma
    - Ptosis
    - Visibility and rippling
    - Less natural appearance
- Hematoma (reported in 1% to 3% of cases)
  - Can present late (14 days)
  - Can present after intense physical activity/trauma to the chest
  - Suggested management
    - Surgical exploration and evacuation of hematoma with replacement of implant if no evidence of infection
    - If left untreated, even a small hematoma after augmentation can lead to complications, including capsular contracture, deformity, and infection.
    - Desire for explantation
  - See above for mastopexy after implant removal.

- Scarring
  - History of keloid scars
  - Incision placement related to complaints regarding scarring
    - IMF incision is often well concealed within IMF
    - Transaxillary scar may be noticeable with arms raised.
    - Hypertrophy or widening of the periareolar scar is the most common complaint with this incision.
- NAC sensory disturbance
  - Risk increases as implant volume increases.
  - Blunt dissection lateral to the lateral edge of the pectoralis major m. reduces the risk for injury to the lateral cutaneous branch of the 4th intercostal n.
- Skin or NAC vascular compromise
  - Increased risk with subglandular position (interruption of perforators from thoracoacromial artery through pectoralis m.)
  - In secondary augmentation-mastopexy procedures, a superior or medially based pedicle is recommended due to unreliability of the inferior pedicle because of atrophy and thinning from the weight of the implants.
- Postoperative lactation and breast-feeding
  - Rates of breast-feeding in women after augmentation mammaplasty is similar to that of child-bearing women who have not had augmentation.
  - Silicone implants are safe with breast-feeding. The silicone levels in breast milk are not higher than levels found in women without silicone implants.

Suggested Readings

Brown, M.H., 2013. Chapter 3: Secondary breast augmentation. In: Neligan, P.C. (Ed.), Plastic Surgery, 3rd ed. Elsevier, pp. 39–66.

Cruz, N.I., Korchin, L., 2010. Breast feeding after augmentation mammoplasty with saline implants. Ann. Plast. Surg. 64 (5), 530–533.

Fine, N.A., 2014. Chapter 14: Breast augmentation. In: Neligan, P.C., Buck, D.W. (Eds.), Core Procedures in Plastic Surgery. Elsevier, pp. 222–232.

Fisher, J., Higdon, K.K., 2013. Chapter 8: Reduction mammaplasty. In: Neligan, P.C. (Ed.), Plastic Surgery, 3rd ed. Elsevier, pp. 152–164.

Glaus, S.W., Tenenbaum, M., 2014. Chapter 27: Breast augmentation. In: Woo, A.S., Shahzad, F., Snyder-Warwick, A.K. (Eds.), Plastic Surgery Case Review. Thieme, pp. 115–118.

Glaus, S.W., Tenenbaum, M., 2014. Chapter 28: Mastopexy/augmentation. In: Woo, A.S., Shahzad, F., Snyder-Warwick, A.K. (Eds.), Plastic Surgery Case Review. Thieme, pp. 119–122.

Hall-Findlay, E.J., 2009. Chapter 119: Breast reduction. In: Guyuron, B., Eriksson, E., Persing, J.A., et al. (Eds.), Plastic Surgery: Indications and Practice. Elsevier, pp. 1575–1590.

Higdon, K.K., Grotting, J.C., 2013. Chapter 7: Mastopexy. In: Neligan, P.C. (Ed.), Plastic Surgery, 3rd ed. Elsevier, pp. 119–151.

Lorenz, P., Bari, A.S., 2013. Chapter 16: Breast reduction. In: Neligan, P.C., Buck, D.W. (Eds.), Core Procedures in Plastic Surgery. Elsevier, pp. 254–262.

Maxwell, G.P., Gabriel, A., 2013. Chapter 2: Breast augmentation. In: Neligan, P.C. (Ed.), Plastic Surgery, 3rd ed. Elsevier, pp. 13–38.

Poppler, L.H., Tenenbaum, M., 2014. Chapter 29: Breast reduction. In: Woo, A.S., Shahzad, F., Snyder-Warwick, A.K. (Eds.), Plastic Surgery Case Review. Thieme, pp. 123–124.

Shestak, K.C., 2014. Chapter 15: Mastopexy. In: Neligan, P.C., Buck, D.W. (Eds.), Core Procedures in Plastic Surgery. Elsevier, pp. 233–253.

Walden, J.L., 2009. Chapter 53: Breast augmentation. In: Aston, S.J., Steinbrech, D.S., Walden, J.L. (Eds.), Aesthetic Plastic Surgery. Elsevier, pp. 661–673.

White, D.J., Maxwell, P.G., 2010. Chapter 67: Reduction mammaplasty. In: Weinzweig, J. (Ed.), Plastic Surgery Secrets Plus, 2nd ed. Mosby, pp. 446–452.

Chapter

Trunk Reconstruction and Pressure Sores

11

General Chest Wall Anatomy

1. The chest wall is composed of a bony shell that protects critical structures (e.g., heart, lungs, liver, kidneys) with a muscular component that assists with respiration as well as stabilization and motion of the upper extremities (see Figure 11.1).

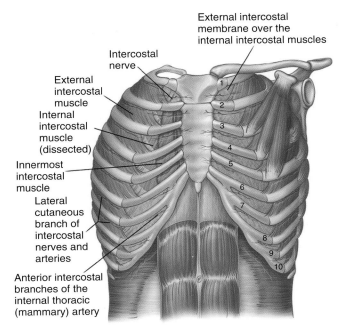

External intercostal membrane over the internal intercostal muscles

Intercostal nerve

External intercostal muscle

Internal intercostal muscle (dissected)

Innermost intercostal muscle

Lateral cutaneous branch of intercostal nerves and arteries

Anterior intercostal branches of the internal thoracic (mammary) artery

Figure 11.1. Anterior chest wall showing the sternum. Note where the costal cartilages articulate with the sternum. In the intercostal space lie different structures: Several kinds of intercostal muscles, intercostal arteries, and associated veins, lymphatics, and nerves. *(Reprinted from Rendina, E.A., Ciccone, A.M., 2007. The intercostal space. Thorac. Surg. Clin. 17 [4], e491–e501; with permission.)*

2. There are 12 paired ribs that make up the bony framework of the chest wall.
   - The first 7 ribs articulate posteriorly with the thoracic vertebrae and anteriorly with the sternum via a true sternocostal joint.
   - The last 5 ribs are often called "false ribs" because they articulate anteriorly with the 7th rib costal cartilage (ribs 8

to 10) or have no anterior articulation and are said to be "floating ribs" (ribs 11 and 12).

3. The sternum contains three bony parts.
   - The manubrium articulates with the first ribs and clavicles.
   - The body articulates with ribs 2 to 7.
   - The xiphoid process is insignificant.

4. Chest wall musculature
   - Intercostal muscles (external, internal, innermost m.) run between ribs, contain neurovascular bundles, and function to increase chest wall volume during inspiration.
     - The neurovascular bundles run between the internal intercostal muscles and the innermost intercostal muscles, just inferior to each rib (see Table 11.1).

Chest Wall Reconstruction

1. Chest wall defects are often the result of tumor resection, deep sternal wound infections, chronic empyemas, and/or trauma.

2. Chest wall defects following tumor extirpation often result in large segmental composite defects.
   - In general, stabilization of the chest wall, in addition to soft-tissue coverage, is required in defects >5 cm or more than 2 to 3 contiguous ribs.
     - Options for skeletal support include mesh (e.g., polypropylene, polytetrafluoroethylene [PTFE]), methylmethacrylate, and acellular dermal matrix.
     - Larger posterior rib defects may be tolerated because of the scapula.

3. Mediastinitis following sternotomy is reported to occur in 0.25% to 5% of cases.
   - Risk factors include diabetes, bilateral internal mammary artery (IMA) harvest, and obesity.

4. Pairolero and Arnold classified sternal wound infections into three types (see Table 11.2).

5. Reconstruction of sternal wounds largely depends on the type of infection, degree of purulence, and presence of bone and/or cartilage infection or necrosis.
   - For type-1 sternal wounds, if the wound is not purulent and the sternal bone is viable, sternal reconstruction with plates and/or wires, followed by flap coverage or closure, is possible.

Table 11.1 Extrathoracic Chest Wall Muscles

MUSCLE	ORIGIN	INSERTION	ARTERY	NERVE	ACTION	USE AND CONSEQUENCE
Trapezius	Midline from the external occipital protuberance, nuchal ligament, medial part superior nuchal line, spinous processes vertebrae C7-T12	At the shoulders, into the lateral third of the clavicle, the acromion process, into the spine of the scapula	Transverse cervical artery	Cranial nerve XI; cervical nerves III and IV receive information about pain	Retraction of scapula	Used for upper chest and neck defects
Latissimus dorsi	Spinous processes of thoracic T6-T12, thoracolumbar fascia, iliac crest, inferior 3 or 4 ribs	Floor of intertubercular groove of the humerus	Subscapular artery, dorsal scapular artery	Thoracodorsal nerve	Pulls the forelimb dorsally and caudally	Lateral and anterior chest wall defect; excellent musculocutaneous collaterals allow significant skin to be taken
Pectoralis major	Anterior surface of medial half of clavicle sternocostal head, anterior surface of the sternum, superior 6 costal cartilages	Intertubercular groove of the humerus	Pectoral branch thoracoacromial trunk and internal mammary, lateral intercostal arteries, lateral thoracic perforators	Lateral and medial pectoral nerve clavicular head: C5/6; sternocostal head: C7/8 T1	Clavicular head; flexes the humerus sternocostal head; extends the humerus; as a whole, adducts and medially rotates the humerus; draws scapula anterioinferiorly	Anterior and midline (sternal defects); used as a pedicle graft based on the primary blood supply or as a turnover flap on secondary supply, possible displacement of the breast and abduction medial rotation loss of arm
Serratus anterior	Fleshy slips from the outer surface of upper 8 or 9 ribs	Costal aspect of medial margin of the scapula	Lateral thoracic artery (upper part), thoracodorsal artery (lower part)	Long thoracic nerve from roots of brachial plexus C5-C7	Protracts and stabilizes scapula, assists in upward rotation	Small muscle best suited as an intrathoracic flap
Rectus abdominis	Pubis	Costal cartilages of ribs 5-7, xiphoid process of sternum	Superior epigastric artery supply and deep inferior epigastric artery	Segmentally by thoracoabdominal nerves T7-T12	Flexion of trunk/lumbar vertebrae postural muscle; assists with breathing, helps to create intra-abdominal pressure	Lower anterior chest wall; some muscle atrophy occurs owing to denervation; if based on superior epigastric, adequate blood flow by way of the IMA required
External oblique	Fleshy digitations from lower 8 costae; broad, thin, and irregularly quadrilateral, its muscular portion occupying the side	Lower iliac crest, inguinal ligament, upper aponeurosis anterior abdominal wall, decussates at the linea alba with contralateral fibers	Lower thoracic intercostal vessels	Intercostal nerves T5-T11, subcostal nerve T12	Rotates torso	Upper abdomen and lower thoracic defects as far as the inframammary fold

Reprinted from Naidu, B.V., Rajesh, P.B., 2010. Relevant surgical anatomy of the chest wall. Thorac. Surg. Clin. 20, 453–463. IMA, Internal mammary artery.

- In general, for type-2 and -3 sternal wound infections, staged reconstruction is required with serial washouts, debridement, and removal of hardware required to obtain a clean wound before flap reconstruction.
- Vacuum-assisted closure (VAC) therapy is often used between serial debridement for assistance with wound control.

6. Common flaps for reconstruction of sternal wounds include
   - Pectoralis major
     - Vascular supply: Thoracoacromial artery (major), IMA perforators (minor, segmental)
     - Can be used as an advancement flap or turnover flap based off of the IMA perforators (requires intact IMA system)
     - Limited coverage of inferior sternal wounds
     - Muscle can be disinserted to allow for additional reach.
   - Rectus abdominis
     - Vascular supply: Superior and inferior epigastric a.
     - Useful for coverage of inferior sternal wounds
     - With ipsilateral IMA harvest sacrificing the superior epigastric artery, the flap can survive off of the 8th intercostal pedicle.

Table 11.2 Classification of Infected Sternotomy Wounds

TYPE I	TYPE II	TYPE III
Occurs within first few days	Occurs within first few weeks	Occurs months to years later
Serosanguineous drainage	Purulent drainage	Chronic draining sinus tract
Cellulitis absent	Cellulitis present	Cellulitis localized
Mediastinum soft and pliable	Mediastinal suppuration	Mediastinitis rare
Osteomyelitis and costochondritis absent	Osteomyelitis frequent, costochondritis rare	Osteomyelitis, costochondritis, or retained foreign body always present
Cultures usually negative	Cultures positive	Cultures positive

Reprinted from Pairolero, P.S., Arnold, P.G., 1985. Chest wall tumors. Experience with 100 consecutive patients. J. Thorac. Cardiovasc. Surg. 90, 367–372.

- Latissimus dorsi
  - Vascular supply: Thoracodorsal a. (major), lumbar perforators (minor, segmental)
  - Useful for lateral chest wall defects
  - May require skin grafts
- Omentum
  - Vascular supply: Gastroepiploic artery (major), short gastrics (minor)
  - Useful for large sternal wounds
  - Requires laparotomy and tunneling of flap through the diaphragm or extrathoracic
  - Requires skin graft (see Figure 11.2)

Abdominal Wall Anatomy

1. The abdominal wall is a hexagonal-shaped structure that functions to
   - Protect critical intra-abdominal structures
   - Stabilize the pelvis during walking, running, and jumping
   - Flex the vertebral column
   - Increase intra-abdominal pressure (e.g., to assist with expiration and defecation)
2. Vascular supply: Deep inferior epigastric a., superior epigastric a., superficial inferior epigastric a., intercostal and lumbar a.
3. Innervation: Nerves travel with the intercostal and lumbar arteries in the plane between the internal oblique (IO) and transversalis muscles.
   - Sensory: Anterior branches of the T7 to L1 intercostal and subcostal nerves
   - Motor: T7 to L2 intercostal nerves, iliohypogastric n., ilioinguinal n.
4. Abdominal wall musculature
   - Rectus abdominis
     - Origin: Pubic symphysis and pubic crest
     - Insertion: Anterior surfaces of 5th to 7th costal cartilages and xiphoid
     - Principle flexor of the abdomen, stabilizes pelvis, protects abdominal organs
   - External oblique
     - Vascular supply: Segmental intercostal a., deep circumflex iliac a., iliolumbar a.
     - Origin: Lower 8 ribs

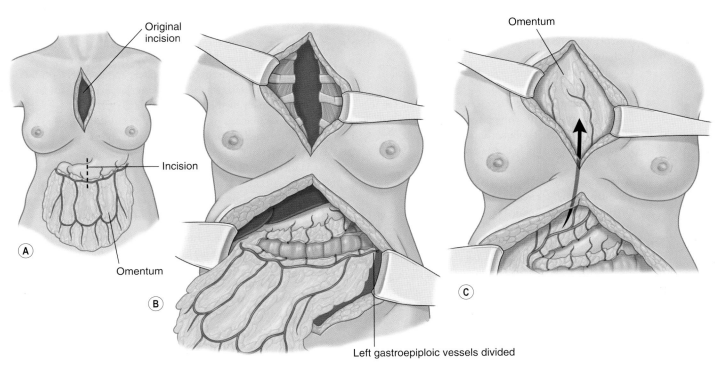

Figure 11.2. Omentum anatomy. *(Reprinted from Neligan, P.C., Song, D.H. [Eds.], 2013. Plastic Surgery, 3rd ed. Elsevier, 239–255.)*

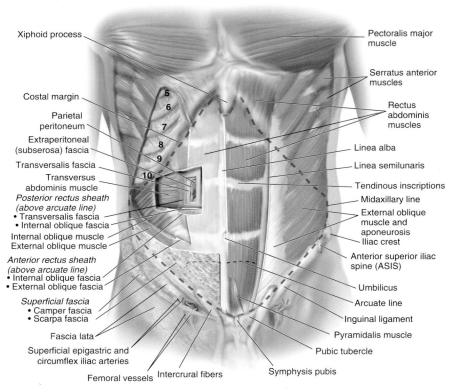

Figure 11.3. Anatomy of the anterior abdominal wall. *(Reprinted from Rosen, M. [Ed.], 2012. Atlas of Abdominal Wall Reconstruction. Saunders, 2–20.)*

- Insertion: Pubic crest; forms the inguinal ligament
- Contributes to the anterior rectus sheath through aponeurosis; most superficial of the lateral abdominal wall muscles
- IO
  - Vascular supply: Intercostal a., circumflex iliac a., iliolumbar a.
  - Origin: Thoracolumbar fascia, iliac crest, inguinal ligament
  - Insertion: Inferior and posterior borders of ribs T10 to T12; pubic crest via the conjoint tendon
  - Deep to the external oblique; above arcuate line, the IO fascia splits to supply the anterior and posterior rectus sheath.
- Transversus abdominis
  - Vascular supply: Intercostal and subcostal a.
  - Origin: Iliac crest, inguinal ligament, inner surface of T6 to T12 costal cartilages
  - Insertion: Posterior rectus sheath (above arcuate line); pubic crest via the conjoint tendon
5. The rectus sheath is located in the midline of the abdominal wall and is formed via the aponeuroses of the abdominal musculature. The components of the anterior and posterior rectus sheath change according to position with respect to the arcuate line (located midway between the umbilicus and pubic symphysis).
  - Above the arcuate line, the anterior rectus sheath is formed by external oblique fascia and part of the IO fascia, whereas the posterior rectus sheath is formed by the IO fascia and transversalis fascia.
  - Below the arcuate line, the anterior rectus sheath is formed by the external and IO fascia and transversus abdominis fascia, whereas the posterior rectus sheath is formed solely by the transversalis fascia.
6. The linea semilunaris or semilunar line marks the junction between the medial border of the external oblique muscle and lateral border of the rectus muscle where the anterior rectus fascia merges with the external oblique aponeurosis (see Figures 11.3-11.5).

Abdominal Wall Reconstruction

1. Abdominal wall defects commonly result from ventral hernia formation, oncologic tumor resection, and abdominal catastrophes.
2. Goals of abdominal wall reconstruction
  - Soft-tissue coverage
  - Reestablish abdominal domain

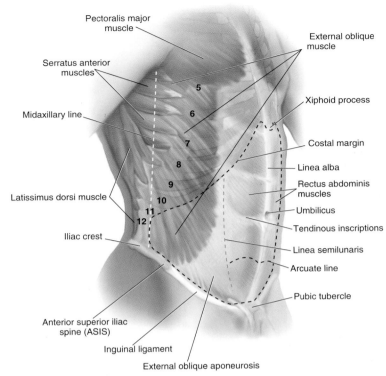

Pectoralis major muscle

Serratus anterior muscles

Midaxillary line

Latissimus dorsi muscle

Iliac crest

Anterior superior iliac spine (ASIS)

Inguinal ligament

External oblique aponeurosis

External oblique muscle

Xiphoid process

Costal margin

Linea alba

Rectus abdominis muscles

Umbilicus

Tendinous inscriptions

Linea semilunaris

Arcuate line

Pubic tubercle

5 6 7 8 9 10 11 12

Figure 11.4. Anatomy of the lateral trunk. *(Reprinted from Rosen, M. [Ed.], 2012. Atlas of Abdominal Wall Reconstruction. Saunders, 2–20.)*

- Prevent hernia recurrence
- Protect abdominal organs

3. To simplify the approach to abdominal wall reconstruction, the fascia and soft-tissue envelope should be considered as two distinct problems, each approached separately.
   - Common approach to fascia defects
     - Components separation
     - Mesh placement
       - Synthetic (e.g., polypropylene)
       - Biologic (e.g., acellular dermal matrix)
     - Autologous fascia/flaps
       - Tensor fascia lata flap
       - Anterolateral thigh flap
   - Common approaches to skin/soft-tissue deficits
     - Regional flaps (e.g., tensor fascia lata [TFL], anterolateral thigh [ALT], rectus femoris)
       - Difficult for epigastric coverage
     - Free flaps (e.g., TFL, ALT, latissimus)
       - May require vein grafting
     - Tissue expansion
       - Useful when a significant skin deficit exists, and the abdominal defect can be approached in staged fashion.

4. Staged reconstruction: Often performed for management of the open abdomen or after abdominal catastrophe
   - Stage 1: Temporary fascia closure (e.g., Vicryl mesh) and VAC therapy
   - Stage 2: Skin grafting of the granulating abdominal wound

   - Generally performed after 2 to 3 weeks of VAC therapy, when the granulation scar is strong enough to prevent evisceration
   - Stage 3: Formal hernia repair and abdominal wall reconstruction after the wound has settled
     - Generally performed 6 to 12 months after skin graft closure

5. Components separation (see Figures 11.6 and 11.7)
   - Mobilization of the rectus abdominis muscles bilaterally by release of the external oblique aponeurosis from the anterior rectus fascia at the linea semilunaris allows for advancement of the rectus muscle component toward the midline.
     - The external oblique is bluntly dissected off of the underlying IO muscle to allow for greater advancement.
     - The posterior rectus sheath can also be incised internally (preferably at a site distant from the location of the anterior release) to allow for an extra 2 to 3 cm of advancement.
     - The IO should not be dissected off of the transversus abdominis muscle to avoid injury to neurovascular bundles.
   - Components separation can allow for primary muscle reapproximation of defects as large as 20 cm at the level of the umbilicus.
   - Fascial repair should be supported by mesh to reduce recurrence in all cases.

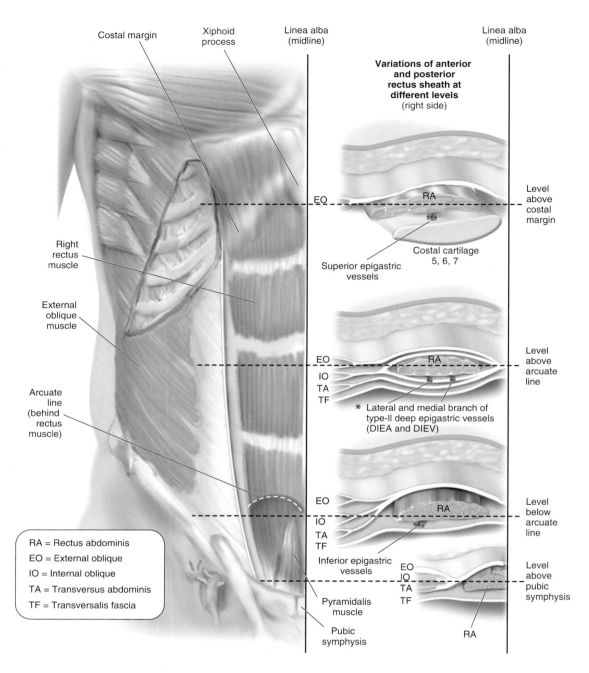

Figure 11.5. Anatomy of the anterior and posterior rectus sheath. *DIEA,* Deep inferior epigastric artery; *DIEV,* deep inferior epigastric vein. (*EO,* External oblique muscle; *IO,* internal oblique muscle; *TA,* transversus abdominis muscle; *TF,* transversalis fascia; *RA,* rectus abdominis muscle; *DIEA,* deep inferior epigastric artery; *DIEV,* deep inferior epigastric vein). (*Reprinted from Rosen, M. [Ed.], 2012. Atlas of Abdominal Wall Reconstruction. Saunders, 2–20.*)

- Underlay with synthetic mesh has been reported to have the lowest recurrence rates; however, synthetic mesh is generally not recommended in contaminated fields. In this case, a biologic mesh (e.g., acellular dermal matrix) should be used because of its inherent ability to incorporate and revascularize.

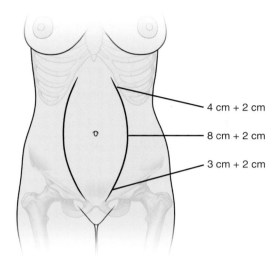

4 cm + 2 cm
8 cm + 2 cm
3 cm + 2 cm

Figure 11.6. Maximal unilateral rectus complex mobility in the upper, middle, and lower abdominal levels, by means of component separation of the external and IO muscles to the posterior axillary line. The additional 2 cm of advancement is gained if the rectus abdominis muscle is separated off of the posterior rectus fascia. *(Reprinted from Neligan, P.C., Buck, D.W. [Eds.], 2013. Core Procedures in Plastic Surgery. Elsevier, 211–221.)*

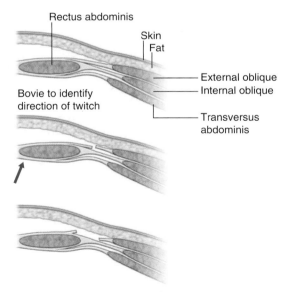

Rectus abdominis

Skin
Fat

Bovie to identify
direction of twitch

External oblique
Internal oblique

Transversus
abdominis

Figure 11.7. Cross-sectional illustration showing external oblique muscle release. *(Reprinted from Neligan, P.C., Buck, D.W. [Eds.], 2013. Core Procedures in Plastic Surgery. Elsevier, 211–221.)*

Reconstruction of the Perineum

1. Defects of the pelvis and perineum can pose challenges to the reconstructive surgeon because of the close proximity to genitalia.
2. Defects of the pelvis and perineum often result from congenital defects, tumor extirpation, trauma, infection, or pressure.
3. Fortunately, many expendable regional flaps are available for use in perineal reconstruction (see Figure 11.8).

Vaginal Reconstruction

1. Acquired vaginal defects most commonly arise from resection of tumors, including primary vaginal tumors, colorectal tumors, and bladder carcinoma.
2. Cordeiro established a useful classification of acquired vaginal defects along with an algorithm for reconstruction (see Figures 11.9-11.11 and Table 11.3).
3. Singapore flaps
    - Vascular supply: Branches of the internal pudendal a. via superficial perineal vessels and posterior labial a.
    - Good for anterior and lateral wall defects; bilateral flaps can be used for total reconstruction
    - Can be sensate by sparing of the superficial perineal n.
    - Advantages: Ease of harvest, thin fasciocutaneous flaps
    - Disadvantages: Relatively small, may be in the field of prior radiation
4. Rectus abdominis myocutaneous (RAM) flaps (vertical: VRAM; oblique: ORAM)
    - Vascular supply: Deep inferior epigastric a.
    - Good for posterior and upper 2/3rds circumferential defects
5. Gracilis myocutaneous flaps
    - Vascular supply: Medial circumflex femoral a. branch off of the profunda femoris a.
    - Bilateral flaps are good for total vaginal reconstruction.
    - Disadvantages: Can be bulky, vertical skin paddle can be unreliable
6. Other flap options
    - Posterior thigh flaps
        - Vascular supply: Descending branch of the inferior gluteal a.
        - Fasciocutaneous flap that can be used for anterior and posterior defects
        - Can be sensate by sparing of the posterior femoral cutaneous n.
    - Gluteal fold flap
        - Sensate flap based off of branches from the superficial perineal vascular network
        - Useful for vulvar or perianal wounds
        - The flap is centered on the infragluteal crease
    - ALT flap
        - Useful for vaginal, vulvar, scrotal, or perineal defects
        - To increase the pedicle length and subsequent reach, the flap can be tunneled underneath the rectus femoris and sartorius muscles.

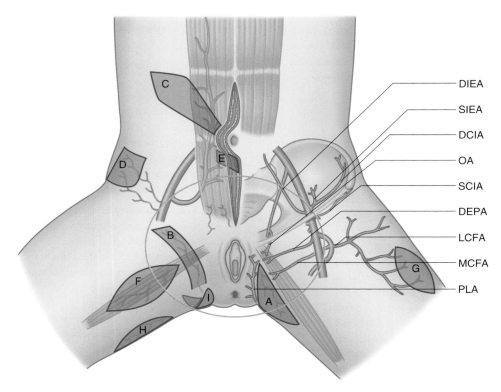

Figure 11.8. The pivot points of the vascular leash of all of the various musculocutaneous, fasciocutaneous, and perforator flaps in the region are all located within a circle, with a radius of 10 cm centered over the perineum. *A,* V-Y flap, from medial thigh or inferior gluteal area. *B,* Pudendal thigh flap. *C,* Rectus abdominis myocutaneous or DIEP (deep inferior epigastric artery) flap. *D,* SIEP (superficial inferior epigastric perforator) flap (or extended SCIA [superficial circumflex iliac artery] flap). *E,* Rectus abdominis musculoperitoneal (RAMP) flap. *F,* Gracilis myocutaneous flap. *G,* ALT (anterior lateral thigh) flap. *H,* Gluteal thigh flap. *I,* Gluteal fold flap. *DCIA,* Deep circumflex iliac artery; *DEPA,* deep external pudendal artery; *DIEA,* deep inferior epigastric artery; *LCFA,* lateral femoral circumflex artery; *MCFA,* medial femoral circumflex artery; *OA,* anterior branch of obturator artery; *PLA,* posterior labial artery (branch of pudendal artery); *SCIA,* superficial circumflex iliac artery; *SIEA,* superficial inferior epigastric artery. *(Reprinted from Guyuron, B., Eriksson, E., Persing, J.A., et al. [Eds.], 2009. Plastic Surgery: Indications and Practice, 1st ed. Elsevier, 213–227.)*

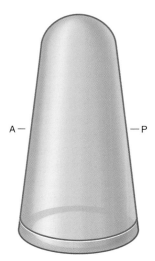

Figure 11.9. Vaginal vault. *A,* Anterior; *P,* posterior. *(Reprinted from Neligan, P.C. [Ed.], 2013. Plastic Surgery, 3rd ed. Elsevier, 326–335.)*

Genital Reconstruction

1. Penile reconstruction
   - In cases of sharp amputation, replantation should be considered.
     - Care should be made to repair the dorsal nerves, veins, and deep dorsal artery.
   - Free radial forearm flap
     - Incorporates an intraflap neourethra reconstruction using the forearm skin paddle
     - Requires implantation of a penile prosthesis
   - Osteocutaneous free fibula flap
     - Presence of vascularized bone obviates the need for a penile prosthesis.
     - A neourethra is formed via full-thickness skin grafting.
2. Gender reassignment surgery
   - Preoperative considerations
     - Psychiatric evaluation to establish a true gender identity disorder

TYPE I: PARTIAL DEFECT

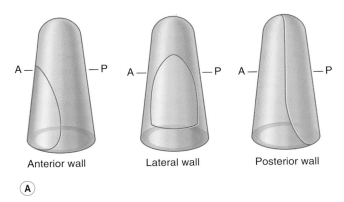

Anterior wall   Lateral wall   Posterior wall

(A)

TYPE II: CIRCUMFERENTIAL DEFECT

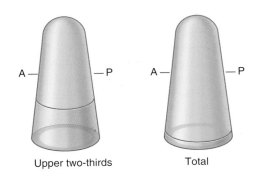

Upper two-thirds   Total

(B)

Figure 11.10. A and **B,** Classification system of acquired vaginal defects. **A,** Type I: Partial defect; **B,** type II: Circumferential defect. *A,* Anterior; *P,* posterior. *(Reprinted from Neligan, P.C. [Ed.], 2013. Plastic Surgery, 3rd ed. Elsevier, 326–335.)*

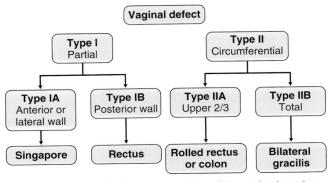

Figure 11.11. Algorithm for reconstruction of the vagina based on defect type. *(Reprinted from Neligan, P.C. [Ed.], 2013. Plastic Surgery, 3rd ed. Elsevier, 326–335.)*

- ■ Confirmation of patient successfully living as the opposite gender for prolonged period of time
- ■ Hormone therapy
- ● Surgery is generally the final phase of transition.
- ● Male-to-female surgical options
  - ■ Penectomy and orchiectomy with vaginoplasty and labioclitoroplasty

Table 11.3 Previously Described flap Options for Vaginal Reconstruction

DEFECT TYPE	FLAP OPTION
IA	Singapore flap (also known as pudendal fasciocutaneous flap)
IB	Pedicled rectus myocutaneous flap
	Pedicled rectus musculoperitoneal flap
	Muscle-sparing rectus myocutaneous flap
IIA/B	Vertical rectus abdominis myocutaneous
	Gracilis
	Singapore flap
	Pedicled jejunum
	Sigmoid colon

Reprinted from Neligan, P.C. (Ed.), 2013. Plastic Surgery, 3rd ed. Elsevier, 326–335.

- ■ Breast augmentation
- ■ Facial feminization procedures
- ● Female-to-male surgical options
  - ■ Penile reconstruction and scrotal reconstruction
  - ■ Mastectomy

Back Reconstruction

1. Defects of the posterior trunk can occur in the setting of congenital defects, following tumor extirpation, and as consequence of spinal surgery and instrumentation.
2. A number of regional muscles can assist with reconstruction of superior back wounds (e.g., trapezius, latissimus, paraspinous/erector spinae, external oblique).
3. Wounds of the lumbosacral spine are more challenging and may require use of gluteal-based flaps or large random-pattern rotation flaps.
4. Midline defects associated with spinal surgery and spinal instrumentation can often be closed using bilateral paraspinous muscle flaps because these muscles are expendable after the fusion.
5. General approach to back wounds
   - ● Debridement of nonviable tissue and local wound control
   - ● Determination of depth of defect, presence of instrumentation, integrity of deep fascia, and exposure of critical structures (e.g., hardware, spine, dura)
   - ● Reconstructive plan based on above factors (see Figures 11.12 and 11.13)
     - ■ Superficial wounds without instrumentation can generally be closed with local wound care and/or VAC therapy.
     - ■ Deep wounds with exposed hardware or critical structures require flap closure.
       - ○ Erector spinae muscle flap
       - ○ Latissimus flap (good for nonfused wounds of the upper back)
       - ○ Trapezius flap
       - ○ Superior gluteal artery flap (good for deep wounds of the lumbosacral region)

○ External oblique flap
○ Omentum
○ Tissue expansion
○ Free flaps (often require vein loops because of limited recipient vessels)

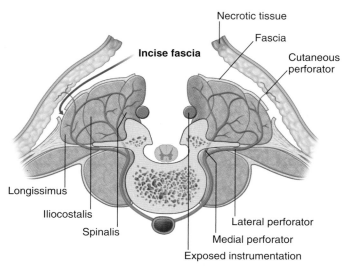

Figure 11.12. Cross section of lumbar spine area. Skin flaps are elevated to expose the thoracolumbar fascia and reach the region of the lateral pedicle entering the erector spinae muscles. The thoracolumbar fascia is incised to allow a medial movement of the muscles. *(Reprinted from Neligan, P.C. [Ed.], 2013. Plastic Surgery, 3rd ed. Elsevier, 256–278.)*

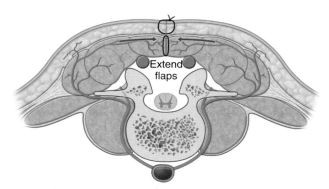

Figure 11.13. The muscles are approximated in the midline. The erector spinae muscles unfurl, changing shape from circular to elliptical. *(Reprinted from Dumanian, G.A., Neligan, P.C. [Eds.], 2013. Plastic Surgery, 3rd ed. Elsevier, 256–278.)*

6. Myelomeningocele
   - Most common neural tube defect worldwide
   - Often associated with motor and sensory defects
   - Characterized by herniation of meninges and cord elements outside of the spinal column
   - Early closure is critical for survival and should be performed within the first 24 to 48 hours of life.

- Requires neurosurgical assistance for dural repair
- Many soft-tissue reconstructive options have been described and generally involve fasciocutaneous or myocutaneous rotation or advancement flaps.
  - One of the most common techniques is bilateral V-Y advancement flaps from the flanks (see Figures 11.14 and 11.15).

Pressure Sores

1. Pressure sores result from prolonged pressure over a bony prominence leading to irreversible tissue ischemia.
   - Muscle is most sensitive to pressure, followed by fat, and finally skin.
   - Other contributing factors to development of these wounds include friction, shear, moisture, and malnutrition.
2. Pressure sores commonly occur in elderly, debilitated patients, patients with spinal cord injury, and patients with prolonged hospitalizations.
3. Pressure sore stages
   - Stage I: Intact, erythematous, nonblanchable skin
   - Stage II: Epidermolysis, blistering, dermal injury
   - Stage III: Destruction into subcutaneous tissue and muscle
   - Stage IV: Destruction to underlying bone, joints, and/or muscle fascia (see Figure 11.16)
4. Preoperative considerations
   - Wound status
     - Debridement of all necrotic debris, including the wound bursa, is a critical first step in pressure sore reconstruction.
     - Establish a clean wound before flap reconstruction.
   - Nutrition
     - Inadequate nutrition is a marker of poor capacity to heal wounds and incisions.
     - Some advocate for albumin >3, prealbumin >15 to 30, and transferrin >200 mg/dL before reconstruction.
   - Age, comorbidities, surgical history (e.g., diabetes, cardiovascular disease, prior surgeries)
   - Smoking status
   - Incontinence
     - Consider bowel diversion through colostomy before reconstruction for challenging perineal wounds.
   - Osteomyelitis
     - Presence of active osteomyelitis is a relative contraindication to flap reconstruction.
     - Bone biopsy is the gold standard for the diagnosis of osteomyelitis.
   - Social support
     - Lack of social support at home may affect patient's ability to care for wounds and/or incisions.
   - Compliance
     - Poor compliance is a contraindication to reconstruction because compliance with postoperative

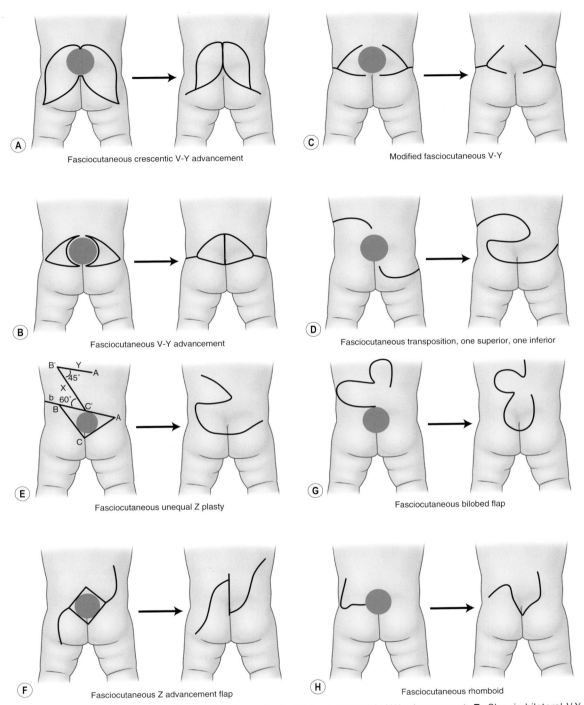

Figure 11.14. Fasciocutaneous flaps in meningomyelocele repair. **A,** Bilateral crescentic V-Y advancement. **B,** Classic bilateral V-Y advancement. **C,** Modified bipedicle V-Y advancement. **D,** Superior and inferior rotational transposition. **E,** Unequal Z plasty. **F,** Z advancement. **G,** Bilobed transposition. **H,** Rhomboid transposition. *(Reprinted from Neligan, P.C. [Ed.], 2013. Plastic Surgery, 3rd ed. Elsevier, 856–876.)*

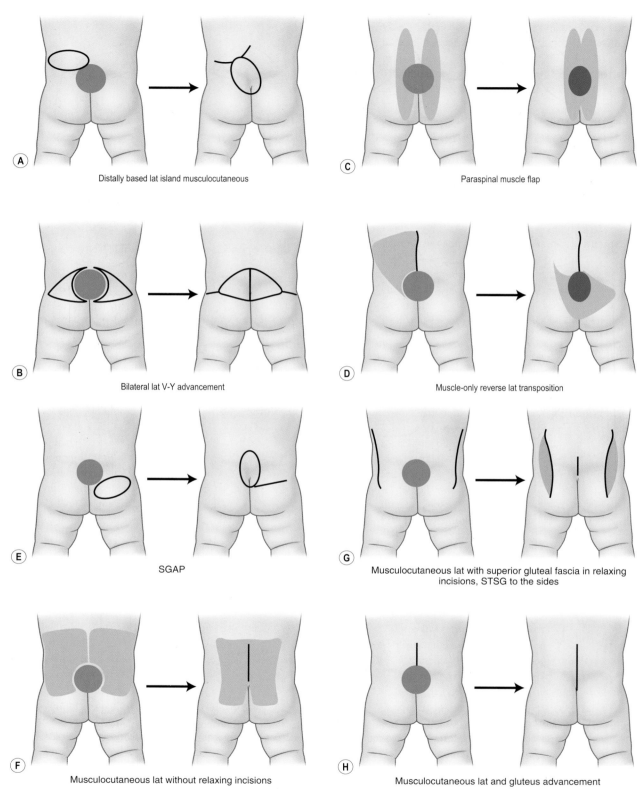

Figure 11.15. Muscle and musculocutaneous flaps in meningomyelocele repair. **A,** Distally based latissimus musculocutaneous advancement. **B,** Bilateral latissimus V-Y musculocutaneous advancement. **C,** Paraspinous muscle advancement or turnover. **D,** Distally based latissimus turnover muscle flap with split-thickness skin graft coverage over flap. **E,** Superior gluteal artery perforator (SGAP) interposition. **F,** Bilateral latissimus musculocutaneous advancement. **G,** Bilateral latissimus musculocutaneous advancement with lateral relaxing incisions covered with split-thickness skin grafts (STSG). **H,** Bilateral latissimus and gluteus maximus interconnected musculocutaneous advancement. *lat,* Latissimus. *(Reprinted from Neligan, P.C. [Ed.], 2013. Plastic Surgery, 3rd ed. Elsevier, 856–876.)*

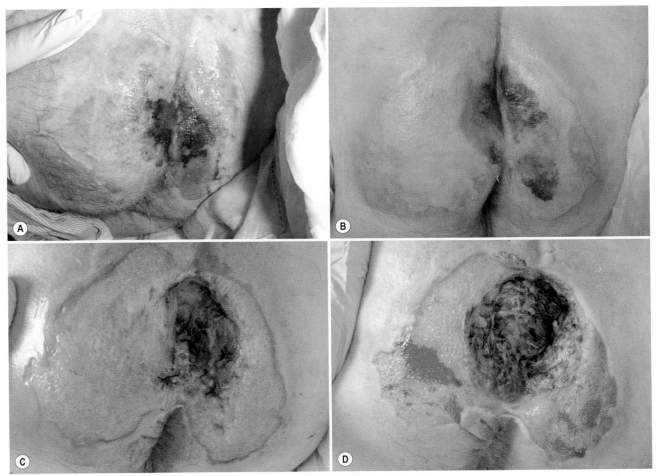

Figure 11.16. The National Pressure Ulcer Advisory Panel staging system. **A,E,** Stage I: Intact skin with nonblanchable redness of a localized area, usually over a bony prominence. Darkly pigmented skin may not have visible blanching; its color may differ from the surrounding area. **B,F,** Stage II: Partial-thickness loss of dermis presenting as a shallow open ulcer with a red pink wound bed, without slough. May also present as an intact or open/ruptured serum-filled blister. This should not be used to describe skin tears, tape burns, perineal dermatitis, maceration, or excoriation. **C,G,** Stage III: Full-thickness tissue loss. Subcutaneous fat may be visible, but bone, tendon, or muscle is not exposed. Slough may be present but does not obscure the depth of tissue loss. May include undermining and tunneling. **D,H,** Stage IV: Full-thickness tissue loss with exposed bone, tendon, or muscle. Exposed bone is sufficient but not necessary to define a stage-IV pressure sore. Slough or eschar may be present on some parts of the wound bed. Often includes undermining or tunneling. May extend into muscle and/or supporting structures (e.g., fascia, tendon, or joint capsule), making osteomyelitis possible. Bone/tendon is visible or directly palpable. **I,** Suspected deep-tissue injury: Purple or maroon localized area of discolored intact skin or blood-filled blister due to damage of underlying soft tissue from pressure and/or shear. The area may be preceded by tissue that is painful, firm, mushy, boggy, warmer, or cooler as compared to adjacent tissue. The wound may evolve and become covered by thin eschar. Evolution may be rapid, exposing additional layers of tissue even with optimal treatment. **J,** Unstageable: Full-thickness tissue loss in which the base of the ulcer is covered by slough (yellow, tan, gray, green, or brown) and/or eschar (tan, brown, or black) in the wound bed. Until the base of the wound is exposed, the true depth, and therefore stage, cannot be determined. *(Reprinted from Kwon, R., Janis, J.E., 2013. Pressure sores. In: Neligan, P.C. [Ed.], Plastic Surgery, 3rd ed. Elsevier, 352.)*

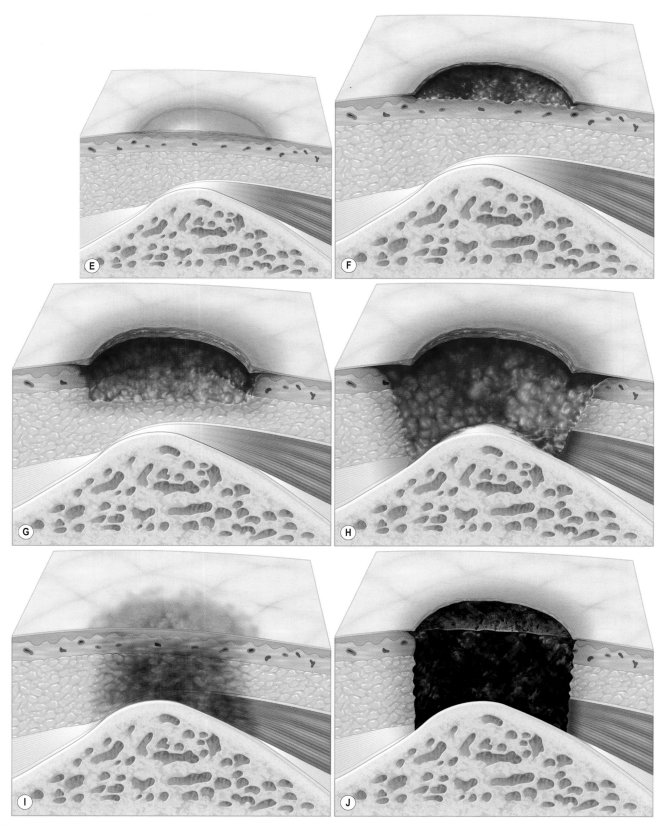

Figure 11.16, cont'd

restrictions and pressure–off-loading regimen is critical to the likelihood of successful reconstruction.

- Spasms
  - Treat spasms postoperatively to prevent undue tension and shear on incisions and flaps (e.g., with benzodiazepines, Baclofen).
- Ambulatory status
  - Nonambulatory patients may be reconstructed with sacrifice of muscle and advancement of myocutaneous flaps.

5. Common flaps by location
   - Sacral pressure sores
     - Gluteal rotation flaps
     - Gluteal V-Y advancement flaps
   - Ischial pressure sores
     - Posterior thigh fasciocutaneous flap
     - Posterior thigh V-Y myocutaneous advancement flap
       - Includes the hamstring muscles
       - Hamstring muscle sacrifice is reserved for nonambulatory patients.
     - Tensor fascia lata flap
   - Trochanteric pressure sores
     - Tensor fascia lata flap
     - Girdlestone procedure
       - Removal of the femoral head with interposition of vastus lateralis muscle

6. Postoperative considerations
   - Pressure relief: Pressure–off-loading mattresses, frequent turning
   - Bed rest, with a limited progressive sitting protocol (typically started after a period of 2 to 4 weeks)
   - Autonomic dysreflexia
     - Presents postoperatively with severe hypertension and bradycardia
     - Often secondary to bladder distension
     - Can be treated with bladder catheterization
   - Recurrence
     - High reported recurrence even in ideal settings. Patient education and careful operative planning is important to allow for the possibility of reelevation and readvancement of prior flaps in the setting of recurrent wounds.

Suggested Readings

Althubaiti, G., Butler, C.E., 2014. Abdominal wall and chest wall reconstruction. Plast. Reconstr. Surg. 133 (5), 688e–701e.

Bauer, J.D., Mancoll, J.S., Phillips, L.G., 2007. Chapter 74: Pressure sores. In: Thorne, C.H. (Ed.), Grabb & Smith, 6th ed. Lippincott Williams & Wilkins, pp. 722–729.

Dumanian, G.A., 2013. Chapter 11: Reconstruction of the soft tissues of the back. In: Neligan, P.C. (Ed.), Plastic Surgery, 3rd ed. Elsevier, pp. 256–278.

Erdmann, D., Meade, R.A., Lins, R.E., et al., 2013. Chapter 12: Back reconstruction. In: Neligan, P.C., Buck, D.W. (Eds.), Core Procedures in Plastic Surgery. Elsevier, pp. 196–210.

Friedman, J.D., 2007. Chapter 72: Reconstruction of the perineum. In: Thorne, C.H. (Ed.), Grabb & Smith, 6th ed. Lippincott Williams & Wilkins, pp. 708–716.

Gottlieb, L.J., Aycock, J.K., 2009. Chapter 20: Reconstruction of the genitalia. In: Guyuron, B., Eriksson, E., Persing, J.A., et al. (Eds.), Plastic Surgery: Indications and Practice, 1st ed. Elsevier, pp. 213–227.

Gottlieb, L.J., Reid, R.R., Lee, J.C., 2013. Chapter 41: Pediatric chest and trunk defects. In: Neligan, P.C. (Ed.), Plastic Surgery, 3rd ed. Elsevier, pp. 856–876.

Kwon, R., Janis, J.E., 2013. Chapter 16: Pressure sores. In: Neligan, P.C. (Ed.), Plastic Surgery, 3rd ed. Elsevier, p. 352.

Manahan, M., Silverman, R.P., 2009. Chapter 21: Chest and abdominal wall reconstruction. In: Guyuron, B., Eriksson, E., Persing, J.A., et al. (Eds.), Plastic Surgery: Indications and Practice, 1st ed. Elsevier, pp. 229–238.

Medalie, D.A., 2012. Chapter 13: Tissue and fascial expansion of the abdominal wall. In: Rosen, M.J. (Ed.), Atlas of Abdominal Wall Reconstruction. Saunders, pp. 224–243.

Naidu, B.V., Rajesh, P.B., 2010. Relevant surgical anatomy of the chest wall. Thorac. Surg. Clin. 20, 453–463.

Netscher, D.T., Baumholtz, M.A., 2009. Chest reconstruction: I. Anterior and anterolateral chest wall and wounds affecting respiratory function. Plast. Reconstr. Surg. 124 (5), 240e–252e.

Netscher, D.T., Baumholtz, M.A., Bullocks, J., 2009. Chest reconstruction II: Regional reconstruction of chest wall wounds that do not affect respiratory function (axilla, posterolateral chest, and posterior trunk). Plast. Reconstr. Surg. 124 (6), 427e–435e.

Rosen, M., 2012. Chapter 1: Clinical anatomy. In: Rosen, M. (Ed.), Atlas of Abdominal Wall Reconstruction. Saunders, pp. 2–20.

Selvaggi, G., Bellringer, J., 2011. Gender reassignment surgery: an overview. Nat. Rev. Urol. 8 (5), 274–282.

Shell, D.H., Vasconez, L.O., de la Torre, J., et al., 2010. Chapter 91: Abdominal wall reconstruction. In: Weinzweig, J. (Ed.), Plastic Surgery Secrets Plus, 2nd ed. Mosby, pp. 587–593.

Singh, N.K., Khalifeh, M.R., 2013. Chapter 13: Abdominal wall reconstruction. In: Neligan, P.C. (Ed.), Plastic Surgery, 3rd ed. Elsevier, pp. 211–221.

Snell, L., Cordeiro, P.G., Pusic, A.L., 2013. Chapter 14: Reconstruction of acquired vaginal defects. In: Neligan, P.C. (Ed.), Plastic Surgery, 3rd ed. Elsevier, pp. 326–335.

Song, D.H., Roughton, M.C., 2013. Chapter 10: Reconstruction of the chest. In: Neligan, P.C., Song, D.H. (Eds.), Plastic Surgery, 3rd ed. Elsevier, pp. 239–255.

Vargo, D., 2012. Chapter 16: Managing the open abdomen. In: Rosen, M.J. (Ed.), Atlas of Abdominal Wall Reconstruction. Saunders, pp. 290–301.

Weinzweig, J., 2010. Chapter 90: Chest wall reconstruction. In: Weinzweig, J. (Ed.), Plastic Surgery Secrets Plus, 2nd ed. Mosby, pp. 587–593.

Zochowski, C.G., Soltanian, H., 2012. Chapter 15: Rotational and free flap closure of the abdominal wall. In: Rosen, M.J. (Ed.), Atlas of Abdominal Wall Reconstruction. Elsevier, Philadelphia, pp. 259–289.

Peripheral Nerve Injuries, Brachial Plexus, and Compression Neuropathies

Chapter 12

General Nerve Anatomy

1. The central nervous system (brain and spinal cord) communicates with the rest of the body via the peripheral nervous system (cranial nerves, spinal nerves with their roots and rami, peripheral nerve trunks/branches, and the autonomic system).

2. The anterior (ventral) and posterior (dorsal) nerve roots arise from rootlets on the spinal cord and merge into the spinal nerves (see Figure 12.1).
   - The anterior primary rami of spinal nerves C5-T1 form the brachial plexus of the upper extremity, whereas the posterior primary rami of the spinal nerves travel to supply the muscle and skin of the posterior neck and trunk.

3. The motor nerve cell body is located within the spinal cord, and the sensory nerve cell body is located in the dorsal root ganglia.

4. Peripheral nerves are surrounded by Schwann cells that create the myelin sheath surrounding myelinated nerve axons.

5. Between each individual Schwann cell is the node of Ranvier that allows for faster propagation of signals down an axon through saltatory conduction.

6. Bundled axon nerve fibers are surrounded by endoneurium and grouped with other neurons by a collagen layer called perineurium. This group of neurons is termed a fascicle.
   - Within a peripheral nerve, the fasicles are also imbedded in loose connective tissue composed of collagen and fibroblasts (the epineurium; see Figure 12.2).

7. The vascular supply of the nerve consists of segmental blood vessels that branch into several vascular plexuses along the epineurium and within the perineurium and endoneurium.
   - This redundancy allows nerve mobilization over extended lengths without disruption of blood supply.

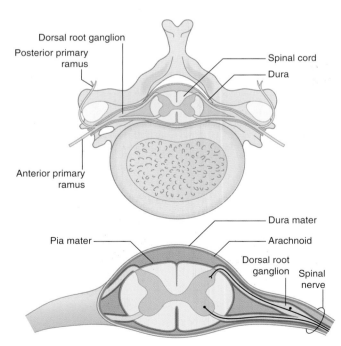

Figure 12.1. The anterior and posterior nerve roots, which emerge from rootlets attached to the spinal cord. *(Reprinted from Neligan, P.C., Chang, J. [Eds.], 2013. Plastic Surgery, vol. 6, 3rd ed. Elsevier, 694–718.)*

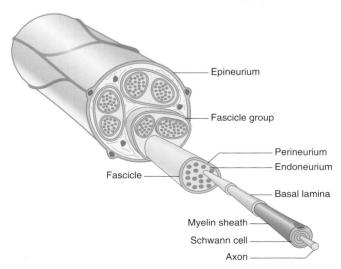

Figure 12.2. Schematic presentation of a peripheral nerve. *(Reprinted from Neligan, P.C., Chang, J. [Eds.], 2013. Plastic Surgery, vol. 6, 3rd ed. Elsevier, 694–718.)*

Nerve Physiology

1. Myelinated nerve fibers have high conduction velocity because the action potentials jump from node of Ranvier to node of Ranvier.
   - Unmyelinated nerve fibers have slower propagation of impulses because they lack myelin and nodes of Ranvier.
2. After nerve injury, the axons and myelin sheath in the distal segment degenerate ("Wallerian degeneration"), whereas the Schwann cells coordinate nerve repair and regeneration by up-regulating the production of neurotrophic factors and their receptors (see Figure 12.3).
   - Wallerian degeneration takes time after injury.
3. Regrowth of nerve occurs via multiple sprouts from the distal part of each viable axon. Within these sprouts is a growth cone that can sample the microenvironment and search for guidance factors/structures to enable targeted growth.

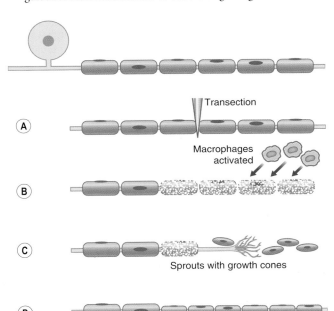

Figure 12.3. A, As the nerve is severed, activated macrophages and Schwann cells will immediately start the removal of myelin and remnants of the disintegrated axon, to allow for a conducive environment for the regenerating axons **(B). C,** Within just a few hours, numerous sprouts emerge from the distal part of each axon and form the sprout growth cone that will guide the regeneration process distally, until nerve regeneration is complete **(D).** *(Reprinted from Neligan, P.C., Chang, J. [Eds.], 2013. Plastic Surgery, vol. 6, 3rd ed. Elsevier, 694–718.)*

Classification of Nerve Injuries

1. Nerve injury can be classified generally into injuries that will temporarily block nerve conduction without loss of axonal architecture (neurapraxia) and those that will result in axonal degeneration distal to the injury (axonotmesis or neurotmesis).
2. Sunderland and Mackinnon modified the Seddon classification to further describe the complexity of nerve injury.

Diagnosis of Nerve Injury

1. Functional evaluation
   - Motor and sensory function should be fully assessed.
2. Electrophysiology testing
   - Must be interpreted with caution in first 3 to 4 weeks because it may take 4-6 weeks for degeneration and denervation to be detected by electrophysiologic studies.
   - Electromyography (EMG) assesses the motor component of a nerve only.
     - Measures resting electrical activity (e.g., abnormal spontaneous activity such as fibrillations and/or positive sharp waves), duration, amplitude, configuration, and motor unit recruitment
     - Abnormal spontaneous activity (e.g., fibrillations) and decreased motor unit recruitment occur with axonal injury.
   - Nerve conduction studies (NCSs) assess sensory (sensory nerve action potentials [SNAPs]) and motor (compound motor action potentials [CMAPs]) components.
     - Measures latency (the time from stimulus to recording), amplitude (evoked response from stimulus), and conduction velocity (calculated across a specific segment)
     - Increased latency, decreased amplitude, and decreased conduction velocity occur with nerve injury. In complete conduction block, no distal response is obtained with proximal stimulation.
     - Preganglionic injuries are associated with loss of sensation but show intact SNAPs and absent CMAPs.

General Nerve Repair Principles

1. Closed nerve injuries should be treated conservatively with observation for signs of recovery.
   - Consideration for electrophysiologic testing should be deferred until at least 4-6 weeks after injury, and many can wait until 3 months.
     - If at 3 months there is no sign of recovery, nerve exploration is warranted.
     - If partial spontaneous recovery is identified within 3 months, regular reevaluation with electrophysiologic testing can occur at 3-month intervals to observe continued recovery.
2. Open nerve injuries should be explored immediately.
   - If the nerve is found to be in continuity, treat as above as if it were a closed injury.
   - If the nerve is discontinuous, attempt immediate repair (unless significant crush injury, wound, or gunshot wound).
3. Nerve repair can occur either immediately or after delay.
   - Direct immediate repair
     - Method of choice, especially if performed within 48 to 72 hours
     - Best outcomes

Table 12.1 Differing Treatments for Different Types of Nerve Injury

TYPE OF NERVE INJURY	NEUROGRAPHY/EMG	EXPLORATION	REVISION	REPAIR OR RECONSTRUCTION
Sharp transection	—	Immediate	Immediate	Immediate
Open wound: Nerve crush injury	4-6 weeks*	Immediate	Immediate	Immediate† Delayed‡
Closed traction injury	4-6 weeks	Delayed	—	3-4 months§
Open wound: Gunshot wound	4-6 weeks*	Immediate	Immediate	Immediate† Delayed‡

Reprinted from Neligan, P.C., Chang, J. (Eds.), 2013. Plastic Surgery, vol. 6, 3rd ed. Elsevier, 694–718.
EMG, Electromyogram.
*If the nerve is in continuity on exploration, can perform neurography/EMG in the same manner as that for closed injuries.
†If there is macroscopic nerve discontinuity on exploration, perform repair or reconstruction after repeated revision to ensure that the wound is tidy.
‡If there is nerve continuity on exploration, treat the nerve injury as a closed injury so that repair or reconstruction is performed only when there is no sign of nerve regeneration (Tinel's sign), for example, for some injuries, exploration after 3-4 months.
§Repair or reconstruction is performed after 3-4 months if there are no clinical signs of nerve regeneration or reinnervation.

- ■ Technically easier than delayed repair
  - ○ Less retraction of nerve ends
  - ○ Less scarring
  - ○ Identification of nerve ends is easier because the nerve can often be stimulated for up to 72 hours after transection.
- • Delayed repair
  - ■ Typically requires a nerve graft
  - ■ Impaired functional outcomes (see Table 12.1)

4. Primary repair must occur without tension; otherwise, consider a nerve graft.
   - • For nerve gaps <3 cm, nerve conduits (e.g., synthetic, vein) can be used.
   - • For nerve gaps >3 cm, nerve grafts are recommended.
     - ■ Common donor grafts: Sural n., posterior interosseous n., lateral antebrachial cutaneous n.
     - ■ Grafts are preferably reversed at the time of placement to decrease the risk of nerve axon regeneration through cut branches on the graft.
5. Nonviable tissue must be resected until healthy fasicles are identified.
6. Alignment of the nerve ends according to their fasicular pattern and topographical arrangement improves outcomes.
7. Nerve ends are commonly coapted with interrupted 9-0 or 10-0 nylon sutures.
   - • Repair can occur at the epineurial or fasicular level.
   - • Grouped fasicular repair is preferred for injuries to the ulnar n. at the wrist.
8. If the proximal stump is absent, or if the nerve injury is "high," and end-to-side nerve repair can be performed in which the distal stump end is coapted to the side of an uninjured nerve.
9. Nerve transfer is a newer technique that has primarily been used with proximal or brachial plexus injuries to provide a source of regenerating axons in close proximity to the end target and preserve motor end plates.
   - • In some cases, these transfers are performed as a "babysitter" to maintain motor end plates while a proximal injury is allowed to recover.

- • Nerve transfers are associated with minimal to no downgrade in donor function and provide better outcomes (see Box 12.1 and Figure 12.4).

BOX 12.1 INDICATIONS FOR NERVE TRANSFER

- Proximal brachial plexus injuries where grafting is not possible
- Proximal peripheral nerve injuries requiring long distance for reinnervation of distal targets
- Severely scarred areas with risk of damage to critical structures
- Segmental nerve loss
- Major upper extremity trauma
- Partial nerve injuries with functional loss
- Delayed presentation with inadequate time for reinnervation of distal targets with grafting
- Sensory nerve deficits in critical regions

Reprinted from Neligan, P.C., Chang, J. (Eds.), 2013. Plastic Surgery, vol. 6, 3rd ed. Elsevier, 719–744.

Brachial Plexus

1. Formed from the anterior primary rami of spinal nerves C5 to T1
2. Motor nerve cell bodies arise from the anterior horn of the spinal cord, whereas the sensory nerve cell bodies are located in the dorsal root ganglion within the intervertebral foramen, immediately outside of the dura mater.
3. The brachial plexus is commonly divided into five anatomic sections: Roots, trunks, divisions, cords, and branches
4. The mixed spinal nerves travel between the anterior scalene m. and the middle scalene m. to form three trunks.
   - • Upper trunk: C5 and C6
   - • Middle trunk: C7
   - • Lower trunk: C8 and T1
5. Beneath the clavicle, each trunk divides into anterior and posterior divisions.

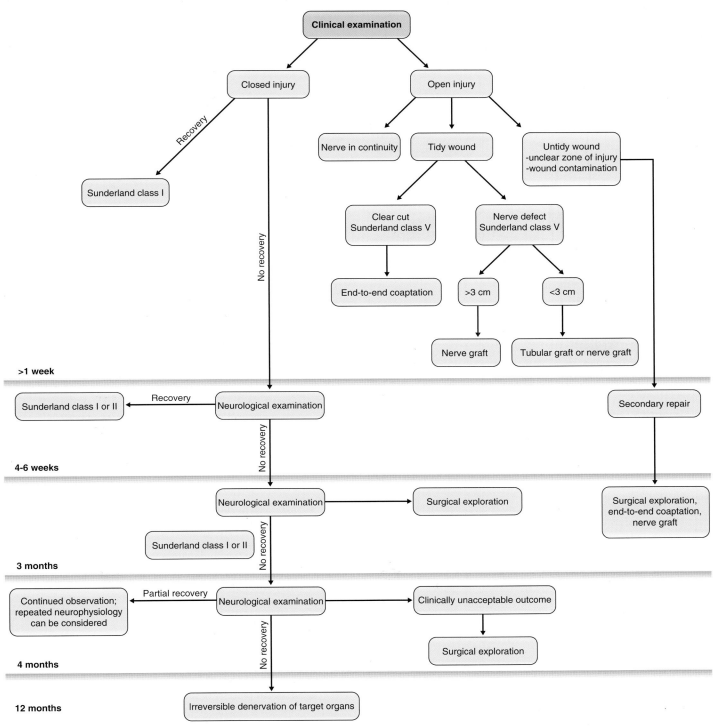

Figure 12.4. Algorithm for open and closed nerve injuries. Flowchart showing timing of surgical exposure and nerve repair. (*Reprinted from Neligan, P.C., Chang, J. [Eds.], 2013. Plastic Surgery, vol. 6, 3rd ed. Elsevier, 694–718.*)

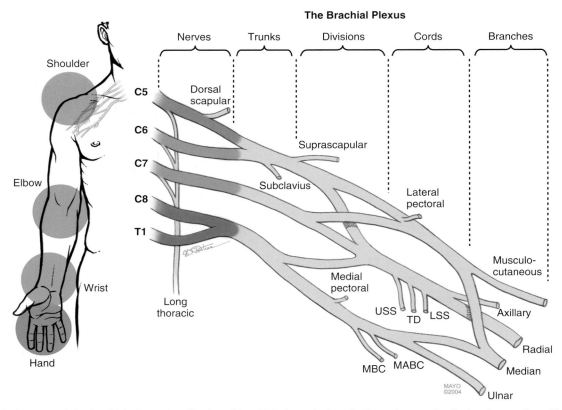

Figure 12.5. Anatomy of the brachial plexus. Localization of brachial plexus lesions is dependent on detailed understanding of brachial plexus anatomy. This illustration is reviewed with patients at the time of their initial evaluation. *LSS,* Lower subscapular nerve; *MABC,* medial antebrachial cutaneous nerve; *MBC,* medial brachial cutaneous nerve; *TD,* thoracodorsal nerve; *USS,* upper subscapular nerve. *(By permission of Mayo Foundation for Medical Education and Research. All rights reserved. Reprinted from Wolfe, S.W., Hotchkiss, R.N., Pederson, W.C., et al. [Eds.], 2011. Green's Operative Hand Surgery, 6th ed. Elsevier, 1235–1292.)*

6. Distal to the clavicle, the nerves exchange fibers to form cords.
   - Lateral cord
     - Formed from the anterior divisions of the upper and middle trunks
     - Passes anterior to the subclavian artery
     - Gives rise to the lateral cord contribution to the median n. and the musculocutaneous n.
   - Medial cords
     - Formed from the anterior division of the lower trunk
     - Passes anterior to the subclavian artery
     - Gives rise to the medial cord contribution to the median n. and the ulnar n.
   - Posterior cord
     - Formed from the posterior divisions of all trunks
     - Passes posterior to the subclavian artery
     - Forms the axillary nerve and the radial nerve (see Figures 12.5 and 12.6)
7. Types of brachial plexus injury
   - Traction injury
     - Includes stretch, rupture, and/or avulsion (see Figure 12.7)
   - Gunshot wound
     - Nerves are often in continuity, and in these patients, spontaneous recovery is possible.

   - High-velocity injuries are less likely to recover spontaneously.
   - Laceration injury
     - Nerves are often in discontinuity, and thus, open laceration injuries require operative exploration and repair when possible.
8. Diagnosis of brachial plexus injury level
   - Complete motor and sensory exam
   - Presence of or progression of Tinel's sign
   - Presence or absence of Horner's syndrome (miosis, ptosis, anhidrosis) suggests avulsion of the C8 to T1 roots.
   - Electrodiagnostic studies: NCSs and EMGs
     - NCSs: Amplitudes of SNAPs and CMAPs are most important; absent CMAPs and absent SNAPs suggest postganglionic lesion (absent motor and sensory), whereas absent CMAPs and present/normal SNAPs suggest preganglionic root avulsion (absent motor, present sensory).
9. Treatment depends on etiology and level of injury and degree of functional deficit.
   - Treatment options can include nerve transfers, tendon transfers, and free functioning muscle transfers.
   - For most closed injuries, a period of observation can be taken to look for spontaneous recovery before surgery.

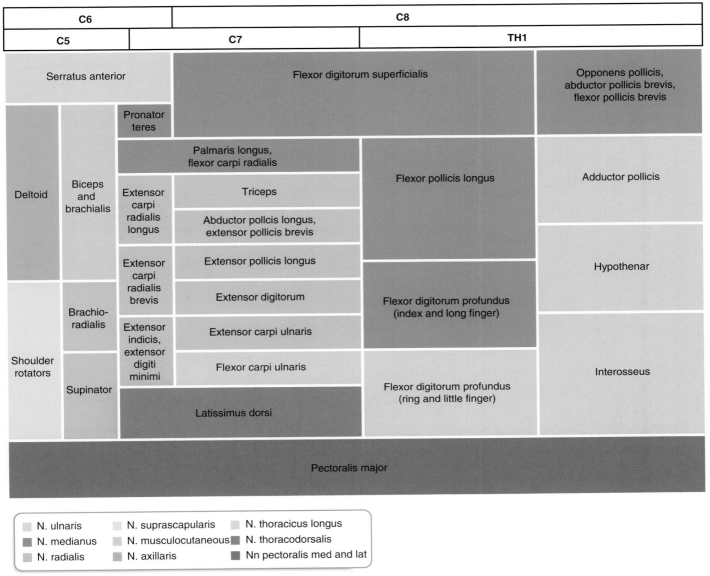

Figure 12.6. The origin of the nerves of the brachial plexus (C5-Th1, top) and their target muscles. *(Reprinted from Neligan, P.C., Chang, J. [Eds.], 2013. Plastic Surgery, vol. 6, 3rd ed. Elsevier, 694–718.)*

- In general, for neonates with traction injuries, if no improvement is observed by 6 months of age, surgical intervention is indicated.

Compression Neuropathies

1. Nerve entrapment occurs commonly, especially in the upper extremity.
2. Double crush phenomenon: Peripheral nerve compression at one site increases the susceptibility to compression at another site along the same nerve (e.g., ulnar nerve compression at the elbow and wrist).
   - May require release of both sites of compression for improvement in symptoms
   - The distal site is often released first.

3. Pathologic changes within the nerve depend on the severity and duration of compression.
   - Progression of nerve entrapment
     - Endoneurial edema and thickening, followed by increased endoneurial pressure and nerve ischemia
       - Results in paresthesias and sensory disturbances
     - Demyelination (localized progressing to diffuse with increased compression) followed by remyelination
       - Results in muscle weakness and increased pressure thresholds
     - Wallerian degeneration: Typically not observed until advanced chronic nerve entrapment occurs
       - Results in anesthesia and muscle atrophy (see Figure 12.8)

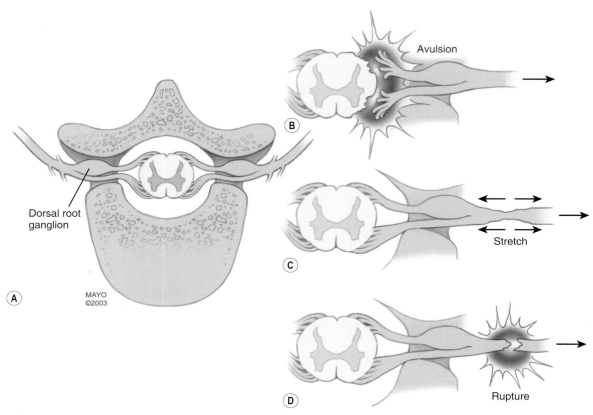

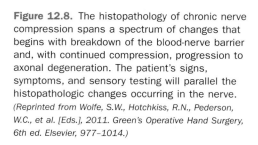

Figure 12.7. A-D, Traction injury to the brachial plexus may cause nerve injuries of varying severity in the same patient. Such injuries include avulsion (preganglionic injury) of nerve roots from the spinal cord (for practical purposes, cannot be repaired), stretch (postganglionic injury) of different magnitudes (some spontaneous recovery possible), and extraforaminal rupture of the nerve or trunk (can be repaired with surgery). *(Reprinted from Wolfe, S.W., Hotchkiss, R.N., Pederson, W.C., et al. [Eds.], 2011. Green's Operative Hand Surgery, 6th ed. Elsevier, 1235–1292. By permission of Mayo Foundation for Medical Education and Research. All rights reserved.)*

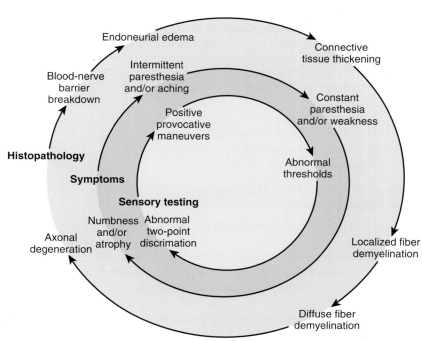

Figure 12.8. The histopathology of chronic nerve compression spans a spectrum of changes that begins with breakdown of the blood-nerve barrier and, with continued compression, progression to axonal degeneration. The patient's signs, symptoms, and sensory testing will parallel the histopathologic changes occurring in the nerve. *(Reprinted from Wolfe, S.W., Hotchkiss, R.N., Pederson, W.C., et al. [Eds.], 2011. Green's Operative Hand Surgery, 6th ed. Elsevier, 977–1014.)*

4. Provocative tests: Useful in eliciting symptoms of nerve compression and identifying potential sites of entrapment (see Table 12.2)

Table 12.2 Provocative Tests for Nerve Entrapment

NERVE	ENTRAPMENT SITE	PROVOCATIVE TEST	CONSERVATIVE MANAGEMENT
Median	Carpal tunnel	Pressure proximal to the carpal tunnel, Phalen's test, reverse Phalen's test (hyperextension of the wrist)	Splint the wrist in neutral position at night
	Proximal forearm	Pressure over the proximal forearm in the region of the pronator teres with the forearm in supination, resisted elbow flexion, pronation, and finger flexion	Use stretching exercises for the pronator teres
Ulnar	Guyon's canal	Pressure proximal to Guyon's canal, reverse Phalen's test	Splint the wrist in neutral position at night
	Cubital tunnel	Elbow flexion and pressure proximal to the cubital tunnel	Educate about the elbow pad, positioning in elbow extension, and decreasing direct pressure on the nerve
Radial (posterior interosseous)	Arcade of Fröhse	Pressure over the supinator, resisted supination, resisted long-finger, and wrist extension	Position in supination and avoid repetitive pronation and supination activities
Radial (sensory)	Forearm	Pressure over the junction of the brachioradialis/extensor carpi radialis tendon, forearm pronation with wrist ulnar flexion	Avoid repetitive pronation and supination activities
Brachial plexus	Supraclavicular	Elevation of arms above the head, pressure over the brachial plexus in the interscalene region	Avoid provocative positions, stretch shortened muscles, and strengthen weakened scapular stabilizers

Reprinted from Wolfe, S.W., Hotchkiss, R.N., Pederson, W.C., et al. (Eds.), 2011. Green's Operative Hand Surgery, 6th ed. Elsevier, 977–1014.

5. Median nerve
   - Sites of compression: Ligament of Struthers, lacertus fibrosis (bicipital aponeurosis), two heads of the pronator teres, transverse carpal ligament (see Figures 12.9 and 12.10)

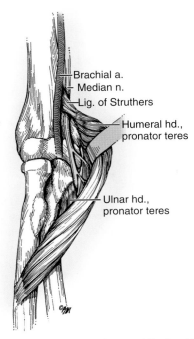

Figure 12.9. The median nerve lies deep and the brachial artery lies superficial to the ligament of Struthers, which forms an accessory origin for the pronator teres. *lig,* Ligament. *(Reprinted from Wolfe, S.W., Hotchkiss, R.N., Pederson, W.C., et al. [Eds.], 2011. Green's Operative Hand Surgery. 6th ed. Elsevier, 977–1014. Copyright Elizabeth Martin.)*

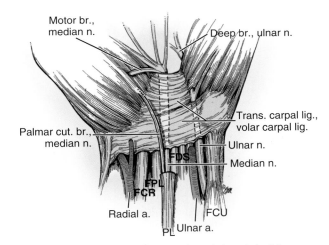

Figure 12.10. The palmar cutaneous branch *(cut. br.)* of the median nerve lies radial to the median nerve and ulnar and to the flexor carpi radialis *(FCR)* tendon. It may pierce either the volar carpal or transverse *(Trans.)* carpal ligament or the antebrachial fascia before it becomes subcutaneous. *FCU,* Flexor carpi ulnaris; *FDS,* flexor digitorum superficialis; *FPL,* flexor pollicis longus; *PL,* palmaris longus. *(Reprinted from Wolfe, S.W., Hotchkiss, R.N., Pederson, W.C., et al. [Eds.], 2011. Green's Operative Hand Surgery, 6th ed. Elsevier, 977–1014. Copyright Elizabeth Martin.)*

- Carpal tunnel syndrome: Compression of the median nerve at the wrist by the transverse carpal ligament
  - Symptoms: Nocturnal pain, numbness, paresthesias, night awakenings
  - Signs: Tinel's, weak abductor pollicis brevis, sensory disturbance, thenar wasting, abnormal electrodiagnostic studies, positive Phalen's test (provocation of symptoms with wrists flexed)
    - Can distinguish from pronator syndrome by preservation of sensory in the palmar cutaneous nerve distribution with carpal tunnel syndrome
  - Treatment
    - Conservative: Splinting, corticosteroid injection
    - Carpal tunnel release: Endoscopic or open
6. Ulnar nerve
  - Sites of compression: Arcade of Struthers, medial intermuscular septum, Osborne's ligament/band, flexor carpi ulnaris origin, anconeus epitrochlearis, Guyon's canal (see Figures 12.11 and 12.12)

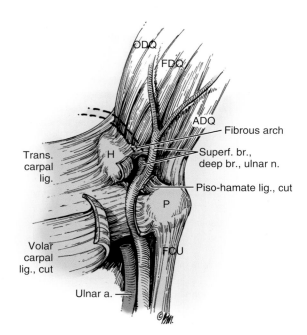

Figure 12.12. The ulnar nerve courses through Guyon's canal between the volar carpal ligament *(lig.)* and the transverse *(Trans.)* carpal ligament. *ADQ,* Abductor digiti quinti; *FCU,* flexor carpi ulnaris; *FDQ,* flexor digiti quinti; *H,* hamate; *ODQ,* opponens digiti quinti; *P,* pisiform; *superf. br.,* superficial branch. *(Reprinted from Wolfe, S.W., Hotchkiss, R.N., Pederson, W.C., et al. [Eds.], 2011. Green's Operative Hand Surgery, 6th ed. Elsevier, 977–1014. Copyright Elizabeth Martin.)*

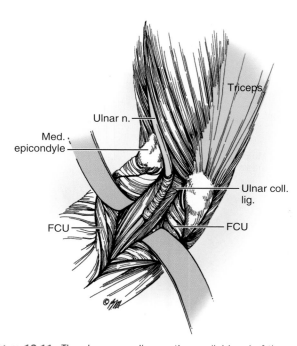

Figure 12.11. The ulnar nerve lies on the medial head of the triceps muscle, enters the cubital tunnel behind the medial *(Med.)* epicondyle, and continues distally beneath the arcade of fascia, where it joins the heads of the flexor carpi ulnaris *(FCU)*. *coll.,* Collateral. *(Reprinted from Wolfe, S.W., Hotchkiss, R.N., Pederson, W.C., et al. [Eds.], 2011. Green's Operative Hand Surgery, 6th ed. Elsevier, 977–1014. Copyright Elizabeth Martin.)*

- Cubital tunnel syndrome: Compression of the ulnar nerve at the elbow
  - Symptoms: Pain, numbness, weak grip
  - Signs: Tinel's at the medial elbow, weak first dorsal interossei muscle, Froment's sign (flexion of the thumb interphalangeal [IP] joint with thumb/index pinch), Wartenberg's sign (abduction of the small finger), provocation of symptoms with the elbow flexion/pressure test, sensory disturbance of the ring and small finger, intrinsic musculature wasting, abnormal electrodiagnostic studies
  - Treatment
    - Conservative: Splinting, physical therapy
    - Surgical decompression: Can be performed alone or with nerve transposition to subcutaneous, intramuscular, or submuscular position

- Ulnar tunnel syndrome: Compression of the ulnar nerve at the wrist within Guyon's canal; can occur secondary to a mass (e.g., ganglion cyst) or ulnar a. aneurysm ("hypothenar hammer syndrome")
  - Symptoms: Paresthesias in the ring and small fingers, ulnar-sided hand pain, decreased grip strength
  - Signs: Similar to cubital tunnel syndrome except with possible Tinel's at the wrist, abnormal electrodiagnostic studies at the wrist level, and/or presence of palpable mass, tumor, or fracture
  - Treatment
    - Release of the pisohamate ligament and volar carpal ligament
7. Radial nerve
   - Sites of compression: Fibrous bands to the radiocapitellar joint, leash of Henry (recurrent radial vessels), proximal edge of the extensor carpi radialis brevis (ECRB), arcade of Fröhse (proximal edge of the supinator), distal edge of the supinator, proximal to the radial styloid between the brachioradialis and extensor carpi radialis longus (ECRL; see Figure 12.13)

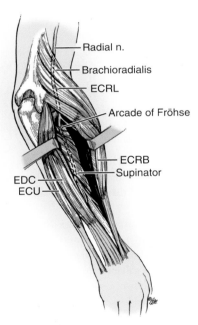

Figure 12.13. Extension of the posterior Thompson approach to the radial tunnel. *ECRB,* Extensor carpi radialis brevis; *ECRL,* extensor carpi radialis longus; *ECU,* extensor carpi ulnaris; *EDC,* extensor digitorum communis. *(Reprinted from Wolfe, S.W., Hotchkiss, R.N., Pederson, W.C., et al. [Eds.], 2011. Green's Operative Hand Surgery, 6th ed. Elsevier, 977–1014. Copyright Elizabeth Martin.)*

- Radial tunnel syndrome: Compression of the radial nerve (posterior interosseus nerve) in the forearm; distinguished from posterior interosseous nerve (PIN) syndrome by lack of motor weakness
  - Symptoms: Lateral proximal forearm pain
  - Signs: Pain along the lateral forearm, provocation of symptoms with resisted elbow extension, forearm pronation, wrist flexion
  - Treatment
    - Surgery is recommended for true PIN syndrome if there is no improvement in muscle function after 3 months.
    - Conservative treatment with rest, physical therapy, and NSAIDs is often successful
- Traumatic radial nerve injury often occurs in setting of supracondylar fractures of the humerus.
  - Treatment
    - Observation because most are neurapraxia injuries
    - No recovery after 3 to 6 months warrants surgical exploration.
8. Common peroneal nerve
   - Sites of compression: Most commonly, the posterior crural intermuscular septum, which compresses the nerve as it courses around the fibular neck and deep to the peroneus longus muscle
     - Can be caused by habitual leg crossing, external compression against a hard object in debilitated or paralyzed patients, trauma, intraneural or extraneural tumors and masses
     - Can also occur in athletes with well-developed lower leg muscles, individuals who spend significant time in a crouched position (e.g., baseball catchers), and patients after massive weight loss secondary to atrophy of the fat pad overlying the fibular head, which predisposes the nerve to external compressive forces
   - Symptoms: Numbness and tingling in the posterior and lateral lower leg and dorsal foot, foot drop
   - Signs: Weak or absent dorsiflexion, abnormal gait, sensory disturbance in the deep peroneal (first web space) and superficial peroneal (dorsum of foot) distribution, Tinel's sign at the fibular neck, exacerbation of symptoms with knee extension, abnormal electrodiagnostic studies

- Treatment
  - Ankle-foot orthotic (AFO) splint for protection and gait assistance
  - Observation for 3 to 4 months in cases where neurapraxia is the likely etiology
  - Surgical decompression is warranted when compression does not improve, is caused by tumors/masses, or in cases of severe compression with evidence of muscle atrophy.
9. Posterior tibial nerve
  - Sites of compression: Tarsal canal or "tarsal tunnel," which is located posterior to the medial malleolus and formed primarily by the talus, calcaneus, and flexor retinaculum
    - Can be caused by external compression from masses, muscle hypertrophy, tenosynovitis, rupture of the medial tendons, and presence of anomalous muscles and/or vasculature (e.g., varicosities, aberrant vascular leashes)
  - Symptoms: Pain, numbness, tingling along the plantar foot; often worse with weight bearing
  - Signs: Sensory disturbance along the medial plantar or lateral plantar nerve distribution, exacerbation of symptoms with dorsiflexion, tenderness to palpation, Tinel's sign over the tarsal canal
  - Treatment
    - Observation and conservative management
    - Trial of cast or walking boot immobilization
    - Surgical release for chronic cases that do not improve and those caused by external compression from tumors or masses

Neuroma

1. Formed after injury to a nerve with aberrant repair, in which regenerating axons from the proximal stump are unable to reenter the distal stump
   - Results in a swelling of the distal end of the proximal stump that contains Schwann cells, fibroblasts, vasculature, and multiple axons
   - Can occur as a "neuroma in continuity" in cases of partial nerve injury with some intact nerve axons
2. Symptoms: Pain, hypersensitivity
3. Signs: Exquisite tenderness with palpation, Tinel's sign, hypersensitivity with history of injury/amputation

4. Treatment
   - Conservative: Hand therapy with desensitization (vibration, massage, and/or transcutaneous nerve stimulation)
   - Resection with primary nerve grafting
   - Resection with iatrogenic injury to proximal stump (crush, cautery) and insertion into deep soft tissues
   - Resection with transfer and coaptation to neighboring nerve ("targeted re-innervation") (see Figure 12.14)

Complex Regional Pain Syndrome (CRPS)

1. Syndrome of regional pain, autonomic dysfunction, atrophy, and functional impairment that develops after trauma/injury to the hand/digits
2. Symptoms: Pain that is out of proportion to the traumatic insult, often with autonomic symptoms (e.g., a red, painful, swollen finger), disuse of the affected extremity, neglect of the extremity (see Figure 12.15)
3. Classification (see Table 12.3)

Table 12.3 Classification of Complex Regional Pain Syndrome

Type 1	Reflex sympathetic dystrophy (pain, functional impairment, autonomic dysfunction, dystrophic changes without clinical peripheral nerve lesion/injury)
Type 2	Causalgia (pain, functional impairment, autonomic dysfunction, dystrophic changes with a diagnosable peripheral nerve injury)
Type 3*	Other pain dysfunction problems (e.g., myofascial pain)

Reprinted from Wolfe, S.W., Hotchkiss, R.N., Pederson, W.C., et al. (Eds.), 2011. Green's Operative Hand Surgery, 6th ed. Elsevier.
*Not discussed in this chapter.

4. Treatment options: Often, multimodal treatment with assistance from hand therapists and pain management specialists
   - Range of motion exercises, stress loading, vibration, massage, transcutaneous nerve stimulation
   - Anticonvulsant and/or antidepressant medications
   - Corticosteroids, gabapentin, lidocaine, and sodium channel blockers have shown some benefit.
   - Peripheral nerve block
   - Nerve decompression

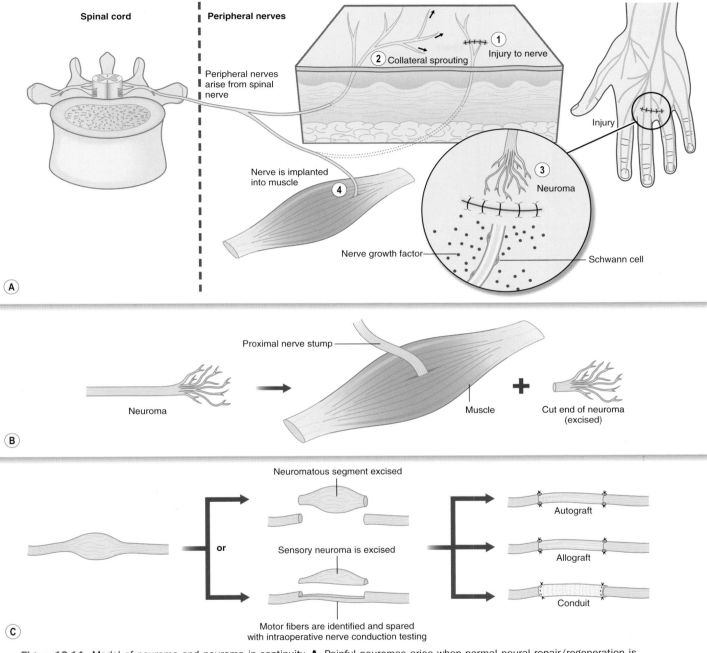

Figure 12.14. Model of neuroma and neuroma in continuity. **A,** Painful neuromas arise when normal neural repair/regeneration is disrupted, such as by intervening scar tissue. **B,** The treatment for painful neuroma is resection of the neuroma with implantation of the proximal nerve stump into a muscle. **C,** Neuroma in continuity is characterized by internal architectural derangement of an intact nerve. The segment containing neuroma can be selectively or totally resected and then repaired using grafting or conduit. *(Reprinted from Neligan, P.C., Chang, J. [Eds.], 2013. Plastic Surgery, vol. 6, 3rd ed. Elsevier, 486.)*

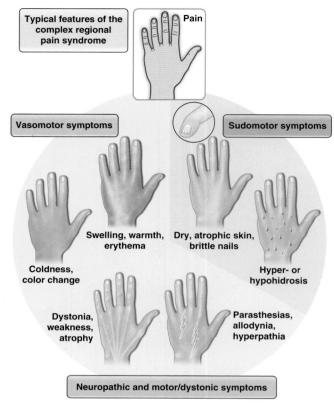

Figure 12.15. Typical features of a patient with complex regional pain syndrome. *(Reprinted from Neligan, P.C., Chang, J. [Eds.], 2013. Plastic Surgery, vol. 6, 3rd ed. Elsevier, 486.)*

Suggested Readings

Bezuhly, M., O'Brien, J.P., Lalonde, D., 2013. Chapter 24: Nerve entrapment syndromes. In: Neligan, P.C., Chang, J. (Eds.), Plastic Surgery, vol. 6, 3rd ed. Elsevier, pp. 503–525.

Birch, R., 2011. Chapter 32: Nerve repair. In: Wolfe, S.W., Hotchkiss, R.N., Pederson, W.C., et al. (Eds.), Green's Operative Hand Surgery, 6th ed. Elsevier, p. 1036.

Boyd, K.U., Fox, I.K., Mackinnon, S.E., 2013. Chapter 33: Nerve transfers. In: Neligan, P.C., Chang, J. (Eds.), Plastic Surgery, vol. 6, 3rd ed. Elsevier, pp. 719–744.

Chuang, D.C.C., 2013. Chapter 36: Brachial plexus injuries: adult and pediatric. In: Neligan, P.C., Chang, J. (Eds.), Plastic Surgery, vol. 6, 3rd ed. Elsevier, pp. 789–816.

Ducic, I., Felder, J.M., 2013. Chapter 23: Complex regional pain syndrome in the upper extremity. In: Neligan, P.C., Chang, J. (Eds.), Plastic Surgery, vol. 6, 3rd ed. Elsevier, p. 486.

Farnebo, S., Thorfinn, J., Dahlin, L.B., 2013. Chapter 32: Peripheral nerve injuries of the upper extremity. In: Neligan, P.C., Chang, J. (Eds.), Plastic Surgery, vol. 6, 3rd ed. Elsevier, pp. 694–718.

Hollis, M.H., Calhoun, J.H., Nerve Entrapment Syndromes of the Lower Extremity. Emedicine.com. Found at: <http://emedicine.medscape.com/article/1234809-overview#aw2aab6b4> Accessed on: October 16, 2014.

Koman, L.A., Poehling, G.G., Smith, B.P., et al., 2011. Chapter 69: Complex regional pain syndrome. In: Wolfe, S.W., Hotchkiss, R.N., Pederson, W.C., et al. (Eds.), Green's Operative Hand Surgery, 6th ed. Elsevier, p. 1959.

Mackinnon, S.E., Novak, C.B., 2011. Chapter 30: Compression neuropathies. In: Wolfe, S.W., Hotchkiss, R.N., Pederson, W.C., et al. (Eds.), Green's Operative Hand Surgery, 6th ed. Elsevier, pp. 977–1014.

Souza, J.M., Cheesborough, J.E., Ko, J.H., et al., 2014. Targeted muscle reinnervation: a novel approach to postamputation neuroma pain. Clini. Orthop. Relat. Res. 472 (10), 2984–2990.

Spinner, R.J., Shin, A.Y., Hebert-Blouin, M.N., et al., 2011. Chapter 38: Traumatic brachial plexus injury. In: Wolfe, S.W., Hotchkiss, R.N., Pederson, W.C., et al. (Eds.), Green's Operative Hand Surgery, 6th ed. Elsevier, pp. 1235–1292.

Verndakis, A.J., Koch, H., Mackinnon, S.E., 2003. Management of neuromas. Clin. Plast. Surg. 30 (2), 247–268.

Wheeler, A.H., Berman, S.A., Complex Regional Pain Syndromes Treatment & Management. Emedicine.com. Found at: <http://emedicine.medscape.com/article/1145318-overview> Accessed on: October 16, 2014.

Lower Extremity Reconstruction and Lymphedema

1. General lower extremity (LE) anatomy
   - Vascular supply (see Figures 13.1 and 13.2)
   - Muscle compartments
     - Thigh
       - Anterior
         - Sartorius m., rectus femoris m., vastus lateralis m., vastus intermedius m., vastus medialis m.
         - Femoral n.
       - Posterior
         - Biceps femoris m., semitendinosus m., semimembranosus m.
         - Sciatic n.
       - Medial
         - Gracilis m., adductor longus m., adductor brevis m., adductor magnus m.
         - Obturator n. (see Figure 13.3)
     - Lower leg
       - Anterior
         - Tibialis anterior m., extensor hallucis longus m., extensor digitorum longus m., peroneus tertius m.
         - Deep peroneal n.
         - Anterior tibial a.
       - Lateral
         - Peroneus longus m., peroneus brevis m.
         - Superficial peroneal n.
       - Deep posterior
         - Tibialis posterior m., flexor hallucis longus m., flexor digitorum longus m., popliteus m.
         - Tibial n.
         - Posterior tibial a.
       - Superficial posterior
         - Gastrocnemius m., plantaris m., soleus m.
         - Sural n. (see Figure 13.4)
     - Foot
       - Medial
         - Abductor hallucis m., flexor hallucis brevis m.
       - Lateral
         - Abductor digiti minimi m., flexor digiti minimi brevis m.
       - Interosseous (4)
       - Central (3)
         - Flexor digitorum brevis m., quadratus plantae m., adductor hallucis m. (see Figure 13.5)
2. LE trauma
   - Classification of injury
     - Gustillo classification
       - Description based on degree of soft-tissue injury and presence of vascular injury
       - Major vascular injury requiring repair is automatically a class IIIC.

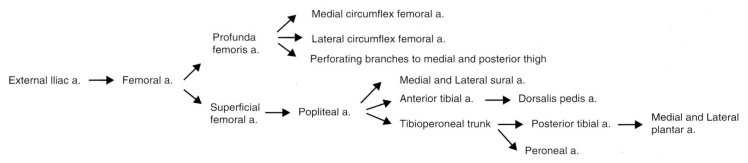

Figure 13.1. Major arterial supply to the lower extremities.

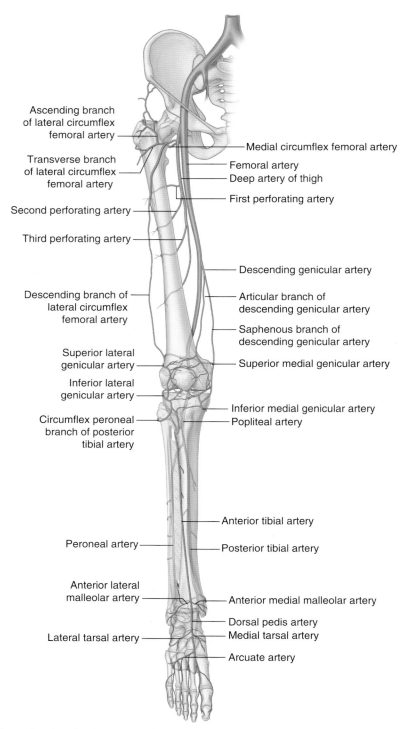

Figure 13.2. Femoral and profunda arteries. *(Reprinted from Neligan, P.C. [Ed.], 2013. Plastic Surgery, 3rd ed. Elsevier, 1–62.)*

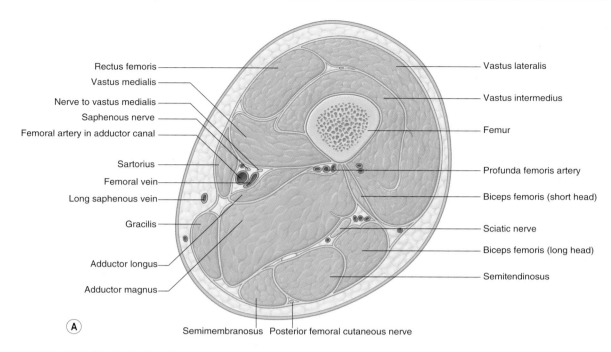

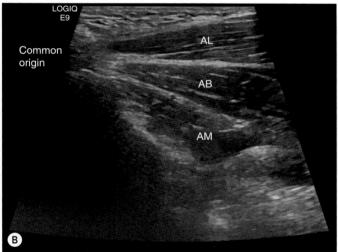

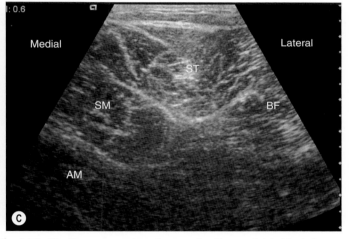

Figure 13.3. Thigh. **A,** Line drawing of the compartmental anatomy of the thigh. The three compartments comprise the medial (adductor), posterior (hamstring flexor), and anterior (extensor). **B,** Transverse sonogram of the medial compartment of the thigh at the level of the pubis. *AL,* Adductor longus; *AB,* adductor brevis; *AM,* adductor magnus. **C,** Transverse sonogram of the posterior compartment of the thigh. *AM,* Adductor magnus; *BF,* biceps femoris; *SM,* semimembranosus; *ST,* semitendinosus. (*A, Reprinted with permission from Standring, S. [Ed.], Gray's Anatomy, 40th ed. Edinburgh, Churchill Livingstone, 2008. B,C, From Allan, P.L., Baxter, G.M., Weston, M.J. [Eds.], 2011. Clinical Ultrasound, 3rd ed. Elsevier, 1137–1157.*)

○ Classes I and II can generally be managed with local wound care.
○ Class III generally requires flap coverage.
  ◆ Classes A, B, and C distinguished according to size of wound and presence of vascular injury
    → A: Wound <10 cm, soft-tissue coverage is usually possible
    → B: Wound >10 cm, regional or free flap needed
    → C: Presence of major vascular injury requiring repair for limb salvage
  ◆ IIIB/C: Often requires initial stabilization with external fixator (see Table 13.1)
■ Byrd classification
  ○ Established based on force of injury and degree of bony comminution
    ◆ Type I: Low-energy, spiral, or oblique fracture with clean wound <2 cm

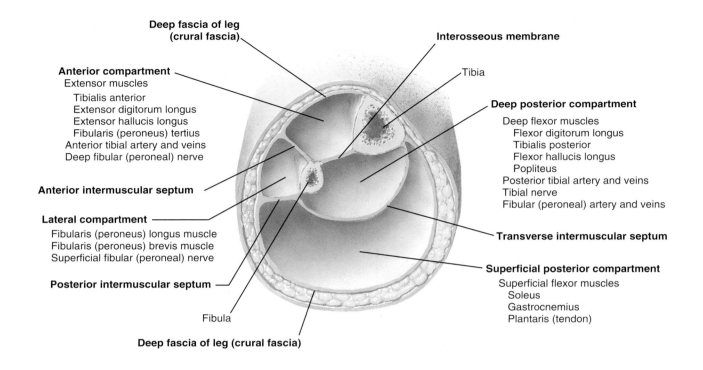

Deep fascia of leg (crural fascia)

Interosseous membrane

Anterior compartment
Extensor muscles
  Tibialis anterior
  Extensor digitorum longus
  Extensor hallucis longus
  Fibularis (peroneus) tertius
  Anterior tibial artery and veins
  Deep fibular (peroneal) nerve

Anterior intermuscular septum

Lateral compartment
  Fibularis (peroneus) longus muscle
  Fibularis (peroneus) brevis muscle
  Superficial fibular (peroneal) nerve

Posterior intermuscular septum

Fibula

Deep fascia of leg (crural fascia)

Tibia

Deep posterior compartment
Deep flexor muscles
  Flexor digitorum longus
  Tibialis posterior
  Flexor hallucis longus
  Popliteus
Posterior tibial artery and veins
Tibial nerve
Fibular (peroneal) artery and veins

Transverse intermuscular septum

Superficial posterior compartment
Superficial flexor muscles
  Soleus
  Gastrocnemius
  Plantaris (tendon)

Cross section just above middle of leg

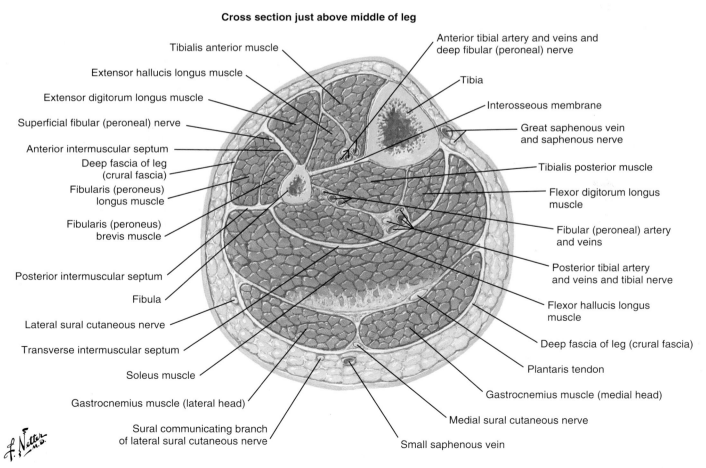

Tibialis anterior muscle

Extensor hallucis longus muscle

Extensor digitorum longus muscle

Superficial fibular (peroneal) nerve

Anterior intermuscular septum

Deep fascia of leg (crural fascia)

Fibularis (peroneus) longus muscle

Fibularis (peroneus) brevis muscle

Posterior intermuscular septum

Fibula

Lateral sural cutaneous nerve

Transverse intermuscular septum

Soleus muscle

Gastrocnemius muscle (lateral head)

Sural communicating branch of lateral sural cutaneous nerve

Anterior tibial artery and veins and deep fibular (peroneal) nerve

Tibia

Interosseous membrane

Great saphenous vein and saphenous nerve

Tibialis posterior muscle

Flexor digitorum longus muscle

Fibular (peroneal) artery and veins

Posterior tibial artery and veins and tibial nerve

Flexor hallucis longus muscle

Deep fascia of leg (crural fascia)

Plantaris tendon

Gastrocnemius muscle (medial head)

Medial sural cutaneous nerve

Small saphenous vein

Figure 13.4. Leg: Cross sections and fascial compartments. *(Netter illustration from www.netterimages.com. Copyright Elsevier Inc. All rights reserved.)*

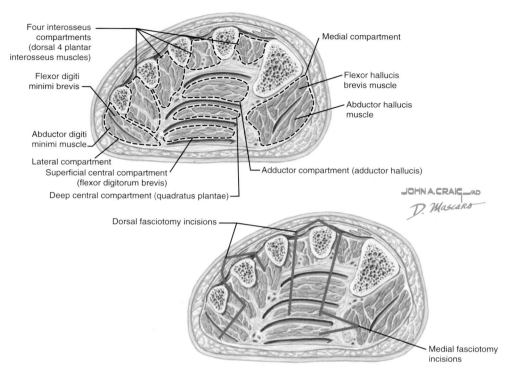

Figure 13.5. Muscles of the foot and ankle. *(Netter illustration from www.netterimages.com. Copyright Elsevier Inc. All rights reserved.)*

Table 13.1 Classification of Open Fractures

WOUND SIZE	CONTAMINATION	BONE INJURY	SOFT-TISSUE INJURY
1. 1 cm	Clean	Simple	Minimal
2. >1 cm	Moderate	Moderate, some comminution	Moderate, some muscle crushing
3. The following injuries are automatically graded as type-3 injuries: • Segmental fracture • Severely contaminated wounds (e.g., farmyard injuries) • Shotgun wounds • High-velocity gunshot wounds			
3a. Usually >10 cm	High	Usually severe	Usually severe, but bone coverage possible
3b. Usually >10 cm	High	Usually severe	Bone coverage impossible, requires soft-tissue reconstruction
3c. Usually >10 cm	High	Usually severe	As 3b, with vascular injury requiring repair

Reprinted from McGrath, L., Royston, S., 2007. Fractures of the tibial shaft (including acute compartment syndrome). Surgery 2003. 21 (9), 231–235.

♦ Type II: Moderate-energy, comminuted, or displaced fracture with >2 cm laceration and moderate muscle contusion
♦ Type III: High-energy, severely displaced, and comminuted fracture or bony defect with extensive skin loss and devitalized muscle
♦ Type IV: Extreme energy, same as class C with degloving or crush injury and/or vascular injury (see Table 13.2)
• General management
  ■ Computed tomography (CT) angiography provides the most rapid method for evaluating LE vasculature.

■ Preferred irrigation–low-pressure pulse lavage (14 PSI) with 1% surgical soap resulted in a more significant clearing of bone-adherent bacteria than other solutions. Osteoclast and osteoblast function were also shown to be preserved more significantly with the use of the 1% soap or detergent solution.
■ Free flaps are often required for large defects because of paucity of available local tissue (IIIB/C).
  ○ According to Godina, preferred timing of free-flap reconstruction is within 72 hours; reports suggest immediate reconstruction requires less dissection and carries less thrombosis and infection risk.

Table 13.2 Byrd Classification of Lower Extremity Fractures

TYPE	ENERGY	FRACTURE	SOFT TISSUE
I	Low	Spiral or oblique	Clean wound, <2 cm
II	Moderate	Comminuted of displaced	>2 cm laceration, moderate muscle contusion
III	High	Severely displaced and comminuted or bony defect	Extensive skin loss and devitalized muscle
IV	Extreme	Severely displaced and comminuted or bony defect	Extensive skin loss and devitalized muscle with degloving, crush, and/or vascular injury

- Free flaps are also preferred for early exposure of hardware (before osseus union) rather than removal of hardware with external fixator.
- Adequate debridement is the key to successful reconstruction in contaminated wounds as well as in the treatment of posttraumatic osteomyelitis.
  - Reconstruction versus amputation
    - Goal: Preserve a limb that will be more functional than an amputation
      - If the extremity cannot be salvaged, the goal is to maintain the maximum functional length.
        - ◆ Minimum of 6 cm is required for adequate prosthetic fitting of below-knee amputation.
          - → Can consider fillet of foot flap to preserve length; otherwise, revision amputation is usually indicated following traumatic LE amputation.
    - Absolute contraindications for reconstruction
      - Tibial nerve disruption
      - Warm ischemia time >8 hours
  - Replantation
    - Contraindications for LE replantation include crush mechanism of injury, warm ischemia time >8 hours, multilevel injury, poor baseline health, and patient of advanced age
  - Vascularized bone flaps versus allogeneic bone grafts
    - Vascularized bone flaps
      - Shorten union time
      - Demonstrate increased osteocyte viability
      - Osteogenesis through osteoinduction versus depending solely on creeping substitution (allogeneic)
      - Indicated for bony defects >6 cm
  - Compartment syndrome
    - Increased pressure in a confined space
      - Requires clinical suspicion
        - ◆ Symptoms/signs
          - → Pain out of proportion (often first sign)
          - → Paresthesias
          - → Poikilothermia
          - → Pallor
          - → Pulselessness (late sign)
          - → Paralysis (late sign)
          - → Tense compartment
            - ▪ Compartment pressure >30 mm Hg
    - Management
      - Fasciotomy

3. Commonly used LE flaps (see Figure 13.6)
   - Sartorius muscle flap
     - Origin: Anterior superior iliac spine
     - Insertion: Anteromedial surface of tibia
     - Function: Flex, laterally rotate, and abduct hip; weak knee flexor
     - Arterial supply: Superficial femoral a. provides segmental blood supply (type-IV muscle).
     - Nerve: Femoral n.
   - Gracilis muscle flap
     - Origin: Ischiopubic ramus
     - Insertion: Medial tibia
     - Function: Flex, medially rotate, and adduct hip; weak knee flexor
     - Arterial supply: Medial circumflex femoral a.
     - Nerve: Obturator n.
   - Anterolateral thigh myocutaneous or perforator flap
     - Arterial supply: Descending branch of lateral circumflex femoral a.
     - Nerve: Lateral femoral cutaneous n.
     - Underlying muscle: Vastus lateralis m.
   - Gastrocnemius flap
     - Origin: Femoral condyles (medial and lateral)
     - Insertion: Calcaneus through achilles tendon
     - Function: Plantarflexion; knee flexion
     - Arterial supply: Sural arteries (medial and lateral)
     - Nerve: Tibial n.
     - Medial muscle: Indicated for medial upper leg 1/3 defects, longer than lateral gastrocnemius, and does not risk damage to the peroneal nerve (see Figure 13.7)
   - Soleus muscle flap
     - Origin: Fibula, medial border of tibia
     - Insertion: Calcaneus through achilles tendon
     - Function: Plantarflexion
     - Arterial supply: Popliteal artery (27.8%) superiorly (anterograde flap), posterior tibial artery (38.8%), or peroneal artery (33.3%) distally (retrograde flap)
     - Nerve: Tibial n.
   - Sural artery flap
     - Arterial supply: Peroneal artery perforators, which emerge 5 cm proximal to medial malleolus; tenous drainage through small valveless comitant veins
     - Flap elevation landmarks: The lesser saphenous vein and sural nerve, which should bisect the cutaneous paddle

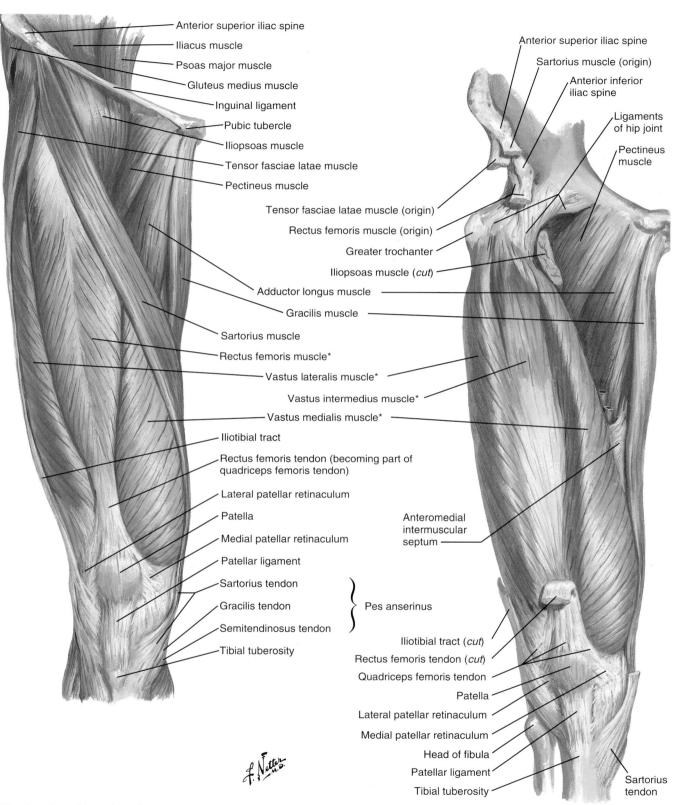

Figure 13.6. Muscles of thigh: Anterior view. *(Netter illustration from www.netterimages.com. Copyright Elsevier Inc. All rights reserved.)*

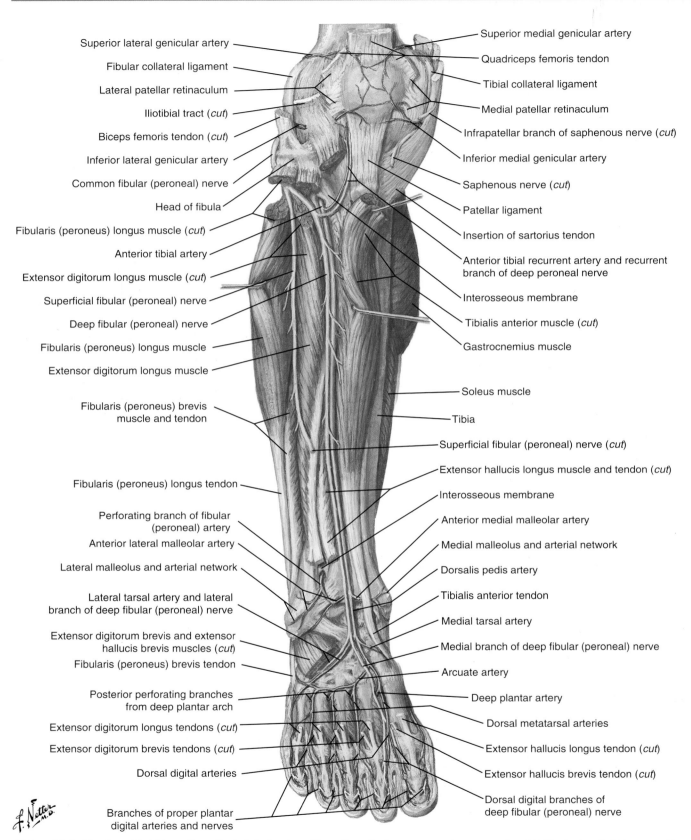

Superior lateral genicular artery

Fibular collateral ligament

Lateral patellar retinaculum

Iliotibial tract (*cut*)

Biceps femoris tendon (*cut*)

Inferior lateral genicular artery

Common fibular (peroneal) nerve

Head of fibula

Fibularis (peroneus) longus muscle (*cut*)

Anterior tibial artery

Extensor digitorum longus muscle (*cut*)

Superficial fibular (peroneal) nerve

Deep fibular (peroneal) nerve

Fibularis (peroneus) longus muscle

Extensor digitorum longus muscle

Fibularis (peroneus) brevis muscle and tendon

Fibularis (peroneus) longus tendon

Perforating branch of fibular (peroneal) artery

Anterior lateral malleolar artery

Lateral malleolus and arterial network

Lateral tarsal artery and lateral branch of deep fibular (peroneal) nerve

Extensor digitorum brevis and extensor hallucis brevis muscles (*cut*)

Fibularis (peroneus) brevis tendon

Posterior perforating branches from deep plantar arch

Extensor digitorum longus tendons (*cut*)

Extensor digitorum brevis tendons (*cut*)

Dorsal digital arteries

Branches of proper plantar digital arteries and nerves

Superior medial genicular artery

Quadriceps femoris tendon

Tibial collateral ligament

Medial patellar retinaculum

Infrapatellar branch of saphenous nerve (*cut*)

Inferior medial genicular artery

Saphenous nerve (*cut*)

Patellar ligament

Insertion of sartorius tendon

Anterior tibial recurrent artery and recurrent branch of deep peroneal nerve

Interosseous membrane

Tibialis anterior muscle (*cut*)

Gastrocnemius muscle

Soleus muscle

Tibia

Superficial fibular (peroneal) nerve (*cut*)

Extensor hallucis longus muscle and tendon (*cut*)

Interosseous membrane

Anterior medial malleolar artery

Medial malleolus and arterial network

Dorsalis pedis artery

Tibialis anterior tendon

Medial tarsal artery

Medial branch of deep fibular (peroneal) nerve

Arcuate artery

Deep plantar artery

Dorsal metatarsal arteries

Extensor hallucis longus tendon (*cut*)

Extensor hallucis brevis tendon (*cut*)

Dorsal digital branches of deep fibular (peroneal) nerve

Figure 13.7. Muscles of leg (deep dissection): Anterior view. (*Netter illustration from www.netterimages.com. Copyright Elsevier Inc. All rights reserved.*)

- Can be transferred as a pedicle flap or free flap; partial flap loss due to venous congestion is the most common complication in a reverse sural artery flap.
  - Fibula flap
    - Arterial supply: Peroneal artery
    - Often used for bony defect reconstruction
    - Can be taken with a skin paddle with osteoseptocutaneous perforators from peroneal artery or harvested with a segment of soleus muscle as an osteomyocutaenous peroneal artery combined flap
  - Medial plantar artery flap
    - Arterial supply: Medial plantar artery
    - Nerve: Medial plantar n. (L4 to 5)
    - Most reliable sensate flap with glabrous skin for coverage of the plantar calcaneus
    - Flap elevation landmarks: Comes from the instep of the foot between the head of the first metatarsal and the midpoint of the heel
  - First dorsal metatarsal artery (FDMA) flap
    - Arterial supply: FDMA from dorsalis pedis a.
    - FDMA is also the most common primary arterial blood supply to the great toe or second toe flap, which is used in toe-to-thumb transfer.

4. Diabetic ulcers
   - Primary etiology: Peripheral neuropathy
   - Not associated with large vessel atherosclerosis
5. Arterial insufficiency
   - Symptoms: Claudication and rest pain
   - Degree of insufficiency often correlates with the ankle–brachial pressure index (ABI).
     - Normal ABI range 0.90 to 1.20
       - Patients with diabetes often have falsely elevated ABIs because of arterial calcifications that make vessels relatively noncompressible.
     - 0.50 to 0.80: Moderate disease, may develop ulcers
     - <0.50: Severe disease, often requires intervention
       - Ulcers associated with an ABI <0.45 generally do not heal without revascularization.
   - Arterial duplex scanning can also be used to evaluate arterial flow.
     - Triphasic waveforms are considered normal flow.
     - Biphasic or triphasic arterial waveforms are usually consistent with sufficient vascularity for wound healing.
     - Monophasic waveforms are associated with extremity ischemia.
       - If there is good amplitude and a narrow waveform complex, monophasic waveforms are not necessarily a contraindication for soft-tissue reconstruction.
   - In patients with arterial calcifications, absolute toe pressures are a better indicator of ischemia than ABIs because digital vessels are frequently spared from calcification.
     - A toe pressure <30 mm Hg indicates ischemia and requires a vascular intervention before soft-tissue reconstruction.

6. Venous stasis ulcers
   - Pathophysiology: Venous valve incompetence → chronic venous hypertension → elevated capillary hydrostatic pressure → fluid and protein leakage into the extracellular space → impaired oxygen transport to tissues → localized cellular necrosis and ulceration
   - Management: Compression of the edematous limb
     - Compression reduces interstitial edema and tissue pressure, which improves oxygen delivery and enhances wound healing.
     - Open wounds are best treated with an absorptive and occlusive dressing.
       - For example, Unna boots
7. Nerve injury/compression (see Figure 13.8)
   - Common peroneal n.
     - Origin: Sciatic n. (L4 to S3)
     - Innervates: Anterior and lateral leg compartments, extensor digitorum brevis
     - Branches
       - Superficial peroneal n.
         - ◆ Motor: Peroneus longus and peroneus brevis m.
         - ◆ Sensory: Anterolateral leg, skin of dorsum of foot (1st dorsal web space spared)
         - ◆ Injury/palsy: Inability to evert foot, numbness along distal anterolateral leg with sparing of 1st web space
       - Deep peroneal n.
         - ◆ Motor: Extensor hallucis longus and brevis m., tibialis anterior, extensor digitorum longus and brevis m., peroneus tertius m.
         - ◆ Sensory: 1st dorsal web space
         - ◆ Injury/palsy: Inability to dorsiflex/foot drop, numbness in 1st dorsal web space
     - Etiology of neuropathy
       - Lateral gastrocnemius harvest
       - Bed rest
       - Hyperflexion of the knee
       - Habitual leg crossing
     - Injury/palsy leads to foot drop and numbness within the 1st web space.
       - Open injury: Urgent exploration with repair or grafting
       - Closed injury: Evaluate with electromyography (EMG) and nerve conduction studies (NCSs) 3 to 4 weeks postinjury, repeat studies in 4 weeks if no improvement, explore for decompression if no improvement in 2 to 3 months (see Figure 13.9).
   - Sural nerve
     - Origin: Comprised of tibial nerve (medial sural cutaneous n.) and common peroneal nerve (lateral sural cutaneous n.)
     - Innervates posterolateral leg, lateral foot, and 5th toe
     - Purely sensory
       - Often harvested as nerve graft

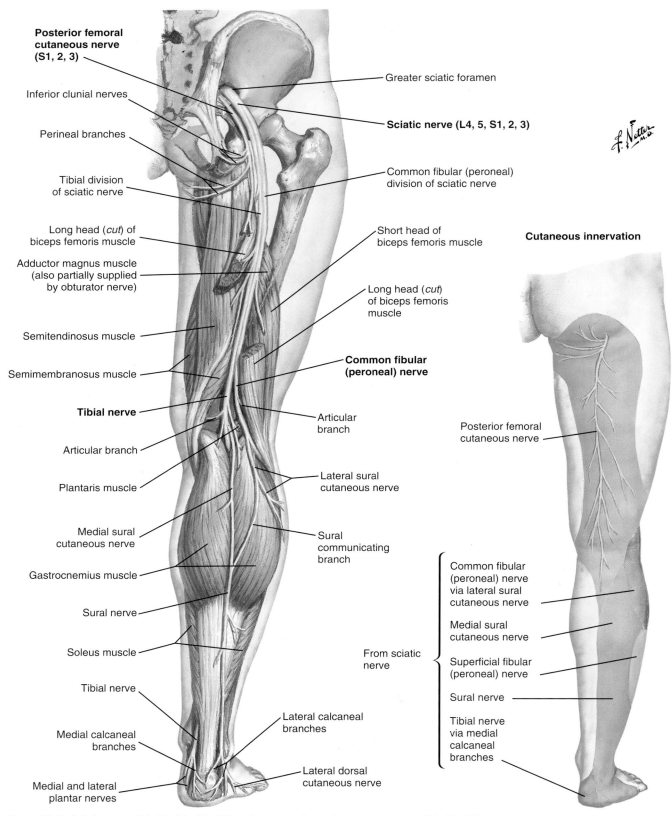

Figure 13.8. Sciatic nerve (L4, L5; S1, S2, S3) and posterior femoral cutaneous nerve (S1, S2, S3). *(Netter illustration from www.netterimages.com. Copyright Elsevier Inc. All rights reserved.)*

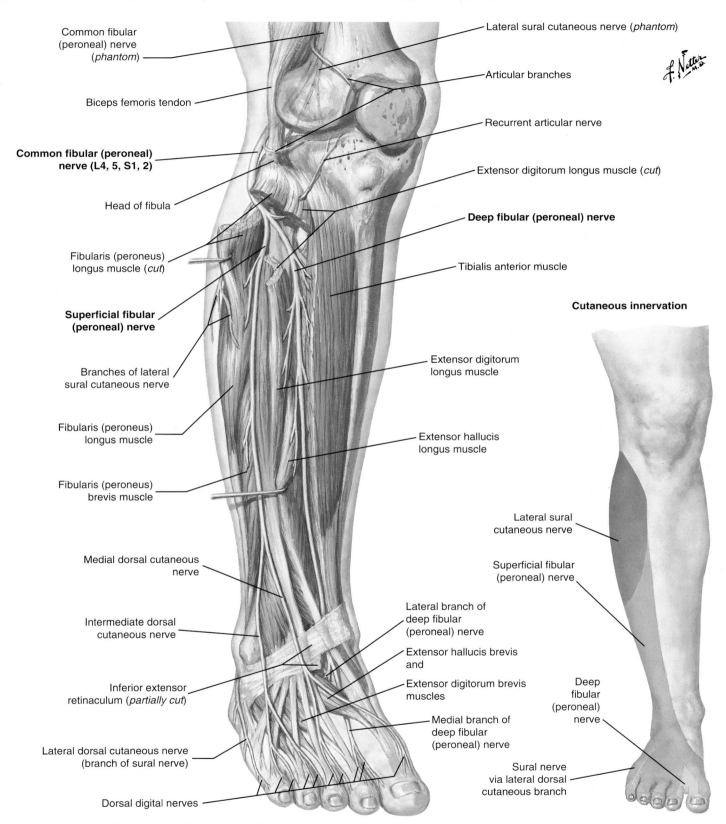

Figure 13.9. Common fibular (peroneal) nerve. (*Netter illustration from www.netterimages.com. Copyright Elsevier Inc. All rights reserved.*)

- Tibial nerve
  - Origin: Sciatic n.
  - Innervates gastrocnemius, popliteus, soleus, plantaris, tibialis posterior, flexor digitorum longus, flexor hallucis longus
  - Branches
    - Medial plantar n.
      - Motor: Abductor hallucis, flexor digitorum brevis, flexor hallucis brevis, 1st lumbrical
      - Sensory: Plantar surface of medial foot, plantar surface of toes 1 to 3, and medial half of toe 4.
      - Injury/palsy: Burning pain and numbness radiating to toes 1 to 3, claw toes
    - Lateral plantar n.
      - Motor: Quadratus plantae, flexor digiti minimi, adductor hallucis, interossei, lumbricals, abductor digiti minimi
      - Sensory: Plantar surface of lateral foot, plantar surface of 5th toe, and lateral half of toe 4
      - Injury/palsy: Burning pain and numbness radiating to toes 4 and 5, claw toes
  - Injury/palsy leads to tarsal tunnel syndrome.
    - Tarsal tunnel is found behind the medial malleolus.
      - Contents include posterior tibial a., tibial n., tendons of the tibialis posterior m., flexor digitorum longus ms., and flexor hallucis longis m.
    - Symptoms: Burning pain and numbness radiating to the toes and heel, claw toes (see Figures 13.10-13.12)
8. Lymphedema
   - Etiology: Inadequate clearance of interstitial fluid → pooling of fluid and protein within the interstitial space → pitting edema (early stage) and nonpitting edema with more fibrotic tissue and adipogenesis (late stage)
   - Diagnosis: Lymphoscintigraphy and exclusion of other causes of peripheral edema (e.g., renal failure, congestive heart failure, venous stasis disease, deep venous thrombosis, etc.)
     - Diagnosis is typically made by thorough history, physical exam, and lymphoscintigraphy.
     - Classic signs
       - Pitting or nonpitting edema
       - Peau d'orange changes in skin
       - Inability to tent skin over toes (Stemmer sign)
       - Blunted appearance of the digits
     - Bilateral LE edema is more likely to be systemic, whereas unilateral edema is more likely to be related to venous insufficiency or lymphedema.
   - Primary lymphedema (less than 1 year old), lymphedema praecox (age of 1 to 35), and lymphedema tarda (older than 35)
   - Secondary lymphedema: Most common cause worldwide is filariasis *(Wucheria bancrofti);* endemic in Africa. The most common cause in western countries is breast-cancer-related lymphedema, which is a sequela of mastectomy, axillary lymph node dissection, and radiation. Radiation, chemotherapy, and obesity are the major risk factors.
   - Management
     - Compression and elevation: Mainstay of management
     - Physical therapy
       - Manual lymphatic drainage
       - Pneumatic pumps
       - Multilayer bandaging
     - Surgical options in carefully selected patients
       - Lymphaticovenous anastomosis
       - Vascularized lymph node flap transfer
       - Excisional surgery including suction lipectomy and debulking procedure or Charles procedure
     - Diuretics are not effective in the treatment of lymphedema.
     - Antibiotics are usually required for the control of infection and cellulitis.

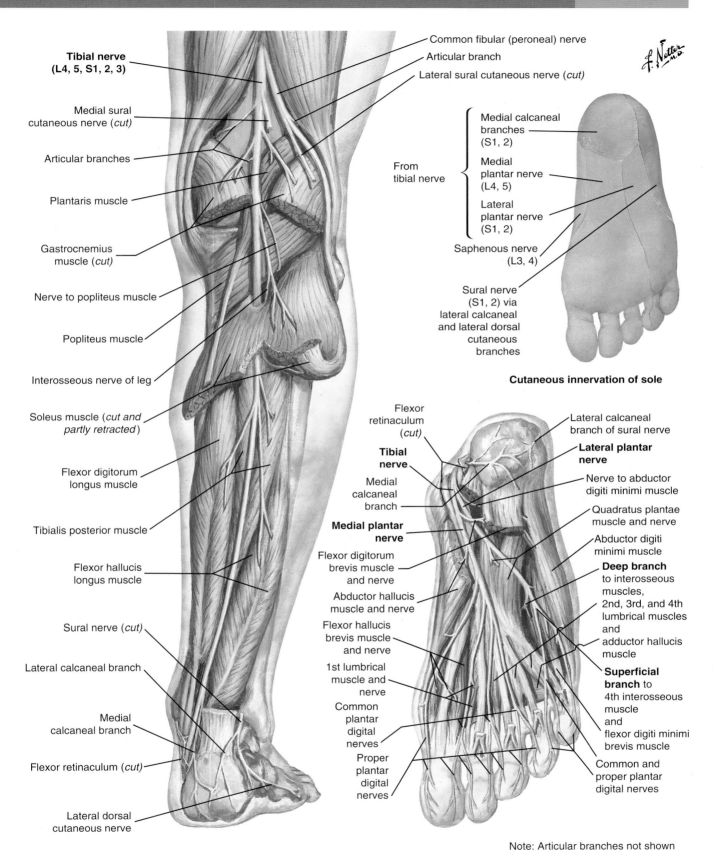

Tibial nerve (L4, 5, S1, 2, 3)

Medial sural cutaneous nerve (*cut*)

Articular branches

Plantaris muscle

Gastrocnemius muscle (*cut*)

Nerve to popliteus muscle

Popliteus muscle

Interosseous nerve of leg

Soleus muscle (*cut and partly retracted*)

Flexor digitorum longus muscle

Tibialis posterior muscle

Flexor hallucis longus muscle

Sural nerve (*cut*)

Lateral calcaneal branch

Medial calcaneal branch

Flexor retinaculum (*cut*)

Lateral dorsal cutaneous nerve

Common fibular (peroneal) nerve

Articular branch

Lateral sural cutaneous nerve (*cut*)

From tibial nerve

{
Medial calcaneal branches (S1, 2)

Medial plantar nerve (L4, 5)

Lateral plantar nerve (S1, 2)
}

Saphenous nerve (L3, 4)

Sural nerve (S1, 2) via lateral calcaneal and lateral dorsal cutaneous branches

Cutaneous innervation of sole

Flexor retinaculum (*cut*)

Tibial nerve

Medial calcaneal branch

Medial plantar nerve

Flexor digitorum brevis muscle and nerve

Abductor hallucis muscle and nerve

Flexor hallucis brevis muscle and nerve

1st lumbrical muscle and nerve

Common plantar digital nerves

Proper plantar digital nerves

Lateral calcaneal branch of sural nerve

Lateral plantar nerve

Nerve to abductor digiti minimi muscle

Quadratus plantae muscle and nerve

Abductor digiti minimi muscle

Deep branch to interosseous muscles, 2nd, 3rd, and 4th lumbrical muscles and adductor hallucis muscle

Superficial branch to 4th interosseous muscle and flexor digiti minimi brevis muscle

Common and proper plantar digital nerves

Note: Articular branches not shown

Figure 13.10. Tibial nerve. *(Netter illustration from www.netterimages.com. Copyright Elsevier Inc. All rights reserved.)*

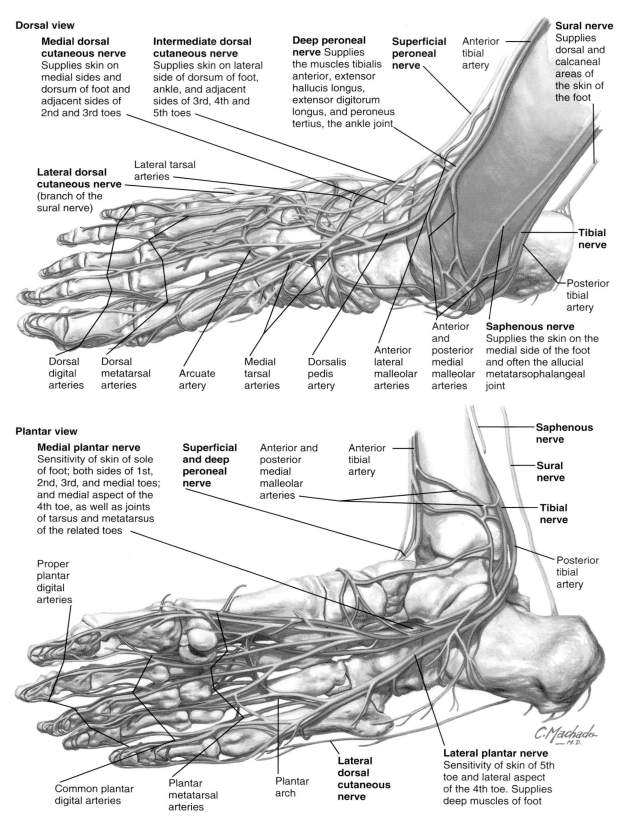

Dorsal view

Medial dorsal cutaneous nerve Supplies skin on medial sides and dorsum of foot and adjacent sides of 2nd and 3rd toes

Intermediate dorsal cutaneous nerve Supplies skin on lateral side of dorsum of foot, ankle, and adjacent sides of 3rd, 4th and 5th toes

Deep peroneal nerve Supplies the muscles tibialis anterior, extensor hallucis longus, extensor digitorum longus, and peroneus tertius, the ankle joint

Superficial peroneal nerve

Anterior tibial artery

Sural nerve Supplies dorsal and calcaneal areas of the skin of the foot

Lateral dorsal cutaneous nerve (branch of the sural nerve)

Lateral tarsal arteries

Tibial nerve

Posterior tibial artery

Dorsal digital arteries

Dorsal metatarsal arteries

Arcuate artery

Medial tarsal arteries

Dorsalis pedis artery

Anterior lateral malleolar arteries

Anterior and posterior medial malleolar arteries

Saphenous nerve Supplies the skin on the medial side of the foot and often the allucial metatarsophalangeal joint

Plantar view

Medial plantar nerve Sensitivity of skin of sole of foot; both sides of 1st, 2nd, 3rd, and medial toes; and medial aspect of the 4th toe, as well as joints of tarsus and metatarsus of the related toes

Superficial and deep peroneal nerve

Anterior and posterior medial malleolar arteries

Anterior tibial artery

Saphenous nerve

Sural nerve

Tibial nerve

Posterior tibial artery

Proper plantar digital arteries

Common plantar digital arteries

Plantar metatarsal arteries

Plantar arch

Lateral dorsal cutaneous nerve

Lateral plantar nerve Sensitivity of skin of 5th toe and lateral aspect of the 4th toe. Supplies deep muscles of foot

C. Machado
—M.D.

Figure 13.11. Anatomy of the foot: Nerves. *(Netter illustration from www.netterimages.com. Copyright Elsevier Inc. All rights reserved.)*

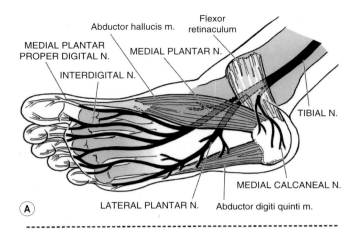

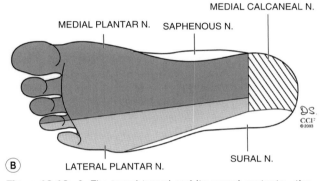

Figure 13.12. A, The tarsal tunnel and its neural contents—the terminal portion of the tibial nerve, medial plantar nerve, lateral plantar nerve, and medial calcaneal nerve—as well as the digital nerves. **B,** The sensory distribution of the five nerves that supply sensation to the sole of the foot. *(Reprinted from Dyck, P.J., Thomas, P.K. [Eds.], 2005. Peripheral Neuropathy, 4th ed. Elsevier, 1487–1510.)*

Suggested Readings

Ali, R.S., Bluebond-Langner, R., Rodriguez, E.D., et al., 2009. The versatility of the anterolateral thigh flap. Plast. Reconstr. Surg. 124 (6 Suppl.), e395–e407.

Baumeister, R.G.D., Chang, D.W., Neligan, P.C., 2013. Chapter 3: Lymphatic reconstruction of the lower extremities. In: Neligan, P.C. (Ed.), Plastic Surgery, 3rd ed. Elsevier, pp. 92–100.

Brem, H., Sheehan, P., Rosenberg, H.J., et al., 2006. Evidence-based protocol for diabetic foot ulcers. Plast. Reconstr. Surg. 117 (7 Suppl.), 193S–209S.

Cheng, M.H., Chen, S.C., Steven, L.H., et al., 2013. Vascularized groin lymph node flap transfer for postmastectomy upper limb lymphedema: flap anatomy, recipient sites, and outcomes. Plast. Reconstr. Surg. 131 (6), 1286–1298.

Cheng, M.H., Huang, J.J., Nguyen, D.H., et al., 2012. A novel approach to the treatment of lower extremity lymphedema by transferring a vascularized submental lymph node flap to the ankle. Gynecol. Oncol. 126 (1), 93–98.

Cheng, M.H., Huang, J.J., Wu, C.W., et al., 2014. The mechanism of vascularized lymph node transfer for lymphedema—natural lymphatico-venous drainage. Plast. Reconstr. Surg. 133 (2), 192e–198e.

Chim, H., Drolet, B., Duffy, K., et al., 2010. Vascular anomalies and lymphedema. Plast. Reconstr. Surg. 126 (2), 55e–69e.

Clemens, M.W., Colen, L.B., Attinger, C.E., 2013. Chapter 8: Foot reconstruction. In: Neligan, P.C. (Ed.), Plastic Surgery, 3rd ed. Elsevier, pp. 189–219.

Colohan, S., Saint-Cyr, M., 2013. Chapter 2: Management of lower extremity trauma. In: Neligan, P.C. (Ed.), Plastic Surgery, 3rd ed. Elsevier, pp. 63–91.

Dellon, A.L., 2013. Chapter 6: Diagnosis and treatment of painful neuroma and of nerve compression in the lower extremity. In: Neligan, P.C. (Ed.), Plastic Surgery, 3rd ed. Elsevier, pp. 151–173.

Fix, R.R., Heinz, T.R., 2010. Chapter 93: Reconstruction of the lower extremity. In: Weinzweig, J. (Ed.), Plastic Surgery Secrets Plus, 2nd ed. Mosby, pp. 610–615.

Follmar, K.E., Baccarani, A., Baumeister, S.P., et al., 2007. The distally based sural flap. Plast. Reconstr. Surg. 119 (6), 138e–148e.

Griffin, J.R., Thornton, J.F., 2003. Low. Extreme. Reconstr. Sel. Readings Plast. Surg. 9, 1–44.

Henry, G.I., Kleiber, G.M., 2013. Chapter 1: Comprehensive lower extremity anatomy. In: Neligan, P.C. (Ed.), Plastic Surgery, 3rd ed. Elsevier, pp. 1–62.

Hijjawi, J.B., Dumanian, G., 2006. The diabetic and the ischemic lower extremity. In: McCarthy, J.G., Galiano, R.D., Boutros, S.G. (Eds.), Current Therapy in Plastic Surgery. Saunders Elsevier, Philadelphia, pp. 658–665.

Hollenbeck, S.T., Toranto, J.D., Taylor, B.J., et al., 2011. Perineal and lower extremity reconstruction. Plast. Reconstr. Surg. 128 (5), 551–563.

Hong, J.P., 2013. Chapter 5: Reconstructive surgery: lower extremity coverage. In: Neligan, P.C. (Ed.), Plastic Surgery, 3rd ed. Elsevier, pp. 127–150.

Hong, J.-P., 2013. Chapter 10: Lower extremity reconstruction. In: Neligan, P.C., Buck, D.W. (Eds.), Core Procedures in Plastic Surgery. Elsevier, pp. 166–184.

Kasabian, A.K., Karp, N.S., 2007. Lower-extremity reconstruction. In: Thorne, C.H., Beasley, R.W., Aston, S.J., et al. (Eds.), Grabb and Smith's Plastic Surgery, 6th ed. Lippincott Williams & Wilkins, Philadelphia, pp. 676–688.

Kovach, S.J., Levin, L.S., 2013. Chapter 7: Skeletal reconstruction. In: Neligan, P.C. (Ed.), Plastic Surgery, 3rd ed. Elsevier, pp. 174–188.

Lin, C.H., Ali, R., Chen, S.C., et al., 2009. Vascularized groin lymph node transfer using the wrist as a recipient site for management of postmastectomy upper extremity lymphedema. Plast. Reconstr. Surg. 123 (4), 1265–1275.

Lu, T.C., Lin, C.H., Lin, C.H., et al., 2011. Versatility of the pedicled peroneal artery perforator flaps for soft-tissue coverage of the lower leg and foot defects. J. Plast. Reconstr. Aesthet. Surg. 64 (3), 386–393.

Mackinnon, S.E., Dellon, A.L., 1988. Tarsal tunnel syndrome. In: Surgery of the Peripheral Nerve. Thieme Publishing Group, New York, pp. 305–317.

Mathes, S.J., 1997. Muscle flaps and their blood supply. In: Aston, S.J., Beasley, R.W., Thorne, C.H. (Eds.), Grabb & Smith's Plastic Surgery, 5th ed. Lippincott-Raven, Philadelphia, pp. 61–72.

Medina, N.D., Kovach, S.J., Levin, L.S., 2011. An evidence-based approach to lower extremity acute trauma. Plast. Reconstr. Surg. 127 (2), 926–931.

Microsurgery Atlas, Techniques and Principles. Found at: <http://www.microsurgeon.org.> Accessed on: July 2, 2014.

Suami, H., Chang, D.W., 2010. Overview of surgical treatments for breast cancer-related lymphedema. Plast. Reconstr. Surg. 126 (6), 1853–1863.

Teo, T.C., 2010. The propeller flap concept. Clin. Plast. Surg. 37 (4), 615–626.

Yazar, S., Cheng, M.H., Wei, F.C., et al., 2006. Osteomyocutaneous peroneal artery perforator flap for reconstruction of composite maxillary defects. Head Neck 28 (4), 297–304.

Congenital Hand Disorders

General Embryology

1. Hand development occurs during the 4th to 8th gestational weeks (see Table 14.1).
   - 3 to 4 weeks' gestation: Upper limb bud formation
   - 4 to 5 weeks' gestation: Proximal-to-distal upper limb development
   - By week 5, the upper limb is formed without digital separation.
   - By week 8, complete development of the upper limb and hand occurs.

Table 14.1 Timing of Hand Formation

TIME AFTER FERTILIZATION	HAND DEVELOPMENT
27 days	Development of arm bud
28-30 days	Further development of arm bud
34-36 days	Elongation of arm bud
34-38 days	Formation of hand paddle
38-40 days	Early separation of digits
44-46 days	Digits separated
Week 9-10	Formation of fingernails begins

Reprinted from Neligan, P.C., Chang, J. (Eds.), 2013. Plastic Surgery, vol. 6, 3rd ed. Elsevier, 526–547.

2. Signaling pathways involved in upper limb development (see Table 14.2)

Classification of Congenital Hand Disorders

1. Type I: Failure of formation of parts
   - Includes cases of longitudinal or transverse arrest
2. Type II: Failure of differentiation (separation) of parts
   - Includes all cases of inadequate separation of parts
     - Syndactyly
     - Camptodactyly
     - Clinodactyly
     - Symbrachydactyly
3. Type III: Duplication disorders
   - Includes all cases of duplication
     - Whole limb duplication and/or mirror hand
     - Polydactyly
     - Triphalangeal thumb
4. Type IV: Overgrowth
   - Includes macrodactyly or hemihypertophy
5. Type V: Undergrowth
   - Includes brachydactyly
   - Thumb hypoplasia
6. Type VI: Constriction band syndrome
7. Type VII: Generalized skeletal deformities
   - Includes all generalized syndromes
     - Apert syndrome
     - TAR syndrome
     - Poland syndrome

Table 14.2 Signaling Pathways During Embryogenesis

SIGNALING CENTER	RESPONSIBLE SUBSTANCE	ACTION	ANOMALY
Apical ectodermal ridge	Fibroblast growth factors	Proximal-to-distal limb development, interdigital necrosis	Transverse deficiency
Zone of polarizing activity	Sonic hedgehog protein	Radioulnar limb formation	Mirror hand
Wnt pathway	Transcription factor Lmx-1	Ventral and dorsal limb axis	Nail-patella syndrome, abnormal nail and pulp arrangement

Reprinted from Wolfe, S.W., Hotchkiss, R.N., Pederson, W.C., et al. (Eds.), 2011. Green's Operative Hand Surgery, 6th ed. Elsevier, 1295–1301.

Radial Deficiencies

1. Deficiencies can range from mild thumb hypoplasia to complete absence of the radius.
2. All forms of radial deficiency warrant systemic evaluation for syndromes or associations (see Table 14.3).

Table 14.3 Syndromes Associated with Radial Deficiency

SYNDROME	CHARACTERISTICS
Holt-Oram	Heart defects; most commonly, cardiac septal defects
TAR	Thrombocytopenia–absent radius syndrome; present at birth but improves over time
VACTERL	Vertebral abnormalities, anal atresia, cardiac abnormalities, tracheoesophageal fistula, esophageal atresia, renal defects, radial dysplasia, lower limb abnormalities
Fanconi's anemia	Aplastic anemia not present at birth; develops at about 6 years of age. Fatal without bone marrow transplant; chromosomal challenge test now available for early diagnosis

Reprinted from Wolfe, S.W., Hotchkiss, R.N., Pederson, W.C., et al. (Eds.), 2011. Green's Operative Hand Surgery, 6th ed., Elsevier, 1371–1403.

3. Hypoplastic thumb
   - Occurs most commonly as part of radial deficiency
   - Blauth classification (see Table 14.4)
     - Correlates with degree of deficiency and necessary treatment

Table 14.4 Thumb Deficiency Classification and Treatment Paradigm

TYPE	FINDINGS	TREATMENT
I	Minor generalized hypoplasia	Augmentation or no treatment
II	Absence of intrinsic thenar muscles, first web-space narrowing, UCL insufficiency	Opponensplasty, first web release, UCL reconstruction
III	Similar findings as Type II, extrinsic muscle and tendon abnormalities, skeletal deficiency A: Stable CMC joint B: Unstable CMC joint	A: Reconstruction B: Pollicization
IV	"Pouce flottant," or floating thumb	Pollicization
V	Absence	Pollicization

CMC, Carpometacarpal; UCL, ulnar collateral ligament.
Reprinted from Wolfe, S.W., Hotchkiss, R.N., Pederson, W.C., et al. (Eds.), 2011. Green's Operative Hand Surgery, 6th ed. Elsevier, 1371–1403.

- Treatment
  - The main determinant for thumb reconstruction and/or pollicization is the presence (Type IIIA) or absence (Type IIIB) of a stable carpometacarpal (CMC) joint.
    - Type-IIIA thumb: The child incorporates thumb into routine use.
      - Reconstruction is warranted
      - Great toe to thumb transfer is an excellent option when most of the metacarpal is present.
    - Type-IIIB thumb: Thumb is ignored by child and grasp actions occur between fingers.
      - Pollicization is the procedure of choice.
        - Movement of the metacarpal and neurovascular (NV) pedicle for a finger
        - Also indicated for Type-IV and -V thumbs
- Options to release/deepen the web space
  - 4-flap Z (4Z) plasty (see Figure 14.1)
  - 5 Z (5Z) plasty or "jumping man" flap (see Figure 14.2)

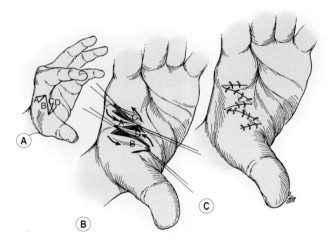

Figure 14.1. The standard four-flap Z (4Z) plasty often used for deepening broader webs such as the thumb web. **A,** Incisions are outlined. **B,** Flaps have been mobilized and crossed. **C,** Closure.
(Copyright, Elizabeth, Martin, 2011. In: Wolfe, S.W., Hotchkiss, R.N., Pederson, W.C., et al. [Eds.], Green's Operative Hand Surgery, 6th ed. Elsevier, 1303–1369.)

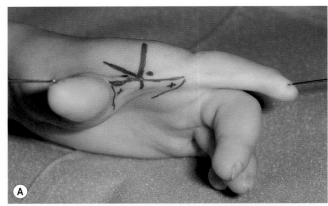

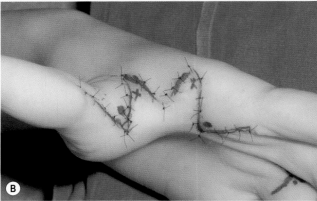

Figure 14.2. A and **B,** Incomplete first web release with 5Z plasty. *(Reprinted from Neligan, P.C., Chang, J. [Eds.], 2013. Plastic Surgery, vol. 6, 3rd ed. Elsevier, 603–633.)*

- Release often involves a combination of full-thickness skin grafts and local flaps.
  - Occasionally, incomplete syndactyly can be closed with local flaps alone.
- Dorsal skin flaps should be used for web-space resurfacing (see Figure 14.3).

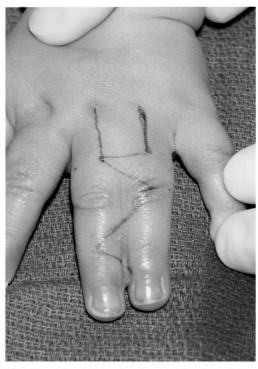

Figure 14.3. A proximally based rectangular flap from the dorsum of the syndactyly is the most frequently used method to reconstruct the commissure. *(Courtesy Shriners Hospitals for Children, Philadelphia. In: Wolfe, S.W., Hotchkiss, R.N., Pederson, W.C., et al. [Eds.], 2011. Green's Operative Hand Surgery, 6th ed. Elsevier, 1303–1369.)*

Syndactyly

1. Failure of differentiation disorder (Type II)
2. Abnormal interconnection between adjacent digits
   - Familial form inherited in an autosomal dominant pattern
3. Classified according to the degree and extent of the interconnection
   - Simple syndactyly involves only skin and fibrous tissue.
   - Complex syndactyly involves skin, fibrous tissue, and bone.
   - Complete syndactyly: The entire length of finger is involved, including the fingertip/nail.
   - Incomplete syndactyly: The fingertip/nail is spared.
   - Complicated syndactyly: Syndactyly that occurs with other anomalies or syndromes (e.g., Apert syndrome)
4. Treatment
   - Separation of border digits by 4 to 6 months of age to limit tethering and growth disturbances
   - Can delay separation of other digits up to 18 months
   - If multiple fingers are involved, release only one side of the digit to prevent vascular compromise.

Camptodactyly

1. Signs: Painless flexion contracture of the small-finger proximal interphalangeal (IP) joint
   - Often progressive
2. Epidemiology
   - Occurs during infancy and adolescence
   - The majority of cases are bilateral.
   - Most often involves the small finger, but other fingers can be affected.
     - Prevalence of finger involvement decreases as you progress to the radial side of the hand.
3. Pathology: Can involve an imbalance of flexion/extension secondary to abnormal lumbrical insertion, tightness of the flexor digitorum superficialis or volar plate, and/or hypoplasia of the finger extensor.

4. Treatment
   - Observation, passive stretching, and splinting
   - Surgery for progressive deformities that are fixed or lead to functional impairment

Clinodactyly

1. Congenital curvature of a digit in the radial-ulnar plane (see Figure 14.4)
   - Most often affects the middle phalanx of the small finger, causing angulation of the distal IP joint.
   - The presence of a C-shaped physis and delta phalanx on imaging is pathognomonic.

2. Epidemiology
   - Familial form is inherited in an autosomal dominant pattern.
   - Nonfamilial form is present in many syndromes and chromosomal abnormalities (e.g., Down syndrome, Apert syndrome).

3. Treatment
   - Observation
   - Surgery is advised for progressive deformities or those with significant angulation (delta phalanx) that can affect functioning of adjacent digits.

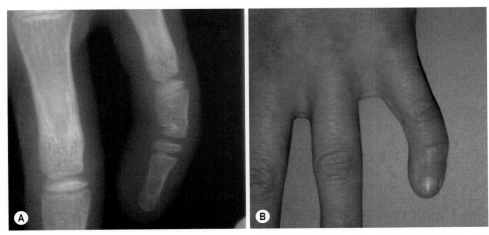

Figure 14.4. Radiograph **(A)** and clinical picture **(B)** of left small finger clinodactyly. *(Reprinted from Wolfe, S.W., Hotchkiss, R.N., Pederson, W.C., et al. [Eds.], 2011. Green's Operative Hand Surgery, 6th ed. Elsevier, 1303–1369.)*

Polydactyly

1. Duplication disorder (Type III)
2. Can be preaxial (radial/thumb) or postaxial (ulnar/small finger)
   - Preaxial duplication is more common in Caucasian patients.
   - Postaxial duplication is more common in patients of African descent.
     - Postaxial duplication in Caucasian patients is often associated with an underlying syndrome or chromosomal abnormality.

3. Postaxial polydactyly
   - Often inherited in an autosomal dominant pattern
   - The supernumerary digit is classified according to degree of development.
     - Type A: Well developed, with articular attachments
       - Requires operative ablation and transfer of the important functional structures to the adjacent finger.
     - Type B: Rudimentary, pedunculated digit, or nubbin
       - Can often be treated with excision or suture ligation at birth.

4. Preaxial polydactyly
   - Most common in Caucasian patients
   - Wassel classification: Thumb duplication (see Table 14.5)

Table 14.5 Classification of Duplicated Thumbs

TYPE	DUPLICATED ELEMENTS
(I)	Bifid distal phalanx
(II)	Duplicated distal phalanx
(III)	Bifid proximal phalanx
(IV)	Duplicated proximal phalanx*
(V)	Bifid metacarpal phalanx
(VI)	Duplicated metacarpal phalanx
(VII)	Triphalangeal component

*Most common type.
Adapted from Wassel, H.D., 1969. The results of surgery for polydactyly of the thumb. A review. Clin. Orthop. Relat. Res. 125, 175-193. Table reprinted from Neligan, P.C., Chang, J. (Eds.), 2013. Plastic Surgery, vol. 6, 3rd ed. Elsevier, 603–633.

- Type IV is most common. Duplicated proximal and distal phalanges with a shared bifid metacarpal head.
  - Treatment requires operative ablation of the radial part, with repositioning and transfer of important functional structures to the ulnar part to construct a properly aligned and functional thumb.
    - The ulnar part is preserved because it is critical to preserve the ulnar collateral ligament (UCL) to stabilize pinch function.
- Type IV: Triphalangeal thumb (see Box 14.1)

BOX 14.1 TRIPHALANGEAL THUMB

- Triphalangeal thumbs can be divided into two distinct forms. The first type has an extra phalanx of variable size within a relatively normal-appearing thumb. The second variety has a fully developed phalanx that lies in the plane of the fingers and is considered a five-fingered hand.
- The inheritance pattern is usually autosomal dominant with variable expressivity and high penetrance. Genetic consultation is warranted.
- The extra phalanx in a triphalangeal thumb may be triangular, trapezoidal, or rectangular in shape. The growth rate of the extra phalanx is variable, and initial treatment consists of observation to assess growth potential.
- A large, wedge-shaped extra phalanx requires fusion of the abnormal phalanx with an adjacent phalanx combined with bone removal. The joint with the greatest motion is preserved and the joint with the least movement is fused.
- A five-fingered hand is treated by pollicization of the nonopposable radial digit.

Reprinted from Wolfe, S.W., Hotchkiss, R.N., Pederson, W.C., et al. (Eds.), 2011. Green's Operative Hand Surgery, 6th ed. Elsevier, 1397.

Mirror Hand (See Figure 14.5 and Box 14.2)

BOX 14.2 MIRROR HAND

- Mirror hand is rare and characterized by symmetric duplication of the limb in the midline. Typically, there is a central digit with three digits on each side and absence of the thumb.
- The forearm often has two ulnae and no radius.
- The etiology has been attributed to transplantation or replication of the zone of polarizing activity from the posterior margin of the limb bud into the anterior region.
- Treatment consists of reduction of the number of digits to four and reconstruction of a thumb from the deleted digits.

Reprinted from Wolfe, S.W., Hotchkiss, R.N., Pederson, W.C., et al. (Eds.), 2011. Green's Operative Hand Surgery, 6th ed. Elsevier, 1321.

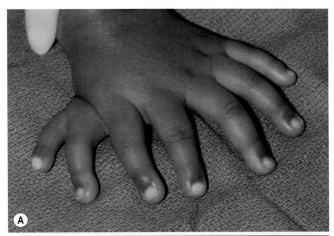

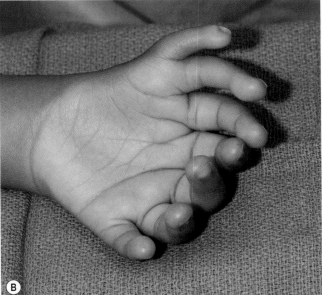

Figure 14.5. A and **B,** One-year-old girl with a left mirror hand and seven digits. *(Courtesy Shriners Hospitals for Children, Philadelphia. In: Wolfe, S.W., Hotchkiss, R.N., Pederson, W.C., et al. [Eds.], 2011. Green's Operative Hand Surgery, 6th ed. Elsevier, 1303–1369.)*

6. Flatt's classification of macrodactly
   - Type I: Macrodactyly and lipofibromatosis of involved nerve; most common form
   - Type II: Macrodactyly and neurofibromatosis
   - Type III: Macrodactyly and hyperostosis (e.g., polyostotic fibrous dysplasia)
   - Type IV: Macrodactyly and hemihypertrophy (e.g., Klippel-Trenaunay syndrome)
7. Treatment options include digital nerve stripping, epiphysiodesis, staged debulking, bulk reduction, and ray amputation as a last resort.

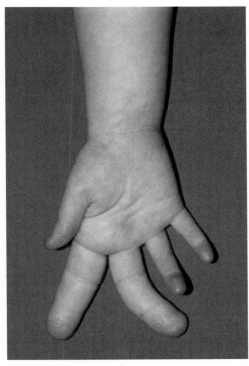

Figure 14.6. Macrodactyly. *(Reprinted from Wolfe, S.W., Hotchkiss, R.N., Pederson, W.C., et al. [Eds.], 2011. Green's Operative Hand Surgery, 6th ed. Elsevier, 1303–1369.)*

Macrodactyly (See Figure 14.6)

1. Overgrowth disorder (Type IV)
2. Characterized by overgrowth of all structures in the involved digit, including bone and soft tissue.
3. Can affect one digit or multiple digits, typically on the radial side of the hand.
4. Two major forms: Static and progressive (more common)
   - Static: Enlarged digit is present at birth and grows proportionately over time.
   - Progressive: Enlargement begins in childhood and the involved digits increase in size throughout growth until physical closure occurs with skeletal maturity.
5. Most commonly an isolated anomaly
   - Can occur with other syndromes, including neurofibromatosis and Klippel-Trenaunay syndrome.

Brachydactyly (See Figure 14.7)

1. Undergrowth disorder (Type V)
2. Characterized by shortening of the digit or ray within the hand.
3. Impact of brachydactyly is dependent on the degree of shortening, number of digits involved, and presence of associated anomalies (e.g., syndactyly, clinodactyly, symphalangism).
   - Treatment of isolated brachydactyly can include lengthening via bone graft, distraction osteogenesis, or toe epiphysis transfer.
     - Surgery is often indicated only for significant functional deficits because lengthening can lead to stiffness or joint contracture of the involved digit.

- For example, lengthening the small and ring fingers to restore power grip, pinch, and opposition
- In this setting, surgery is typically performed between 8 and 12 months of age.

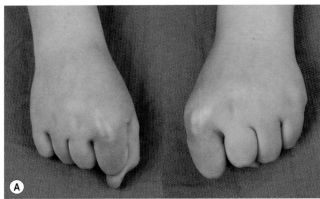

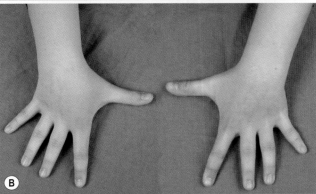

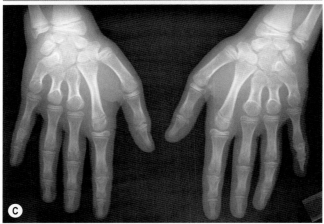

Figure 14.7. Ten year old with isolated bilateral short long-, ring-, and small-finger metacarpals. **A,** Loss of knuckle contour on fist formation. **B,** Shortened long, ring, and small fingers apparent on hand opening. **C,** X rays with shortened long-, ring-, and small-finger metacarpals. *(Courtesy Shriners Hospitals for Children, Philadelphia. In: Wolfe, S.W., Hotchkiss, R.N., Pederson, W.C., et al. [Eds.], 2011. Green's Operative Hand Surgery, 6th ed. Elsevier, 1303–1369.)*

Central Hand Deficiencies

See Figure 14.8, Table 14.6, and Box 14.3.

Table 14.6 Characteristics of a Cleft Hand

TYPICAL CLEFT HAND	ATYPICAL CLEFT HAND (SYMBRACHYDACTYLY)
Autosomal dominant; limbs involved	Sporadic limb involvement (not the feet)
"V"-shaped cleft	"U"-shaped cleft
No finger "nubbins"	Finger nubbins may occur
Syndactyly (especially the first web)	

Reprinted from Wolfe, S.W., Hotchkiss, R.N., Pederson, W.C., et al. (Eds.), 2011. Green's Operative Hand Surgery, 6th ed. Elsevier, 1303–1369.

BOX 14.3 CENTRAL HAND DEFICIENCIES

- True cleft hand is distinct from atypical cleft hand, which is recognized as part of the teratologic sequence of symbrachydactyly.
- Cleft hand is commonly inherited as an autosomal dominant trait and is associated with split hand/split foot (SHSF) and ectrodactyly, ectodermal dysplasia, and cleft lip/palate (EEC) syndrome.
- Surgery is considered for a variety of indications, including progressive widening of the cleft secondary to transverse lying bones, a narrowed first web space, and the widened cleft.
- Indications for early surgery are separation of syndactyly between digits of unequal length, especially the thumb and index finger, and removal of the transverse bones that result in progressive widening of the cleft.
- In cases of thumb–index finger syndactyly, the first web space requires reconstruction. The technique depends on the severity of the syndactyly. Complete syndactyly can be released and the cleft closed in a single setting. The skin from the cleft is rotated into the first web space to create supple tissue.

Reprinted from Wolfe, S.W., Hotchkiss, R.N., Pederson, W.C., et al. (Eds.), 2011. Green's Operative Hand Surgery, 6th ed. Elsevier, 1337.

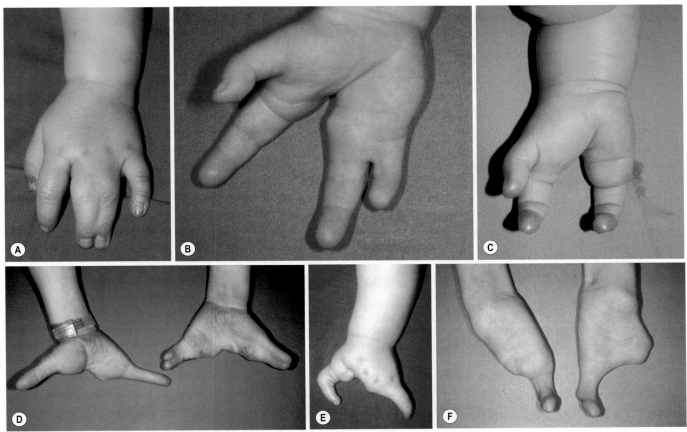

Figure 14.8. A-F, These images illustrate the Manske and Halikis classification and also some aspects of the teratologic sequence in cleft hand. **A,** Type-I hand with a normal web space between the thumb and index finger. A very minor cleft is present between the second and third rays as is syndactyly between the third and fourth rays. **B,** Type-IIA hand in which the thumb web space is mildly narrowed. Note the suppression of the central ray with a deep cleft and minor syndactyly between the ring finger and the little finger. **C,** Type-IIB cleft hand with a severely narrowed first web space and deletion of the third and fourth rays. **D,** Type-III cleft hand (untreated) on the right side and Type-IV cleft hand on the left. On the right side, the thumb and index fingers have untreated syndactyly that completely obliterates the first web space. The central ray is absent, and the fourth and fifth rays are also syndactylized. **E,** Type-IV cleft hand with a merged web space. The two border rays are present, but the index ray and other central rays are suppressed, and the first web space merges with the cleft. **F,** Bilateral Type-V cleft hands. The thumb web space and the thumb are absent, and only the ulnar digit remains. *(Reprinted from Wolfe, S.W., Hotchkiss, R.N., Pederson, W.C., et al. [Eds.], 2011. Green's Operative Hand Surgery, 6th ed. Elsevier, 1303–1369.)*

Amniotic Band Syndrome (See Figure 14.9)

1. A Type-VI congenital hand disorder
2. Characterized by complete or incomplete circumferential constrictions that can lead to amputation, near amputation with distal edema, or ischemia.
   - Can see secondary acrosyndactyly of the involved digits with distal fusion and a proximal sinus between them.
3. Embryology
   - Sporadic disorders
   - Most commonly affect the central long fingers
   - Risk factors: Prematurity, low birth weight, young multigravida mothers, and oligohydramnios
4. Pathology: Entrapment of developing embryonic tissue by amniotic bands
5. Treatment
   - Mild constriction rings: Excision and Z plasty
   - Acrosyndactyly: Follow standard techniques for release of syndactyly, with excision of the proximal sinus.
   - If overt distal ischemia is present, emergent surgical release may be appropriate and amputation required.

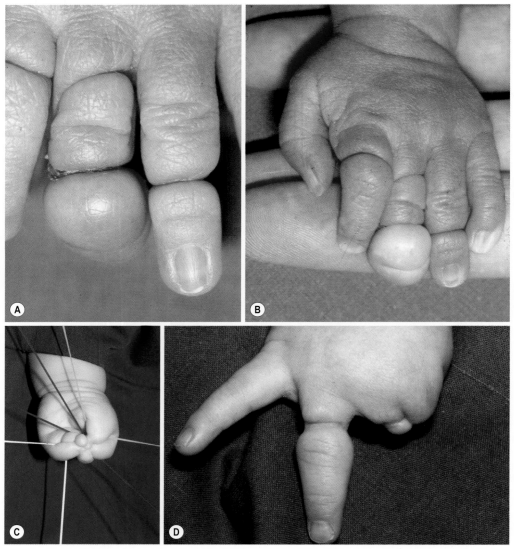

Figure 14.9. Manifestations of the amniotic disruption sequence. **A,** Typical ring constrictions of digits. **B,** Pallor of the finger distal to the ring constriction in a neonate. **C,** Acrosyndactyly with the digits fused at their distal parts and proximal cutaneous clefts. **D,** Amputation secondary to constriction rings. *(Reprinted from Wolfe, S.W., Hotchkiss, R.N., Pederson, W.C., et al. [Eds.], 2011. Green's Operative Hand Surgery, 6th ed. Elsevier, 1303–1369.)*

Apert Syndrome

1. Generalized congenital skeletal/hand disorders (Type VII)
2. Apert syndrome (acrocephalosyndactyly): Combination of bicoronal craniosynostosis, midfacial hypoplasia, and severe complex syndactyly of the hands and feet
3. Pathology: Mutation of the fibroblast growth factor receptor Type-2 gene *(FGFR2)*
4. Often characterized by complex, complete syndactyly of the index, long, and ring fingers (see Figure 14.10).
5. Classification of the Apert hand deformity (see Table 14.7)

Table 14.7 Classification of the Apert Hand Deformity

	FIRST WEB	CENTRAL MASS	FOURTH WEB
Type I: "Obstetrician" or "spade" hand	Incomplete simple syndactyly	Digital mass flat in the palmar plane, good MPJs with variable degree of symphalangism at the IPJs	Incomplete simple syndactyly
Type II: "Mitten" or "spoon" hand	Complete simple syndactyly	The digital mass forms a palmar concavity with splaying of the metacarpals proximally, tight fusion of the fingertips distally, and synonychia of the central digital mass	Complete simple syndactyly
Type III: "Hoof" or "rosebud" hand	Complete complex syndactyly	The thumb is incorporated into the mass, which is tightly cupped; synonychia of all digits apart from the small finger; skeletal abnormalities of the index ray, complicated by paronychial infections and maceration of the palmar skin	Simple syndactyly, usually with synostosis of the fourth and fifth metacarpals

IPJ, *Interphalangeal joint*; MPJ, *metacarpophalangeal joint*.
Reprinted from Upton, J., 1991. Apert syndrome: classification and pathologic anatomy of limb abnormalities. Clin. Plast. Surg. 18, 321–355.

6. Treatment: Must be performed in concert with the craniofacial anomalies
   - Goal: Complete separation of the digits and correction of the thumb deformity before two years of age to allow for growth and development
   - Release of the thumb and creation of an adequate first web space is often the first priority, followed by staged release of the finger syndactylies.
     - The distal bifurcation of digital arteries and nerves often seen in the Apert hand makes separation difficult.

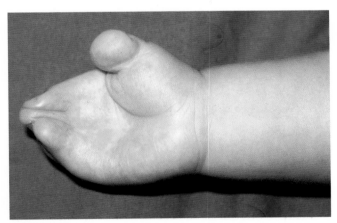

Figure 14.10. Complex multiple syndactyly associated with Apert syndrome. The hand deformity includes complex syndactyly of the index, long, and ring fingers, simple syndactyly between the ring and small fingers, and an incomplete first web space. *(Reprinted from Wolfe, S.W., Hotchkiss, R.N., Pederson, W.C., et al. [Eds.], 2011. Green's Operative Hand Surgery, 6th ed. Elsevier, 1303–1369.)*

Poland Syndrome

1. Generalized congenital skeletal/hand disorder (Type VII)
2. Characterized by absence of the sternal head of pectoralis major muscle and symbrachydactyly (short, fused fingers), often affecting the index, long, and ring fingers (see Figure 14.11).
   - Can also have severe hypoplasia of the chest wall and hand, including breast hypoplasia, aplasia of the pectoralis minor m. and latissimus dorsi m., skeletal thoracic wall abnormalities, and cleft hand.
   - The severity of the hand and chest-wall disorders do not correlate.
3. Treatment of the hand deformity depends on the severity of the disorder.
   - Can include syndactyly release and web-space deepening.

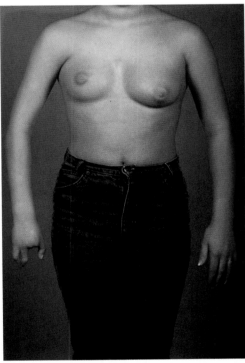

Figure 14.11. Symbrachydactyly and pectoralis major anomaly and smaller breast on the right side. *(Reprinted from Neligan, P.C., Chang, J. [Eds.], 2013. Plastic Surgery, vol. 6, 3rd ed. Elsevier, 603–633.)*

"Congenital" Trigger Fingers

1. Not truly "congenital" and may be present at birth or up to age 3.

2. Can involve any digit, although the thumb is 10 times more likely to be involved.
3. May be difficult to diagnose in infants because they tend to carry their hands with fingers in the clinched position.
4. Characterized by fixed flexion contracture of the IP joint, with a palpable nodule over the flexor pollicis longus tendon ("Notta's node").
   - Presence of Notta's node distinguishes trigger finger from camptodactyly in the small finger.
5. Treatment: Observation or splinting in children younger than 1 year of age; surgical release of the A1 pulley in children older than 3 years.
   - Surgical release of trigger thumb is highly successful, whereas trigger finger release may require additional resection of a slip of the flexor digitorum superficialis tendon if triggering is persistent.

Suggested Readings

Hovius, S.E.R., 2013. Chapter 28: Congenital hand IV: Disorders of differentiation and duplication. In: Neligan, P.C., Chang, J. (Eds.), Plastic Surgery, vol. 6, 3rd ed. Elsevier, China, pp. 603–633.

Kay, S.P., McCombe, D.B., Kozin, S.H., 2011. Chapter 40: Deformities of the hand and fingers. In: Wolfe, S.W., Hotchkiss, R.N., Pederson, W.C., et al. (Eds.), Green's Operative Hand Surgery, 6th ed. Elsevier, Philadelphia, pp. 1303–1369.

Kozin, S.H., 2003. Upper-extremity congenital anomalies. J. Bone. Joint. Surg. Am. 85, 1564–1576.

Kozin, S.H., 2011. Chapter 41: Deformities of the thumb. In: Wolfe, S.W., Hotchkiss, R.N., Pederson, W.C., et al. (Eds.), Green's Operative Hand Surgery, 6th ed. Elsevier, Philadelphia, pp. 1371–1403.

Kozin, S.H., 2011. Chapter 39: Embryology of the upper extremity. In: Wolfe, S.W., Hotchkiss, R.N., Pederson, W.C., et al. (Eds.), Green's Operative Hand Surgery, 6th ed. Elsevier, Philadelphia, pp. 1295–1301.

Tonkin, M., Oberg, M., 2013. Chapter 25: Congenital hand I: Embryology, classification, and principles. In: Neligan, P.C., Chang, J. (Eds.), Plastic Surgery, vol. 6, 3rd ed. Elsevier, China, pp. 526–547.

Upton, J., Taghinia, A., 2013. Chapter 27: Congenital hand III: Disorders of formation—thumb hypoplasia. In: Neligan, P.C., Chang, J. (Eds.), Plastic Surgery, vol. 6, 3rd ed. Elsevier, China, pp. 572–602.

Hand Masses, Vascular Disorders, and Dupuytren's Contracture

Hand Masses

1. Excluding cutaneous malignancies, the majority of hand masses are benign (~95%).
   - Ganglion cysts are the most common mass found on the hand and wrist.
   - Cutaneous malignancies are the most common malignant masses found on the hand and wrist (accounting for 90% of all hand malignancies).
     - Squamous cell carcinoma > basal cell carcinoma > melanoma
   - Enchondroma is the most common bone tumor found in the hand.
   - Although rare, chondrosarcoma is the most common malignant bone tumor found in the hand.
   - Epitheliod sarcoma is the most common malignant soft-tissue sarcoma found in the hand.
2. Evaluation of hand masses
   - Thorough history and physical examination
     - Include examination of regional nodal basins if concerned for malignancy
   - Imaging studies
     - X ray: Useful for evaluation of bony definition
     - Computed tomography (CT) scan: Better bony resolution than plain radiographs, useful for anatomical evaluation of soft-tissues and when plain radiographs are equivocal
     - Magnetic resonance imaging (MRI): Better soft-tissue resolution than CT scan, useful for determining the exact location of gross involvement
     - Ultrasound: Useful in determining if lesion is cystic or solid
     - Bone scan: Useful in assessing for bony metastases or osteomyelitis
   - Tissue biopsy
     - Aspiration or core needle biopsy: Useful for lesions with a cystic component

- Core needle biopsy: Useful for cell sampling of a lesion before formal excision or to assist in determining best method of treatment
- Incisional biopsy: Useful for lesions that are too large to be excised completely without affecting adjacent structures
- Excisional biopsy: Complete excisional biopsy is the preferred method but may not be the best primary diagnostic approach (e.g., when excision could compromise function or cosmesis).
  - Careful consideration of incision placement is critical in the event that further resection is necessary (e.g., most incisions should be placed longitudinally).
- When performing a biopsy for an unknown diagnosis, the extremity should not be exsanguinated.

Common Benign Hand Masses

1. Ganglion cyst (see Figure 15.1)
   - Most common soft-tissue mass in the hand and wrist
   - Etiology: Mucoid degeneration
   - Characterized by pseudocysts (not epithelial lined) that are closely connected to a joint or tendon sheath and filled with mucinous material
   - Most common locations (in order of frequency)
     - Dorsal wrist: Emanates from scapholunate ligament
     - Volar wrist: Emanates from radioscaphocapitate ligament or scaphotriquetral ligament
       - Often in close proximity to radial artery and venae comitantes
     - Flexor tendon sheath
     - Dorsal distal interphalangeal (DIP) joint: Mucous cysts
   - Treatment
     - Aspiration and corticosteroid injection
       - High recurrence rate
     - Excision of the cyst stalk and debridement of the origin

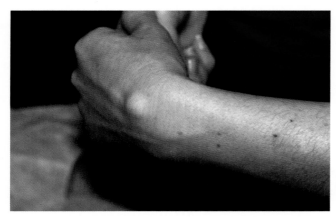

Figure 15.1. Ganglion cyst. The cyst is a mucinous-filled structure associated with joint capsules, tendons, and tendon sheaths. The etiology of these cystic structures is presumed to be secondary to synovial herniation and trauma. *(Reprinted from Neligan, P.C., Chang, J., [Eds.], 2013. Plastic Surgery, vol. 6, 3rd ed. Elsevier, 311.)*

2. Mucous cyst (see Figure 15.2)
   - Ganglion cyst that originates from the DIP joint and is present on the dorsal aspect of the distal phalanx
   - Frequently associated with arthritis of the DIP joint and osteophyte formation
   - If the mucous cyst affects the germinal matrix, it can cause nail plate grooving.
     - Cyst treatment will resolve nail plate issues.
   - Treatment
     - Elevation of the terminal extensor tendon, debridement of the cyst origin at the DIP joint, and removal of any associated osteophytes

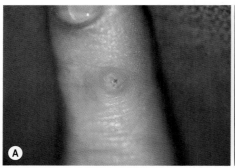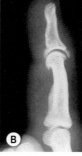

Figure 15.2. Mucous cyst. **A,** Ganglions found on the dorsal proximal interphalangeal joint associated with osteoarthritis are termed mucous cysts. **B,** To treat this clinical entity completely, must perform excision of the cyst along with excision of osteophytes. *(Reprinted from Neligan, P.C., Chang, J., [Eds.], 2013. Plastic Surgery, vol. 6, 3rd ed. Elsevier, 311.)*

3. Epidermal inclusion cyst (see Figure 15.3)
   - Often caused by penetrating trauma and located on the tactile surfaces of the hands
   - As it grows in size, it can cause pressure erosion of the underlying bone.
   - Treatment: Excision is the mainstay of treatment.
     - Complete cyst wall removal reduces risk for recurrence.
     - In cases of significant pressure erosion of bone, bone grafting may be necessary.

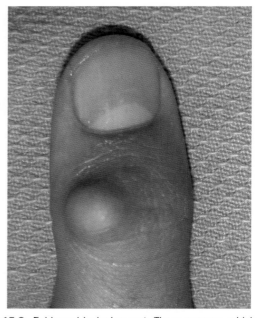

Figure 15.3. Epidermal inclusion cyst. These masses, which originate from an invagination of epithelium, can follow trauma, injection, or an incision. The epithelium is internalized, resulting in subcutaneous keratin deposition. *(Reprinted from Neligan, P.C., Chang, J., [Eds.], 2013. Plastic Surgery, vol. 6, 3rd ed. Elsevier, 311.)*

4. Lipoma
   - Very common benign fatty tumor
   - Lipomas in the hand may cause peripheral nerve compression with growth.
   - Most commonly located within the thenar eminence of the hand
   - MRI is useful for differentiating lipomas from other hand masses.
   - Treatment: Resection, especially if symptomatic or enlarging
5. Giant cell tumor (see Figure 15.4)
   - Benign nodular tumor found on the tendon sheath
     - Most commonly found on the palmar surface of the index and long fingers.
     - Second most common soft-tissue tumor of the hand and fingers
   - Signs: Nontender, firm, enlarging nodular mass that does not transilluminate
   - Histology: Proliferating histiocytes with multinucleated giant cells

- Treatment: Marginal excision
  - High recurrence rate, even with excision

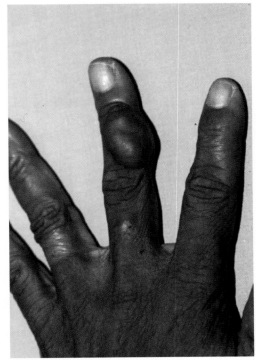

Figure 15.4. Giant cell tumor (pigmented villonodular synovitis). A benign tumor containing multinucleated giant cells and xanthoma cells found in synovial fluid-producing sites such as joints, capsular ligaments, and tendon sheaths. *(Reprinted from Neligan, P.C., Chang, J., [Eds.], 2013. Plastic Surgery, vol. 6, 3rd ed. Elsevier, 311.)*

6. Pyogenic granuloma (see Figure 15.5)
   - Benign reactive vascular tumor frequently found on the upper arms and hands
   - Characterized by a rapidly growing, reddish nodule that is friable and frequently ulcerates and bleeds
   - Treatment: Excision of the lesion with a margin of normal appearing tissue, shaving of the lesion, and coagulation of the tumor base

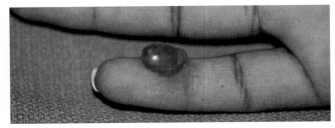

Figure 15.5. Pyogenic granuloma. Rapidly progressing benign vascular lesion commonly found in the finger. Etiology is unknown. *(Reprinted from Neligan, P.C., Chang, J., [Eds.], 2013. Plastic Surgery, vol. 6, 3rd ed. Elsevier, 311.)*

7. Schwannoma (see Figure 15.6)
   - Most common benign, solitary, peripheral nerve tumor
   - Characterized by asymptomatic masses along the course of a peripheral nerve that are mobile in the transverse direction
     - Typically without sensory or motor deficits, although paresthesias can occur
   - MRI often demonstrates a homogenous "egg-shaped" lesion within the nerve.
   - Treatment: Enucleation without disruption of the nerve fascicles

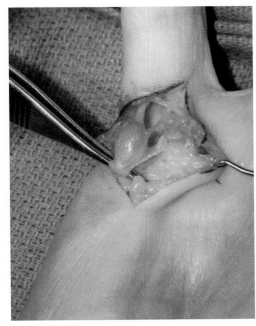

Figure 15.6. Schwannoma/neurilemmoma. This soft-tissue mass arises from Schwann cells and is typically found on the volar surface of the hand and forearm. *(Reprinted from Neligan, P.C., Chang, J., [Eds.], 2013. Plastic Surgery, vol. 6, 3rd ed. Elsevier, 311.)*

8. Enchondroma
   - Most common primary bone tumor
   - Arises from cartilage and most commonly occurs in the proximal phalanx, followed by the metacarpals and/or the middle phalanges
   - X rays typically demonstrate a well-defined radiolucency within the metaphysis or diaphysis, often with a sclerotic rim and/or scalloping of the endosteal cortex.
   - Enchondromas can lead to pathologic fractures.
   - Treatment: Curettage of the lesion and fracture repair when necessary

9. Osteoid osteoma
   - Benign, bone-forming tumor of osteoblast origin
   - Typically affects the distal radius, carpus, and/or phalanges
   - Characterized by a persistent, painful hand mass that is relieved by nonsteroidal antiinflammatory drugs (NSAIDs)
   - X rays typically demonstrate bone sclerosis around a central lucency.
   - Treatment: Observation and NSAIDs; curettage or surgical resection may be curative
10. Osteochondroma (see Figure 15.7)
    - Most common bone tumor in the pediatric population
    - Arises from the bony surface near the epiphysis and contains bone with a cartilage cover
    - Characterized by a firm, fixed, painless mass near joints
      - Can occasionally cause pain with activity, or paresthesias, depending on location
    - May present with a solitary mass or multiple masses
      - Familial pattern inherited in an autosomal dominant manner and presents with multiple osteochondromas
      - Solitary lesions are typically benign, whereas the risk of malignant transformation is greatest for familial osteochondromas.
    - Treatment
      - Observation
        - Indicated for small, asymptomatic osteochondromas with a benign appearance on imaging studies
      - Surgical resection
        - Indicated for large, symptomatic osteochondromas (e.g., pain, functional limitations, sensory deficits, etc.) or any osteochondroma that has a malignant appearance on imaging studies (e.g., thick cartilage cap, growth, etc.)

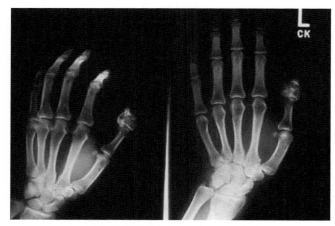

Figure 15.7. Osteochondroma. The most common benign bone tumor. Seen here in the distal phalanx of the thumb, it is a benign bone prominence with a cartilage cap. *(Reprinted from Neligan, P.C., Chang, J., [Eds.], 2013. Plastic Surgery, vol. 6, 3rd ed. Elsevier, 311.)*

Malignant Hand Masses

1. Cutaneous malignancy
   - Most common malignant masses found on the hand and wrist
     - Squamous cell carcinoma > basal cell carcinoma > melanoma
   - See Chapter 24 for more specific information on cutaneous malignancies.
   - General treatment guidelines for cutaneous malignancies of the hand: Wide local excision with negative margins
     - Mohs micrographic surgery may be useful at anatomically sensitive areas.
     - Amputation at the level of the joint proximal to the lesion is often indicated when the tumor involves bone or the nail bed.
     - Sentinel lymph node biopsy may be indicated depending on pathologic features, depth, and tumor characteristics.
2. Epithelioid sarcoma
   - Most common soft-tissue sarcoma in the hand
   - Characterized by a painless nodule on the volar aspect of the hand that can ulcerate
   - High risk of proximal spread and metastasis to lymph nodes
   - Treatment: Wide excision or amputation and adjuvant radiation therapy
     - Sentinel lymph node biopsy may be necessary.
     - Adjuvant chemotherapy is considered for recurrent or metastatic disease.
3. Chondrosarcoma
   - Most common primary malignant bone tumor of the hand
   - Arises from cartilage cells near joints or can develop from malignant transformation of benign cartilaginous tumors (e.g., enchondromas or osteochondromas)
   - Most commonly affects the metacarpals and proximal phalanges of men older than 60.
   - Characterized by slow-growing, firm, painful masses
   - X rays demonstrate poorly defined lesions with lytic areas and stippled calcifications.
   - Most common site of metastasis: Lung
   - Treatment: Excision or amputation depending on the location and size
4. Osteosarcoma
   - Most common pediatric bone tumor, although rarely affects the hands in children
   - Hand osteosarcoma typically affects the proximal phalanges and metacarpals of patients older than 40.
   - Characterized by painful, rapidly enlarging masses
   - X rays demonstrate intramedullary lesions with sclerotic and lytic areas and overlying periosteal elevation ("sunburst").
   - Treatment: Excision or amputation with adjuvant or neoadjuvant chemotherapy
5. Ewing sarcoma
   - Rare, malignant bone tumor that most commonly affects the metacarpals or phalanges

- Histology reveals characteristic sheets of small, round cells.
- Characterized by pain, swelling, and systemic symptoms (fever, leukocytosis)
- X rays demonstrate a characteristic "onion skin" pattern along the cortex.
- Treatment: Chemotherapy (neoadjuvant and adjuvant) and surgical excision
  - Ewing sarcomas are also radiosensitive, although radiation is rarely used for hand tumors.
6. Synovial sarcoma
  - Aggressive, malignant tumor that arises from a joint, tendon, or bursae
  - Characterized by a painful mass near a joint that can have a period of slow or rapid growth
  - Most commonly affects the carpus in the hand
  - High rate of lymph node metastases (~25%)
  - Treatment: Wide surgical excision or amputation with adjuvant radiation therapy

Vascular Tumors of the Hand

1. Vascular aneurysm
  - Typically arises following blunt trauma
    - Example: Hypothenar hammer syndrome
      - Arises from repeated blunt trauma to hypothenar region of the hand and ulnar artery (e.g., hand usage of manual laborers, carpenters, etc.)
      - May have an associated ulnar neuropathy from compression of the ulnar nerve within Guyon's canal or digital ischemia from spasm ulnar artery thrombus or distal emboli
  - Characterized by a gradually enlarging mass that may be associated with pain and ischemia
  - Gold standard for diagnosis is an angiogram
  - May be true aneurysm or false aneurysm (pseudoaneurysm)
    - True aneurysm contains all three vessel wall layers: Intima, media, adventitia
    - Pseudoaneurysm results from an arterial wall injury with extravascular hematoma that organizes and forms a false lumen lined only by endothelium.
  - Treatment: Recommendations are generally dependent on the location of the aneurysm and the source artery involved.
    - Perform an Allen's test preoperatively to evaluate for superficial palmar arch patency and the dominant source of hand perfusion.
    - Aneurysm excision and arterial repair or reconstruction with vein graft are indicated when the source artery is critical to hand perfusion.
    - Aneurysm excision and ligation of source artery are indicated when the source artery is not critical to hand perfusion.
2. Vascular malformation (VM)
  - Arises from disorders in the embryologic development of the vascular system

- Characterized by a lesion that is present at birth, grows proportionally with the child, and never involutes
- Categorized based on vascular flow: Low or high
  - High-flow VM
    - Contains an arterial component (e.g., arterial malformation, arteriovenous malformation)
      - Painless mass that is not compressible
      - May lead to distal ischemia or high-output cardiac failure
  - Low-flow VM
    - Venous malformation
      - Most common low-flow VM
      - Bluish discoloration, compressible, painful, secondary to thrombus formation or dependent position
    - Lymphatic malformation
      - Enlarges as a result of fluid accumulation, cellulitis, or inadequate drainage
      - Propensity for infection
      - May cause bone hypertrophy
  - Treatment: Options include selective embolization, ligation, and surgical excision.
    - High-flow VM: Preoperative embolization followed by surgical excision are often recommended.
3. Hemangioma (see Figure 15.8)
  - Vascular tumor that frequently appears within the first 4 weeks of life
    - Affects females more commonly than males
  - Characterized by a red, spongy lesion with a rapid growth phase, followed by involution
    - In general, 70% of hemangiomas will involute by 7 years of age.
    - A noninvoluting variant is possible.

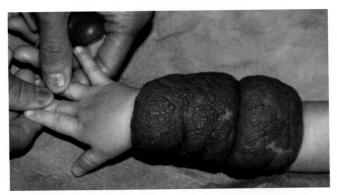

Figure 15.8. Hemangiomas present as (1) superficial in the cutaneous form; (2) deep, which represents cavernous lesions; or (3) a mixture of both. Not present at birth, they are characterized by a rapid growth phase during the first year. Expected involution is 50% by 5 years of age and 70% by 7 years of age, respectively. *(Reprinted from Neligan, P.C., Chang, J., [Eds.], 2013. Plastic Surgery, vol. 6, 3rd ed. Elsevier, 311.)*

- Diagnosis: Often made through history, physical examination, and growth patterns
  - MRI and CT scan are useful for evaluation and demonstrate a well-defined vascular tumor.
- Treatment options
  - Initial observation
  - Involution may be induced by steroid administration or propranolol treatment.
  - Surgical excision indicated for persistent bleeding, when tumor location or growth impairs function or cosmesis, or if patient develops a platelet-consumptive coagulopathy (Kasabach-Merritt syndrome)
  - Laser ablation is also a possibility.
4. Glomus tumor (see Figure 15.9)
  - Benign lesion containing cells of a glomus apparatus (an afferent vessel, a Sucquet-Hoyer canal, and multiple vascular shunts beneath the nail bed and within the glabrous skin)

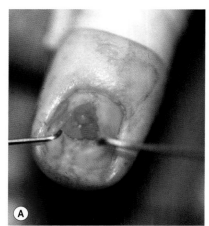

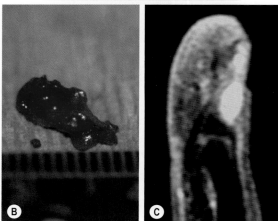

Figure 15.9. Glomus tumor. A benign tumor of the neuromyoarterial apparatus responsible for controlling skin circulation, presenting in a subungual location. **A,** Glomus tumor in situ. **B,** Glomus tumor excised. **C,** MRI scan of glomus tumor distal phalanx. *(Reprinted from Neligan, P.C., Chang, J., [Eds.], 2013. Plastic Surgery, vol. 6, 3rd ed. Elsevier, 311.)*

- Characterized by pinpoint, paroxysmal pain, and cold insensitivity
- Diagnosis
  - Subcutaneous nodules, most commonly in the subungual region, that are painful with cold exposure and/or focal pressure (Love's sign)
    - Pain is often ablated with proximal tourniquet insufflation (Hildreth's sign).
    - May have a violaceous discoloration of the nail bed
  - X ray demonstrates a scalloped, osteolytic lesion of the distal phalanx.
  - MRI demonstrates a high-signal-intensity lesion of the distal phalanx.
- Treatment: Excision
5. Acquired arteriovenous fistula
  - Arises after trauma or surgical intervention (e.g., radial artery cannulation)
  - Characterized by communication between an artery and a vein that results in vascular shunting of blood flow into the low-resistance venous system and bypassing of the higher-resistance capillary system
  - May result in an enlarging mass with a palpable thrill or bruit or ischemia secondary to vascular steal or shunting
  - Treatment: Resection of the fistula with arterial repair and/or reconstruction in the setting of unstable fistulas or those with ischemic sequelae

Other Vascular Disorders of the Hand

1. CREST (calcinosis, Raynaud's phenomenon, esophageal dysmotility, sclerodactyly, and telangiectasia) syndrome
   - Also known as systemic sclerosis or scleroderma
   - Hand involvement is characterized by cutaneous calcinosis, Raynaud's phenomenon (exaggerated vasoconstriction of the digital vasculature in the settings of stress and cold temperatures), taut shiny skin, and finger ulcerations.
   - Treatment
     - Large, painful calcium deposits can be excised, but surgical debridement should be conservative and include good local wound care.
     - Digital sympathectomy or arterial bypass may help alleviate symptoms; however, amputation may be indicated with large ulcerations/wounds or persistent progressive ischemia.
2. Buerger's disease
   - Also known as thromboangiitis obliterans
   - Characterized by recurring progressive inflammation and thrombosis of small vessels in the hands and feet secondary to tobacco use (e.g., heavy smoking and smokeless tobacco)
   - Signs: Severe pain, cold sensitivity, digital ischemia and discoloration, and ulcerations
   - Treatment: Smoking cessation

3. Compartment syndrome
   - Arises from increased pressure within soft-tissue compartments, resulting in ischemia and necrosis of compartmental contents (e.g., muscle, nerves)
   - Tissue necrosis from compartment syndrome can lead to significant functional deficits, systemic organ failure (e.g., renal failure from myoglobinemia), neurologic deficit, and amputation.
   - In the upper extremity, the most common causes include fractures (e.g., distal radius fracture, supracondylar humerus fracture), crush injuries, contusions, gunshot wounds, tight circumferential casts/dressings, extravasation, postischemia-reperfusion edema, and arterial injuries.
   - Compartments of the upper extremity
     - Forearm: Volar, dorsal, mobile wad
       - Deep muscles of the volar compartment are most commonly affected first (e.g., flexor digitorum profundus).
     - Hand: Hypothenar, thenar, adductor, 4 dorsal interossei, 3 palmar interossei, and the carpal canal
   - Signs of compartment syndrome: The "5 Ps"
     - Pain
       - Out of proportion to the injury or exam
       - With passive stretch (most sensitive sign)
     - Palpable swelling and tense compartments
     - Paresthesias
     - Paralysis
     - Pulselessness
       - Late finding
   - Diagnosis
     - History, physical examination, and high index of clinical suspicion
     - Compartment pressure measurements
       - Absolute value above 30 mm Hg
       - In patients with low diastolic blood pressure: Compartment pressure measurements within 30 mm Hg of the diastolic blood pressure
   - Treatment: Emergent fasciotomy
     - With arterial injury and repair in the forearm, consider prophylactic fasciotomy because of anticipated ischemia-reperfusion swelling.
     - Forearm: Volar and dorsal incisions
     - Hand: Longitudinal incisions over radial side of 1st metacarpal, dorsal aspect of 2nd and 4th metacarpals, ulnar side of 5th metacarpal, carpal tunnel release
   - Complications
     - Volkmann's ischemic contracture: Muscle necrosis resulting in irreversible muscle contractures in the forearm
     - Treatment: Depending on severity, ranges from splinting and tendon lengthening to tendon transfers and/or free functional muscle transfer

Dupuytren's Contracture

1. A benign, progressive fibromatosis of the palmar and digital fascia
2. Genetic predilection with an autosomal dominant pattern of inheritance with variable penetrance
   - Highest incidence in men of Northern European descent
   - May be associated with repetitive trauma, alcohol abuse, hepatic disease
3. Typically affects the metacarpophalangeal (MCP) joint first, followed by the proximal interphalangeal (PIP) joint (see Table 15.1)
   - Ring finger > small finger > thumb > long finger > index finger

Table 15.1 Fascial Anatomy of Dupuytren's Disease

DISEASED STRUCTURE	ANATOMIC ORIGIN	CLINICAL SIGNIFICANCE
Palmar Cords		
Pretendinous cord	Pretendinous band	MCP joint flexion contracture
Vertical cord	Vertical fibers of McGrouther or septa of Legueu and Juvara	Causes painful triggering
Palmodigital Cords		
Spiral cord	Pretendinous band, spiral band, lateral digital sheet, Grayson's ligament	Displaces the neurovascular bundle medially and superficially (spiral nerve)
Natatory cord	Natatory ligament (distal fibers)	Web-space adduction contracture
Digital Cords		
Central cord	Pretendinous cord (digital extension)	PIP joint flexion contracture
Retrovascular cord	Retrovascular band of thomine	PIP and DIP joint flexion contracture; prevents full correction of PIP joint contracture
Lateral cord	Lateral digital sheet (often closely associated with pretendinous and natatory cord)	PIP and DIP joint flexion contracture; displaces neurovascular bundle medially
Abductor digiti minimi cord	Abductor digiti minimi tendon	PIP joint flexion contracture
Thumb and First Web-Space Cords		
Proximal commissural cord	Proximal commissural ligament	First web adduction contracture
Distal commissural cord	Distal commissural ligament	First web adduction contracture
Thumb pretendinous cord	Pretendinous band	MCP joint flexion contracture

DIP, *distal interphalangeal*; MCP, *Metacarpophalangeal*; PIP, *proximal interphalangeal*.
Reprinted from Neligan, P.C., Chang, J., (Eds.), 2013. Plastic Surgery, vol. 6, 3rd ed. Elsevier, 347.

4. Occasionally associated with other benign, progressive fibromatoses
   - Plantar fibromatosis: Ledderhose's disease
   - Penile fibromatosis: Peyronie's disease
5. Characterized by the transformation of normal palmar and digital fascial structures into diseased cords with high levels of type-III collagen and myofibroblasts
6. Signs: Characteristic progression from pitting/dimpling of the palm and nodule formation to fibrotic cord development and contracture of the MCP and PIP joints
   - Patients may present with overt flexion contractures and Garrod's nodules (knuckle pads over the dorsum of the PIP joint).
     - Garrod's nodules more common in bilateral disease and patients with other associated fibromatoses
7. Treatment: Generally dependent upon severity of disease; high rate of recurrence
   - Steroid injection may have a role in the treatment of painful palmar nodules
   - Collagenase injection
     - Has become a first-line treatment for many surgeons
     - Indications for injection are the same for surgery: MCP flexion contracture >30 degrees or any flexion contracture of the PIP joints.

Table 15.2 Surgical Options for the Treatment of Dupuytren's Disease

SURGICAL TECHNIQUE	DESCRIPTION
Fasciotomy	Division of diseased cords without excision
Local fasciectomy	Removal of segment of diseased cord
Regional fasciectomy	Removal of all diseased fascia as well as local region of grossly normal tissue
Radical fasciectomy	Removal of the entire palmar and digital fascia
Open-palm technique (McCash)	Division of the palmar aponeurosis without closure of the skin deficit created
Dermatofasciectomy	Removal of the diseased fascia as well as the overlying skin; closure typically obtained with the use of a full-thickness skin graft

Reprinted from Neligan, P.C., Chang, J., (Eds.), 2013. Plastic Surgery, vol. 6, 3rd ed. Elsevier.

- Results are relatively good with treatment of MCP joint contractures but poor with treatment of PIP joint contractures.
- Complications: Localized skin tears/reactions, edema, pain, flexor tendon rupture
- Surgery
  - Indications: MCP flexion contracture >30 degrees or any flexion contracture of the PIP joint
  - Techniques (see Table 15.2)
  - Palmar fasciectomy is the preferred surgical technique.
- Complications
  - Injury to the neurovascular bundle
    - The neurovascular bundle is pulled to a more volar position primarily by the spiral cord, placing it at risk for direct injury during surgery.
    - Release of flexion contracture and placement of the digit in extension can put excessive stretch on the bundle, resulting in ischemia. In this instance, remove the splint and allow fingers to be in a more flexed position.
  - Complex regional pain syndrome
    - A spectrum of posttraumatic pain that is characterized by regional pain combined with autonomic dysfunction, atrophy, and functional impairment
    - Classed in 3 stages
      - Stage I (0 to 3 months): Pain out of proportion to injury, hyperesthesia, edema and stiffness, erythema, hyperhidrosis
      - Stage II (3 to 9 months): Pain, stiffness, edema, warmth, cyanosis, hair loss, decreased moisture, osteopenia secondary to disuse
      - Stage III (9 to 18 months): Decreased pain, increased stiffness, dry, cool, pale skin

Suggested Readings

Athanasian, E.A., 2011. Chapter 65: Bone and soft-tissue tumors. In: Wolfe, S.W., Hotchkiss, R.N., Pederson, W.C., et al. (Eds.), Green's Operative Hand Surgery, 6th ed. Elsevier, pp. 2141–2196.

Beckert, B.W., Molnar, J.A. Malignant Hand Tumors. Emedicine.com. Found at: <http://emedicine.medscape.com/article/1286560-overview.> Accessed on: September 10, 2014.

Finkel, R., Kasdan, M., 2010. Chapter 110: Surgical treatment of vascular tumors of the hand. In: Wiesel, S.W. (Ed.), Operative Techniques in Orthopaedic Surgery, 1st ed. Wolters Kluwer/Lippincott Williams & Wilkins, pp. 2992–3003.

Haase, S.C., Chung, K.C., 2011. Chapter 64: Skin tumors. In: Wolfe, S.W., Hotchkiss, R.N., Pederson, W.C., et al. (Eds.), Green's Operative Hand Surgery, 6th ed. Elsevier, pp. 2121–2140.

Hurst, L., 2011. Chapter 5: Dupuytren's contracture. In: Wolfe, S.W., Hotchkiss, R.N., Pederson, W.C., et al. (Eds.), Green's Operative Hand Surgery, 6th ed. Elsevier, pp. 141–158.

Kleinert, H.E., Burget, G.C., Morgan, J.A., et al., 1973. Aneurysms of the hand. Arch. Surg. 106 (4), 554–557.

Koman, L.A., Poehling, G.G., Smith, B.P., et al., 2011. Chapter 59: Complex regional pain syndrome. In: Wolfe, S.W., Hotchkiss, R.N., Pederson, W.C., et al. (Eds.), Green's Operative Hand Surgery, 6th ed. Elsevier, pp. 1959–1988.

Koman, L.A., Smith, B.P., Smith, T.L., et al., 2011. Chapter 66: Vascular disorders. In: Wolfe, S.W., Hotchkiss, R.N., Pederson, W.C., et al. (Eds.), Green's Operative Hand Surgery, 6th ed. Elsevier, p. 2197.

Leversedge, F.J., Moore, T.J., Peterson, B.C., et al., 2011. Education objectives: compartment syndrome of the upper extremity. J. Hand Sur. 36 (3), 544–559.

Lin, S.J., Molnar, J.A., Benign Hand Tumors. Emedicine.com. Found at: <http://emedicine.medscape.com/article/1286448-overview.> Accessed on: September 10, 2014.

Sacks, J.M., Azari, K.K., 2010. Chapter 141: Tumors. In: Weinzweig, J. (Ed.), Plastic Surgery Secrets Plus, 2nd ed. Mosby, pp. 912–923.

Sacks, J.M., Azari, K.K., Oates, S., et al., 2013. Chapter 15: Benign and malignant tumors of the hand. In: Neligan, P.C., Chang, J. (Eds.), Plastic Surgery, vol. 6, 3rd ed. Elsevier, p. 311.

Hand Fractures and Dislocations

Chapter 16

General Treatment of Metacarpal and Phalangeal Fractures

1. Metacarpal and phalangeal fractures are the most common fractures in the upper extremity.
2. Diagnosis requires a thorough history, physical examination, and radiographic images.
   - Specifically, look for open lacerations, digital shortening, malrotation (see Figures 16.1 and 16.2), scissoring, gross deformity, and angulation (see Figure 16.3), which affects hand motion/function.

3. Most fractures can be treated nonoperatively; however, the unique anatomy of the hand and associated muscular attachments can result in displacement, rotation, misalignment, and significant functional deficits.

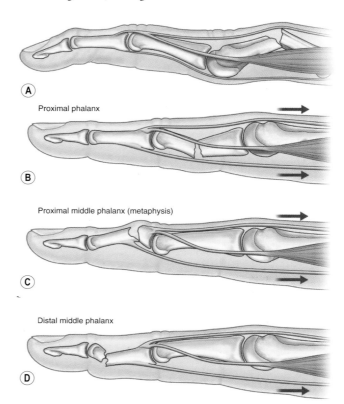

Figure 16.3. Angular deformity associated with fractures of the metacarpal and phalanges. **A,** Metacarpal fractures typically have apex dorsal angulation secondary to the location of the interosseous muscles, whereas the proximal phalanx fractures **(B)** have an apex volar angulation. The angulation of middle phalanx fractures is dependent on the location of the fracture, relative to the insertion of the FDS tendon: Fractures proximal to the insertion **(C)** will have apex dorsal angulation, whereas those distal **(D)** will have apex volar angulation. *(Reprinted from Neligan, P.C., Chang, J. [Eds.], 2013. Plastic Surgery, 3rd ed. Elsevier, 138–160.)*

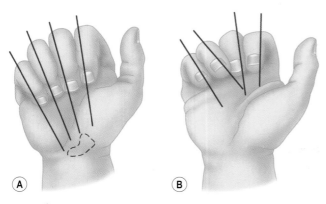

Figure 16.1. Malrotation of metacarpal or phalangeal fracture must be corrected. **A,** Normally, all fingers point toward region of scaphoid when fist is made. **B,** Malrotation at fracture causes affected finger to deviate. *(Reprinted from Canale, S.T., Beaty, J.H. [Eds.], 2013. Campbell's Operative Orthopedics, 12th ed. Mosby, 3305–3365.)*

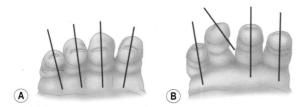

Figure 16.2. Observing plane of fingernails helps in detecting malrotation at fracture; compare with opposite hand. **A,** Normal alignment of fingernails. **B,** Alignment of fingernails with malrotation of ring finger. *(Reprinted from Canale, S.T., Beaty, J.H. [Eds.], 2013. Campbell's Operative Orthopedics, 12th ed. Mosby, 3305–3365.)*

4. General indications for fixation of these fractures are shown in Table 16.1

Table 16.1 Indications for Fixation of Metacarpal and Phalangeal Fractures

- Irreducible fractures
- Malrotation (spiral and short oblique)
- Intra-articular fractures
- Subcapital fractures (phalangeal)
- Open fractures
- Segmental bone loss
- Polytrauma with hand fractures
- Multiple hand or wrist fractures
- Fractures with soft-tissue injury (vessel, tendon, nerve, skin)
- Reconstruction (i.e., osteotomy)

Reprinted from Wolfe, S.W., Hotchkiss, R.N., Pederson, W.C., et al. (Eds.), 2011. Green's Operative Hand Surgery, 6th ed. Elsevier, pp. 239–290.

5. Numerous fixation techniques are available, although many fractures can be adequately fixed with percutaneous pinning (see Table 16.2).

Distal Phalanx Injuries

1. Mallet finger (see Figure 16.4): Disruption, either tendinous or bony, of the terminal extensor tendon at or distal to the distal interphalangeal joint (DIPJ)

Table 16.2 Fracture Stabilization Techniques

TECHNIQUE	INDICATIONS	ADVANTAGES	DISADVANTAGES
Kirschner pins	Transverse Oblique Spiral Longitudinal	Available and versatile Easy to insert Minimal dissection Percutaneous insertion	Lacks rigidity May loosen May distract fracture Pin tract infection Requires external support Splint and therapy awkward
Intraosseous wires	Transverse fractures (phalanges) Avulsion fractures Supplemental fixation (butterfly fragment) Arthrodesis	Available Low profile Relatively simple	May cut out (especially osteopenic bone)
Composite wiring	Transverse Oblique Spiral	More rigid than Kirschner pins Low profile Simple and available	Pin or wire migration Secondary removal (sometimes) Exposure may be significant
Intramedullary device	Transverse Short oblique	No special equipment Easy to insert No pin protrusion Minimal dissection	Rotational instability Rod migration
Interfragmentary fixation	Long oblique Spiral	Low profile Rigid	Special equipment Little margin for error
Plates and screws	Multiple fractures with soft-tissue injury or bone loss Markedly displaced shaft fracture (especially border metacarpals) Intra-articular and periarticular fractures Reconstruction for nonunion or malunion	Rigid (stable) fixation Restore or maintain length	Exacting technique Special equipment Extensive exposure May require removal Refracture after plate removal Bulky
External fixation	Restore length for comminution or bone loss Soft-tissue injury or loss Infection Nonunion	Preserves length Allows access to bone and soft tissue Percutaneous insertion Direct manipulation of fracture avoided	Pin tract infections Osteomyelitis Overdistraction: Nonunion Neurovascular injury Fractures through pin holes Loosening

Reprinted from Wolfe, S.W., Hotchkiss, R.N., Pederson, W.C., et al. (Eds.), 2011. Green's Operative Hand Surgery, 6th ed. Elsevier, pp. 239–290.

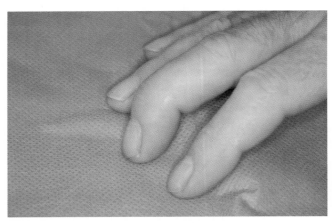

Figure 16.4. Hanging fingertip (mallet finger). *(Reprinted from Neligan, P.C., Buck, D.W. [Eds.], 2013. Core Procedures in Plastic Surgery. Elsevier, 414–426.)*

- Etiology: Forced flexion of the DIPJ due to an impaction force to tip of extended finger
- Characterized by a painful, swollen DIPJ, with the fingertip resting in flexion without active DIP extension
- Treatment
  - Extension splinting of the DIPJ for 6 to 8 weeks; keep proximal interphalangeal (PIP) joint free
  - Operative repair is indicated with volar subluxation, >50% articular surface involvement, and/or >2 mm articular gap. Can be performed with
    - Pin fixation
    - Dorsal blocking pin
    - Open reduction internal fixation (ORIF)
  - Terminal tendon reconstruction in chronic injuries (>12 weeks)
  - DIP arthrodesis is reserved for treatment of chronically painful, arthritic DIP joints.
- Complications
  - Extensor lag
  - Swan-neck deformity
2. Jersey finger: Avulsion of the flexor digitorum profundus (FDP) tendon from its insertion at the base of the distal phalanx
   - Etiology: Forced DIPJ extension of an actively flexed DIPJ (i.e., athlete grasping a moving object such as a jersey, etc.)
     - The ring finger is involved in most cases because it is the most prominent fingertip exposed to the force of gripping.
   - Characterized by pain, tenderness over the volar distal finger, with the finger in extension relative to others, and no active DIPJ flexion.

- Leddy-Packer classification (see Table 16.3)
  - Based on the level of tendon retraction and presence of fracture
  - One of the only classification systems where the lowest type (type I) is associated with the worst pathology
  - Type II is the most common.

Table 16.3 Leddy-Packer Classification of Flexor Digitorum Profundus Avulsion Injury (Jersey Finger)

LEDDY-PACKER TYPE	DESCRIPTION	TREATMENT
Type I	FDP tendon retracted to palm. Leads to disruption of the vascular supply	Prompt surgical treatment within 10 to 14 days to avoid need for tendon graft
Type II	FDP retracts to level of PIP joint (caught on A3 pulley)	Can repair within 3 months without need for tendon graft; however, over time can convert to type-1 injury
Type III	Large avulsion fracture limits retraction to the level of the DIP joint (caught on A4 pulley)	Can often be repaired at any time without need for tendon graft, even if after 3 months
Type IV	Osseous fragment and simultaneous avulsion of the tendon from the fracture fragment (retraction of the tendon into palm)	If tendon separated from fracture fragment, first fix fracture via ORIF, then reattach tendon as for type-I and -II injuries

DIP, *Distal interphalangeal;* FDP, *flexor digitorum profundus;* ORIF, *open reduction and internal fixation;* PIP, *proximal interphalangeal.*

- Treatment (see Figure 16.5)
  - Types I, II: Direct tendon repair or tendon reinsertion with a dorsal button
    - Indications: Acute injuries (<4 weeks)
    - Complications: Advancement of the FDP tendon >1 cm can lead to DIP contracture or quadrigia (functional shortening of FDP tendon, leading to a flexion lag of adjacent fingers).
  - Types III, IV: ORIF of the fracture fragment with a K wire, screw, or pull-out wire
  - Two-stage flexor tendon grafting indicated in patients with chronic injuries and full passive range of motion (PROM).
  - DIPJ arthrodesis: Salvage procedure in patients with chronic injuries and limited range of motion (ROM)

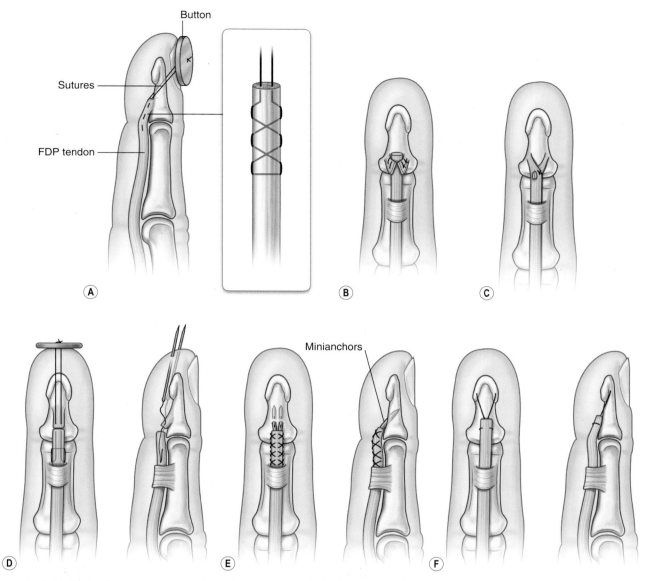

Figure 16.5. Methods of making a tendon-to-bone junction in zone 1. **A,** A conventional method of anchoring the flexor digitorum profundus (FDP) tendon to the bone by pull-out sutures through the nail tied over a button. Alternative ways to anchor the distal tendon stump to the bone by **(B)** directly suturing the stump to the residual FDP tendon, **(C)** looping the tendon through the bone, **(D)** pull-out suturing over the fingertip, **(E)** using minianchors, and **(F)** looping the sutures through a transverse hole in the bone. *(Reprinted from Neligan, P.C. [Ed.], 2013. Plastic Surgery, 3rd ed. Elsevier, 179–210.)*

3. Distal phalanx fractures and DIPJ fracture dislocations
   - Most commonly encountered fracture in the hand
   - Classified into three types: Tuft, shaft, and intra-articular
     - Tuft fractures: Typically a result of a crush injury and often associated with a nail-bed laceration
   - Treatment
     - Tip or tuft fracture
       - Address subungual hematoma: Remove nail plate and repair nail bed as necessary; replace nail plate to splint eponychial fold.
       - Splint immobilization of fracture

   - Shaft fracture
     - Closed reduction and splinting
       - Indicated in nondisplaced transverse fractures
       - Reduction can be blocked by nail matrix.
     - Closed reduction percutaneous pinning (CRPP)
       - Considered in displaced transverse fractures and longitudinal fractures
     - ORIF with or without autologous bone grafting is indicated for fracture nonunion.

- Intra-articular fracture/DIPJ fracture dislocation (see Figure 16.6)
  - Bony "mallet finger" (see above)
  - Inability to reduce dorsal DIPJ dislocations is most likely due to interposition of the volar plate or FDP tendon in open injuries

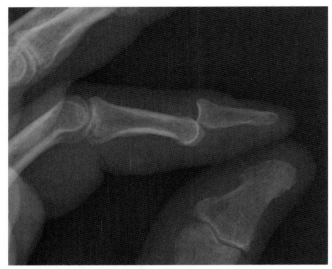

Figure 16.6. Radiograph of DIP dorsal dislocation of index finger. *(Reprinted from Neligan, P.C. [Ed.], 2013. Plastic Surgery, 3rd ed. Elsevier, 138–160.)*

Proximal Phalanx/Proximal Interphalangeal Joint (PIPJ) Injuries

1. PIPJ dislocation/fracture dislocation (see Figure 16.9)
   - Dorsal dislocations are more common than volar dislocations.
   - Dorsal dislocation results in injury to the volar plate and if left untreated can become a swan-neck deformity (hyperextension of the PIPJ and flexion of the DIPJ), secondary to weakened volar plate with dorsal migration of the lateral bands.
   - Volar dislocation results in injury to the central slip and if left untreated can become a boutonniere deformity (flexion of the PIPJ and hyperextension of the DIPJ) secondary to volar migration of the lateral bands.
   - Treatment
     - Dislocation
       - Closed reduction and buddy taping to adjacent finger for 3 to 6 weeks
         - Indicated if dislocation is reducible
         - Inability to obtain reduction in dorsal dislocations is often related to volar plate obstruction in closed injuries and the FDP tendon in open injuries.
         - Inability to obtain reduction in volar dislocations is often related to central slip obstruction.

- Dorsal fracture dislocation (see Figures 16.7 and 16.8)
  - Dorsal extension block splinting
    - Indicated for fractures that involve <30% to 40% of the articular surface and require <30 degrees of flexion to maintain reduction
  - ORIF or CRPP
    - Indicated if >30 degrees of flexion is required to maintain reduction or if the fracture involves >30% to 40% of the articular surface (see Figure 16.10)
  - Force-coupler dynamic splinting or hemi-hamate reconstruction
    - Indicated for more complex injuries, including those with comminution

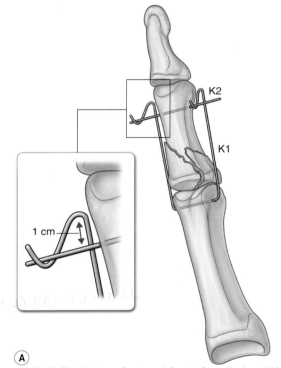

Figure 16.7. A, Fabrication of external fixator from K wires (K1, K2).

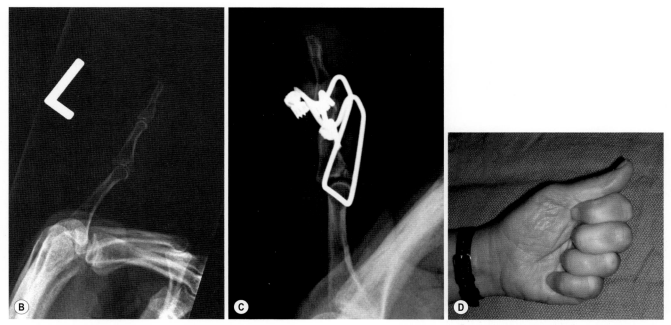

Figure 16.7, cont'd. Preoperative radiograph **(B)** of PIP fracture dislocation involving the small finger. **C,** Radiograph with external fixator in place, allowing motion. **D,** Postoperative results in flexion. *(Reprinted from Neligan, P.C. [Ed.], 2013. Plastic Surgery, 3rd ed. Elsevier, 138–160.)*

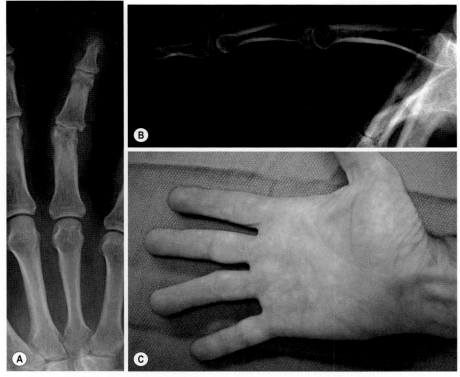

Figure 16.8. Technique of hemi-hamate replacement arthroplasty. **A,** Preoperative posterioanterior (PA) and **(B)** lateral radiographs and clinical photographs in extension **(C)** and flexion **(D).**

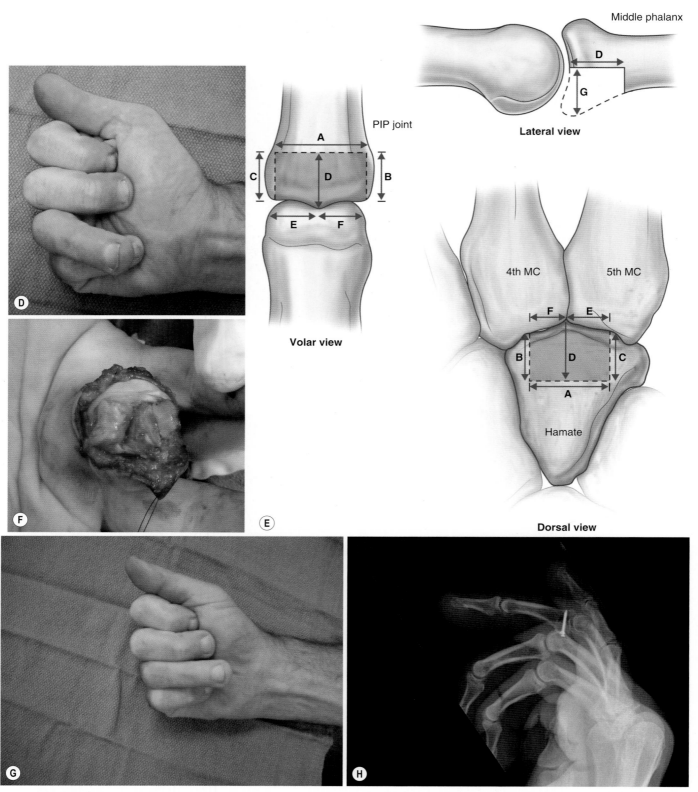

Figure 16.8, cont'd. E, Diagram of configuration of hemi-hamate graft. **F,** Intraoperative photograph of graft secured (note articular wear on the head of the proximal phalanx due to delay in presentation). **G,** Postoperative clinical photograph; **H,** lateral radiograph. *MC,* Metacarpal.
(Reprinted from In Neligan, P.C. [Ed.], 2013. Plastic Surgery, 3rd ed. Elsevier, 138–160.)

- Volar plate arthroplasty
  - ◆ Often reserved for chronic injuries that involve <60% of the articular surface
- ○ PIPJ arthrodesis
  - ◆ Reserved as a salvage procedure for chronic injuries with chronic pain and for PIPJ arthritis
- ■ Volar fracture dislocation: Treatment similar to dorsal dislocations
  - ○ Extension splinting for injuries involving <40% of the articular surface
  - ○ ORIF or CRPP in unstable injuries or those involving >40% of the articular surface

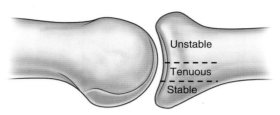

Figure 16.10. Stability of PIP fracture dislocations. Fractures involving <30% of the articular surface are typically stable, those involving 30% to 50% are tenuous, and those involving >50% are unstable and have resultant dorsal subluxation. *(Reprinted from Neligan, P.C. [Ed.], 2013. Plastic Surgery, 3rd ed. Elsevier, 138–160.)*

2. Proximal and middle phalanx fractures (see Figure 16.11)
   - Treatment is dependent on fracture stability and pattern.
   - Splint immobilization (~2 to 3 weeks) followed by protected motion with buddy taping
     - ■ Indicated for stable, nondisplaced fractures without malrotation
   - ORIF or CRPP
     - ■ Indicated for fractures with malrotation; oblique and/or spiral fractures that are inherently unstable; fractures with angulation, shortening >2 mm, or articular step-off; unstable condylar fractures

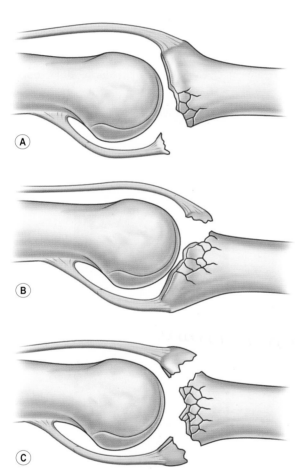

Figure 16.9. Classification of PIPJ fracture dislocations. **A,** Volar base fracture resulting in dorsal subluxation of the middle phalanx. **B,** Dorsal base fracture resulting in volar subluxation of the middle phalanx. **C,** Pilon-type fracture with dorsal and volar base fractures and comminuted, depressed central articular surface. *(Reprinted from Neligan, P.C. [Ed.], 2013. Plastic Surgery, 3rd ed. Elsevier, 138–160.)*

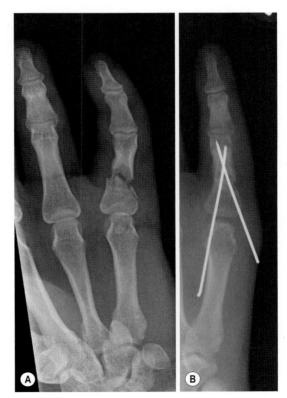

Figure 16.11. Preoperative and postoperative PA radiograph of proximal phalanx shaft **(A,B)** and base **(C,D)** fractures treated with K wires *(vertical lines)*. *(Reprinted from Neligan, P.C. [Ed.], 2013. Plastic Surgery, 3rd ed. Elsevier, 138–160.)*

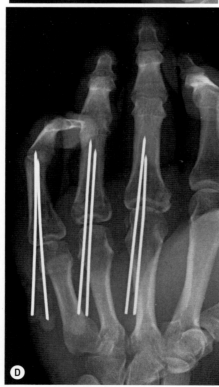

Figure 16.11, cont'd.

Metacarpal Phalangeal Joint (MCPJ) Injuries

1. MCPJ dislocation
   - Dorsal dislocations are most common, with the border digits being most commonly involved (see Figure 16.12).
   - Occurs from hyperextension force with rupture of the volar plate
   - Classification: Simple versus complex
     - Simple: Reducible dislocation
       - ○ Can be treated with closed reduction and splinting
     - Complex: Irreducible dislocation, often secondary to obstruction from the volar plate (most common); in the index finger, obstruction can also occur from the lumbrical (radial) and flexor (ulnar) tendons; in the small finger, obstruction can also occur from the lumbrical and flexor tendons (radial) and the flexor digiti minimi (ulnar)
   - Treatment: Open reduction in irreducible dislocations

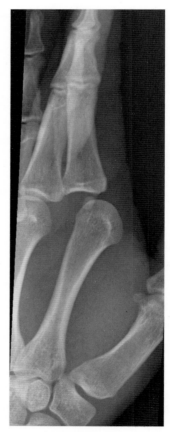

Figure 16.12. Radiograph of MCP dorsal dislocation. *(Reprinted from Neligan, P.C. [Ed.], 2013. Plastic Surgery, 3rd ed. Elsevier, 138–160.)*

2. MCJ fracture dislocation
   - Often results from fights, crush injuries, motor vehicle accidents
   - Examine for rotation deformity (scissoring), angulation, shortening, carpometacarpal joint (CMCJ) dislocation, and "fight bite"
     - Angulation is better compensated for in the ring and small fingers (up to 40 to 50 degrees) compared to the index and long fingers (10 to 15 degrees) because the CMCJ of these digits allows for greater compensatory motion.
   - Treatment: Depends on stability, rotation, and angulation/shortening
     - Closed reduction
       - Indicated in simple dislocations with stable fracture pattern, no rotation, and acceptable angulation/shortening (see Table 16.4)

Table 16.4 Acceptable Angulation and Shortening of Finger Metacarpal Fractures

	ACCEPTABLE SHAFT ANGULATION (DEGREES)	ACCEPTABLE SHAFT SHORTENING (mm)	ACCEPTABLE NECK ANGULATION
Index finger	10	2-5	10-15
Long finger	20	2-5	10-15
Ring finger	30	2-5	30-40
Small finger	40	2-5	50-60

   -
       - Performed with the wrist flexed, to relax the flexor tendons, and application of distal pressure to the base of the proximal phalanx (see Figure 16.13)
     - ORIF or CRPP
       - Indicated for complex dislocations and/or fractures with intra-articular involvement, rotation (scissoring), shortening, displacement, multishaft fractures, or unacceptable angulation
         - Can be opened volarly or dorsally. The volar approach is more direct but places the neurovascular structures at risk. The dorsal approach may require splitting of the volar plate.
     - MCPJ arthrodesis
       - Indicated in persistent MCPJ injuries with chronic pain, arthritis, and decreased ROM
         - Appropriate positioning for arthrodesis
           → Thumb: 15 degrees of flexion
           → Index: 25 degrees of flexion
           → Long: 30 degrees of flexion
           → Ring: 35 degrees of flexion
           → Small: 40 degrees of flexion

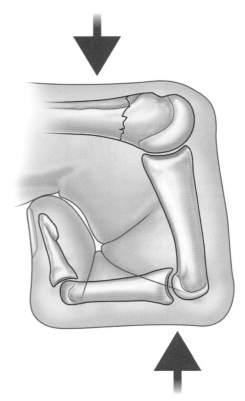

Figure 16.13. The Jahss maneuver for reduction of a metacarpal neck fracture. The DIP and PIP joints are flexed and dorsal pressure is applied to the PIP joint *(top arrow)*, while counter pressure is applied to the metacarpal shaft proximal to the fracture *(bottom arrow)*. (Reprinted from Neligan, P.C. [Ed.], 2013. Plastic Surgery, 3rd ed. Elsevier, 138–160.)

4. Metacarpal fractures
   - Often occur from a direct blow
   - Many can be treated nonoperatively if stable
   - Consider open wounds over the MCPJ with associated fractures "fight bites" and treat accordingly until proven otherwise.
   - Metacarpal base fractures
     - 5th metacarpal base fracture (also known as "reverse Bennett" or "baby Bennett" fracture) (see Figure 16.14)
       - Results in proximal and dorsal subluxation of the metacarpal shaft
       - The proximal fragment is held in place by the intermetacarpal ligaments, whereas the distal fragment and digit is displaced secondary to pull the extensor carpi ulnaris, flexor carpi ulnaris, and the abductor digiti minimi.

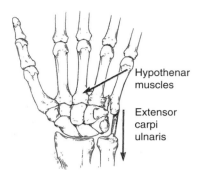

Figure 16.14. Deforming forces of 5th metacarpal base fractures. The hypothenar muscles and extensor carpi ulnaris muscle act in different force vectors to produce a characteristic displacement of fractures of the 5th metacarpal base. Note how the intermetacarpal ligament between the 4th and 5th metacarpal bases stabilizes the baby Bennett fragment. *(Reprinted with permission from Niechajev, I., 1985. Dislocated intra-articular fracture of the base of the fifth metacarpal: a clinical study of 23 patients. Plast. Reconstr. Surg. 75, 406–410.)*

- Hypothenar muscles
- Extensor carpi ulnaris

> - Treatment: ORIF or CRPP
> - Metacarpal shaft fractures
>   - Often stable and amenable to nonoperative management
>   - Indications for operative treatment include open fractures, malrotation, unacceptable angulation
>   - ORIF or CRPP
>   - K-wire fixation
>   - Lag screw fixation requires an oblique fracture, with a fracture length that is twice the diameter of the bone.
>   - Dorsal plate fixation indicated when multiple shaft fractures are present
> - Metacarpal neck fractures
>   - Neck fracture of the 5th metacarpal is also known as a "boxer's fracture"
>   - Treatment is dependent on the presence of malrotation and angulation.
>   - Closed reduction and immobilization (with MCPJ flexed and IPJ extended) are often adequate.
>   - Jahss maneuver for reduction (see Figure 16.13): Flexion of the DIPJ, PIPJ, and MCPJ, with dorsal pressure over the flexed PIP and simultaneous volar force over the apex of the fracture
>   - ORIF or CRPP indicated with unacceptable angulation, rotation, and intra-articular fractures.
> - Metacarpal head fractures
>   - Requires anatomic reduction and stabilization
>   - Rigid fixation is preferred, often with screws

Thumb Injuries

1. Thumb distal and proximal phalanx and metacarpal fractures are managed similarly to those of the fingers (see above).
   - The thumb metacarpal can tolerate significant rotation and angulation because of the motion allowed at the thumb CMCJ.

2. Ulnar collateral ligament (UCL) injury (also known as "gamekeeper's thumb" or "skier's thumb")
   - Results from tear of the UCL, characterized by instability of the thumb with grip, radial deviation, and pain
   - The UCL is composed of two structures
     - The proper collateral ligament, which resists radial deviation of the flexed thumb
     - The accessory collateral ligament and volar plate, which resist radial deviation of the extended thumb
     - Laxity of the thumb in both flexion and extension is consistent with a complete tear of the UCL.
   - Diagnosis: The thumb MCPJ is stressed with a radial deviation force in neutral and in flexion, and the degree of "opening" and/or variation between injured and uninjured sides is recorded.
   - "Stener lesion" (see Figure 16.15): Complete avulsion of the UCL (with or without a bony fragment), with proximal retraction and interposition of the adductor aponeurosis precluding primary healing
     - Requires operative repair

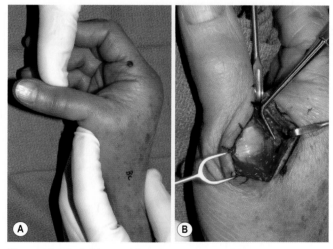

Figure 16.15. A 64-year-old woman presents with marked pain and instability at the ulnar aspect of the MCP joint. **A,** Stress testing of the ulnar collateral ligament reveals marked laxity with greater than 35° of rotational deformity. **B,** At the time of surgical exploration, a Stener lesion is identified. The bony insertion of the ulnar collateral ligament can be seen sitting on top of the aponeurosis of the adductor pollicis muscle (fragment at the end of dental probe). *(Reprinted From Carlsen, B.T., Moran S.L., 2009. J. Hand Surg. 34 [5], 945–952.)*

   - Treatment
     - Nonoperative immobilization is acceptable in incomplete UCL tears that have <20-degree side-to-side variation of instability.
     - Operative repair is indicated in injuries with >20-degree side-to-side variation instability or >35 degrees of opening due to a Stener lesion.

3. 1st metacarpal base fractures/fracture dislocations (also known as "Bennett" or "Rolando" fractures; see Figures 16.16 and 16.17)
   - Etiology: Axially directed force through the partially flexed thumb metacarpal shaft
   - Bennett fracture: A two-part fracture with a proximal volar lip fragment that is stable and a distal fragment that subluxates radially, proximally, and dorsally
     - Displacement of the distal segment is secondary to the combined pull of the thumb extensors, the abductor pollicis longus, and the adductor pollicis longus.
   - Rolando fracture: An intra-articular metacarpal base fracture with a Y or T shape or one that is comminuted
   - Treatment
     - CRPP is often adequate with ORIF reserved for irreducible fractures.

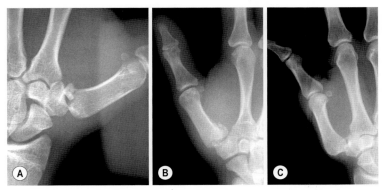

Figure 16.16. Gedda classified the Bennett fractures into 3 types. **A,** Type 1 represents a fracture with a large single ulnar fragment and subluxation of the metacarpal base. **B,** Type 2 represents an impaction fracture without subluxation of the thumb metacarpal. **C,** Type 3 represents those injuries presenting with a small ulnar avulsion fragment in association with metacarpal dislocation. *(Reprinted From Carlsen, B.T., Moran, S.L., 2009. J. Hand Surg. 34 [5], 945–952.)*

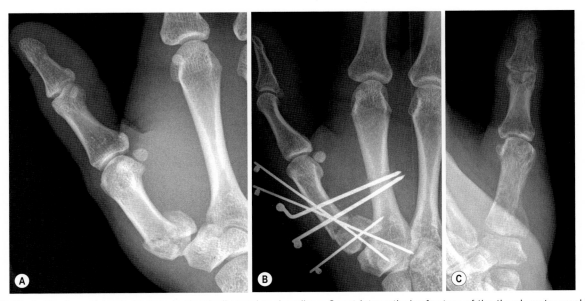

Figure 16.17. A, The term Rolando fracture is classically used to describe a 3-part intra-articular fracture of the thumb metacarpal base with a Y- or T-fracture pattern, as seen in this radiograph. **B,** A radiograph of the same fracture after transosseous K-wire fixation. Such fractures often require transmetacarpal pinning to stabilize and suspend the metacarpal shaft during the healing process. **C,** A Robert's view of the same thumb 3 months postoperatively, showing adequate articular congruity. *(Reprinted From Carlsen, B.T., Moran, S.L., 2009. J. Hand Surg. 34 [5], 945–952.)*

General Complications of Metacarpal and Phalangeal Fractures

1. Stiffness: Most phalangeal fracture patients will have residual stiffness.
   - Stiffness related to adhesions from plates and screws to extensor tendons may benefit from hardware removal and tenolysis.
2. Infection often occurs at pin sites. Treatment includes antibiotics and possible hardware removal if the fracture site is stable or if the hardware is loose or grossly infected.
3. Malunion: Most commonly occurs as abnormal angular or rotational deformities
   - Angular deformities: Frequently treated with opening or closing wedge osteotomies
     - Opening wedge osteotomies require bone grafting.
   - Rotational deformities are typically treated with osteotomies, rigid fixation, and early motion.
4. Nonunion: Rare with metacarpal or phalangeal fractures.
   - Treatment is similar to the principles for long-bone reconstruction and nonunions and includes debridement and bone grafting and/or vascularized bone grafting.

Suggested Readings

Blazar, P., 2009. Chapter 79: Finger instabilities and ligamentous injuries. In: Guyuron, B., Eriksson, E., Persing, J.A. (Eds.), Plastic Surgery: Indications and Practice. Saunders/Elsevier, China, pp. 1033–1043.

Bushnell, B.D., Draeger, R.W., Crosby, C.G., et al., 2008. Management of intra-articular metacarpal base fractures of the second through fifth metacarpals. J. Hand Surg. 33 (4), 573–583.

Calandruccio, J.H., 2013. Chapter 67: Fractures, dislocations, and ligamentous injuries. In: Canale, S.T., Beaty, J.H. (Eds.), Campbell's Operative Orthopedics, 12th ed. Mosby, pp. 3305–3365.

Carlsen, B.T., Moran, S.L., 2009. Thumb trauma: Bennett fractures, Rolando fractures, and ulnar collateral ligament injuries. J. Hand Surg. 34 (5), 945–952.

Day, C.S., Stern, P.J., 2011. Chapter 8: Fractures of the metacarpals and phalanges. In: Wolfe, S.W., Hotchkiss, R.N., Pederson, W.C., et al. (Eds.), Green's Operative Hand Surgery, 6th ed. Elsevier, pp. 239–290.

Egeland, B.M., Sebastin, S.J., Chung, K.C., 2012. Chapter 7: Acute repair of zone 1 flexor digitorum profundus avulsion. In: Chung, K.C. (Ed.), Operative Techniques: Hand and Wrist Surgery, 2nd ed. Saunders, pp. 55–63.

Hammert, W.C., 2013. Chapter 7: Hand fractures and joint injuries. In: Neligan, P.C., Chang, J. (Eds.), Plastic Surgery, 3rd ed. Elsevier, pp. 138–160.

Merrell, G., Slade, J.F., 2011. Dislocation and ligament injuries in the digits. In: Wolfe, S.W., Hotchkiss, R.N., Pederson, W.C., et al. (Eds.), Green's Operative Hand Surgery, 6th ed. Churchill Livingstone, Philadelphia, pp. 291–332.

Neligan, P.C., Buck, D.W., 2013. Core Procedures in Plastic Surgery. Chapter 21: Flexor tendon injury and reconstruction. Elsevier, pp. 358–374.

Neligan, P.C., Buck, D.W., 2013. Core Procedures in Plastic Surgery. Chapter 24: Extensor tendon injuries. Elsevier, pp. 414–426.

Oak, N., Lawton, J.N., 2013. Intra-articular fractures of the hand. In: Lawton, J.N., Chung, K.C. (Eds.), Hand Clin. 29 (4), 535–549.

Strauch, R.J., 2011. Chapter 6: Extensor tendon injury. In: Wolfe, S.W., Hotchkiss, R.N., Pederson, W.C., et al. (Eds.), Green's Operative Hand Surgery, 6th ed. Elsevier, pp. 159–188.

Nail-Bed Injuries, Soft-Tissue Amputations, and Replantation

General Fingernail and Nail-Bed Anatomy

1. Perionychium
   - Nail plate
   - Nail bed
   - Surrounding skin (nail fold, paronychium, hyponychium)
2. Paronychium: The lateral skin that surrounds the nail bed and nail
3. Hyponychium: The skin and keratin along the distal edge of the nail bed
4. Eponychium: The skin proximal and dorsal to the nail fold
5. Lunula: The white part of the proximal nail that corresponds to the distal extent of the germinal matrix
6. Matrix: The nail-plate growth centers
   - Germinal matrix
     - Accounts for almost 90% of nail-plate production
     - Soft tissue deep to nail plate at lunula and nail fold
     - Insertion of the terminal extensor tendon is approximately 1 to 1.5 mm proximal to the germinal matrix.
   - Sterile matrix
     - Accounts for 10% of nail production
     - The soft tissue located deep to the nail plate, distal to the lunula/germinal matrix
     - Responsible for adherence of nail plate to nail bed (see Figure 17.1)

Nail Growth and Physiology

1. Nail-plate growth is estimated to be 3 to 4 mm per month; complete nail-plate growth takes ~6 months.
   - Factors that speed the rate of nail-plate growth: Longer digits, summer months, persons <30 years old, and nail biting
2. The nail has a natural convex curvature from proximal to distal because more of the nail-plate substance is produced proximally.
3. Nail growth occurs in the germinal matrix, sterile matrix, and dorsal roof of the nail fold.
   - The germinal matrix produces cells that migrate distally and dorsally in a column toward the nail plate. As they abut the nail plate, they flatten and elongate. Initially, the nuclei of these cells are retained and produce the white color associated with the lunula. As they move distal, they become nonviable cells and lose their nuclei.
   - The sterile matrix provides some nail growth but primarily contributes strength and thickness to the nail plate. In addition, it plays a significant role in adherence of the nail plate to the nail bed.
   - The dorsal roof of the nail fold produces nail-plate cells similar to those of the germinal matrix and has a significant role in producing the shiny appearance of the nail (see Figure 17.2).

Nail-Bed Injuries

1. Subungual hematoma
   - Most commonly caused by crush injury
   - Signs: Pain and bleeding underneath nail with discoloration, signifying an injury to the nail bed
   - Treatment
     - <50% of the nail involved or hematoma with nail-plate edges intact: Percutaneous drainage (trephination) with battery microcautery or heated paper clip
     - >50% of the nail involved or disruption of the nail edges: Nail-plate removal and nail-bed repair (see Figure 17.3)
2. Nail-bed lacerations
   - Signs: Subungual hematoma >50% of the nail if nail plate intact or avulsion of nail plate and portion of the underlying nail bed with obvious injury
   - Commonly associated with distal phalanx fractures
   - Treatment: Nail-plate removal with nail-bed repair
     - If distal phalanx fracture is present, it may require management.
     - If significant avulsion injury and loss of nail matrix is present, may require nail-matrix graft from adjacent injured finger or second toe.
   - Nail-bed repair can be performed with 6-0 absorbable sutures or 2-octylcyanoacrylate (Dermabond).
   - After repair, splint the eponychial fold to prevent fold adhesions and obstruction of nail growth.
     - Can be performed with the original nail plate, aluminum foil, or nonadherent gauze

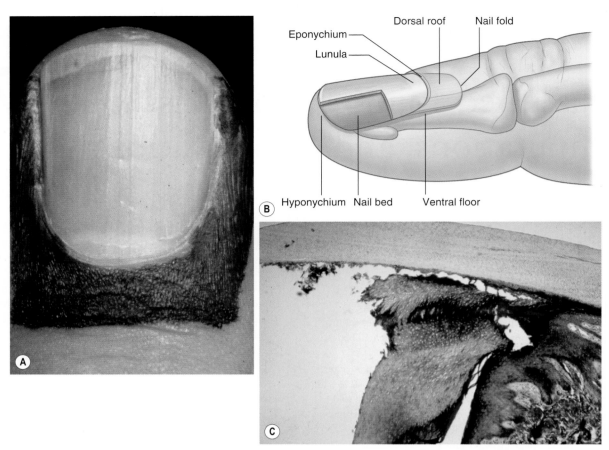

Figure 17.1. A, The nail, the sterile and germinal matrices, and the surrounding tissue marked here compose the perionychium. **B,** A lateral view of the nail bed showing the ventral floor (germinal matrix), the nail bed (sterile matrix), and the dorsal roof of the nail fold. **C,** The keratinous plug is shown at the hyponychium. *(Reprinted from Neligan, P.C., Chang, J. [Eds.], 2013. Plastic Surgery, vol. 6, 3rd ed. Elsevier, 117–134. © Southern Illinois University School of Medicine.)*

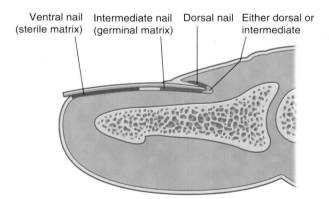

Figure 17.2. Components of the nail are produced in three areas. *(Reprinted from Neligan, P.C., Chang, J. [Eds.], 2013. Plastic Surgery, vol. 6, 3rd ed. Elsevier, 117–134. © Southern Illinois University School of Medicine.)*

3. Complications of nail-bed injury
   - Nonadherence (onycholysis)
     - Most common nail deformity after trauma
     - Secondary to nail-bed scarring
     - Treatment: Scar excision and primary closure or split-thickness sterile matrix graft from the adjacent nail bed or toe
   - Hook nail deformity
     - Secondary to inadequate bony support from the dorsal tuft of the distal phalanx
     - Nail growth hooks volarly over the fingertip
     - Treatment: Removal of redundant nail bed or advancement flap of volar fingertip tissue with no tension (see Figure 17.4)
   - Pincer nail deformity
     - Excess transverse curvature of the nail plate that is progressive and ultimately leads to an unesthetic, painful nail
     - Treatment: Elevation of the nail plate with dermal grafting (see Figure 17.5)

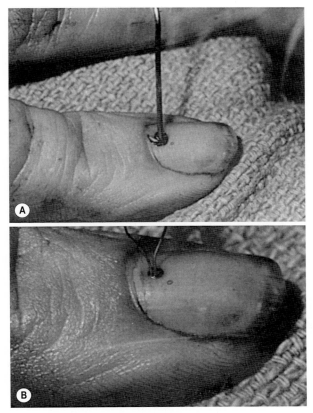

Figure 17.3. A, Time-honored method of burning a hole through the nail with a heated paperclip. **B,** The authors' preferred method of burning a hole through the nail with an ophthalmic battery-powered cautery. *(Reprinted from Sommer, N.Z., Brown, R.E., 2011. The perionychium. In: Wolfe, S.W., Hotchkiss, R.N., Pederson, W.C., et al. [Eds.], Green's Operative Hand Surgery, 6th ed. Elsevier, 333–353.)*

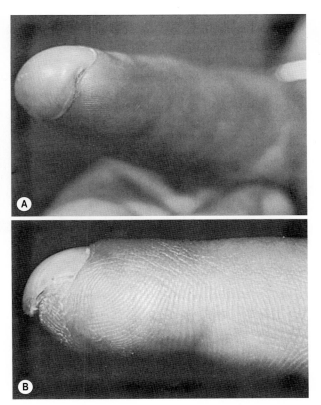

Figure 17.4. A, Hook nail deformity caused partially by some loss of bony support but primarily by the nail bed being pulled over the tip to close the amputation. **B,** Loss of bony support to hold the nail bed flat. *(Reprinted from Sommer, N.Z., Brown, R.E., 2011. The perionychium. In: Wolfe, S.W., Hotchkiss, R.N., Pederson, W.C., et al. [Eds.], Green's Operative Hand Surgery, 6th ed. Elsevier, 333–353.)*

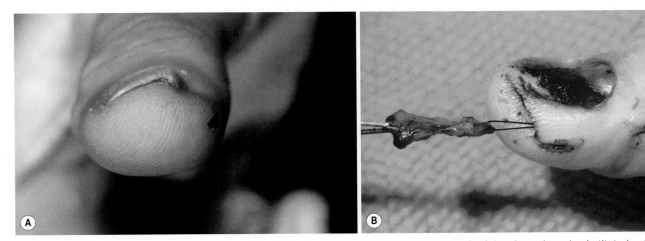

Figure 17.5. A, Unilateral pincer nail. **B,** The perionychium is freed from the bone, and a graft of dermis or dermal substitute is placed into the tunnel to flatten the nail bed.

Continued

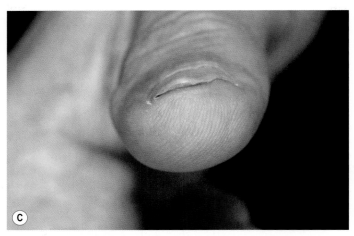

Figure 17.5, cont'd. C, 1 year after correction. *(Reprinted from Neligan, P.C., Chang, J. [Eds.], 2013. Plastic Surgery, vol. 6, 3rd ed. Elsevier, 117–134. © Southern Illinois University School of Medicine.)*

- Split nail deformity
  - Scarred nail matrix after injury
  - Treatment
    - Germinal matrix scar: Excision of scar tissue, full-thickness matrix graft from second toe
    - Sterile matrix scar: Excision of scar tissue, split-thickness matrix graft from second toe
    - Eponychial fold adhesion: Incision and eponychial flap

Fingertip Soft-Tissue Injuries

1. In general, treatment options depend on wound size, location and orientation of injury, and presence or absence of exposed critical structures (e.g., bone, tendon, vasculature).
   - Volar soft-tissue loss ≤1 cm²: Secondary intention
     - May have superior restoration of sensation and function compared to other options
   - >1-cm defect, without exposed bone or tendon: Skin graft
     - Full-thickness grafts give better restoration of sensation.
     - Split-thickness grafts will contact more, which may be advantageous in certain instances.
   - Large defects or defects with exposed tendon or bone: Local flaps (see Figure 17.6)

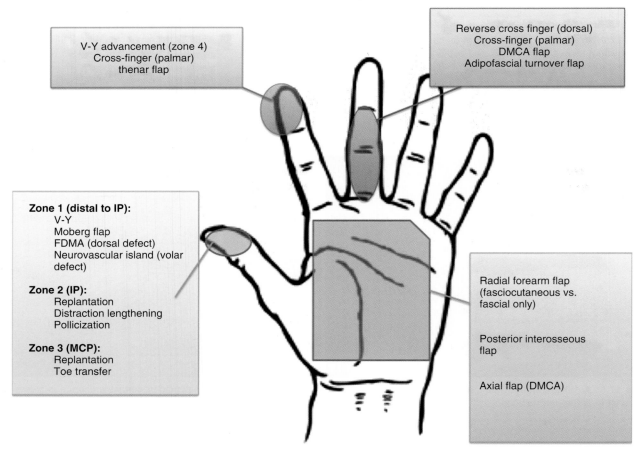

Figure 17.6. Schematic of soft-tissue reconstructive procedures based on location of the primary defect. *DMCA,* Dorsal metacarpal artery; *FDMA,* first dorsal metacarpal artery; *IP,* interphalangeal. *(Reprinted from Biswas, D., Wysocki, R.W., Fernandez, J.J., et al., 2014. Local and regional flaps for hand coverage. J. Hand Surg. Am. 39 [5], 992–1004.)*

2. Common local flaps
   - Bilateral V-Y advancement flaps (Kutler flap)
     - Useful with volar oblique amputations (see Figure 17.7)
   - Volar advancement (Atasoy-Kleinert/Tranquilli-Leali)
     - Useful with dorsal oblique amputations
     - Good for coverage of distal phalanx and support of the nail bed
     - Generally cannot be advanced >5 to 10 mm
     - May be at increased risk for contracture of the distal interphalangeal (DIP) joint (see Figure 17.8)
   - Thenar flap
     - Useful for young patients with volar defects of the index or long finger
     - Requires second stage for flap division, inset, and donor site closure
     - Older patients may be at increased risk for finger stiffness and/or joint contracture (see Figure 17.9)
   - Cross-finger flap
     - Useful for volar defect of over middle phalanx of adjacent finger
     - Skin graft over donor site (see Figure 17.10)
   - Reverse cross-finger flap
     - Useful for dorsal defect over middle phalanx of adjacent finger

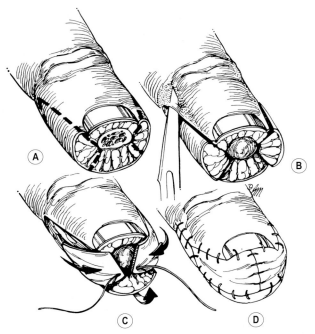

Figure 17.7. Kutler lateral V-Y technique. *(Reprinted from Jebson, P.J.L., Louis, D.S., 2005. Amputations. In: Green, D.P., Hotchkiss, R.N., Pederson, W.C., Wolfe, S.W. [Eds.], Green's Operative Hand Surgery, 5th ed. Churchill Livingstone, New York, 1943.)*

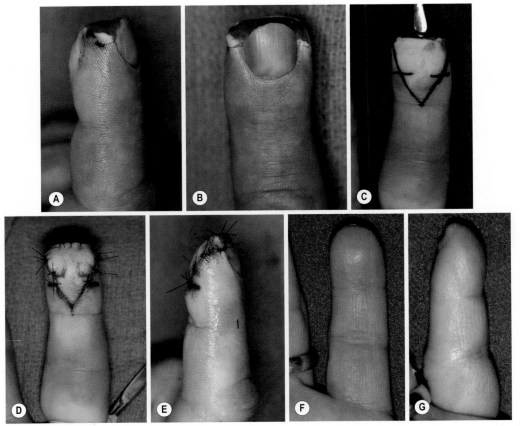

Figure 17.8. Patient presenting with a transverse fingertip injury. **A,B,** More than 50% of the nail bed remains. **C-E,** A V-Y advancement flap is used to treat this defect. **F,G,** The patient demonstrates a fully sensate, pain-free digit at final follow-up. *(Reprinted from Biswas, D., Wysocki, R.W., Fernandez, J.J., et al., 2014. Local and regional flaps for hand coverage. J. Hand Surg. Am. 39 [5], 992–1004.)*

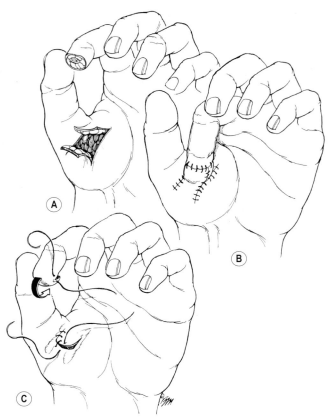

Figure 17.9. Thenar H flap. *(Reprinted from Jebson, P.J.L., Louis, D.S., 2005. Amputations. In: Green, D.P., Hotchkiss, R.N., Pederson, W.C., Wolfe, S.W. [Eds.], Green's Operative Hand Surgery, 5th ed. Churchill Livingstone, New York, 1947.)*

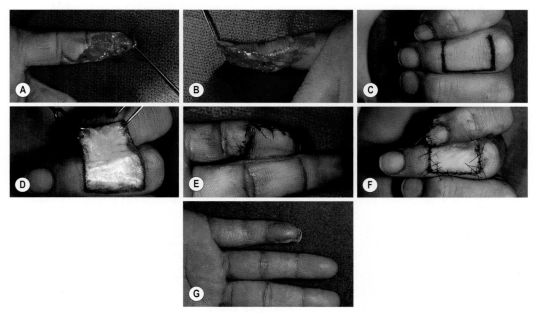

Figure 17.10. A,B, Patient sustained a soft-tissue injury with extensive palmar tissue loss over the middle and distal phalanx of the little finger. **C,D,** A cross-finger flap was harvested from the dorsal middle phalanx of the ring finger and **(E)** was inset into the defect; **(F)** the donor site was covered with a skin graft. The flap was divided at 2 weeks, and the patient reported a fully sensate digit with no appreciable flexion contractures of the proximal interphalangeal (PIP) or DIP with excellent cosmesis **(G).** *(Reprinted from Biswas, D., Wysocki, R.W., Fernandez, J.J., et al., 2014. Local and regional flaps for hand coverage. J. Hand Surg. Am. 39 [5], 992–1004.)*

- Adipofascial flap and skin graft used for coverage of defect; donor site closed with skin flap (see Figure 17.11)
- Adipofascial turn down flap
  - Open skin as an "H", elevate flap from proximal to distal, turn flap over to cover defect, close skin incision and, perform split-thickness skin graft (STSG) to recipient site.
- Free toe pulp flap
  - Useful for providing bulk and sensation to volar finger pad injuries (especially in musicians)
  - Often used in setting of failed secondary intention healing
  - Toe pulp harvested from the great toe or medial aspect of second toe

Thumb Soft-Tissue Injuries

1. First dorsal metacarpal artery flap
   - Useful for
     - Volar tip defects that are 2 × 3 cm in size
     - Midthumb defects
     - Coverage of exposed flexor pollicis longus
   - Donor site is the first ray, which must lie outside of the zone of injury (see Figure 17.12).
2. Littler neurovascular island flap
   - Useful for defects where first dorsal metacarpal artery flap is unavailable

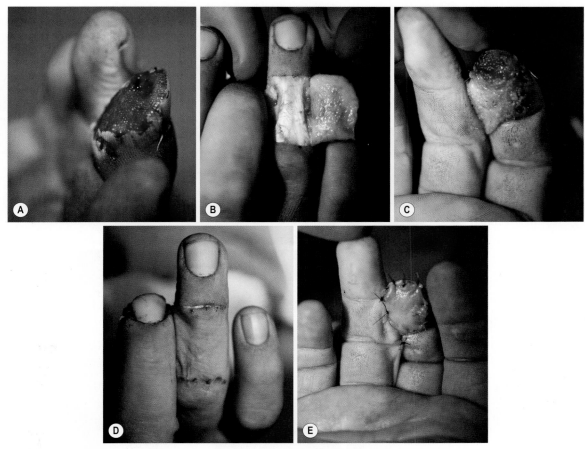

Figure 17.11. A, Patient presented with a fingertip defect with volar soft-tissue loss of the middle finger. **B,** A reverse cross-finger flap was performed to provide coverage by using donor tissue overlying the dorsum of the ring finger, first by elevating a 3-sided, full-thickness skin flap only to the level of the dermis, with the hinge on the ulnar aspect of the flap. The paratenon was preserved overlying the extensor mechanism atop the middle phalanx of the ring finger. **C,** A 3-sided flap consisting of fat and subcutaneous tissue was then elevated in the opposite direction, with its hinge on the radial side of the donor site and rotated to cover the volar defect of the middle finger. **D,** The original skin flap was then sutured to cover the donor site and a full-thickness skin graft was applied to cover the rotated subcutaneous flap at the recipient site **(E)**. *(Reprinted from Biswas, D., Wysocki, R.W., Fernandez, J.J., et al., 2014. Local and regional flaps for hand coverage. J. Hand Surg. Am. 39 [5], 992–1004.)*

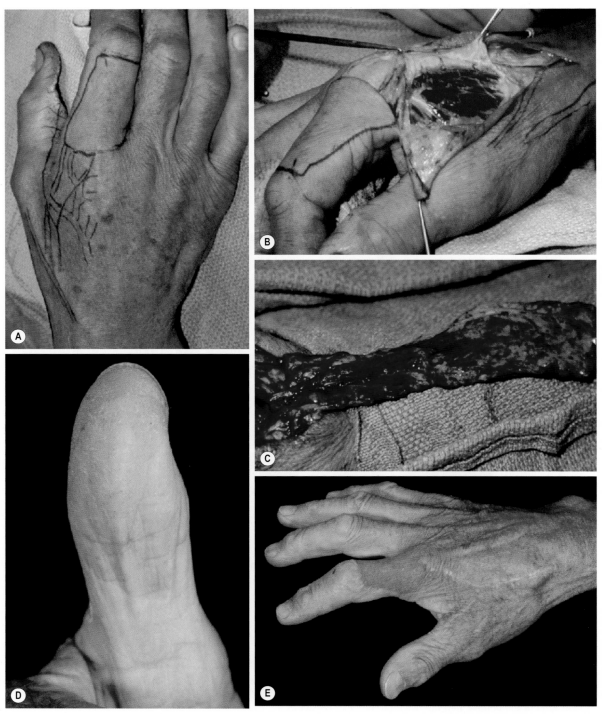

Figure 17.12. A, First dorsal metacarpal artery flap is designed over the dorsal aspect of the index finger. **B,C,** First dorsal metacarpal artery lies within the fascia of the first dorsal interosseous muscle. The pedicle is elevated with the fascia and care is taken to keep the superficial veins to allow appropriate drainage of the flap. **D,E,** Final appearance of the defect on the thumb and donor site. *(Reprinted from Neligan, P.C., Chang, J. [Eds.], 2013. Plastic Surgery, vol. 6, 3rd ed. Elsevier, 117–134.)*

- Donor site is the dorsoulnar aspect of the long or ring finger.
- Disadvantages: Small flap, poor donor site, venous congestion, requires significant cortical reorientation (see Figure 17.13)

3. Moberg flap
   - Useful for 1- to 1.5-cm tip defects of the thumb
   - Characterized by a volar, rectangular advancement flap
   - Risk of interphalangeal (IP) joint contracture in defects >1 to 1.5 cm (see Figure 17.14)

4. First web-space free flap
   - Useful for large volar thumb defects (~6 × 3 cm) or defects when local flaps are not available
   - Donor site is the lateral aspect of the great toe and the medial aspect of the second toe.
   - Vascular supply: First dorsal metatarsal a. (off of the dorsalis pedis a.)

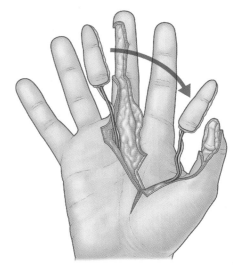

Figure 17.13. The Littler neurovascular island flap uses the skin subcutaneous tissue and neurovascular bundle from the nondominant side of the long or ring fingers. The dissection is carried down into the palm and the flap is transposed to the defect on the thumb. *(Reprinted from Neligan, P.C., Chang, J. [Eds.], 2013. Plastic Surgery, vol. 6, 3rd ed. Elsevier, 117–134.)*

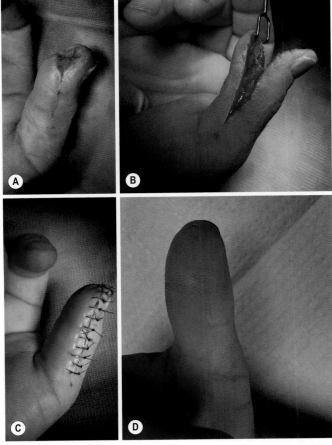

Figure 17.14. A, Patient presents with a chronic soft-tissue defect of the volar tip of the thumb and **(B,C)** underwent a Moberg advancement. **D,** Postoperatively, the patient experienced excellent cosmesis with full extension of the IP joint. *(Reprinted from Biswas, D., Wysocki, R.W., Fernandez, J.J., et al., 2014. Local and regional flaps for hand coverage. J. Hand Surg. Am. 39 [5], 992–1004.)*

Replantation (See Box 17.1)

1. Relative indications for replantation
   - Amputations of the thumb
     - Thumb contributes significantly to overall hand function.
     - Can consider vein grafting to avoid zone of injury
     - Length is more important than function; thus, in injuries with severe muscle belly damage, the interphalangeal joint can be fused.
     - If the thumb is not salvageable, consider pollicization or great-toe-to-thumb transfer.
       - Pollicization preferred in proximal amputations
       - Great toe flap preferred in amputations distal to the metacarpal phalangeal joint.
   - Multidigit amputations
   - Single-digit amputations distal to the flexor digitorum superficialis tendon insertion
   - Pediatric patients

2. Relative contraindications
   - Crush injuries or severe avulsion injuries
     - Avulsions have a large zone of injury, including traction injury to vasculature; thus, often require vein grafting or adjacent digital artery transfer when replantation attempted in this setting.
   - Single-digit amputations involving the index or long finger
   - Single-digit amputations in manual laborers who wish to return to work quickly
     - Revision amputation will allow faster return to work.
   - Single-digit amputations proximal to the flexor digitorum superficialis tendon insertion
   - Warm ischemia >6 hours proximal to the carpus or >12 hours for any digit
     - May be able to tolerate 12 to 24 hours of cold ischemia

3. Transport the amputated part dry inside of a plastic bag that is placed in a saline ice slurry (see Figure 17.15).

BOX 17.1 CRITICAL POINTS: REPLANTATION

Indications/Contraindications
- See the "Critical Points" box in the section "Patient Selection."

Preoperative Evaluation
- Level of injury and number of digits
- Type of injury (sharp vs. crush vs. avulsion)
- General condition/stability of patient
- Radiographic evaluation of the amputated part and residual limb
- Patient's vocation, avocations, expectations

Pearls
- Take the amputated part to the operating room before the patient arrives to begin identifying vessels and nerves and debriding.
- May insert the distal fixation in part
- Keep the part cool on ice in a sterile container.
- Plan to vein-graft arteries early if there is any question of injury.
- Avoid tension on the skin closure.

Technical Points/Sequence of Replantation
- Locate and tag vessels and nerves (6-0 Prolene or hemoclips).
- Debride soft tissues after the identification of vessels and nerves.
- Shorten and fix the bone.
- Repair the extensor tendons.
- Repair the flexor tendons.
- Anastomose the arteries.
- Repair the nerves.
- Anastomose the veins (two for every artery repair).
- Obtain skin coverage.

Pitfalls
- Make absolutely certain that the vessel for anastomosis is not damaged or stretched (perform a vein-graft if there is any question).
- Shortening of bone may allow primary vessel repair.
- Avoid tight wound closure or tight dressing.

Postoperative Care
- Keep patient warm.
- Watch volume status: Keep blood pressure and urine output at adequate levels.
- Heparinize with a crush or avulsion injury or with a problem involving blood flow in operating room.
- Monitor digital temperature and observe capillary refill, color, and turgor for signs of arterial insufficiency or venous congestion.

Reprinted from Wolfe, S.W., et al. [Eds.], 2011. Green's Operative Hand Surgery, 6th ed. Elsevier, p. 1592.

Early care of amputated part

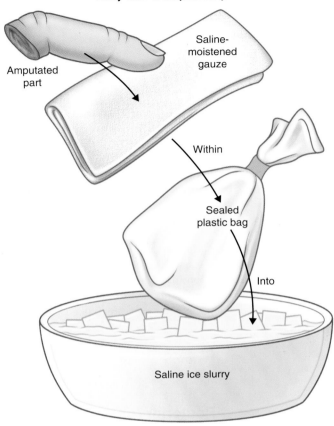

Amputated part

Saline-moistened gauze

Within

Sealed plastic bag

Into

Saline ice slurry

Figure 17.15. Wrap the amputated part in moist gauze placed in a plastic bag chilled in an ice-water mixture. Direct contact of the part with the ice must be avoided. *(Reprinted from Neligan, P.C., Chang, J. [Eds.], 2013. Plastic Surgery, vol. 6, 3rd ed. Elsevier, 228–249.)*

4. Methods for multidigit replantation
   - Part by part: Perform replant by structure, rather than digit by digit.
     - Typical order includes bone, extensor/flexor tendons, arteries, nerves, and veins.
       - Neural repair: Use a maximum of 4 sutures to prevent neuroma formation.
   - Digit by digit: Perform replant one digit at a time, rather than replant based on structure.
     - Preferred approach when warm ischemia times differ between digits
     - The digit in the best condition is replanted first.
     - Digits may be replanted either orthotopically (in same location) or heterotopically (in different location) depending on functional circumstances.
       - In severely injured hands, the functional goals are restoration of 3-point pinch grip, functional thumb, and two opposing fingers.
       - Heterotopic replantation is preferred if ulnar digits are all in poor condition.

Suggested Readings

Biswas, D., Wysocki, R.W., Fernandez, J.J., et al., 2014. Local and regional flaps for hand coverage. J. Hand Surg. Am. 39 (5), 992–1004.

Dzwierzynski, W.W., 2013. Chapter 11: Replantation and revascularization. In: Neligan, P.C., Chang, J. (Eds.), Plastic Surgery, vol. 6, 3rd ed. Elsevier, pp. P228–P249.

Goldner, R.D., Urbaniak, J.R., 2011. Chapter 48: Replantation. In: Wolfe, S.W., Hotchkiss, R.N., Pederson, W.C., et al. (Eds.), Green's Operative Hand Surgery, 6th ed. Elsevier, pp. 1585–1601.

Neumeister, M.W., Zook, E.G., Sommer, N.Z., et al., 2013. Chapter 6: Nail and fingertip reconstruction. In: Neligan, P.C., Chang, J. (Eds.), Plastic Surgery, vol. 6, 3rd ed. Elsevier, pp. 117–134.

Sommer, N.Z., Brown, R.E., 2011. Chapter 10: The perionychium. In: Wolfe, S.W., Hotchkiss, R.N., Pederson, W.C., et al. (Eds.), Green's Operative Hand Surgery, 6th ed. Elsevier, pp. 333–353.

Zienowicz, R.J., Harris, A.R., Mehan, V., 2010. Chapter 121: Fingertip injuries. In: Weinzweig, J. (Ed.), Plastic Surgery Secrets Plus, 2nd ed. Elsevier, pp. 787–793.

Carpal Injuries and Hand Arthritis

Carpal Anatomy

1. The distal radioulnar joint (DRUJ) allows for supination and pronation of the hand.
2. The proximal carpal row consists of the scaphoid, lunate, triquetrum, and pisiform and allows for wrist extension, flexion, and radial/ulnar deviation.

- The proximal row articulates primarily with the distal radius through the scaphoid and lunate.
3. The distal carpal row consists of the trapezium, trapezoid, capitate, and hamate and forms the fixed unit of the hand along with the second and third metacarpals (see Figure 18.1).

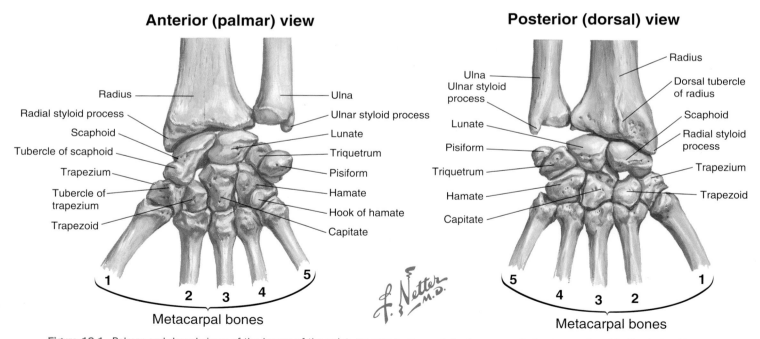

Anterior (palmar) view

Radius
Radial styloid process
Scaphoid
Tubercle of scaphoid
Trapezium
Tubercle of trapezium
Trapezoid
Ulna
Ulnar styloid process
Lunate
Triquetrum
Pisiform
Hamate
Hook of hamate
Capitate

1 2 3 4 5

Metacarpal bones

Posterior (dorsal) view

Ulna
Ulnar styloid process
Lunate
Pisiform
Triquetrum
Hamate
Capitate
Radius
Dorsal tubercle of radius
Scaphoid
Radial styloid process
Trapezium
Trapezoid

5 4 3 2 1

Metacarpal bones

Figure 18.1. Palmar and dorsal views of the bones of the wrist. *(Reprinted with permission from www.netterimages.com. Copyright Elsevier Inc. All Rights Reserved.)*

4. The extrinsic carpal ligaments help to anchor the proximal row with the distal radius and ulna.
   - The proximal row is anchored to the distal radius and ulna by the strong extrinsic palmar radiocarpal ligaments and the palmar portion of the triangular fibrocartilage complex (TFCC), as well as the dorsal intercarpal ligament (from scaphoid to triquetrum) and the dorsal radiocarpal ligament.
5. The intrinsic carpal ligaments are strong structures that link the carpal bones together, and/or the carpal rows together. The two most important intrinsic carpal ligaments are the scapholunate (SL) ligament and the lunotriquetral (LT) ligament. Disruptions of these ligaments lead to carpal instability.
   - The SL ligament allows synchronous motion of the scaphoid and lunate
     - It is U-shaped with a dorsal, proximal, and palmar component. The dorsal component is the strongest and most important for stability.
   - The LT ligament anchors the lunate and triquetrum together and allows less motion than the SL ligament (see Figure 18.2).

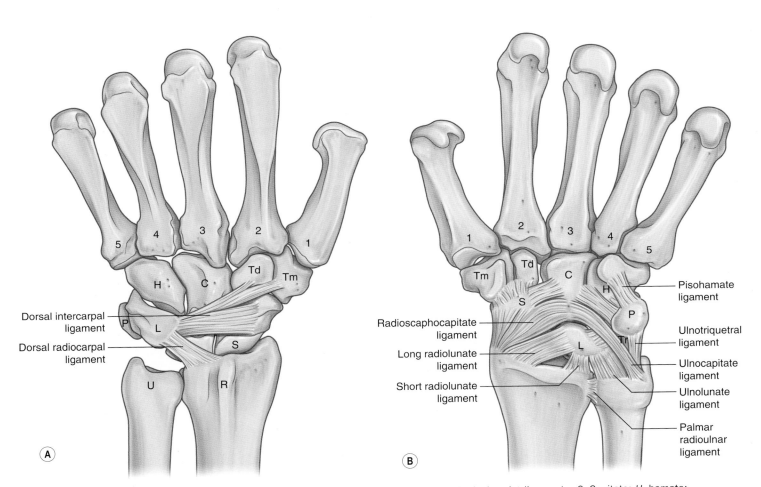

Figure 18.2. A, Dorsal extrinsic wrist ligaments; **B,** volar extrinsic wrist ligaments; **C,** intrinsic wrist ligaments. *C,* Capitate; *H,* hamate; *L,* lunate; *P,* pisiform; *R,* radius; *S,* scaphoid; *Td,* trapezoid; *Tm,* trapezium; *Tr,* Triquetrum; *U,* ulna. *(Reprinted from Neligan, P.C., Chang, J. [Eds.], 2013. Plastic Surgery, vol. 6, 3rd ed. Elsevier, 1–46.)*

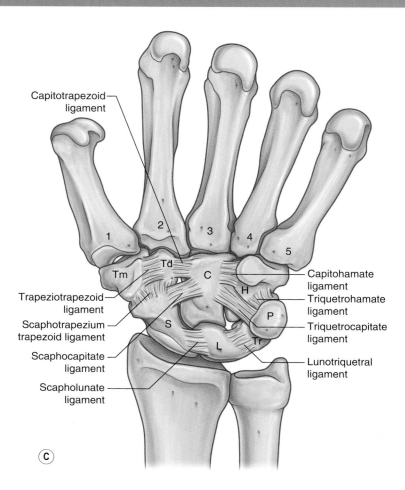

Capitotrapezoid ligament

Capitohamate ligament

Triquetrohamate ligament

Triquetrocapitate ligament

Lunotriquetral ligament

Trapeziotrapezoid ligament

Scaphotrapezium trapezoid ligament

Scaphocapitate ligament

Scapholunate ligament

C

Figure 18.2, cont'd.

6. The distal radius slopes 22 degrees in the radioulnar plane and 12 degrees in the dorsal/palmar plane.
7. The ulna should complete the smooth curve of the articular surface of the radius. The relationship of the ulna to this imaginary curve is called ulnar variance.
    - Ulnar positive variance: The ulna extends distal to this imaginary curve.
        - Associated with ulnar impaction syndrome (ulnar-sided wrist pain)
    - Ulnar negative variance: The ulna is short of this imaginary curve.
        - Associated with Kienböck's disease (avascular necrosis of the lunate)
8. Gilula's lines: Imaginary curves within the carpus that indicate normal extracarpal and intracarpal architecture (see Figure 18.3).
    - Disruptions of these lines suggest ligamentous or bony carpal abnormalities.

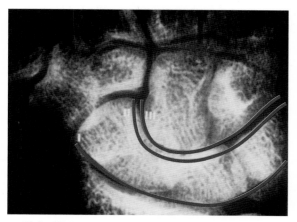

Figure 18.3. Gilula's lines, showing the greater arc and lesser arc of the carpal bones. *(Reprinted from Hentz, V.R., Chase, R.A., 2001. Hand Surgery: A Clinical Atlas. WB Saunders, Philadelphia.)*

Common Carpal Ligament Injuries

1. SL dissociation
   - Results from an injury to, or tear of, the SL ligament or scaphoid fracture
   - Characterized by pain and swelling over the radial dorsal wrist with widening of the gap between the scaphoid and lunate on plain X ray ("Terry Thomas" sign)
     - Must compare with unaffected hand
     - A gap >2 mm is suggestive of an injury.
   - Disrupts the synchrony between the scaphoid and lunate, allowing the scaphoid to flex and lunate to extend
     - As the scaphoid flexes, the cortex of the distal scaphoid pole projects as a ring on radiographs ("cortical ring sign").
     - On physical exam, a clunk can be palpated as the scaphoid is subluxed and relocated with radioulnar deviation of the wrist ("Watson scaphoid shift test").
     - A DISI (dorsal intercalated segment instability) deformity develops with SL injury as the lunate assumes a dorsally tilted posture and the scaphoid flexes. This can be identified on lateral X ray by an increased SL angle.
   - Treatment options
     - Immobilization for 3 to 4 weeks is generally acceptable for partial tears
     - Open repair of the ligament is indicated with acute, complete tears or partial tears with persistent pain after immobilization.
     - For chronic SL injuries, severe arthritis can develop, creating an SL advanced collapse (SLAC) wrist deformity.
       - ○ Characterized by radioscaphoid, capitolunate, and scaphocapitate arthritis. In severe cases, the capitate can become impacted between the scaphoid and lunate.
       - ○ Treatment: Proximal row corpectomy (removal of the scaphoid, lunate, and triquetrum) or "4-corner fusion" (removal of the scaphoid with fusion of the lunate, triquetrum, hamate, and capitate)
2. LT ligament injury
   - Characterized by wrist swelling and pain, with a disruption in Gilula's line from a step-off between the lunate and the triquetrum
   - Disrupts the synchrony of the lunate and triquetrum, allowing the lunate to flex with the scaphoid
     - On physical examination, pain and instability with "ballottement" or "shucking" of the lunate and triquetrum suggests injury.
     - A VISI (volar intercalated segment instability) deformity develops as the lunate tilts volarly.
   - Treatment options
     - The ligament is often too short to repair primarily; thus, pinning of the LT interval is often performed, with or without ligament reconstruction.

3. Perilunate dislocation
   - Caused by wrist hyperextension and supination with ligamentous injuries around the lunate, which progress from radial to ulnar
     - When all of the ligaments are torn, the lunate can dislocate volarly into the carpal tunnel through the space of Poirer ("spilled tea cup sign" on lateral X ray).
   - Characterized by a high-energy injury, with wrist swelling, pain, and potentially acute carpal-tunnel-syndrome symptoms
   - Can also develop with scaphoid fracture and/or other carpal fractures (see Figures 18.4 and 18.5)

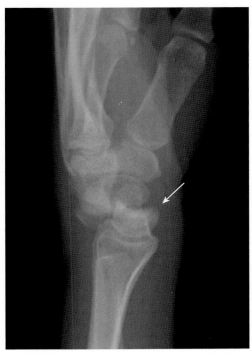

Figure 18.4. *Arrow,* A perilunate dislocation, when the lunate stays in its fossa, whereas the rest of the wrist subluxes dorsally. *(Reprinted from Neligan, P.C. [Ed.], 2013. Plastic Surgery, 3rd ed. Elsevier, 161–178.)*

   - Follows a natural progression of injury around the lunate complex
     - Mayfield classification (see Figure 18.6)
   - Treatment
     - Closed reduction and splinting in the emergency room to relieve carpal tunnel symptoms (especially if no operating room is available)
     - Urgent operative fixation and carpal tunnel release

Common Wrist/Carpal Fractures

1. Distal radius fracture
   - The most common fracture of the human skeleton
   - Often caused by a fall onto an outstretched hand

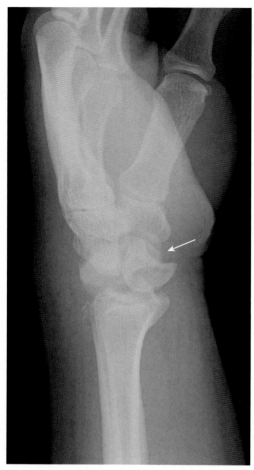

Figure 18.5. *Arrow,* The telltale spilled tea cup sign, an indication of lunate dislocation. *(Reprinted from Neligan, P.C. [Ed.], 2013. Plastic Surgery, 3rd ed. Elsevier, 161–178.)*

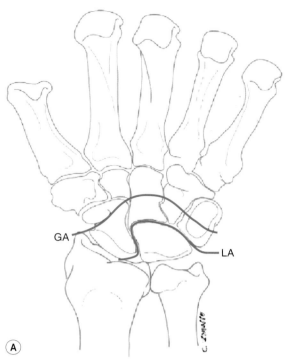

Ⓐ

Figure 18.6. Mayfield classification. Mayfield described a classification system based on a progressive sequence of injuries. He further classified these injuries into greater arc *(GA)* or lesser arc *(LA)* injuries. **A,** Greater arc injuries involve a fracture of any bone in the sequence—the radial styloids, scaphoid, capitate, hamate, or triquetrum. Lesser arc injuries do not involve a fracture and are only ligamentous injuries. **B,** Mayfield's stages I to IV showing a progressive sequence of injuries ending with a complete perilunate dislocation *(arrow).* (**A,** *Reprinted from Sauder, D.J., Athwal, G.S., Faber, K.J., et al., 2007. Perilunate injuries. Orthop. Clin. North. Am. 38, 279–288;* **B,** *Reprinted from Kozin, S.H., 1998. Perilunate injuries: diagnosis and treatment. J. Am. Acad. Orthop. Surg. 6, 114–120.)*

- Characterized by pain, swelling, limited motion, and gross deformity of the wrist
- Treatment options
  - Cast immobilization is indicated for nondisplaced or minimally displaced fractures, especially in elderly patients.
  - Open reduction internal fixation (ORIF)
    - General indications for ORIF: Displaced fractures, comminuted fractures, intra-articular fractures with displacement or >2 mm of cortical step-off, radial shortening >3 mm, and/or dorsal tilt >10 degrees.
    - Most commonly performed with volar locking plates
- Extensor pollicis longus (EPL) tendon rupture can occur after distal radius fracture.
  - Secondary to attrition through disruption of tendon vascularity
  - Treated with extensor indicis proprius tendon transfer

2. Scaphoid fracture
   - The most common carpal fracture
   - The scaphoid can be divided into three segments: Distal pole, waist, and proximal pole
     - Single, dominant, vascular supply that enters the distal pole and travels retrograde to supply the proximal pole via the dorsal carpal branch of the radial artery
       - In addition, a minor secondary supply also enters distally via the superficial palmar branch of the radial artery.
       - This retrograde vascular supply portends a higher risk of nonunion or avascular necrosis with more proximal fractures.
   - Scaphoid fractures are often caused by a fall onto an outstretched hand.
   - Characterized by pain in the anatomic snuff box
   - Fractures may not be visualized on initial plain radiographs
     - Computed tomography (CT) is useful to evaluate for fracture in the acute period if concern for fracture is high and initial films are negative.

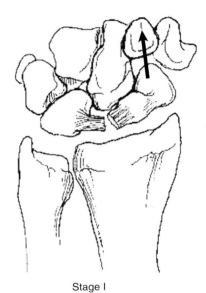

Stage I

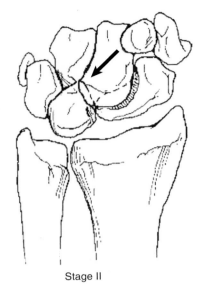

Stage II

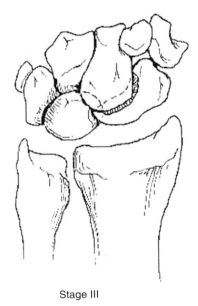

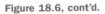
(B)   Stage III

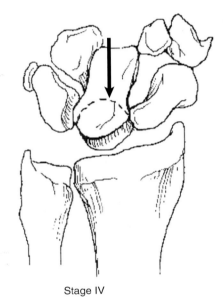

Stage IV

Figure 18.6, cont'd.

- Treatment options
  - Long arm thumb spica cast immobilization for 6 to 8 weeks
    - ○ Indicated for nondisplaced, distal pole fractures
    - ○ For proximal pole fractures, immobilization is often recommended for 6 months.
  - ORIF
    - ○ Indicated in distal pole fractures displaced >1 mm, unstable transverse or oblique wrist fractures, and/or most proximal pole fractures.
    - ○ Often performed with compression screw fixation (see Table 18.1)
- Scaphoid nonunion or malunion ("humpback deformity") can occur after scaphoid fracture.
  - Higher risk with more proximal fractures

- Can progress to arthritis and SNAC (scaphoid nonunion advanced collapse) wrist deformity.
- Occurs often with missed scaphoid fractures in young athletic patients.
- Treatment: Bone grafting
  - ○ Nonvascularized bone grafting (e.g., iliac crest, distal radius) can be used for treatment of severe humpback deformity.
  - ○ Vascularized bone grafting (e.g., retrograde distal radius bone flap, medial femoral condyle flap) is indicated for most nonunions.
3. Other carpal fractures (in order of frequency)
- Triquetrum fractures
  - Patients present with pain over the triquetrum.
  - Dorsal lip fractures are the most common.

Table 18.1 Algorithm for Acute Scaphoid Fracture Management

TYPE OF FRACTURE	TREATMENT
Stable Fractures, Nondisplaced	
Tubercle fracture	Short arm cast for 6 to 8 weeks
Distal third fracture/incomplete fracture	Short arm cast for 6 to 8 weeks
Waist fracture	• Long arm thumb spica cast for 6 weeks, short arm cast for 6 weeks or until CT confirmed healing • Percutaneous or open internal fixation
Proximal pole fracture, nondisplaced	Percutaneous or open internal fixation
Unstable Fractures	
• Displacement >1 mm • Lateral intrascaphoid angle >35 degrees • Bone loss or comminution • Perilunate fracture/dislocation • Dorsal intercalated segmental instability alignment	Dorsal percutaneous/open screw fixation

Reprinted from Wolfe, S.W., Hotchkiss, R.N., Pederson, W.C., et al. (Eds.), 2011. Green's Operative Hand Surgery, 6th ed. Elsevier, 639–707.

■ Treatment: Most can be treated with cast immobilization for 4 to 6 weeks.
• Trapezium fractures
  ■ Often associated with other fractures (e.g., distal radius, metacarpals)
  ■ Often result from an impaction force of the thumb metacarpal into the trapezium
  ■ Trapezial ridge fractures can occur from a direct blow (e.g., from a baseball).
  ■ Treatment: Nondisplaced ridge fractures may be treated with cast immobilization; however, displaced fractures of the trapezium require open reduction and internal fixation (e.g., compression screw, K wire).
• Hamate fractures
  ■ Relatively rare, although fractures of the hook of the hamate are more common in athletes (e.g., baseball players, golfers, tennis and racquet ball players)
  ■ The hook protrudes from the base of the hamate into the hypothenar musculature and is at risk for direct force.
  ■ Characterized by chronic pain at the base of the hypothenar eminence, which is worse with grasping, and occasionally ulnar nerve paresthesias
  ■ Hook of hamate fractures require special carpal tunnel views on X ray for visualization.
  ■ Treatment: Nondisplaced, acute fractures can be treated with cast immobilization; however, displaced or chronic fractures are often treated with excision of the hook of hamate fragment.

Osteoarthritis of the Hand and Wrist

1. Osteoarthritis (OA) of the small joints of the hand is relatively common and can cause significant pain, deformity, or stiffness.
   • The distal interphalangeal (DIP) joints are most commonly involved, followed by the proximal interphalangeal (PIP) joints, and metacarpal phalangeal (MCP) joints.
   • The treatment of small-joint arthritis centers on optimal medical management (especially for inflammatory arthritis), patient selection, and relative active and passive joint motion.
   • The primary surgical procedures for the stiff arthritic finger are arthroplasty and arthrodesis.
     ■ Arthroplasty requires adequate soft tissue and ligamentous support for stability.
       ○ Silicone and pyrolytic carbon implants available
         ◆ Silicone lacks stability, especially with side-to-side force, when compared to pyrolytic carbon implants, and has a high rate of implant fatigue.
         ◆ Pyrolytic carbon implants have high revision rates.
     ■ Arthrodesis: Indicated for painful, unstable, or deformed digits with loss of motor control or inadequate bony stock to support a prosthesis or digits with intractable pain that have failed all other conservative measures (see Figure 18.7)

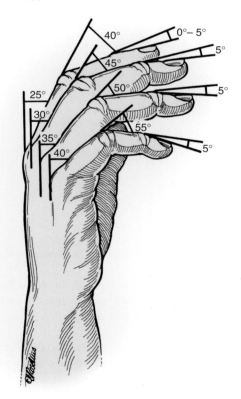

Figure 18.7. Recommended preferred positions for arthrodesis of finger joints. *(Reprinted from Wolfe, S.W., Hotchkiss, R.N., Pederson, W.C., et al. [Eds.], 2011. Green's Operative Hand Surgery, 6th ed. Elsevier, 389–406. Copyright Elizabeth Martin.)*

2. Basilar/first carpometacarpal (CMC) joint arthritis
   - The thumb accounts for 50% of all hand function.
   - Arthritis of the trapeziometacarpal joint is very common and prevalence increases with age.
   - Many patients will remain asymptomatic and symptoms do not necessarily correlate with findings on plain radiographs.
     - Patients typically complain of difficulty opening jars or pain with pinch grip. Stiffness and pain at rest are typically present in late-stage disease.
   - Diagnosis and staging of the disease can be made using plain radiographs (see Table 18.2).

Table 18.2 Eaton Classification

STAGE	RADIOGRAPHIC CHARACTERISTICS
Stage I	Normal or slightly widened trapeziometacarpal joint Trapeziometacarpal subluxation up to $\frac{1}{3}$ of articular surface Normal articular contours
Stage II	Decreased trapeziometacarpal joint space Trapeziometacarpal subluxation up to $\frac{1}{3}$ of articular surface Osteophytes or loose bodies <2 mm
Stage III	Decreased trapeziometacarpal joint space Trapeziometacarpal subluxation >$\frac{1}{3}$ of articular surface Osteophytes or loose bodies ≥2 mm Subchondral cysts or sclerosis
Stage IV	Involvement of the scaphotrapezial joint or less commonly the trapeziotrapezoid or trapeziometacarpal joint of the index

Data from Eaton, R.G., Littler, J.W., 1973. Ligament reconstruction for the painful thumb carpometacarpal joint. J. Bone Joint Surg. Am. 55 (8), 1655–1666.

- Treatment is focused on patients with significant pain, thumb weakness, and instability, which can lead to functional deficits. Options include
  - Conservative treatments: Nonsteroidal anti-inflammatory drugs (NSAIDs), splinting, corticosteroid injections
    - First-line treatment
  - Arthroscopy
    - Often reserved for early-stage-I disease that has failed conservative treatment
    - Synovectomy, debridement, and capsulorrhaphy of the volar beak ligament can all be performed.
  - Arthroplasty
    - Often reserved for stage-II to -IV disease, with loss of articular cartilage
    - Performed with either trapeziectomy alone or in combination with ligament reconstruction and flexor carpi radialis (FCR) tendon interposition (ligament reconstruction tendon interposition [LRTI] CMC arthroplasty).

- Regardless of technique, postoperative spica cast or splint immobilization of the thumb is critical to preserve length and prevent subsidence.
  - Arthrodesis
    - Usually preferred over arthroplasty for patients <50 years old with arthritis of the trapeziometacarpal joint only, who wish to maintain grip and pinch strength
    - Also indicated when other reconstructions have failed
    - Fuse the thumb in 35 degrees of radial and palmar abduction with 15 degrees of pronation and 10 degrees of extension.
3. Carpal arthritis
   - Often caused by avascular necrosis of the scaphoid or lunate or secondary to trauma (e.g., chronic SL injury, distal radius fracture, SNAC or SLAC wrist, etc.)
   - Characterized by significant pain, stiffness, and functional limitations
   - Treatment options are directed at eliminating pain and include
     - Radial styloidectomy
       - Reserved for patients with arthritis confined to the radial styloid
     - Denervation of the wrist through partial neurectomy of the anterior interosseus nerve and posterior interosseus nerve (PIN)
     - Proximal row corpectomy
       - Indicated when the capitate and lunate fossa of the radius are spared from arthritic changes
       - Removal of the scaphoid, lunate, and triquetrum ("proximal row") converts the wrist into a hinge joint through articulation of the capitate with the radius.
     - 4-corner fusion
       - Indicated in advanced stages of SLAC or SNAC wrist, with involvement of the lunocapitate joint
       - Involves scaphoidectomy with fusion of the lunate, capitate, triquetrum, and hamate
     - Total wrist arthrodesis
       - Reserved for cases of advanced arthritis with involvement of the midcarpal joint and lunate fossa or as a salvage procedure when other reconstructive options have failed
       - Involves fusion of the radiocarpal, midcarpal, and third CMC joints with a dorsal plate or intramedullary pin

Rheumatoid Arthritis (RA) of the Wrist and Hand

1. Systemic autoimmune disorder that affects 1% of adults, with a female predilection and genetic component
2. Characterized by synovial inflammation of the joints of the hand and wrist, resulting in joint destruction, deformity, and functional disability
   - RA can also be associated with extra-articular disease including soft-tissue nodules, vasculitis, pericarditis,

peripheral neuropathy, conjunctivitis, and pulmonary disease.

3. Diagnosis is largely clinical and based on established criteria (see Table 18.3).
   - The presence of anemia, rheumatoid factor (RF), and elevated erythrocyte sedimentation rate (ESR) is suggestive of disease.
   - RF is a marker for RA and also correlates with severity of disease.

Table 18.3 Diagnostic Criteria for Rheumatoid Arthritis

CRITERION	DETAILS
1. Morning stiffness	1 hour
2. Soft-tissue swelling	3 or more joints
3. Soft-tissue swelling	Symmetric
4. Soft-tissue swelling of hand	MCP, PIP, wrist joints
5. Subcutaneous nodules	Rheumatoid nodules
6. Seropositivity	Rheumatoid factor
7. Typical radiographic findings	Periarticular erosions/osteopenia, hand or wrist

Reprinted from Neligan, P.C., Chang, J. (Eds.), 2013. Plastic Surgery, vol. 6, 3rd ed. Elsevier.
MCP, *Metacarpal phalangeal*; PIP, *proximal interphalangeal.*

4. Joint involvement follows a predictable pattern: MCP, PIP, and wrist joint involvement first, followed by knees, hips, shoulders, and elbows.
   - Unlike in OA, the DIP joints are often spared.
5. Wrist involvement
   - Progresses from inflammation to carpal instability, ulnar translocation of the carpus, caput ulnae (dorsal dislocation of the ulnar head, carpal supination, and volar subluxation of the extensor carpi ulnaris [ECU]), extensor tendon synovitis and rupture, and ankylosis or instability.
6. Finger involvement
   - MCP joint: Progresses to volar subluxation and ulnar deviation
   - PIP joint: Progresses to swan-neck deformity or boutonniere deformity (see Figures 18.8 and 18.9)
7. Management of RA is often multimodal and involves NSAIDs, corticosteroids, and disease-modifying antirheumatic drugs (DMARDs) (e.g., methotrexate, azathiropine, anti-TNF[alpha] agents, etanercept, and infliximab) as well as surgery for specific indications.
8. The goals of surgery for RA include pain reduction, cessation of disease progression, and improved function and appearance.
   - In general, stage and perform surgery first on proximal joints and then proceed distally.

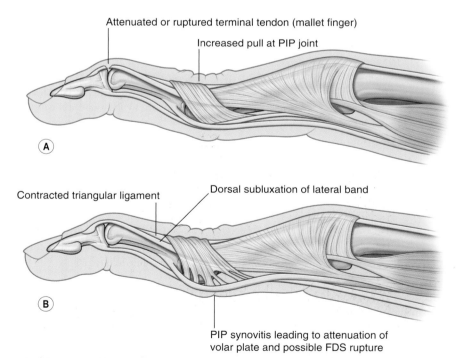

Attenuated or ruptured terminal tendon (mallet finger)

Increased pull at PIP joint

A

Contracted triangular ligament

Dorsal subluxation of lateral band

B

PIP synovitis leading to attenuation of volar plate and possible FDS rupture

Figure 18.8. A, Swan-neck deformity originating from a mallet finger, with subsequent increased extension force at the PIP joint. **B,** Swan-neck deformity originating at the PIP joint, with volar plate attenuation and possible FDS rupture due to PIP synovitis, and subsequent dorsal subluxation of the lateral bands. *FDS, Flexor digitorum superficialis; PIP, proximal interphalangeal. (Reprinted from Neligan, P.C., Chang, J. [Eds.], 2013. Plastic Surgery, vol. 6, 3rd ed. Elsevier.)*

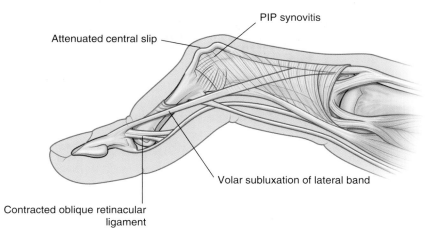

PIP synovitis

Attenuated central slip

Volar subluxation of lateral band

Contracted oblique retinacular ligament

Figure 18.9. Boutonniere deformity secondary to synovitis at the PIP joint, with attenuation of the central slip, and subsequent volar subluxation of the lateral bands. *(Reprinted from Neligan, P.C., Chang, J. [Eds.], 2013. Plastic Surgery, vol. 6, 3rd ed. Elsevier.)*

- Preoperatively, cervical spine radiographs in flexion and extension must be obtained to evaluate for atlantoaxial instability, which is common in RA patients.
9. Treatment options include
   - Synovectomy: Removal of painful inflammatory pannus and synovitis unresponsive to medical treatment
   - Distal ulna resection ("Darrach" procedure): Indicated for caput ulna syndrome with extensor tendon ruptures or intractable pain with DRUJ instability
     - Can lead to worsening of ulnar drift of the carpus because the ulnar stop has been removed
   - Wrist arthrodesis: Indicated for severe disease and instability
   - MCP/PIP arthroplasty: Indicated for pain and loss of function due to MCP deformity
     - Silicone is preferred in RA patients because of soft-tissue laxity and joint instability.
     - Pyrocarbon implants can be used for MCP arthroplasty but should be limited to young patients with stable soft tissues.
   - MCP/PIP arthrodesis: Indicated in patients who desire effective pain relief and will accept the loss in motion or those with retractable pain despite other procedures
   - Treatment of swan-neck deformity depends on the severity of joint disease, presence of intrinsic tightness, and relative motion of the PIP joint.
     - Options include splinting (early disease with full PIP flexion and no intrinsic tightness), intrinsic release, sublimus sling procedure, PIP arthrodesis, and PIP arthroplasty.
   - Tendon ruptures
     - Caused by attrition of tendon from tendon friction over a bony prominence, synovitis of the tendon, or vascular disruption of the tendon.
     - Most common tendons to rupture are the extensor tendons on the ulnar aspect of the hand secondary to caput ulnae (e.g., "Vaughn-Jackson syndrome": rupture of extensor digiti minimi [EDM] and extensor digitorum

communis [EDC] to the small, ring, and long fingers), the EPL tendon, and the flexor pollicis longus (FPL) tendon (from a "Mannerfelt lesion": Volar osteophyte of the scaphoid).
      - ○ Compression of the PIN can mimic EPL rupture (distinguished by absence of tenodesis effect with true rupture).
     - Treatment follows traditional tendon repair principles, with addition of osteophyte removal and Darrach procedure in caput ulna.
   - Trigger finger
     - Caused by synovitis and nodule formation of the flexor tendons
     - Treatment involves corticosteroid injection and flexor tenosynovectomy with removal of intratendinous nodules.
     - Never release the A1 pulley in rheumatoid arthritis patients because this can worsen the patient's ulnar drift.

Other Inflammatory Disorders of the Wrist and Hand (see Table 18.4)

1. Scleroderma
   - A rare autoimmune connective tissue disease characterized by systemic sclerosis of multiple tissues including the skin, blood vessels, heart, lung, gastrointestinal tract, and kidneys
   - Can present as limited cutaneous disease or CREST (calcinosis, Raynaud's phenomenon, esophageal dysmotility, sclerodactyly, and telangiectasia) syndrome
   - Finger deformities are related to contracture of skin with development of flexion contractures and ulcerations.
     - Most common lesion is PIP flexion contracture
     - Treat soft-tissue loss conservatively, with topical antimicrobials and minimal debridement.
     - For severe PIP contracture with intact skin, arthrodesis may be indicated, and phalanx shortening may be required to relieve pressure on overlying skin.
     - Occasionally, amputation is required.

Table 18.4 Characteristics of Other Rheumatologic Conditions of the Hand

CONDITION	SEROLOGY	RADIOGRAPHS	EXAMINATION
Psoriatic arthritis	Negative	Erosions Resorption Osteolysis Periostitis Ankylosis (PIP) Juxta-articular bone formation "Pencil in cup" (DIP)	Psoriasis Nail abnormalities, dactylitis PIP flexion contracture Opera glass hand swan-neck deformity
SLE	ANA Anti-DNA, antiphospholipid antibody Leucopenia Hemolytic anemia Thrombocytopenia	Preservation of joints Secondary OA	Deformity similar to that seen in RA Malar rash Discoid rash Serositis Other
Scleroderma	ANA Anticentromere Antitopoisomerase I Anti-RNA polymerase	Tuft resorption Secondary OA	Cutaneous telangiectasia Raynaud's Cutaneous sclerosis Ischemic ulceration Joint contracture due to skin contracture
Gout	Hyperuricemia Negatively birefringent crystals (synovial analysis)	Sclerotic joint margins Overhanging edges Erosion from tophi (late) Joint destruction (late)	Red, hot, swollen joint MTP of great toe involvement Tophi

Reprinted from Neligan, P.C., Chang, J. (Eds.), 2013. Plastic Surgery, vol. 6, 3rd ed. Elsevier.
ANA, *Antinuclear antibody;* DIP, *distal interphalangeal;* MTP, *metatarsophalangeal;* OA, *osteoarthritis;* PIP, *proximal interphalangeal;* RA, *rheumatoid arthritis;* SLE, *systemic lupus erythematosus.*

2. Gout
   - Hyperuricemia that progresses to recurrent bouts of acute arthritis
   - Gout affects 1% of adults, with a male predilection.
   - Risk factors: Obesity, alcoholism, hypertension, renal disease, cyclosporine, and hydrochlorothiazide
   - Triggers include stress, fevers, surgery, dehydration, alcohol, oatmeal, mushrooms, lentils, and spinach.
   - Characterized by an exquisitely painful, edematous, and erythematous joint
     - Diagnosed by arthrocentesis with presence of monosodium urate crystals
   - As the disease progresses, systemic symptoms (fever, chills, sweats) and chronic polyarticular arthritis with tophi development are common.
     - Radiographic findings in chronic gout include bony erosions with sclerotic margins.
   - Treatment is largely medical and includes NSAIDs (e.g., indomethacin), colchicine, and corticosteroids for acute attacks and colchicine or the xanthine oxidase inhibitor allopurinol for prophylaxis.
     - Surgery is reserved to selective arthrodesis for intractable joint pain or functional deficit and complete excision of painful, debilitating tophi.

Suggested Readings

Amadio, P.C., Shin, A.Y., 2011. Chapter 12: Arthrodesis and arthroplasty of small joints of the hand. In: Wolfe, S.W., Hotchkiss, R.N., Pederson, W.C., et al. (Eds.), Green's Operative Hand Surgery, 6th ed. Elsevier, pp. 389–406.

Barron, O.A., Catalano, L.W., 2011. Chapter 13: Thumb basal joint arthritis. In: Wolfe, S.W., Hotchkiss, R.N., Pederson, W.C., et al. (Eds.), Green's Operative Hand Surgery, 6th ed. Elsevier, pp. 407–426.

Carlsen, B.T., Bakri, K., Al-Mufarrej, F.M., et al., 2013. Chapter 20: Osteoarthritis of the hand and wrist. In: Neligan, P.C., Chang, J. (Eds.), Plastic Surgery, vol. 6, 3rd ed. Elsevier, pp. 411–448.

Chang, J., Valero-Cuevas, F., Hentz, V.R., et al., 2013. Chapter 1: Anatomy and biomechanics of the hand. In: Neligan, P.C., Chang, J. (Eds.), Plastic Surgery, vol. 6, 3rd ed. Elsevier, pp. 1–46.

Chung, K.C., Haase, S.C., 2013. Chapter 8: Fractures and dislocation of the wrist and distal radius. In: Neligan, P.C., Chang, J. (Eds.), Plastic Surgery, vol. 6, 3rd ed. Elsevier, pp. 161–177.

Geissler, W.B., Slade, J.F., 2011. Chapter 18: Fractures of the carpal bones. In: Wolfe, S.W., Hotchkiss, R.N., Pederson, W.C., et al. (Eds.), Green's Operative Hand Surgery, 6th ed. Elsevier, pp. 639–707.

Nelson, D.L., Gellman, H., Distal Fractures of the Radius Treatment & Management. Emedicine.com. Found at: http://emedicine.medscape.com/article/1245884-treatment Accessed on October 20, 2014.

Sammer, D.M., Chung, K.C., 2013. Chapter 19: Rheumatologic conditions of the hand and wrist. In: Neligan, P.C., Chang, J. (Eds.), Plastic Surgery, vol. 6, 3rd ed. Elsevier, pp. 371–410.

Wolfe, S.W., 2011. Chapter 17: Distal radius fractures. In: Wolfe, S.W., Hotchkiss, R.N., Pederson, W.C., et al. (Eds.), Green's Operative Hand Surgery, 6th ed. Elsevier, pp. 561–638.

Yao, J., Ahubhav, J., 2010. Chapter 44: Carpus: perilunate and greater arc injuries. In: Slutsky, D.J. (Ed.), Principles and Practice of Wrist Surgery, 1st ed. Saunders, pp. 473–484.

Tendon Injuries and Reconstruction

Flexor Tendon Anatomy (see Figures 19.1-19.4)

1. There are 12 flexor tendons in the hand and forearm. Common flexor group arises near the medial epicondyle. Most are median n. innervated, except the flexors to the 4th and 5th digits and interossei.
   - Finger flexors
     - Flexor digitorum superficialis (FDS)
       - Separate muscle belly origin, allowing independent finger motion
       - Tendons superficial to the flexor digitorum profundus (FDP) tendons up to their bifurcation into slips at the metacarpophalangeal (MCP) joint, where they travel around the FDP tendon, dive deep, rejoin to form Camper's chiasm, and insert onto the middle phalanx
       - Flexes the proximal interphalangeal (PIP) joint
     - FDP
       - Common muscle belly origin
         - Because of this common origin, shortening of FDP tendon or overtightening of repair can lead to decreased grip strength and decreased flexion of the uninjured digits ("quadrigia" effect).
       - Inserts into the volar aspect of the distal phalanx
       - Flexes the distal interphalangeal (DIP) joint
       - Lumbrical muscles originate from FDP tendon in the palm.
         - Proximal migration of the FDP after injury leads to lumbrical contracture and paradoxical extension of the PIP joint when attempting to flex the MCP joint ("lumbrical plus" deformity). Can address through division of the lumbrical
     - Flexor pollicis longus (FPL)
       - Arises from the midaspect of the radial shaft and interosseous membrane
       - The only tendon inside the flexor sheath of the thumb; inserts onto the distal phalanx
       - Flexes the thumb interphalangeal (IP) joint
   - Wrist flexors
     - Flexor carpi radialis (FCR)
       - Inserts onto the base of the 2nd and 3rd metacarpals
     - Flexor carpi ulnaris (FCU)
       - Inserts onto the base of the 5th metacarpal, hook of hamate, and pisiform
       - Overlies ulnar artery and nerve
         - Laceration to FCU is concerning for injury to the ulnar a. and n.
     - Palmaris longus (PL)
       - Absent in ~15% to 20%
       - Ends in the fan-shaped palmar fascia
       - Lies volar to median nerve traveling within carpal canal
       - Lacerations to PL are concerning for median nerve laceration.
   - Intrinsic flexors
     - Interossei muscles act as prime flexors of the MCP joints and extensors of the IP joints through their pull on the lateral bands (see Figure 19.5).

2. Flexor tendon healing
   - Nutrition of flexor tendons occurs through the synovial sheath, insertion, and vincula, which provide blood vessels directly to the tendon proper (see Figure 19.6).

3. Flexor tendon zones: Divisions of the flexor tendon anatomy within the hand that have important implications in fundamentals of repair (see Figure 19.7)

4. Carpal canal anatomy: Contains 9 tendons (4 FDS, 4 FDP, and 1 FPL) and the median nerve. Anatomic relationships within the canal are consistent; knowledge of these relationships is important when repairing injuries in this zone (zone 4).
   - FDS tendons to the ring and middle finger lie most volar, followed by the FDS tendons to the index and small fingers deep to this.
   - FDP tendons lie on the dorsal floor of the carpal canal.
   - FPL tendon lies radial, deep, and adjacent to the scaphoid and trapezium

General Flexor Tendon Repair Principles

1. Indications and contraindications to flexor tendon repair (see Box 19.1)
2. Primary tendon repair with atraumatic techniques is critical to minimize the risk for postrepair adhesions.

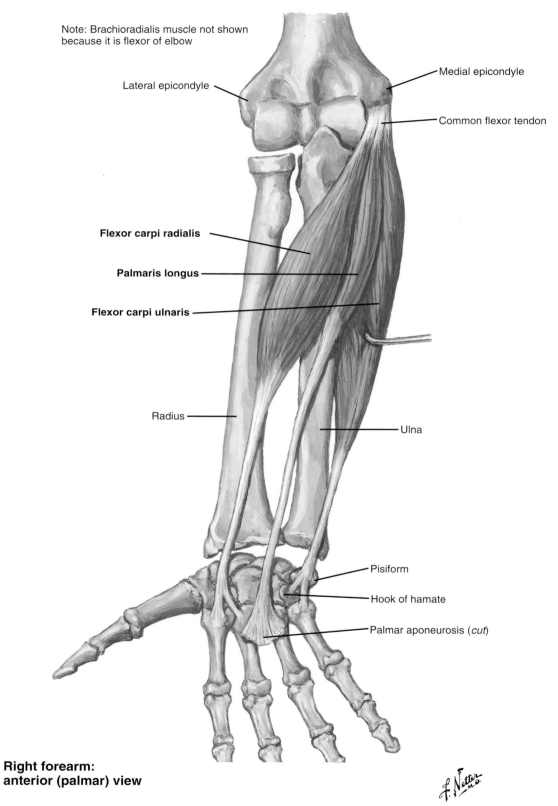

Note: Brachioradialis muscle not shown
because it is flexor of elbow

Lateral epicondyle

Medial epicondyle

Common flexor tendon

Flexor carpi radialis

Palmaris longus

Flexor carpi ulnaris

Radius

Ulna

Pisiform

Hook of hamate

Palmar aponeurosis (*cut*)

**Right forearm:
anterior (palmar) view**

Figure 19.1. The anatomy of the flexor muscles: Superficial to deep. *(Reprinted with permission from www.netterimages.com. © Elsevier Inc. All Rights Reserved.)*

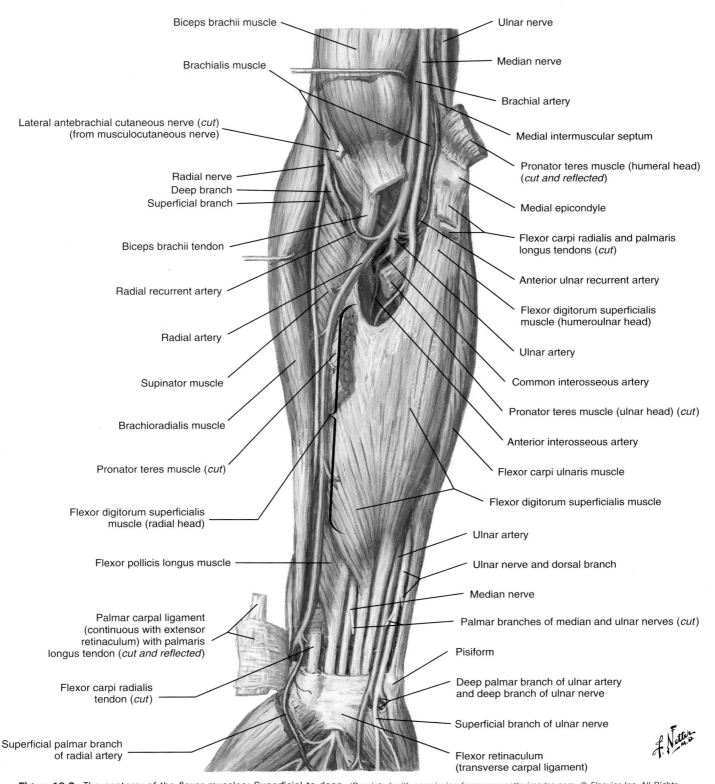

Biceps brachii muscle

Brachialis muscle

Lateral antebrachial cutaneous nerve (*cut*)
(from musculocutaneous nerve)

Radial nerve
Deep branch
Superficial branch

Biceps brachii tendon

Radial recurrent artery

Radial artery

Supinator muscle

Brachioradialis muscle

Pronator teres muscle (*cut*)

Flexor digitorum superficialis
muscle (radial head)

Flexor pollicis longus muscle

Palmar carpal ligament
(continuous with extensor
retinaculum) with palmaris
longus tendon (*cut and reflected*)

Flexor carpi radialis
tendon (*cut*)

Superficial palmar branch
of radial artery

Ulnar nerve

Median nerve

Brachial artery

Medial intermuscular septum

Pronator teres muscle (humeral head)
(*cut and reflected*)

Medial epicondyle

Flexor carpi radialis and palmaris
longus tendons (*cut*)

Anterior ulnar recurrent artery

Flexor digitorum superficialis
muscle (humeroulnar head)

Ulnar artery

Common interosseous artery

Pronator teres muscle (ulnar head) (*cut*)

Anterior interosseous artery

Flexor carpi ulnaris muscle

Flexor digitorum superficialis muscle

Ulnar artery

Ulnar nerve and dorsal branch

Median nerve

Palmar branches of median and ulnar nerves (*cut*)

Pisiform

Deep palmar branch of ulnar artery
and deep branch of ulnar nerve

Superficial branch of ulnar nerve

Flexor retinaculum
(transverse carpal ligament)

Figure 19.2. The anatomy of the flexor muscles: Superficial to deep. (*Reprinted with permission from www.netterimages.com. © Elsevier Inc. All Rights Reserved.*)

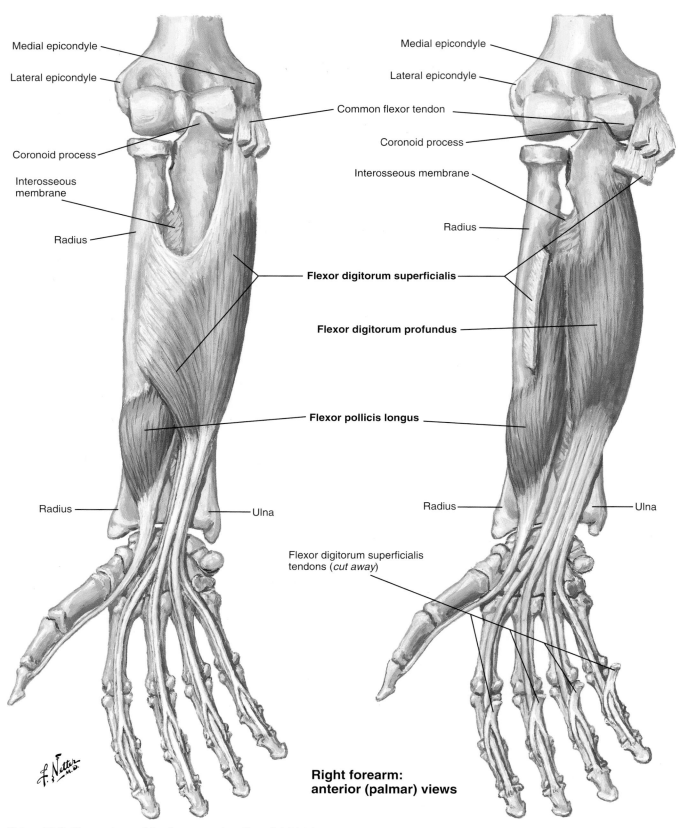

Medial epicondyle

Lateral epicondyle

Coronoid process

Interosseous membrane

Radius

Radius — Ulna

Medial epicondyle

Lateral epicondyle

Common flexor tendon

Coronoid process

Interosseous membrane

Radius

Flexor digitorum superficialis

Flexor digitorum profundus

Flexor pollicis longus

Radius — Ulna

Flexor digitorum superficialis tendons (*cut away*)

Right forearm: anterior (palmar) views

Figure 19.3. The anatomy of the flexor muscles: Superficial to deep. *(Reprinted with permission from www.netterimages.com. © Elsevier Inc. All Rights Reserved.)*

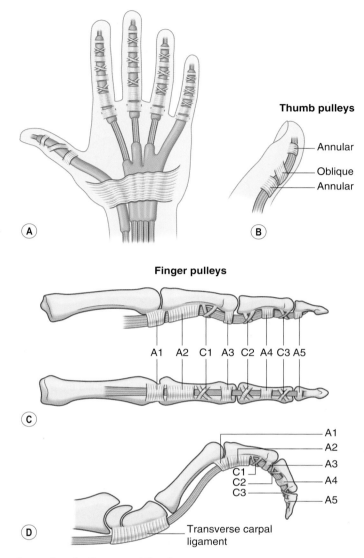

Figure 19.4. The flexor tendon pulley system for fingers and thumb. *(Redrawn after Chase, R.A., 1984. Atlas of Hand Surgery, vol. 2. WB Saunders, Philadelphia.)*

Thumb pulleys
- Annular
- Oblique
- Annular

Finger pulleys

A1 A2 C1 A3 C2 A4 C3 A5

A1
A2
A3
C1
C2
A4
C3
A5

Transverse carpal ligament

3. Strength of the tendon repair is affected by
   - Number of core suture strands across the repair site
     - Strength proportionate to the number of strands
   - Tension of the repair
     - Relevant to gap formation and stiffness
   - Suture characteristics
     - Tendon–suture locking technique, diameter of suture locks, suture caliber and material
   - Holding capacity of the tendon
   - Early mobilization and range of motion may also increase the strength of repair.
4. Recommended repair technique: A 3-0 or 4-0 core coated nylon or woven/braided polyester suture (4 to 6 strands) on a tapered needle (with approximately 1 cm of tendon purchase), with a locking tendon–suture junction and a 6-0 nylon epitendinous suture

- Epitendinous sutures can add strength to the repair site and smooth the approximation of tendon ends to help resist gapping during tendon movement.
5. Partial tendon lacerations
   - Lacerations <50% to 60% of the tendon do not require repair.
   - Trim frayed edges to prevent a trigger site within the annular pulley system.
6. Annular pulley disruptions
   - In the fingers, the A2 and A4 pulleys are the largest and most important to hand function.
     - Complete laceration of the A2 pulley leads to decreased motion at the PIP joint, with an increased moment arm and power.

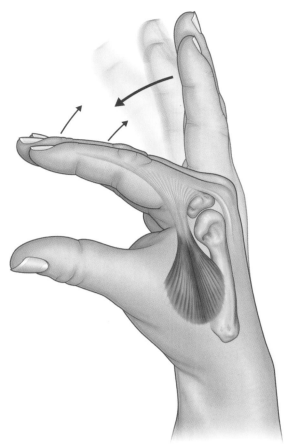

Figure 19.5. All interossei act as prime flexors of the metacarpophalangeal joints because they pass palmar to the joint axis. Extensions into the lateral bands result in extension of the IP joints. *(From Chase, R.A., 1973. Atlas of Hand Surgery, vol. 1. WB Saunders, Philadelphia.)*

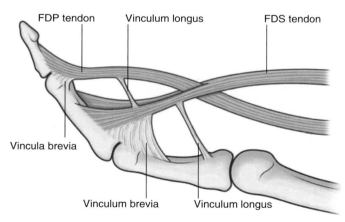

Figure 19.6. Insertions and relative positions of the flexor digitorum superficialis *(FDS)* and flexor digitorum profundus *(FDP)* tendons and vincula. Each of the FDS and FDP tendons has two vincula, one short and one long. The relationships of the FDS and FDP tendons are complex in the middle part of the proximal phalanx under the A2 pulley (zone 2C). *(Reprinted from Neligan P.C., Buck D.W. [Eds.], 2014. Core Procedures in Plastic Surgery, Elsevier, 358-374.)*

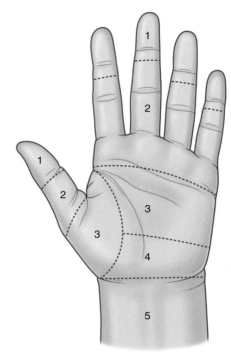

Figure 19.7. Division of the flexor tendons into 5 zones according to anatomical structures of the flexor tendons, presence of the synovial sheath, and the transverse carpal ligament. *(Reprinted from Neligan, P.C., Buck, D.W. [Eds.], 2014. Core Procedures in Plastic Surgery. Elsevier, 358–374.)*

BOX 19.1 PRIMARY FLEXOR TENDON REPAIRS

Indications
- Clean-cut tendon injuries
- Tendon cut with limited peritendinous damage; no defects in soft-tissue coverage
- Regional loss of soft-tissue coverage or fractures of phalangeal shafts (borderline indications)
- Within several days or at most 3 or 4 weeks after tendon laceration

Contraindications
- Severe wound contamination
- Bony injuries involving joint components or extensive soft-tissue loss
- Destruction of a series of annular pulleys and lengthy tendon defects
- Experienced surgeons unavailable

Reprinted from Neligan, P.C., Buck, D.W. (Eds.), 2014. Core Procedures in Plastic Surgery. Elsevier, 358–374.

- Incision of the A2 pulley up to ½ or 2/3rds its length, or release of the entire A4 pulley, can be tolerated without significant functional deficits.
  - May be required for assistance with repair
- In the thumb, A1 and oblique pulleys are most important to function.

7. Common complications of tendon repairs
   - Adhesions
     - Can develop from traumatic technique during repair, excessive scarring, and prolonged immobilization

- Adhesions of the flexor tendons will prevent extension, but allow continued flexion of the involved finger.
- Treatment: Tenolysis
  - Rupture
    - Most commonly occurs within 1 to 2 weeks and at suture knots
    - Can often be primarily repaired if occurs within the first few weeks (up to 1 month) after the initial surgery
    - Secondary tendon grafts, or staged reconstruction with Hunter rods, may be required in the presence of delayed rupture, multiple surgical failures, and retraction or excessive scarring.
      - One-stage tendon grafting is contraindicated in joints with absent passive range of motion.
8. Early postoperative motion of repaired tendons is critical for prevention of adhesions and strengthening the repair.
   - Motion typically begins 2 to 5 days after repair.
   - Indications for prolonged immobilization include tendon repairs in children (often immobilized at 3 to 3.5 weeks), noncompliant patients, and tendon injury associated with underlying fractures.
   - Early postoperative motion protocols
     - Early passive motion
       - Allows active extension with passive flexion ("Kleinert" method)
     - Early active motion
       - Under supervision, allows active extension and active flexion.
     - Combined passive-active motion

Flexor Tendon Injuries

1. Zone-1 injury
   - Affects the FDP tendon only
   - Characterized by inability to flex the DIP
   - Tendon may be held out to length by vinculum
   - Distal injuries often require pull-out suture over buttons or bone-anchor screws because distal tendon stump is too short (<~1 cm) for direct end-to-end suture repair.
   - Proximal zone injuries are usually amenable to direct suture repair.
   - Take care to preserve the A4 pulley.
   - Avulsion and fracture/avulsion injuries of the FDP tendon ("jersey finger" injuries) require special consideration (see Chapter 16: Hand Fractures and Dislocations)
2. Zone-2 injury
   - Often involves both FDP and FDS tendons
   - May disrupt the vincula, with retraction of the proximal tendon ends into the palm
     - Flexion of the MCP and PIP joints may bring the tendon end into sight; otherwise, a counter incision in the palm is necessary.

- Adequate exposure requires Bruner incisions and windows or releases within the synovial sheath and/or pulley system.
  - Attempts to preserve the A2 pulley (at least $\frac{1}{3}$ to $\frac{1}{2}$) are important, functionally.
  - If the A2 pulley is lacerated completely, it can be reconstructed with a free tendon graft or fascia graft (e.g., extensor retinaculum or tensor fascia lata).
- Many surgeons advocate repairing both FDP and FDS tendons.
3. Zones-3 to 5 injury
   - Repair techniques almost identical to those for zone 2
   - Injuries in zones 3 to 5 have better prognosis because of a richer vascular supply and less constricting tissue overlying the tendons (i.e., pulleys).
     - Zone-5 repairs have the best outcomes because of the greater area allowed for tendon gliding.
     - Zone-4 injuries are often associated with concomitant injuries to the median n.
   - Spaghetti wrist
     - Wrist laceration/injury with transection of a majority of tendons, vessels, and nerves (at least 10 out of 15 of these structures, excluding the palmaris)
     - May require lengthy repair, with intermittent deflation and reinflation of the tourniquet during surgery to allow episodic hand perfusion
       - Often allow 20 to 30 minutes of perfusion between 2-hour intervals of tourniquet ischemia.
4. FPL injury
   - Repair techniques and principles similar to those for repair of the FDP tendon in the fingers
   - Proximal tendon end frequently retracts into the thenar musculature.
   - Closed injuries can occur with fracture and/or rupture from attrition (e.g., scaphoid malunion).
5. Stenosing tenosynovitis ("trigger" finger/thumb)
   - Characterized by entrapment of the flexor tendon at the A1 pulley, resulting in pain and catching, popping, or "locking" of the involved digit during flexion and extension
     - Occasionally, the digit can become locked in the flexed position and require passive extension of the digit with the uninvolved hand.
     - May be associated with a painful, palpable nodule along the flexor tendon
   - Caused by hypertrophy of the A1 pulley or occasionally intratendinous swelling
   - Treatment: Initial treatment is conservative with splinting and corticosteroid injection. Surgical release of the A1 pulley (open or percutaneous) can be performed in severe cases (active locking) and for triggering that has failed conservative treatment.

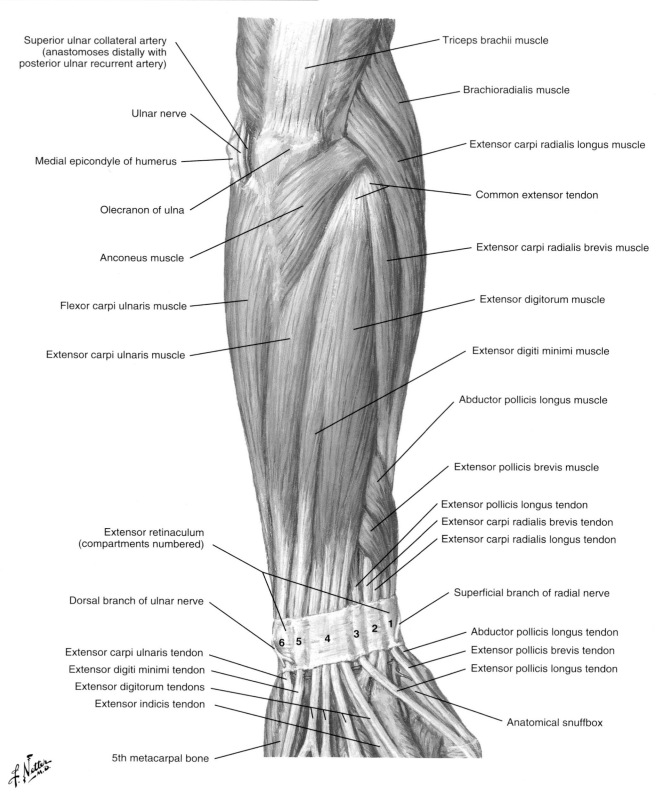

Superior ulnar collateral artery
(anastomoses distally with
posterior ulnar recurrent artery)

Ulnar nerve

Medial epicondyle of humerus

Olecranon of ulna

Anconeus muscle

Flexor carpi ulnaris muscle

Extensor carpi ulnaris muscle

Extensor retinaculum
(compartments numbered)

Dorsal branch of ulnar nerve

Extensor carpi ulnaris tendon
Extensor digiti minimi tendon
Extensor digitorum tendons
Extensor indicis tendon

5th metacarpal bone

Triceps brachii muscle

Brachioradialis muscle

Extensor carpi radialis longus muscle

Common extensor tendon

Extensor carpi radialis brevis muscle

Extensor digitorum muscle

Extensor digiti minimi muscle

Abductor pollicis longus muscle

Extensor pollicis brevis muscle

Extensor pollicis longus tendon
Extensor carpi radialis brevis tendon
Extensor carpi radialis longus tendon

Superficial branch of radial nerve

Abductor pollicis longus tendon
Extensor pollicis brevis tendon
Extensor pollicis longus tendon

Anatomical snuffbox

Figure 19.8. The anatomy of the extensor muscles: Superficial to deep. *(Reprinted with permission from www.netterimages.com. © Elsevier Inc. All Rights Reserved.)*

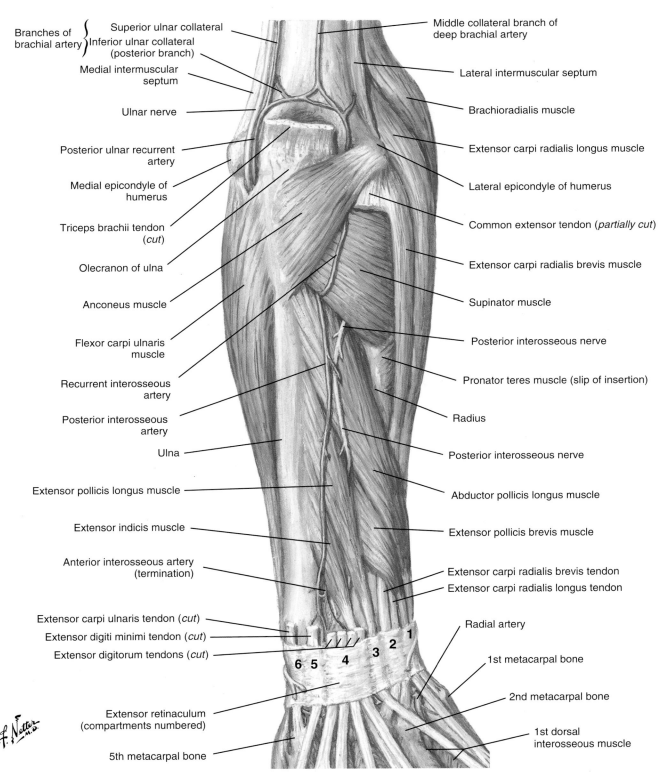

Figure 19.9. The anatomy of the extensor muscles: Superficial to deep. *(Reprinted with permission from www.netterimages.com. © Elsevier Inc. All Rights Reserved.)*

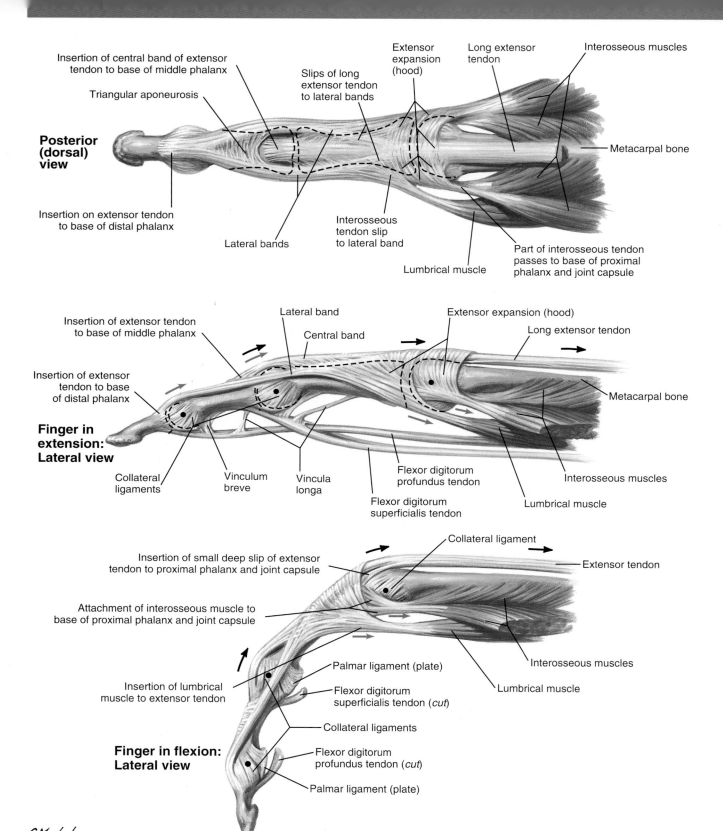

Posterior (dorsal) view

Insertion of central band of extensor tendon to base of middle phalanx

Triangular aponeurosis

Slips of long extensor tendon to lateral bands

Extensor expansion (hood)

Long extensor tendon

Interosseous muscles

Metacarpal bone

Insertion on extensor tendon to base of distal phalanx

Lateral bands

Interosseous tendon slip to lateral band

Lumbrical muscle

Part of interosseous tendon passes to base of proximal phalanx and joint capsule

Finger in extension: Lateral view

Insertion of extensor tendon to base of middle phalanx

Insertion of extensor tendon to base of distal phalanx

Lateral band

Central band

Extensor expansion (hood)

Long extensor tendon

Metacarpal bone

Collateral ligaments

Vinculum breve

Vincula longa

Flexor digitorum profundus tendon

Flexor digitorum superficialis tendon

Interosseous muscles

Lumbrical muscle

Finger in flexion: Lateral view

Insertion of small deep slip of extensor tendon to proximal phalanx and joint capsule

Collateral ligament

Extensor tendon

Attachment of interosseous muscle to base of proximal phalanx and joint capsule

Insertion of lumbrical muscle to extensor tendon

Palmar ligament (plate)

Flexor digitorum superficialis tendon (*cut*)

Collateral ligaments

Flexor digitorum profundus tendon (*cut*)

Palmar ligament (plate)

Interosseous muscles

Lumbrical muscle

C. Machado M.D.

Figure 19.10. The extensor mechanism of the fingers. *Black arrows* indicate pull of long extensor tendon; *red arrows* indicate pull of interosseous and lumbrical muscles; *dots* indicate axis of rotation of joints. (Reprinted with permission from www.netterimages.com. © Elsevier Inc. All Rights Reserved.)

1. The extensor muscles are located on the dorsum of the hand and forearm and are all innervated by the radial n.
2. The common extensor tendon arises from the lateral epicondyle of the humerus.
3. The extensor retinaculum prevents bowstringing of the extensor tendons across the wrist.
4. Unlike the flexor tendons, the extensor tendons do not lie within synovial sheaths.
5. Extension of the phalanges is dependent on the extrinsic extensors at the MCP joints, and the extrinsic and intrinsic muscles at the IP joints.
   - The sagittal bands help to centralize the extensor tendons over the MCP joint to maximize function and prevent hyperextension.
   - At the level of the proximal phalanx, the extensor tendons split into the central band and two lateral bands that merge with the intrinsic muscles to form the extensor apparatus.
   - The central slip inserts at the base of the middle phalanx, whereas the terminal tendon inserts at the base of the distal phalanx.
   - The extensor pollicis longus (EPL) inserts on the base of the thumb distal phalanx, whereas the extensor pollicis brevis (EPV) inserts on the base of the proximal phalanx.
6. The extensor digitorum tendons arise from a common muscle belly, and only the index (extensor indices pollicis) and small fingers (extensor digiti minimi [EDM]) have independent extensors.
7. The extensor digitorum tendons are interconnected by intertendinous bridges (juncturae) that can provide some backup finger extension (albeit weak) in the setting of proximal extensor tendon injury.
   - Testing each finger individually against resistance can overcome this backup and uncover an extensor tendon injury.
8. There are 6 dorsal extensor compartments at the wrist; knowledge of their location and contents is important.
   - Extensor compartment 1: Abductor pollicis longus (APL) and EPB
     - APL tendon can have multiple slips.
     - May have septations between APL and EPB
     - Dorsal sensory branch of the radial n. lies superficial to extensor compartment 1
   - Extensor compartment 2: Extensor carpi radialis longus (ECRL) and extensor carpi radialis brevis (ECRB)
     - Insert on the 2nd and 3rd metacarpal base, respectively
     - ECRB is the prime wrist extensor (because of insertion).
   - Extensor compartment 3: EPL
     - Crosses wrist above extensor compartment 2 and then reorients around Lister's tubercle to the thumb
     - Vulnerable to rupture (e.g., distal radius fractures)
     - Laceration or rupture of the EPL prevents extension of the thumb IP and ability to "lift" the thumb off of a tabletop.
   - Extensor compartment 4: Extensor digitorum communis (EDC) and extensor indicis proprius (EIP)
     - EIP rests ulnar and deep to the EDC tendon to the index finger.
     - Posterior interosseus n. lies deep to extensor compartment 4.
   - Extensor compartment 5: EDM
     - Typically has 2 tendon slips
     - Rests ulnar and deep to the EDC tendon to the small finger
   - Extensor compartment 6: Extensor carpi ulnaris (ECU)
     - ECU functions as a wrist extensor, part of the triangular fibrocartilage complex (TFCC), and major stabilizer of the distal radioulnar joint (DRUJ).
9. The intrinsic extensors
   - The palmar interossei arise from the medial side of the 2nd, 4th, and 5th metacarpal, cross volar to the MCP joint, and join the extensor apparatus at the level of the proximal phalanx.
     - Function to adduct the fingers, flex the MCP joint, and extend the IP joints
   - The dorsal interossei arise from the adjacent sides of the 5 metacarpal bones and join the extensor apparatus.
     - Function to abduct the fingers, flex the MCP joint, and extend the IP joints
   - The lumbrical muscles arise from the radial side of the FDP tendons at the level of the metacarpal and join the extensor apparatus on the radial side.
     - Function primarily as IP extenders
10. Extensor tendon zones: Divisions of the extensor tendon anatomy within the hand that have important implications in fundamentals of repair (see Figure 19.11)

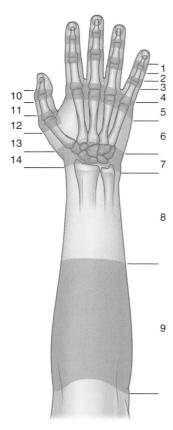

Figure 19.11. The zones of extensor tendon injuries. *(Reprinted from Neligan, P.C., Buck, D.W. [Eds.], 2014. Core Procedures in Plastic Surgery. Elsevier, 309–341.)*

General Extensor Tendon Repair Principles

1. Suture techniques are dependent on the location of the injury because the tendons become thin and flat distally.
2. Injuries proximal to zone 6 can be repaired in similar fashion as that for flexor tendons because of their size (core suture plus epitendinous suture).
3. Minimal changes in tendon length can cause significant alterations in range of motion because the excursion amplitude of extensor tendons is limited.
4. Closed ruptures of the extensor tendon at the level of the DIP and PIP joints are often treated conservatively.
5. Lacerations in zone 5 (over the MCP joints) are frequently caused by "fight bites" and are prone to infection.
   - Treatment: Surgical debridement, antibiotics, splinting, and primary or delayed tendon repair
6. Because of the superficial nature of the extensor tendons, complex injuries to the dorsal hand can involve skin, tendon, and bone.
   - Adequate debridement of nonviable tissue is the critical first step.

- After nonviable tissue has been debrided, fractures must be stabilized and soft-tissue coverage provided before tendon reconstruction.
  - Many surgeons aim for soft-tissue coverage within 72 hours.
- Complete primary tendon repair if it is possible; if not, tendon reconstruction is required and can be performed at the time of soft-tissue coverage by primary grafting or transfers.
- With advent of microsurgery, many surgeons perform single-stage bone fixation, tendon reconstruction, and soft-tissue coverage.
  - The anterolateral thigh flap has become a workhorse flap for this indication.
7. Common extensor tendon repair complications
   - Adhesions
     - Treatment includes hand therapy and splinting, followed by tenolysis.
     - Occasionally capsulotomies, collateral ligament release, and/or flexor tendon tenolysis are also necessary for range-of-motion improvements.
   - Rupture
     - Sagittal band ruptures result in subluxation of the extensor tendon at the MCP joint.
   - Swan-neck deformity
     - Characterized by DIP flexion and PIP hyperextension
     - Often caused by an untreated "mallet finger" or volar plate laxity
     - Treatment options: Fowler tenotomy (central slip release), tendon reconstruction, tenodesis of the FDS (when volar plate laxity is the cause)
   - Boutonniere deformity
     - Characterized by DIP hyperextension and PIP flexion
     - Caused by disruption of the central slip or volar subluxation of the lateral bands
     - Treatment options: Acute treatment of central slip injuries includes splinting in extension; treatment of boutonniere is challenging and includes extensor tendon tenotomy, tendon relocation or grafting, and central slip reconstruction.
8. As with flexor tendons, postoperative therapy is critical to successful treatment of these injuries.
   - Mallet injuries (zone 1) and closed ruptures of the central slip (zone 3) require strict immobilization.
   - Immobilization is also considered for injuries proximal to the extensor retinaculum (zones 8 and 9).
   - Early controlled dynamic motion is often recommended for injuries in zones 3 to 5.

Extensor Tendon Injuries

1. Zone-I injury
   - Characterized by flexion at the DIP joint without active extension (mallet finger)
   - Causes include laceration and/or avulsion.

- Treatment: Closed injures are treated with splinting of the DIP in extension for 8 weeks continuously, followed by nighttime splinting for 2 to 6 weeks.
    - Treat open injuries open.
        - In most cases, skin-only laceration repair with splinting will allow healing strong enough for extension function.
    - In avulsion injuries with bone fragments > one third of the articular surface, K-wire fixation can be used.
    - Alternative options include extension block pinning.

2. Zone-II injury
   - Characterized by inability to extend the DIP joint
   - Caused primarily by lacerations or crush injuries
   - Treatment: Explore acute lacerations to rule out tendon involvement.
       - Partial lacerations (<50% tendon substance) do not require repair.
       - Complete lacerations (or partial lacerations >50%) require suture repair.
       - Avoid significant shortening of the tendon to prevent flexion of the DIP.

3. Zone-3 injury
   - Characterized by flexed PIP without active PIP extension
   - Caused by disruption of the central slip through both closed and open injuries
   - Can lead to boutonniere deformity if not properly treated
       - As the lateral bands migrate volarly, they will lead to flexion contracture of the PIP joint with hyperextension of the DIP.
   - Treatment options: Extension splinting of the PIP, K-wire fixation with the joint in extension, tendon reinsertion with bone anchors
       - In open injuries, exploration is warranted.
       - Clean injuries can be repaired primarily with sutures.
       - Do not have staged reconstruction for contaminated injuries or those with significant tendon loss.

4. Zone-4 injury
   - The extensor becomes broader over the proximal phalanx, resulting in many partial lacerations.
   - Tendon injuries in zone 4 are often associated with proximal phalanx fractures.
   - The tendon is in close proximity to the proximal phalanx in this zone; therefore, adhesions are relatively common and may require secondary tenolysis.
   - Treatment: Surgical repair and early active motion

5. Zone-5 injury
   - At this level, the extensor mechanism includes the tendon and the sagittal bands.
       - The tendon is relatively broad, so complete lacerations are uncommon.
   - Commonly caused by human bite injuries ("fight bite")
   - Treatment: Surgical exploration and washout, especially if "fight bite" is suspected
       - If the injury occurred with a clinched fist, the tendon injury commonly occurs proximal to the skin tear, and

the proximal tendon end will be found proximal with the hand in the open position.
   - Concomitant sagittal band injuries can be treated conservatively with buddy taping or splinting in cases with stable tendon injuries, partial lacerations, or closed/spontaneous ruptures; in cases with unstable tendon injuries or old sagittal band injuries, suture repair is recommended.

6. Zone-6 injury
   - In this zone, the tendon is often of similar caliber to a flexor tendon and thus can be repaired in similar fashion: With a core suture and an epitendinous suture.
   - Early active motion protocols will reduce tendon adhesions.

7. Zone-7 injury
   - Injuries in this zone typically involve open lacerations with multiple tendon involvement or closed rupture associated with underlying fractures or arthritis (e.g., EPL rupture associated with distal radius fractures or rheumatoid arthritis).
   - Open lacerations at this level often require opening of the extensor retinaculum for exposure and repair.
   - Concomitant nerve injury is also common; repair if present.
   - Treatment: Surgical repair with core and epitendinous sutures
       - Closed ruptures of the EPL tendon often cannot be repaired primarily because of the possibility for unacceptable tendon shortening in these cases; therefore, primary tendon transfer (EIP to EPL) is preferred.

8. Zones-7 and 9 injury
   - Often associated with injuries to the musculotendinous junctions and muscle bellies
   - Treatment: Surgical repair of tendons and/or fascial layers with brief postoperative immobilization (3 to 4 weeks) is recommended.
       - Concomitant nerve injuries must be repaired as well.

9. de Quervain's disease
   - Characterized by entrapment of the APL and EPB tendons at the 1st extensor compartment, resulting in radial-sided wrist pain and swelling, which is worse with thumb motion
   - Caused by tension on the tendons in the 1st extensor compartment, which produces friction with subsequent swelling and/or narrowing of the compartment
   - Diagnosed by localized pain and swelling over the 1st dorsal compartment, ~1 cm proximal to the radial styloid, and severe pain when the wrist is forced into ulnar deviation with the thumb adducted into the palm (positive "Finkelstein's" test)
       - Differential diagnosis: 1st carpometacarpal arthritis, intersection syndrome
   - Treatment: Initial treatment is conservative with rest, splinting, and corticosteroid injection. Surgical release of the 1st dorsal compartment for recurrent disease
       - Must ensure release of all tendon slips and septae within the compartment to optimize success of surgical release.

10. Intersection syndrome
    - Characterized by pain and swelling overlying the 2nd extensor compartment (ECRL and ECRB) in the location where the APL and EPB cross over (or "intersect") this compartment.
    - Caused by friction and swelling of the 2nd extensor compartment associated with activities requiring repetitive wrist motion (e.g., rowing, weightlifting)
    - Diagnosed by localized pain, swelling, and crepitus 4 cm proximal to the wrist joint
    - Treatment: Initial treatment is conservative with splinting and corticosteroid injection into the 2nd extensor compartment. Surgical release of the 2nd extensor compartment is indicated for recurrent or persistent disease.

Tendon Grafting (see Box 19.2)

> **BOX 19.2 TENDON GRAFTING AND STAGED RECONSTRUCTION**
>
> **Indications**
> - Tendon injuries not treated within about 1 month after injuries
> - Rupture of the tendon repairs at primary or delayed primary stages
> - Tendon injuries not indicated for primary repair
> - Badly scarred digits are indicative for staged tendon reconstruction
>
> **Essential Requirements**
> - Supple passive motion of the hand
> - Soft-tissue conditions: Good
> - Sufficient time passed after initial tendon injury: 3 months
>
> **Contraindications**
> - Joint motion very limited (but may be suitable for staged reconstruction)
> - Presence of soft-tissue wounds or defects and fractures not well healed

Reprinted from Neligan, P.C., Chang, J. (Eds.), Plastic Surgery, vol. 6, 3rd ed. Elsevier, 178–209.

1. Most common tendon donor sites
    - PL
        - From ipsilateral limb
        - Useful for palm-to-fingertip grafts
        - Absent in 15% of hands
        - Take care to protect median n. during harvest
    - Plantaris
        - Can obtain graft up to 25 cm; useful for long distal forearm-to-fingertip grafts
        - Absent in 7% to 20% of limbs
        - Care must be taken to protect tibial n. during harvest
    - Toe extensors
        - Extensor digitorum longus tendons to the 2nd to 4th toes
    - Other potential options
        - EIP, FDS to the 5th finger, ECRL or ECRB, Allograft tendon

2. Technical considerations
    - Depending on the location and size of the distal and proximal tendon stumps, the graft can be secured through varying techniques.
        - Distally, can be sewn directly to residual stump, buried under an osteoperiosteal flap, or secured over a button.
        - Proximally, either at the palm or in the forearm, the graft is secured to the native stump through a Pulvertaft weave (see Figure 19.12)

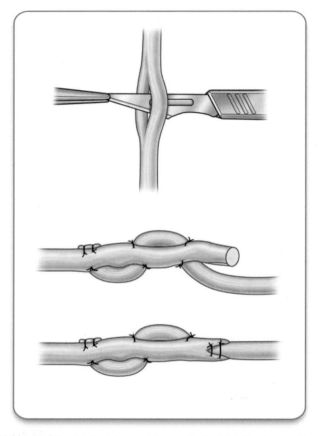

Figure 19.12. Skin incision and the method of free tendon grafting to reconstruct the function of digital flexion. As many annular pulleys as possible are preserved. The junction is placed at either palm or distal forearm. The graft is weaved with the digital flexor through holes in the tendons created by a knife. *(Reprinted from Neligan, P.C., Chang, J. [Eds.], 2013. Plastic Surgery, vol. 6, 3rd ed. Elsevier, 178–209.)*

    - Postoperatively, immobilization is recommended for at least 3 weeks followed by graded motion protocols.
3. Staged tendon reconstruction
    - Indications: Severely scarred digits
    - Stage 1: Excision of tendon and scar, preservation or reconstruction of pulleys, and insertion of a Hunter rod (Silicone tendon implant)
        - The Hunter rod will stimulate formation of a pseudosheath
    - Stage 2: The Hunter rod is replaced with a tendon graft
        - Typically occurs 3 months after the first stage.

Tendon Transfers

1. Indications
   - Paralyzed muscle secondary to peripheral nerve, brachial plexus, or spinal cord injury
   - Direct muscle or tendon injury (open and closed rupture/injuries)
   - Restore balance to hands affected by neurological disease
2. Basic principles of tendon transfer (see Box 19.3)

BOX 19.3 BASIC PRINCIPLES OF TENDON TRANSFERS

Soft-tissue equilibrium
Full passive range of motion of involved joints
Adequate amplitude of donor muscle
Adequate excursion of donor muscle
Direct line of pull
Single function for each transferred tendon
Synergy of transfer

Reprinted from Neligan, P.C., Buck, D.W. (Eds.), 2014. Core Procedures in Plastic Surgery. Elsevier, 393–413.

3. Technical considerations
   - The timing of transfers can be classified as early, conventional, or late
     - Early: Performed simultaneously with peripheral n. repair, or before the expected time of reinnervation of the muscle to act as an internal splint and serve as a temporary substitute for the paralyzed muscle until reinnervation occurs
     - Conventional: Performed after failed reinnervation (typically 3 months after the expected time of reinnervation)
     - Late: Performed for chronic deficits, beyond 3 months from time of expected reinnervation.
   - List in order of priority (and approach in this way) the specific functions of the hand that need to be restored.
   - Success depends on preventing scarring or adhesions along the path of the transferred tendon and a patient who will be compliant with postoperative restrictions and therapy.
   - Transfers should only act across one joint and perform a single function.
   - Use Pulvertaft weave tendon junctures when possible.
   - The power of the transferred muscle tendon is typically downgraded one level after the transfer procedure; therefore, place the transferred tendon at slightly greater resting tension than that in the donor site.
   - The potential excursion of the donor muscle–tendon unit must be sufficient to restore the lost function.
     - Finger flexor excursion amplitude: 7 cm
     - Finger extensor excursion amplitude: 5 cm
     - Wrist flexor/extensor excursion amplitude: 3.3 cm.
     - The tenodesis effect may increase the effective amplitude of a tendon transfer by 2.5 cm.

Radial Nerve Palsy

1. Functional deficits
   - Wrist extension
   - Finger extension at the MCP joints
   - Thumb extension and radial abduction
2. Tendon transfers for radial n. palsy

Table 19.1 Tendon Transfers for Radial Nerve Palsy

STANDARD FCU TRANSFER	FCR TRANSFER	BOYES SUPERFICIALIS TRANSFER
PT to ECRB	PT to ECRB	PT to ECRB
FCU to EDC	FCR to EDC	FDS of ring finger to EDC middle, ring, and small fingers
PL to EPL	PL to EPL	FDS middle finger to EIP and EPL
		FCR to APL and EPB

Reprinted from Neligan, P.C., Buck, D.W. (Eds.), 2014. Core Procedures in Plastic Surgery. Elsevier, 393–413.
APL, Abductor pollicis longus; ECRB, extensor carpi radialis brevis; EDC, extensor digitorum communis; EIP, extensor indicis proprius; EPB, extensor pollicis brevis; EPL, extensor pollicis longus; FCR, flexor carpi radialis; FCU, flexor carpi ulnaris; FDS, flexor digitorum superficialis; PL, palmaris longus; PT, pronator teres.

Low Median Nerve Palsy

1. Distal to innervation of the extrinsic forearm flexors (thus, extrinsic flexors are intact)
2. Functional deficits
   - Loss of thumb opposition
   - Numbness over the thumb, index, and long fingers and radial half of the ring finger
3. Tendon transfer for low median n. palsy (opponensplasty)
   - EIP-to–abductor pollicis brevis (APB) transfer
   - Bunnell transfer: Ring-finger FDS to APB
     - Contraindicated if concomitant injury to FDS, combined low median/high ulnar n. palsy (ring-finger FDS is only remaining ring-finger flexor), or low median/low ulnar n. palsy (ring-finger FDS needed to correct clawing)
   - Huber transfer: ADM to APB
   - Camitz transfer: PL to APB

High Median Nerve Palsy

1. Injury proximal to innervation of the extrinsic forearm flexors
2. Functional deficits
   - Thumb flexion at IP joint
   - Thumb opposition
   - Index and long-finger flexion at PIP and DIP
3. Tendon transfers for high median n. palsy
   - Thumb flexion: BR to FPL
   - Opposition: See above.

- Finger flexion: Side-to-side tenodesis of index and long-finger FDP to the ulnar innervated FDP (ring and small)
  - ECRL tendon transfer to FDP, or index and long, can also be performed, especially if power flexion is required.

Ulnar Nerve Palsy

1. Low ulnar n. palsy: Injury distal to innervation of the ring and small-finger FDP and FCU
2. High ulnar n. palsy: Injury proximal to innervation of the ring and small-finger FDP and FCU
3. Functional deficits
   - Clawing
     - Hyperextension of the MCP joint, flexion at the PIP and DIP joints ("Duchenne" sign) secondary to flexor/extensor imbalance
     - Involves only the ring and small fingers in low ulnar n. palsy but will affect all four fingers in combined median and ulnar n. palsy
   - Loss of key pinch
     - Secondary to paralysis of the adductor pollicis, $\frac{1}{2}$ of the flexor pollicis brevis (FPB), and the 1st dorsal interosseous m.
     - Compensatory activation of FPL, producing IP flexion ("Froment's" sign) and MCP hyperextension ("Jeanne's" sign) with forceful pinch
   - Ulnar deviation of the small finger ("Wartenberg's" sign)
     - Secondary to paralysis of the 3rd palmar interosseous m. and unopposed action of the EDM
   - Weak flexion of the ring- and small-finger DIP
   - Weak wrist flexion (high ulnar n. palsy)
4. Tendon transfers for ulnar n. palsy
   - Correction of clawing: ECRB extended with tendon grafts to the radial lateral bands ("Brand" transfer: ECRB, extensor route, 4-tailed graft, or extensor-to-extensor 4-tailed [EE4T] transfer)
     - Can also use ECRL ("Brand EF4T" transfer: ECRL, flexor route, 4-tailed graft), PL, FCR, Zancolli lasso procedure (FDS tendon is split into two slips that are wrapped around the A1 pulleys and secured to each other), or Stiles-Bunnell transfer (FDS split into two slips and secured to radial lateral bands).
   - Restore key pinch (thumb adduction): ECRB extended with tendon graft to adductor pollicis
     - Use of the ring-finger FDS, BR, ECRL, and EIP has also been described.
   - Correct ulnar deviation of small finger: Ulnar half of EDM passed volar and sutured to the insertion of the radial collateral ligament of the MCP or looped under the A2 pulley and secured to itself
   - Restore flexion of ring- and small-finger DIP: Side-to-side tenodesis of the ring- and small-finger FDP tendons to the middle-finger FDP tendon (median n. innervated).

Combined Nerve Palsy

1. Low median/Low ulnar
   - Most common combined nerve injury (extrinsic flexors intact)
   - Typically a result of open laceration/"spaghetti wrist"
   - Characterized by sensory loss over the palmar aspect of the hand, claw hand, and Wartenberg's sign
   - Goals of reconstruction
     - Restore thumb adduction for key pinch: ECRB with tendon graft to adductor tubercle of the thumb metacarpal
       - Ring-finger FDS is also an option
     - Restore opposition: EIP transfer to the APB tendon
     - Correction of finger clawing: ECRL or PL transfer extended by 4 tendon grafts to the radial lateral bands or A2 pulleys (e.g., Brand EP4T transfer)
     - Sensory restoration: If nerve repair or nerve graft has failed, can consider superficial radial n. transfer to the distal median n.
2. High median/high ulnar
   - Characterized by findings in low/low injury (above), with no active flexion of the fingers or thumb
   - Transfers often performed in stages
   - Goals of reconstruction
     - Restore finger and thumb flexion
       - Thumb: Brachioradialis (BR) transfer to FPL
       - Fingers: ECRL transfer with grafts to the four FDP tendons
     - Restore key pinch: ECRB with graft to adductor tubercle/adductor pollicis insertion
     - Restore opposition: EIP transfer to the APB tendon
     - Correct clawing: If above transfers have been performed, there are no expendable wrist extensors for correction of clawing. If above transfers have not been performed, transfer of the ECRB to the intrinsics has been described.
     - Restoration of wrist flexion: ECU to FCU

Tendon Transfers for Muscle Spasticity

1. Classically involves patients with spasticity syndromes (e.g., cerebral palsy)
2. Goals of treatment: Improve digital contractures, assist with hand hygiene by getting digits out of fixed flexed position within the palm
3. Common deformities
   - Thumb-in-palm deformity: One of the most important factors affecting good hand function in these patients (see Table 19.2)

Table 19.2 Classifications of Thumb-in-Palm Deformity

TYPE	DESCRIPTION	INVOLVED ELEMENTS
1	Simple metacarpal adduction contracture	Spastic adductor and 1st dorsal interosseous
2	Metacarpal adduction contracture with MP flexion deformity	Spastic adductor, 1st dorsal interosseous, FPB
3	Metacarpal adduction contracture with MP hyperextension/instability	Spastic adductor, 1st dorsal interosseous, EPB
4	Metacarpal adduction contracture, MP and IP flexion deformities	Spastic adductor, 1st dorsal interosseous, FPL

Reprinted from Wolfe, S.W., Hotchkiss, R.N., Pederson, W.C., et al. (Eds.), 2011. Green's Operative Hand Surgery, 6th ed. Elsevier, 1139–1172.
EPB, *Extensor pollicis brevis*; FPB, *flexor pollicis brevis*; FPL, *flexor pollicis longus*; IP, *interphalangeal*; MP, *metacarpophalangeal.*

- Fist-in-palm deformity: Classically treated with FDS to FDP transfer (superficialis-to-profundus [STP] transfer).
  - FDS and FDP tendons identified in the distal forearm
    - The FDP tendons are sutured together distally, and the FDS tendons are sutured together proximally if there is little digital function.
  - The FDS tendons are transected distally, and the FDP tendons are transected proximally.
  - The FDS tendons are then sutured side to side to the FDP tendons.

Common Tendon Transfers for Reconstruction after Trauma

1. Closed EPL rupture after distal radius fracture
   - Classically occurs at Lister's tubercle
   - Etiology: Ischemia of tendon secondary to tenosynovial edema and attrition over the radial cortex
   - Treatment: EIP-to-EPL transfer
2. Restoration of finger extension after trauma
   - Etiology: Complex dorsal hand trauma with soft-tissue damage and tendon loss
   - Treatment: Similar transfers used in radial n. palsy (FCU, FCR, or FDS of long and ring fingers to EDC)
3. Laceration or rupture of FPL
   - Treatment: Ring-finger FDS to FPL
4. Volar crush or avulsion injuries involving the extrinsic flexor muscles
   - Treatment: ECRL with grafts to all 4 FDP tendons or free functioning muscle transfer (e.g., gracilis)

Free Functioning Muscle Transfers

1. Indicated when no simpler alternative is available
2. Complex procedure that requires strict patient compliance and meticulous microsurgical technique

3. The transplanted muscle must be able to generate sufficient force to power the desired function.
4. The transplanted muscle must be placed at the same resting tension as that in the donor site.
5. Requirements for free functional muscle transfer (see Box 19.4)

BOX 19.4 REQUIREMENTS FOR FREE FUNCTIONAL MUSCLE TRANSFER

- Available, undamaged motor nerve, artery, and vein at the site of muscle transplantation
- Adequate skin coverage for the distal half of the muscle
- Supple joints and gliding tendons
- Good hand sensibility and intrinsic function
- Adequate antagonist muscle function
- Good patient motivation
- No simpler solution for patient's problem

Adapted from Anastakis D., Manktelow R., 2005. Free functioning muscle transfers. In: Green's operative hand surgery, 5th ed. Elsevier, Philadelphia.

Suggested Readings

Carlson, M.G., 2011. Chapter 35: Cerebral palsy. In: Wolfe, S.W., Hotchkiss, R.N., Pederson, W.C., et al. (Eds.), Green's Operative Hand Surgery, 6th ed. Elsevier, pp. 1139–1172.

Davis, T.R.C., 2011. Chapter 34: Median and ulnar nerve palsy. In: Wolfe, S.W., Hotchkiss, R.N., Pederson, W.C., et al. (Eds.), Green's Operative Hand Surgery, 6th ed. Elsevier, pp. 1093–1138.

Harvey, I., Borschel, G.H., 2013. Chapter 35: Free-functioning muscle transfer in the upper extremity. In: Neligan, P.C., Chang, J. (Eds.), Plastic Surgery, vol. 6, 6th ed. Elsevier, pp. 777–788.

Ingari, J.V., Green, D.P., 2011. Chapter 33: Radial nerve palsy. In: Wolfe, S.W., Hotchkiss, R.N., Pederson, W.C., et al. (Eds.), Green's Operative Hand Surgery, 6th ed. Elsevier, pp. 1075–1092.

Jones, N.F., 2013. Chapter 34: Tendon transfers in the upper extremity. In: Neligan, P.C., Chang, J. (Eds.), Plastic Surgery, vol. 6, 3rd ed. Elsevier, pp. 745–776.

Magerle, K., Germann, G., 2013. Chapter 10: Extensor tendon injuries. In: Neligan, P.C., Chang, J. (Eds.), Plastic Surgery, vol. 6, 3rd ed. Elsevier, pp. 210–227.

Neligan, P.C., Buck, D.W., 2013. Core Procedures in Plastic Surgery. Chapter 19: Essential anatomy of the upper extremity. Elsevier, pp. 309–341.

Neligan, P.C., Buck, D.W., 2013. Core Procedures in Plastic Surgery. Chapter 20: Examination of the upper extremity. Elsevier, pp. 342–357.

Neligan, P.C., Buck, D.W., 2013. Core Procedures in Plastic Surgery. Chapter 21: Flexor tendon injuries and reconstruction. Elsevier, pp. 358–374.

Neligan, P.C., Buck, D.W., 2013. Core Procedures in Plastic Surgery. Chapter 22: Nerve transfers. Elsevier, pp. 375–392.

Neligan, P.C., Buck, D.W., 2013. Core Procedures in Plastic Surgery. Chapter 23: Tendon transfers in the upper extremity. Elsevier, pp. 393–413.

Neligan, P.C., Buck, D.W., 2013. Core Procedures in Plastic Surgery. Chapter 24: Extensor tendon injuries. Elsevier, pp. 414–426.

Seiler, J.G., 2011. Chapter 7: Flexor tendon injury. In: Wolfe, S.W., Hotchkiss, R.N., Pederson, W.C., et al. (Eds.), Green's Operative Hand Surgery, 6th ed. Elsevier, pp. 189–206.

Strauch, R.J., 2011. Chapter 6: Extensor tendon injury. In: Wolfe, S.W., Hotchkiss, R.N., Pederson, W.C., et al. (Eds.), Green's Operative Hand Surgery, 6th ed. Elsevier, pp. 159–188.

Tang, J.B., 2013. Chapter 9: Flexor tendon injury and reconstruction. In: Neligan, P.C., Chang, J. (Eds.), Plastic Surgery, vol. 6, 3rd ed. Elsevier, pp. 178–209.

Taras, J.S., Kaufman, R.A., 2011. Flexor tendon reconstruction. In: Wolfe, S.W., Hotchkiss, R.N., Pederson, W.C., et al. (Eds.), Green's Operative Hand Surgery, 6th ed. Elsevier, pp. 207–238.

Wolfe, S.W., 2011. Chapter 62: Tendinopathy. In: Wolfe, S.W., Hotchkiss, R.N., Pederson, W.C., et al. (Eds.), Green's Operative Hand Surgery, 6th ed. Elsevier, pp. 2067–2088.

Chapter

Wound Healing and Tissue Expansion 20

1. Wound healing phases
   - Hemostasis: Platelet plug, fibrin clot, vasoconstriction. α granules in the platelets release cytokines such as platelet-derived growth factor (PDGF), transforming growth factor (TGF), and basic fibroplast growth factor (bFGF).
   - Inflammatory: Activated to cleanse and prepare wound for healing
     - Polymorphonuclear (PMN) leukocytes: Initial 24 to 48 hours. Act as defensive units, phagocytosing bacteria and foreign debris from the wound to prevent infection
       - Phagocytosed by macrophages and destroyed
     - Macrophage: Dominant cell between 48 and 72 hours (key regulatory cell). Functions to phagocytose bacteria and dead tissue. Secretes collagenases and cytokines responsible for proliferation of fibroblasts, resulting in collagen production, and endothelial cells, resulting in angiogenesis
   - Proliferative/fibroplastic: 3 to 5 days after injury, fibroblasts migrate into the wound and become predominant cell type. They begin to lay down new collagen. At first, type 3 is greater than type 1 but is eventually replaced by type 1 to the normal ratio (4:1, T1:T3).
     - It is during this time that the greatest rate of collagen synthesis occurs in the wound.
     - Contraction begins and continues into remodeling phase.
   - Remodeling begins day 21. Cross-linking and organization of collagen fibers (procollagen is cleaved into collagen)
     - Net amount of collagen is constant because there is an equal amount of degradation and synthesis.
     - Wound becomes stronger because of cross-linking.
       - Maximum tensile strength is achieved after ~12 weeks.
         - 80% by 60 days
2. Wound healing process
   - Epithelial cell migration: Initiated by loss of contact inhibition and occurs from the periphery of the wound and adnexal structures
     - Cell division occurs in 48 to 72 hours, resulting in a thin epithelial cell bridge across the wound.
     - Epidermal growth factors play a key role.
     - Can be delayed by retinoids (Accutane/isotretinoin)
       - Can be stimulated by tretinoin (Retin-A)
         - Promotes epithelialization by stimulating mitotic activity and decreasing the turnover of follicular epithelial cells
         - Often used as a pretreatment in patients undergoing chemical peeling and laser skin resurfacing to accelerate wound healing
   - Myofibroblasts: Involved in wound contraction and play no role in epithelialization
   - Collagen deposition is seen in the remodeling phase of wound healing.
   - Fibronectin produced by fibroblasts serves as an adhesion molecule, anchoring cells to collagen or proteoglycan substrates.
   - Release of cytokines from platelets plays an important role in the initiation of the hemostatic initial phase.
3. Growth factors involved in wound healing process (see Table 20.1)
4. Important nutrients for wound healing
   - Vitamin C: Collagen cross-linking via the hydroxylation of proline and lysine to hydroxyproline and hydroxylysine, respectively
     - Lack of cross-linking results in impaired collagen synthesis and a decrease in collagen tensile strength. Collagen-containing tissues, such as skin, dentition, bone, and blood vessels, are therefore affected, leading to the development of scurvy.
       - Hallmark signs of scurvy: Hemorrhaging in any organ (ie, petechiae, swollen gums), loss of dentition, and a lack of osteoid formation
       - Seen in patients who are severely malnourished, have a history of alcoholism, or have restrictive diets for medical, social, or economic reasons
   - Folate and vitamin B6 (pyridoxine) are integral in DNA synthesis and cellular proliferation.
   - Vitamin A is an essential factor in epithelialization and fibroblast proliferation.
     - Impairment of wound healing caused by use of corticosteroids can be reversed by the oral administration of vitamin A (retinoic acid), 15,000 IU daily, for 7 days.
   - Vitamin E is a strong antioxidant and immune modulator.

Table 20.1 Partial List of Growth Factors Present in the Wound Site

GROWTH FACTOR ABBREVIATION	GROWTH FACTOR	CELLULAR SOURCE	TARGET CELLS	BIOLOGIC ACTIVITY
CTGF	Connective tissue growth factor	Fibroblasts, endothelial cells	Fibroblasts	Downstream of TGF-β_1
EGF	Epidermal growth factor	Platelets, macrophages, keratinocytes	Keratinocytes, fibroblasts, endothelial cells	Proliferation, chemotaxis
FGF-1, FGF-2, FGF-4	Fibroblast growth factor-1, -2, and -4	Macrophage, fibroblasts, endothelial cells	Keratinocytes, fibroblasts, endothelial cells, chondrocytes	Angiogenesis, proliferation, chemotaxis
FGF-7 (KGF-1), FGF-10 (KGF-2)	Fibroblast growth factor-7 (keratinocyte growth factor-1), fibroblast growth factor-10 (keratinocyte growth factor-2)	Fibroblasts	Keratinocytes	Proliferation, chemotaxis
IGF-1/Sm-C	Insulin-like growth factor-1/ somatostatin-C	Fibroblasts, macrophages, serum	Fibroblasts, endothelial cells	Proliferation, collagen synthesis
IL-1α and IL-1β	Interleukin-1α and -1β	Macrophages, neutrophils	Macrophages, fibroblasts, keratinocytes	Proliferation, collagenase synthesis, chemotaxis
PDGF	Platelet-derived growth factor	Macrophage, platelets, fibroblasts, endothelial cells, vascular smooth-muscle cells	Neutrophils, macrophages, fibroblasts, endothelial cells, vascular smooth-muscle cells	Chemotaxis, proliferation, matrix production
TGF-α	Transforming growth factor-α	Macrophages, platelets, keratinocytes	Keratinocytes, fibroblasts, endothelial cells	Proliferation
TGF-β_1 and -β_2	Transforming growth factor-β_1 and β_2	Macrophages, platelets, fibroblasts, keratinocytes	Inflammatory cells, keratinocytes, fibroblasts	Chemotaxis, proliferation, matrix production (fibrosis)
TGF-β_3	Transforming growth factor-β_3	Macrophages	Fibroblasts	Antiscarring
TNF-α	Tumor necrosis factor-α	Neutrophils	Macrophages, keratinocytes, fibroblasts	Activation of growth factor expression
VEGF	Vascular endothelial cell growth factor	Macrophages, keratinocytes, fibroblasts	Endothelial cells	Angiogenesis

Modified from Lorenz, H.P., Longaker, M.T., 2000. Wounds: biology, pathology, and management. In: Norton, J., Barie, P., Bollinger, R., et al. (Eds.), Surgery: Basic Science and Clinical Evidence, 2nd ed. Springer, New York, 191–208.

- Zinc is one of the most important micronutrients because it acts as a cofactor for numerous metalloenzymes and proteins.
  - Essential for proper protein (like collagen) and nucleic acid synthesis
- Silicone/silicone sheeting
  - Exact mechanism of action unknown
  - Most widely accepted hypothesis is that there is an increase in hydration resulting from occlusion
    - Studies have either ruled out or not supported alteration of cytokine levels, direct chemical effects, increased oxygen tension, or pressure.
  - Some postulate that their effect is associated with the generation of an increased static electronegative field by the silicone.
  - To be effective, it must be worn for at least 12 hours/day for 3 months or longer.
5. Systemic factors affecting wound healing (see Table 20.2)
   - Diabetes mellitus adversely affects healing by altering circulation, attenuating inflammation, reducing tissue oxygenation, and adversely affecting glucose metabolism, resulting in stress hyperglycemia.

- Malnutrition, including caloric, protein, vitamin, and mineral insufficiency, impairs the immune system, prevents tissue repair, and may lead to progression or recurrence of a wound.
- Aging is associated with reduced production of collagen and angiogenesis and a diminished response to environmental stresses.
- By reducing inflammation, steroids impair angiogenesis, fibrogenesis, and wound contraction; reduce wound strength; and delay healing.
- Other factors such as infection, smoking, poor tissue oxygenation, radiation, chemotherapy, and the presence of foreign bodies or cancer within a wound are also associated with poor healing.
- Anemia, even to severe levels, when circulation is maintained has not been found to impair wound healing.
6. Collagens
   - Type 1: Mature skin, tendon, bone
   - Type 2: Hyaline cartilage, eye
   - Type 3: Papillary dermis, arteries, intestinal walls, uterus, hypertrophic/keloid scars
   - Type 4: Basement membrane

Table 20.2 Factors that May Impair Normal Healing and Lead to Chronic Nonhealing Wounds

ETIOPATHOLOGY		EXAMPLES
Vascular	Arterial	Arteriosclerosis, arterial aneurysm, fat embolism with arterial obstruction, hypertension (Martorell ulcer)
	Lymphatic	Lymphatic edema, lymphangiodysplasia
	Venous	Chronic venous insufficiency, necrotizing thrombophlebitis
	Mixed arteriovenous	Combined arteriosclerosis with venous insufficiency, arteriovenous malformations/dysplasia; steal phenomenon (e.g., arteriovenous shunts, vascular compression/obstruction; due to tumors, enlarged lymphatic nodes, etc.)
	Vasculitis	Wegener's granulomatosis, Churg-Strauss vasculitis, Henoch-Schönlein purpura, Sneddon syndrome, systemic lupus erythematosus, rheumatoid arthritis, Felty syndrome, Takayasu arteriitis, polyarteritis nodosa, Kawasaki syndrome, pyoderma gangrenosum, necrobiosis lipoidica diabeticorum, thromboangiitis obliterans (Buerger's disease), allergic reactions
	Vasculopathic syndromes	Raynaud's syndrome, systemic scleroderma, CREST, Klippel-Trenaunay syndrome, proteus syndrome, CLOVES syndrome, Kasabach-Merritt syndrome
Physical, chemical, and biological causes	Pressure	Immobility, intra- and postoperative bedding, tight shoes and casts, compression therapy
	Trauma	Lacerations, any type of soft-tissue and bone injury, vascular rupture
	Thermal	Burns/frostbite, electrical injury (electrical current/high voltage/lightning)
	Radiation	Radiation therapy
	Chemical-toxic	Extravasation, chemical burns (acids/bases), sclerotherapy
	Infections	Erysipelas, necrotizing fasciitis, septic cutaneous embolism, osteomyelitis, complications after cutaneous infection
		Herpes simplex, cytomegalovirus, human immunodeficiency virus, syphilis, leprosy, tuberculosis
		Tropical ulcers, parasitic and vermicular infections
Neuropathic	Posttraumatic	Spinal lesions with palsy, peripheral nerve injury
	Congenital	Spina bifida, syringomyelia, multiple sclerosis, neurological syndromes
	Systemic neuropathic diseases	Diabetes mellitus, ethylene oxide toxic neuropathy, degenerative central and peripheral neuropathies
		Poliomyelitis, leprosy, tabes dorsalis
Hemopathological	Systemic diseases	Polycythemia vera, sickle-cell anemia, other anemias, thalassemia, thrombocythemia vera, thrombocytopenic purpura, increased blood viscosity (paraneoplastic, paraproteinemia, hyperglobulinemia, leukemia), complication after blood transfusion
	Disturbed hemostasiology	Factor V Leiden syndrome, antiphospholipid syndrome, disturbed fibrinolysis, factor-XIII deficiency syndrome, antithrombin-III deficiency, proteins C and S deficiency, Marcumar necrosis, disseminated intravascular coagulation, necrosis due to vitamin K antagonist therapy
Neoplastic diseases	Cutaneous tumors	Basal and squamous cell carcinoma, melanoma, Bowen syndrome, Marjolin ulcer (scar carcinoma), tumors with cutaneous metastasis or penetration (e.g., Paget syndrome)
Therapeutic modalities		Steroids, vaccination ulcer (BCG), cytostatic drugs, NSAIDs, extravasation of various drugs
Systemic diseases		Hepatic and/or renal insufficiency, immunosuppression, sarcoidosis, homocysteinemia, hemochromatosis
Other causes		Alcoholism, obesity, gout, smoking, advanced age, malnutrition (e.g., vitamin, protein, and micronutrient deficiency; scurvy); psychiatric diseases with self-harming, neglect, intravenous drug abuse; foreign bodies/projectiles with fistulas

Reprinted from Neligan, P.C, Chang, J. (Eds.), 2013. Plastic Surgery, 3rd ed. Elsevier.
BCG, *Bacillus Calmette-Guérin;* CLOVES, *congenital lipomatous overgrowth, vascular malformations, epidermal nevi, and spinal/skeletal;*
CREST, *calcinosis, Raynaud's syndrome, esophageal dysmotility, sclerodactyly, and telangiectasia;* NSAIDs, *nonsteroidal anti-inflammatory drugs.*

- Type 5: Found within the basement membrane in lesser amounts than type-4 collagen
7. Negative pressure wound therapy (NPWT) effects on wound
   - The most likely mechanism by which NPWT expedites healing is deformation of the wound.
     - Causes both macrodeformation and microdeformation of a wound

- Macrodeformation maintains approximation of the tissues, preventing loss of domain and facilitating earlier closure by delayed primary or secondary intention.
- Microdeformation at the interface of the sponge and wound bed changes cell shape, which then affects gene transcription via the cytoskeleton (mechanotransduction).

- ◆ These microdeformational forces stimulate cellular proliferation and angiogenesis in the wound.
- NPWT prevents desiccation of the wound.
  - The semiocclusive polyurethane drape maintains a favorable, moist wound environment.
- NPWT decreases matrix metalloproteinase activity in the wound.
  - Elevated matrix metalloproteinases inhibit wound healing and neovascularization.
- NPWT decreases exudate of the wound by removing excess fluid through suction.
  - Removes toxic inflammatory mediators and proteinases
  - Improves the diffusion of oxygen and nutrients to the wound
- Contraindication: Gross bacterial infection

8. Skin substitutes
- Integra: Bilayer dermal replacement product that is composed of a biodegradable bovine collagen glycosaminoglycan (GAG; collagen-GAG) matrix underlayer with a silicone outer layer
  - FDA on-label indication is for burn reconstruction.
  - Has been used in reconstruction of wounds with exposed bone without periosteum, exposed cartilage without perichondrium, and exposed tendon without paratenon
  - The collagen-GAG matrix serves as scaffolding for the ingrowth of cells and neovascularization.
    - ○ After 2 to 4 weeks, the silicone outer later is removed and a thin split-thickness skin graft completes the reconstruction by providing epithelial cells over the neovascularized dermal replacement.
  - Advantages: Availability of large quantities, simple and reliable to use, pliability and cosmetic appearance of the resulting cover, less wound contraction
- Biobrane: Temporary; constructed of an inner layer composed of nylon and collagen, covered by an outer silicone film
  - Useful as temporary coverage of burn wounds, where it helps prevent evaporative loss (due to the silicone outer layer) and subsequent wound desiccation
  - Reported to decrease wound pain and provide a barrier to bacterial infection
  - Removed either before permanent grafting or after epithelialization of the wound has occurred.
- Dermagraft: Dermal substitute composed of neonatal foreskin fibroblasts cultured on a polyglactin mesh; generally used in the treatment of diabetic foot ulcers, where it often is combined with meshed skin grafts
- TransCyte: Similar to Biobrane but has an added biologic layer derived from neonatal fibroblasts that are seeded onto the nylon matrix to produce type-1 collagen, fibronectin, and glycosaminoglycans
  - Removed either before skin grafting or after epithelialization of the wound
  - Has been shown to decrease pain and time to epithelialization

- Apligraf: Permanent, constructed of type-1 bovine collagen and cultured neonatal human fibroblasts and keratinocytes
  - Generally used in the treatment of venous ulcers and diabetic foot ulcers
  - Long-term durability makes it an inappropriate choice in situations with a full-thickness defect with exposed vital structures.
- Cultured epidermal autografts: Patient's own keratinocytes expanded in tissue culture (2 to 3 weeks)
  - No donor site limitations
    - ○ Useful with significant burns and limited donor site availability
  - No dermal matrix tissue used; thus, the graft lacks the elastic quality of normal skin or even split-thickness skin grafts
    - ○ Results in stiff wounds with limited motion in the face and around joints
  - The lack of a dermis results in very slow basement membrane formation, producing frequent blistering and shearing
  - Use is somewhat limited by high cost and delay in availability because the tissue is cultured.
  - Low resistance to infection (10^2 bacteria will result in infection)
- Acellular dermal matrices: Cadaveric (or porcine) dermis that is processed to be acellular and nonimmunogenic and then freeze-dried for preservation.
  - Provides a substrate for tissue ingrowth; however, it does not bring in any blood supply
  - Use described in the literature for abdominal wall reconstruction, lower eyelid reconstruction, breast reconstruction, lining of breast implant capsules, and cleft palate repair

9. Dressings
- Silver ions kill a broad spectrum of bacteria. No resistant organisms have been identified, and it is nontoxic to human cells.
- Alginates absorb up to 20 times their weight and are used to exudate wounds.
- Films and transparent dressings are waterproof and would be impermeable to bacterial contamination.
- Hydrogels are generally waterproof and would prevent bacterial contamination.

10. Extravasation injuries
- Cytotoxic and hyperosmolar agents may result in local tissue necrosis.
  - Doxorubicin (Adriamycin) associated with severe soft-tissue necrosis and warrants close follow-up for early surgical debridement, if needed.
    - ○ Dilution with saline or hyaluronidase may be helpful.
- High-volume injuries may cause compartment syndrome and limb ischemia.
  - Higher-risk groups include children, the elderly, and intensive care/chronically ill patients.

- Interventions standard to all extravasation injuries, include splinting, elevation, local dressings, and close serial examination
11. Enzymatic debriding agents
    - Main drawbacks: Not sufficient for significant levels of necrotic tissue burden
    - These ointments can cause burning and they may be diluted with a hydrogel to reduce pain.
        - Papain is a potent digestant of nonviable protein material but does not affect healthy tissues.
            - Urea increases the digestive potency of papain.
            - Dressings containing silver ions inactivate papain.
        - Collagenases are another class of commonly used enzymatic debridement agents.
            - Work slowly
12. Effects of radiation on skin
    - Permanent and may present either acutely or in delayed fashion, even years after the original radiation insult
    - The mechanism of injury: Through free radical production, which directly damages the DNA
        - Acute changes: Erythema and edema of the skin, vasodilation with endothelial edema, and lymphatic obliteration
        - Chronic changes: Capillary thrombosis and subsequent inadequate tissue oxygenation/development of nonhealing ulcers
13. Abnormal scarring (2:1 ratio, T1:T3 collagen)
    - Keloid scars: Scarring with hypertrophy beyond original borders
        - May develop months after injury, seldom regresses, and is not associated with contractures
        - More frequent in darker-skinned individuals
        - Extremely high recurrence rate (up to 80% for excision alone)
        - Radiation therapy effective method to prevent keloid scarring
            - External beam irradiation decreased recurrence rates of 12% to 27%, but this may be associated with pigmentary changes
        - Other methods (intralesional injection of corticosteroids, interferon, retinoic acid, and 5-fluorouracil) have recurrence rate of 50%.
            - Intralesional corticosteroid relieves symptoms of itching and burning.
        - Pressure therapy has been found to be helpful in decreasing keloid recurrence but requires ongoing treatment for 3 to 10 months, which may not be acceptable.
            - Mode of action (MOA): Local tissue hypoxia, reduced fibroblast proliferation, and reduced collagen synthesis
            - Required pressure: 24 and 30 mm Hg
        - Commonly found on deltoid, upper back, chest, and earlobes
        - Histopathology: Extensive, random collagen fibers in bundles. Fibroblasts have increased proliferation rates

and decreased apoptosis (when compared with those from hypertrophic scars), decreased density of blood vessels, relatively acellular absent myofibroblasts, elevated TGF-β.
    - Hypertrophic scars: Boundaries of original scar maintained
        - Develop soon after the injury (within 6 to 8 weeks).
        - Can worsen up to 6 months but subside with time
        - Can produce contractures and have a predilection to occur over the flexor surface of joints
        - Histopathology: Increased density of blood vessels, increased myofibroblasts
    - Both hypertrophic and keloid scars are raised, erythematous, and often pruritic.
14. Wound dehiscence
    - Early wound dehiscence (immediate postoperative period) may be caused by patient movement.
    - Late wound dehiscence is often due to underlying seroma, although infection and skin necrosis can occur.
15. Hyperbaric oxygen
    - Proven utility in conditions such as osteomyelitis, necrotizing infections, ischemia reperfusion injury, and diabetic lower extremity (LE) wounds
    - No proven utility in the treatment of extravasation injury, pressure sores, or pyoderma gangrenosum
16. Chronic wounds: Interruption in the natural sequence of wound healing involving a highly regulated cascade of events among many cell types, soluble factors, and matrix components; prolonged inflammatory phase
    - The chronic wound microenvironment: Imbalance between matrix-degrading enzymes and their inhibitors
        - Metalloproteinase levels are elevated, resulting in extracellular matrix degradation.
        - Proinflammatory cytokines are elevated, which leads to an increase in protease activity and a decrease in protease inhibitor and growth factor levels.
            - Results in decreased matrix deposition, which prevents epithelization and healing
        - Tissue oxygen tension is abnormally low in the central aspect of chronic wounds.
17. Tissue expansion (TE)
    - Results in increased cell division through stretch-induced signal transduction pathways involving growth factors, the cytoskeleton, and protein kinases
        - Net result is an increase in protein synthesis, keratinocyte growth, and new skin production to restore resting tension
    - Cells in adjacent, nonexpanded areas are not affected, expanded cells do not undergo apoptosis followed by cellular replacement, and expansion of the intracellular cytoskeleton alone does not result in increased tissue generation.
    - Several experimental animal studies have shown increased flap survival following TE, similar to that seen with the delay effect. It has been shown to occur with both random-patterned and island flaps.

- Large bundles of compacted collagen fibrils have been demonstrated within the expanded dermis, and the total collagen content of the flap is increased, although the dermis is thinner.
- TE also results in an increase in the total surface area of the flap; however, tensile strength and elasticity are decreased.
- Histopathologic examination demonstrates thinning of the dermis, but the stratum spinosum of the epidermis becomes thickened.
- Creep: Mechanical stretching changes the orientation of elastic fibers and collagen.
- Stress relaxation: During a period of time when skin is stretched to a certain length, the amount of force necessary to maintain that length is decreased.

18. Scalp reconstruction with TE
    - In patients with nearly 50% scalp loss, TE will provide the optimal functional and aesthetic outcome.

- TE increases the amount of locally available tissue, preserves sensation, and maintains hair follicles and adnexal structures.
- When performing expansion, place the largest tolerated expander(s) in the subgaleal plane.
    - Rectangular and crescent-shaped prostheses provide more expansion than circular devices.
- To account for tissue recoil, continue expansion until the expanded flap is ~20% larger than the expected defect.
- Disadvantages: Prolonged time to complete the expansion process (up to 3 months is not uncommon), need for at least two operations, and a high rate of complication (6% to 48%)
    - Common problems include infection, prosthesis exposure or extrusion, hematoma, flap necrosis, skull erosion, alopecia, and wide scars. (see Figure 20.1 and Table 20.3)

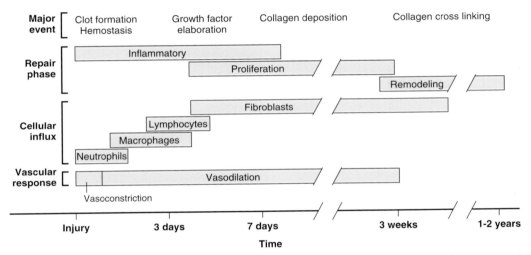

Figure 20.1. The temporal patterns of repair phase, cellular influx, and vascular response during wound repair. The time points are approximate, and overlap occurs during these repair events. *(Reprinted from Lorenz, H.P., Longaker, M.T., 2000. Wounds: Biology, Pathology, and Management. Springer-Verlag, New York.)*

Table 20.3 Diagnostic Criteria for Distinction between Hypertrophic Scars and Keloids

	HYPERTROPHIC SCAR	KELOID
Clinical symptoms	Remain within the boundaries of the wound Rarely more than 1 cm in thickness or width Form scar contractures Less pruritic and painful Occur after injury only: Disruption of skin continuity, burns Generally arise within 4 weeks, grow intensely for several months, then regress often within 1 year Occur on points with excessive tensile forces: Across joint surfaces, sternum, neck, palm, and soles after injury Regress spontaneously	Grow beyond the wound borders Size variations; growth may be widespread, vertical, or both No contractures Pruritic and painful Spontaneous appearance without skin injury possible Appear within several months after initial scar, then gradually proliferate indefinitely Occur often on the chest, shoulders, trunk, back of the neck, and earlobes; rarely on the palms or soles Do not regress spontaneously
Histological features	Fine and thin collagen fibers oriented parallel to the epidermis Nodules with increased fibroblast density Presence of α-smooth-muscle actin-expressing myofibroblasts is typical	Large and thick collagen fibers; closely packed collagen fibrils; increased ratio of type-2 to type-3 collagen Increased fibroblast density in enlarging borders, acellular in keloid center Lack of α-smooth-muscle actin-expressing myofibroblasts

Reprinted from Neligan, P.C., Chang, J. (Eds.), 2013. Plastic Surgery, 3rd ed. Elsevier.

Suggested Readings

Buchanan, E.P., Lorenz, H.P., 2009. Chapter 3: Wound healing, including fetal skin healing. In: Guyuron, B., Eriksson, E., Persing, J.A., et al. (Eds.), Plastic Surgery: Indications and Practice, 1st ed. Elsevier.

Buck, D.W., Galiano, R.D., 2013. Chapter 3: Wound care. In: Thorne, C.H., Chung, K.C., Gosain, A.K., et al. (Eds.), Grabb and Smith Plastic Surgery. 7th ed. Wolters Kluwer, pp. 58–75.

Desai, K.K., Hahn, E., Pulikkotill, B., et al., 2012. Negative pressure wound therapy. Clin. Plast. Surg. 39 (3), 311–324.

Gantwerker, E.A., Hom, D.B., 2012. Skin: histology and physiology of wound healing. Clin. Plast. Surg. 39 (1), 85–97.

Gurtner, G.C., Wong, V.W., 2013. Chapter 2: Wound healing: abnormal and normal. In: Thorne, C.H., Chung, K.C., Gosain, A.K., et al. (Eds.), Grabb and Smith Plastic Surgery. 7th ed. Wolters Kluwer, pp. 42–57.

Hsu, A., Mustoe, T.A., 2010. Chapter 1: The principles of wound healing. In: Weinzweig, J. (Ed.), Plastic Surgery Secrets Plus. Mosby, pp. 3–7.

Leedy, J.E., Janis, J.E., Rohrich, R.J., 2005. Reconstruction of acquired scalp defects: an algorithmic approach. Plast. Reconstr. Surg. 116 (4), 54e–72e.

Marks, M.W., Argenta, L.C., 2013. Chapter 27: Principles and applications of tissue expansion. In: Neligan, P.C., Chang, J. (Eds.), Plastic Surgery, 3rd ed. Elsevier, pp. 622–653.

Mirastschijski, U., Jokuszies, A., Vogt, P.M., 2013. Chapter 15: Skin wound healing. In: Neligan, P.C., Chang, J. (Eds.), Plastic Surgery, 3rd ed. Elsevier, pp. 26–296.

Sen, C.K., Roy, S., 2013. Chapter 14: Wound healing. In: Neligan, P.C., Chang, J. (Eds.), Plastic Surgery, 3rd ed. Elsevier, pp. 240–266.

Soft-Tissue and Hand Infections

Bites

1. Human bites
   - Generally polymicrobial: *Staphylococcus aureus, Streptococcus, Corynebacterium, Eikenella corrodens,* and anaerobics
   - *Eikenella* species unique to human bites
     - Treat with penicillin including ampicillin and amoxicillin
     - *Eikenella* species are resistant to clindamycin.
   - Note that fight bites require operative exploration and washout because bacteria can be inoculated into joint spaces and spread proximally by extensor tendon motion.
2. Dog bites
   - Immediately irrigate wounds with saline and wash with soap and/or Betadine
   - Leave puncture wounds open to heal by secondary intent.
   - Lacerations can be repaired after copious irrigation if wound appears clean.
   - Penicillin antibiotics most commonly used
   - Must be concerned about rabies
     - If a known animal, it should be quarantined for at least 10 days.
     - If an unknown animal, rabies prophylaxis is indicated.
       - Rabies prophylaxis
         - If prior vaccination: Wash wound thoroughly and provide booster vaccine.
         - If no prior vaccination: Wash wound thoroughly, administer rabies vaccine and rabies immunoglobulin.
3. Cat bites
   - Cat bites tend to result in puncture wounds that can seal quickly; therefore, incision and drainage is recommended.
   - High rate of infection from cat bites
   - Many infections are polymicrobial; however, *Pasteurella multocida* is unique to cat bites.
     - *Pasteurella* is resistant to cephalexin and cefazolin.
     - Treat with amoxicillin-clavulanate or fluoroquinolone and clindamycin for penicillin-allergic patients.
     - Preferred treatment for pediatric patients is trimethoprim-sulfamethoxazole (Bactrim) and clindamycin.
4. Snake bites
   - The majority of snakebites are from pit vipers.
   - Treat with immediate immobilization to prevent spread of venom, tetanus prophylaxis, broad-spectrum antibiotics, and observation for venom inoculation (worsening edema, pain, ecchymosis, altered mental status, coagulopathy, compartment syndrome).
   - Antivenin is indicated for progressive injury or symptoms.
     - If nonurgent, skin test first for hypersensitivity reaction is preferred.
   - Avoid debridement and/or tourniquet application
5. Spider bites
   - Brown recluse spider
     - Venom inoculation causes a dermonecrotic reaction: Blistering, ischemia, ulceration at the bite site.
     - Treat with Dapsone.
       - Watch for hematologic side effects.
   - Black widow spider
     - Venom is a neurotoxin that causes severe muscle pain and cramping. Late findings include abdominal pain, tremors, emesis, excessive salivation, and shock.
     - Treat with calcium gluconate and benzodiazepines (e.g., diazepam).
     - Spider antivenin can be used in immunocompromised patients.
6. Scorpion stings
   - Stings are typically self-limiting in adults.
   - Symptoms include severe localized pain and hyperesthesia and can progress to blurry vision, strabismus, dyspnea, dysphagia, incontinence, fevers, and muscle contraction.
   - Treat initially with cold compresses and observation.
   - In children, symptoms can be more severe.
     - Treat with admission, monitoring, and potentially intubation for airway protection.
   - Avoid debridement and tourniquet application.
7. Special considerations
   - Tetanus prophylaxis
     - If prior vaccination
       - Tetanus-prone wound (contaminated, etc.): Administer tetanus booster if last dose occurred more than 5 years before new injury.

○ Non-tetanus-prone wound (clean): Administer tetanus booster if last dose occurred more than 10 years from new injury.
- If no prior vaccination
  ○ Tetanus immunoglobulin

Necrotizing Soft-Tissue Infections

1. Necrotizing fasciitis: A progressive soft-tissue infection affecting skin, subcutaneous tissue, and fascia and sparing muscle
   - Extremely high mortality and rapid progression
   - Can result from minor trauma or hematogenous spread
     - Most patients have predisposing morbidity, placing them at risk.
       ○ Immunocompromised
       ○ Diabetes
       ○ Renal failure
       ○ Substance abuse
     - Head and neck infections can result from pharyngeal abscesses, tonsillar abscesses, and dental abscesses.
   - Requires emergent debridement of all devitalized tissue
2. Classification
   - Type 1 (75% of cases): Polymicrobial, mixed aerobic and anaerobic infections (non-group-A *Streptococcus*)
     - Treat with ampicillin-sulbactam, clindamycin, ciprofloxacin, or gentamicin.
   - Type 2: Monomicrobial, group-A *Streptococcus* (*Streptococcus pyogenes*)
     - Treat with clindamycin and penicillin.
3. Progression of infection
   - Initial cellulitis stage: Tenderness, erythema, edema, warm skin, fever
     - May have increased white blood cells (WBCs), thrombocytopenia, hyperkalemia
   - Cellulitis progresses to ischemia with severe pain, crepitus, and bullae formation.
   - Final stage characterized by frank necrosis, anesthesia, and "dishwater" drainage.
4. Principles of management
   - Fluid resuscitation
   - Intravenous antibiotics
   - Emergent surgical debridement
     - Include fasciotomies in setting of compartment syndrome.
     - Many require multiple trips to the operating room for serial debridement.
   - Hyperbaric oxygen is indicated as an adjunct to surgical debridement for patients with persistent or extensive necrosis.
   - Negative pressure wound therapy (NPWT) is often used as a bridge to reconstruction after debridement.
5. Fournier's gangrene
   - A necrotizing soft-tissue infection of the perineum
   - Risk factors: Diabetes, alcoholism, smoking, leukemia, immunocompromised
   - Rapid progression and high mortality
   - Treat as above and include antibiotic coverage for anaerobic clostridium species.

Other Common Soft-Tissue Infections

1. Methicillin-resistant *Staphylococcus aureus* (MRSA)
   - Increasingly common flora, especially in the nares
   - More virulent and resistant to penicillins and cephalosporins
   - Suspect in patient with persistent infection in setting of penicillin antibiotic treatment.
     - Treat with vancomycin, linezolid, trimethoprim-sulfamethoxazole (Bactrim), or clindamycin.
   - Nasal mupirocin (Bactroban) can be used to decolonize patients who are noted to be carriers by nasal culture.
2. Orbital cellulitis
   - Signs
     - Edema of the upper and lower eyelids
     - Erythema and cellulitis in the periorbital region
     - Proptosis
     - Pain with globe movement
   - Diagnosis: Computed tomography (CT) scan
   - Treatment: Broad-spectrum intravenous antibiotics and operative drainage
3. Purpura fulminans
   - Signs: Acute onset of hemorrhagic bullae formation, desquamation, bilateral symmetric gangrene, and shock
   - Rapid progression, with high mortality
     - Most common pathogens are *Neisseria meningitides* and MRSA
   - Typically involves pediatric patients
   - Treatment: Supportive care, broad-spectrum intravenous antibiotics, and activated protein C
     - Delay surgery until demarcation occurs, except in the setting of acute wound infection or compartment syndrome.
4. Hidradenitis suppurativa
   - A defect of the follicular epithelium causing follicle occlusion, rupture, and formation of abscesses and sinus tracts, which leads to chronic apocrine gland inflammation and secondary bacterial infections
   - Commonly affects hair-bearing regions with apocrine glands and skin folds (e.g., axilla, groin, perineum).
   - Most common pathogens are *Staphylococcus aureus* and *Streptococcus viridans*.
   - Treatment: Antibiotics and incision and drainage of acute abscesses followed by wide excision of all involved skin and sinus tracts with healing by secondary intent or grafting
5. Toxic shock syndrome
   - Signs: Fever, hypotension, diffuse macular rash, and desquamation of the palms and soles 2 weeks after onset of symptoms
   - Can occur after surgery, trauma, or retained foreign bodies (e.g., nasal packing, tampons, etc.)

- Most common pathogens are *Staphylococcus aureus* and group-A *Streptococcus pyogenes*.
  - Streptococcal toxic shock syndrome characterized by severe disproportionate pain, with potential progression to coagulopathy and organ failure
- Treatment: Supportive care and antibiotics

6. Wound infections
   - Can develop after surgery, trauma, injury
   - Risk factors can include host (diabetes, malnutrition, obesity, ischemia, steroid use, immunosuppression), wound (presence of nonviable tissue, foreign bodies, contamination), and procedural (length of operation) characteristics.
     - Of the wound factors, contamination portends the highest risk.
   - Treatment: Drainage and/or debridement, antibiotics, supportive care

Hand Infections

1. Hand abscess
   - Often complex due to deep communication with anatomic hand spaces
     - Horseshoe abscess: Communication of flexor sheath infection with Parona space in the distal forearm
       - Parona space: Potential space in the distal forearm that joins the radial and ulnar bursa, superficial to the pronator quadratus, and contiguous with the midpalmar and thenar space
       - Treat with aggressive debridement of the digit and Parona space (can access through an extended carpal tunnel incision).
     - Collar button abscess: Tracks from dorsal to volar within the web space via the palmar fascia
       - Hallmark sign: Finger abduction away from the affected web space
       - Treat with dorsal and volar incision and drainage and intravenous antibiotics (see Figure 21.1).
2. Flexor tenosynovitis
   - Kanavel's signs: Fusiform swelling, partially flexed finger posturing, pain over the flexor sheath, pain with passive extension
   - Most common pathogens are *Staphylococcus aureus* or *Eikenella corrodens* through human bite injuries.
   - Treatment: Intravenous antibiotics, irrigation of the flexor tendon sheath
     - Can access flexor sheath through incisions at the A1 and A5 pulley or distal flexor crease (see Figure 21.2)
3. Septic arthritis
   - Infection of the joint space
   - Signs: Joint edema, pain with motion and joint impaction, erythema, limited motion
   - Diagnosis: Aspiration of the joint
     - Elevated synovial fluid WBC count (>50,000 to 100,000) with predominance of neutrophils is the most sensitive marker of septic arthritis.

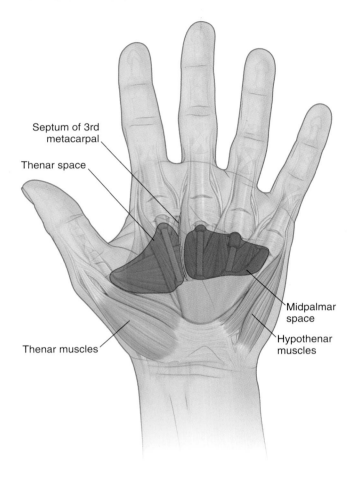

Figure 21.1. Deep spaces of the hand. (*Reprinted from Neligan, P.C., Chang, J. [Eds.], 2013. Plastic Surgery, 3rd ed. Elsevier, 333–345.*)

- Most common pathogens are *Staphylococcus aureus* and *Streptococcus viridians*.
  - Treat with penicillin or 1st-generation cephalosporin.
- Other potential organisms
  - *Neisseria* species
    - Often develops without history of trauma (hematogenous spread).
    - Gram positive diplococci on gram stain of joint fluid
    - No incision and drainage necessary because *Neisseria* does not destroy joint cartilage
    - Treatment: Aspiration of joint fluid, intravenous 3rd-generation cephalosporin (e.g., ceftriaxone)
  - *Serratia* species
    - Often affects patients with history of diabetes, immunosuppression, or intravenous drug abuse
  - Tuberculosis infections can masquerade as tenosynovitis or arthritis.
    - Diagnosis is made by the presence of rice bodies on imaging studies.
4. Paronychia
   - Infection of the nail fold
   - Often present without any specific history of trauma or exposure

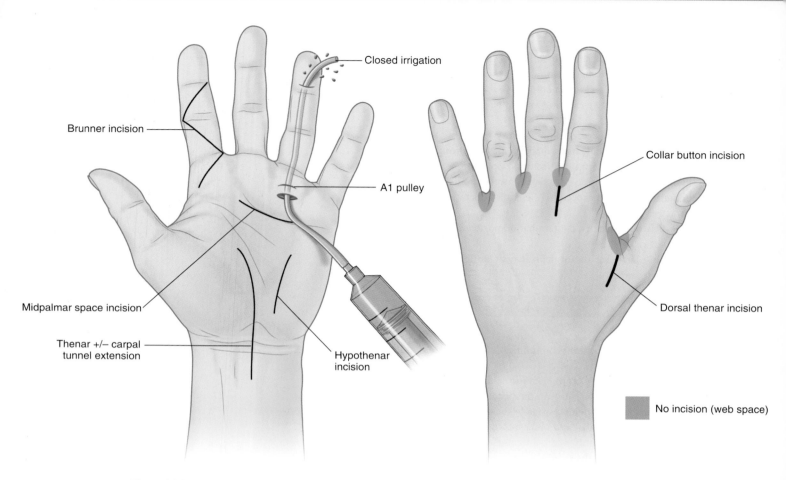

Figure 21.2. Hand incisions. *(Reprinted from Neligan, P.C., Chang, J. [Eds.], 2013. Plastic Surgery, 3rd ed. Elsevier, 333–345.)*

- Treatment
  - Acute paronychia: Removal of a segment of the nail plate and antibiotics
    - May require incision within the nail fold for drainage
    - Most common pathogens are *Staphylococcus aureus* and *Streptococcus*.
  - Chronic paronychia: Removal of a segment of the nail plate and antifungal medication
    - May require marsupialization of the paronychia with healing by secondary intent if antifungal medication fails
    - Most common pathogen is candida.
5. Felon (see Figure 21.3)
   - Infection of the volar pad of a finger after a traumatic puncture injury
     - Complex infections because of the multiple fibrous septae within the finger pads
   - Signs: Severe pain, swelling
   - Treatment: Incision and drainage (with care to divide the fibrous septae) and antibiotics

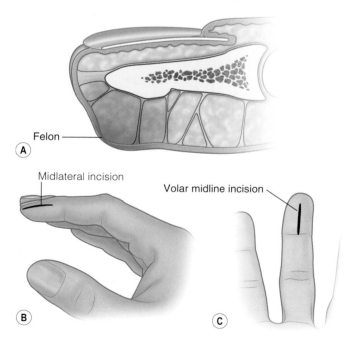

Figure 21.3. A, Anatomy of a felon; **B,C,** options for felon incisions. *(Reprinted from Neligan, P.C., Chang, J. [Eds.], 2013. Plastic Surgery, 3rd ed. Elsevier, 333–345.)*

Table 21.1 General Recommendations for Hand Infections

INFECTION	LIKELY ORGANISM(S)	INITIAL ANTIBIOTIC THERAPY*	SURGICAL THERAPY
Cellulitis	*Staphylococcus* or *Streptococcus*	Cephalexin. Use clindamycin or trimethoprim-sulfamethoxazole (Bactrim) for suspected MRSA	Only indicated for associated abscess
Abscess	*Staphylococcus*	Vancomycin. Add piperacillin-tazobactam (Zosyn) for diabetic/immunocompromised patients	Immediate drainage (no closure), soaks, and motion 1 day after surgery
Flexor tenosynovitis	*Staphylococcus*, anaerobes, polymicrobial	Ampicillin-sulbactam (Unasyn). Replace Unasyn with Zosyn for diabetic/immunocompromised patients and add vancomycin if suspect possible MRSA	Consider 12- to 24-hour observation for early signs; otherwise, drainage of flexor sheath (no closure), soaks, and motion 1 day after surgery
Septic arthritis	*Staphylococcus*	Vancomycin. Add ceftriaxone if suspect *Neisseria gonorrhoeae*	Immediate drainage (no closure), soaks, and motion 1 day after surgery
Animal bite	*Pasteurella multocida* is classic, but *Staph*, *Strep*, and anaerobes are common	Unasyn or oral (PO) equivalent. If penicillin allergic, consider fluoroquinolone and clindamycin	Clean thoroughly in ER and observe closely for signs of deep infection. Cat teeth inoculate the deep tissues, so consider incising the puncture site to facilitate drainage. Dog teeth tear local tissues; wound will usually drain spontaneously
Human bite	*Eikenella corrodens* is classic, but *Staph*, *Strep*, and anaerobes are common	Unasyn or PO equivalent. If penicillin allergic, consider fluoroquinolone and clindamycin	Clean thoroughly in ER and observe closely for signs of a deep infection (e.g., abscess, FTS, etc.). "Fight bites" require immediate drainage, even in the absence of overt infection
Necrotizing fasciitis	*Streptococcus* or polymicrobial	Vancomycin *and* clindamycin *and* piperacillin-tazobactam (Zosyn)	Emergent radical debridement(s), hemodynamic monitoring, possible amputation
Gas gangrene	*Clostridium perfringens*, *Strep pyogenes*, *Staph aureus*, *Vibrio vulnificus*, polymicrobial	Vancomycin *and* clindamycin *and* piperacillin-tazobactam (Zosyn). Consider high-dose penicillin.	Emergent radical debridement(s), hemodynamic monitoring, possible amputation

Reprinted from Cameron, J.L., Cameron, A.M. (Eds.), 2014. Current Surgical Therapy, 11th ed. Saunders, 724–732.
FTS, *Flexor tenosynovitis.*
*Antibiotic coverage should be adjusted once cultures are back to decrease the creation of antibiotic-resistant organisms and to minimize drug side effects to the patient.

6. Herpetic whitlow
   - A lesion on the finger or thumb secondary to the herpes simplex virus
   - Signs: Pain, multiple vesicles on an erythematous base
   - Risk factors: Immunocompromised patients
   - Diagnosis: Tzanck smear shows giant cells.
   - Treatment: Acyclovir (oral or topical) only; surgical incision or debridement may result in superinfection or encephalitis.
7. Sweet syndrome
   - Also known as acute febrile neutrophilic dermatosis.
   - Signs: Fever and painful erythematous skin lesions that primarily appear on the arms, neck, face, and back
   - Diagnosis: Biopsy reveals neutrophilic infiltration of the dermis and epidermis.
   - Treatment: Corticosteroid administration
8. Atypical mycobacterial infections
   - Resulting from exposure to ocean water, aquatic life, or marine environments
   - Most common pathogen is *Mycobacterium marinum.*
   - Signs: Tenosynovitis signs without pain
9. *Vibrio vulnificus* infections
   - Infections resulting from exposure to water, raw aquatic life, or puncture wounds from fish and/or stingrays
   - Signs: Pain, cellulitis, severe edema, and hemorrhagic bullae formation
   - Can progress to bacteremia and systemic symptoms
   - High mortality rate
   - Treatment: Intravenous fluoroquinalone (or a 3rd-generation cephalosporin with a tetracycline) and supportive care (see Table 21.1)

Suggested Readings

Brinster, N.K., Liu, V., Hafeez, D., et al. (Eds.), 2011. Dermatopathology. Saunders.

Dodds, S.D., 2010. Chapter 11: Hand infections and injection injuries. In: Trumble, T.E., Rayan, G.M., Budoff, J.E., et al. (Eds.), Principles of Hand Surgery and Therapy, 2nd ed. Elsevier, pp. 193–200.

Masden, D.L., Forthman, C.L., 2014. Hand infections. In: Cameron, J.L., Cameron, A.M. (Eds.), Current Surgical Therapy, 11th ed. Saunders, pp. 724–732.

O'Neal, P.B., Itani, K.M., 2014. Necrotizing skin and soft tissue infections. In: Cameron, J.L., Cameron, A.M. (Eds.), Current Surgical Therapy, 11th ed. Saunders, pp. 745–750.

Bidic, S.M., Schaub, T., 2013. Chapter 16: Infections of the hand. In: Neligan, P.C., Chang, J. (Eds.), Plastic Surgery, 3rd ed. Elsevier, pp. 333–345.

Shenoy, E.S., Hooper, D.C., 2013. Chapter 38: Skin and soft tissue infections. In: Parsons, P.E., Wiener-Kronish, J.P. (Eds.), Critical Care Secrets, 5th ed. Mosby, pp. 262–270.

Slavin, E.M., 2013. Chapter 184: Skin and soft-tissue infections. In: Adams, J.G. (Ed.), Emergency Medicine Clinical Essentials, 2nd ed. Saunders, pp. 1550–1554.

Durand, M.L., 2015. Chapter 118: Periocular infections. In: Bennett, J.E., Dolin, R., Blaser, M.J. (Eds.), Principles and Practice of Infectious Diseases, 8th ed. Saunders, pp. 1432–1438.

Evans, D.C., Steinberg, S.M., 2011. Chapter 135: Infections of skin, muscle, and soft tissue. In: Vincent, J.L., Abraham, E., Moore, F.A., et al. (Eds.), Textbook of Critical Care, 6th ed. Saunders, pp. 1028–1035.

Norris, R.L., Auerbach, P.S., Nelson, E.E., et al., 2012. Chapter 22: Bites and stings. In: Townsend, C.M., Beauchamp, R.D., Evers, B.M., et al. (Eds.), Sabiston Textbook of Surgery, 19th ed. Saunders, pp. 548–562.

Fagan, S., Chai, J., Spies, M., et al., 2012. Chapter 43: Exfoliative diseases of the integument and soft tissue necrotizing infections. In: Herndon, D.N. (Ed.), Total Burn Care, 4th ed. Elsevier, pp. 471–481.

Burns and Burn Reconstruction

Initial Evaluation

1. Burn severity or "degree": Described based on depth of injury
   - First degree ("superficial" partial thickness): Superficial, erythema, sometimes painful, epidermal integrity intact
   - Second degree ("deep" partial thickness): Blisters, erythema, edema, very painful, epidermis violated, injury is into dermis
   - Third degree (full thickness): Charred or translucent, "white" color, mild pain, pin prick absent
2. Burn volume: Described by total body surface area (TBSA) involved
   - "Rule of nines" (see Figure 22.1)
   - Lund and Browder method (see Figure 22.2)
3. Burn center referrals
   - Outcomes of burns better at high-volume centers
   - Criteria for referral to an accredited burn center (American Burn Association) (see Box 22.1)

Burn Physiology

1. The three zones of a burn
   - Zone of coagulation: Central area of nonviable tissue
   - Zone of stasis: Threatened area with initial perfusion that can progress to ischemia
     - Progression can be prevented with adequate resuscitation
   - Zone of hyperemia: Outer area of viable tissue (see Figure 22.3)
2. Burns >30% TBSA are associated with a systemic inflammatory response and general down-regulation of the immune system, including
   - Diminished activation of complement and decrease in levels of circulating immunoglobulins (levels may take 2 to 4 weeks to recover as patient condition improves)
   - Up-regulation of proinflammatory cytokines TNF-α, interleukin-1 (IL-1), IL-8, and integrins that promote neutrophil chemotaxis, extravasation, and tissue necrosis
   - Reduced B-lymphocyte function, T-helper-cell function, and cytotoxic T-lymphocyte function
     - Contributes to delayed allograft rejection, suppression of graft versus host disease, and skin hypersensitivity
   - Increased T-suppressor function

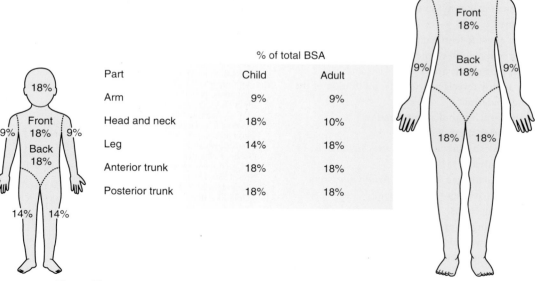

Part	% of total BSA	
	Child	Adult
Arm	9%	9%
Head and neck	18%	10%
Leg	14%	18%
Anterior trunk	18%	18%
Posterior trunk	18%	18%

Figure 22.1. Estimation of burn size using the "rule of nines." *BSA,* Body surface area.

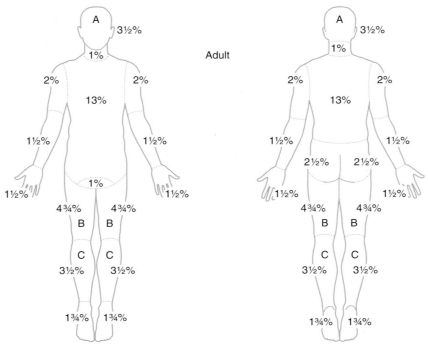

Age	0–1	1–4	5–9	10–14	15
A – ½ of head	9½%	8½%	6½%	5½%	4½%
B – ½ of one thigh	9½%	8½%	6½%	5½%	4½%
C – ½ of one leg	9½%	8½%	6½%	5½%	4½%

Figure 22.2. Estimation of burn size using the Lund and Browder method. *(Reprinted from Herndon, D.N. [Ed.], 2012. Total Burn Care. Elsevier, 93–102.)*

BOX 22.1 BURN CENTER REFERRAL CRITERIA

1. Partial-thickness burns >10% TBSA
2. Burns that involve the face, hands, feet, genitalia, perineum, or major joints
3. Full-thickness burns in any age group
4. Burns caused by electric current including lightning
5. Chemical burns
6. Inhalation injury
7. Burn injury in patients with preexisting medical disorders that could complicate management, prolong recovery, or affect mortality
8. Any patient with burns and concomitant trauma (such as fractures) in whom the burn injury poses the greatest risk of morbidity or mortality. In such cases, if the trauma poses the greater immediate risk, the patient may be stabilized in a trauma center before transfer to a burn center
9. Burned children in a hospital without qualified personnel or equipment for the care of children
10. Burn injury in a patient who will require special social, emotional, or rehabilitative intervention

Adapted from American Burn Association, 2011. Advanced Burn Life Support Course Provider Manual. American Burn Association, Chicago, IL, 25–26.
TBSA, Total body surface area.

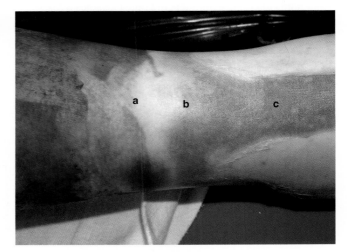

Figure 22.3. Jackson's three zones of injury on an ankle burn. **a,** Zone of coagulation; **b,** zone of stasis; **c,** zone of hyperemia. *(Reprinted from Herndon, D.N. [Ed.], 2012. Total Burn Care, 4th ed. Elsevier, 125–130.)*

Burn Management

1. Fluid resuscitation
   - High-volume resuscitation is warranted in burns >20% TBSA
   - Parkland formula
     - $(4 \text{ mL/kg}) \times (\text{weight in kg}) \times (\% \text{ TBSA})$ = total fluid to be infused over 24-hour period.
     - Give half of this in the first 8 hours from the time that the burn injury occurred (not from time of presentation).
     - Give remaining half during the next 16 hours.
   - Titrate fluid resuscitation to urine output.
     - Adults: ½ cc/kg/hr
     - Pediatrics: 1 cc/kg/hr
     - Urine output can be falsely elevated with elevated urine glucose (glycosuria), thereby overestimating a patient's fluid status.
       - When following urine output in these patients, obtain a urinalysis to check for the presence of glucose.
2. Supportive care
   - Systemic prophylactic antibiotics and steroids have not been shown to improve outcomes.
     - Antibiotics are indicated in the presence of cellulitis, purulent drainage, and active infection.
       - Most common organisms are methicillin-resistant *Staphylococcus aureus, Pseudomonas,* and *Klebsiella.*
       - Initial coverage using broad-spectrum antibiotics (e.g., vancomycin and piperacillin-tazobactam) followed by culture-directed therapy
   - Children are at high risk for hypoglycemia in the first 24 hours following a burn due to limited hepatic glycogen stores.
   - Most common cause of death is bronchopneumonia.
3. Burn nutrition
   - Large burns are associated with hypermetabolism.
   - Elevated daily protein requirement for burn patients
     - Adults: 1 to 2 g/kg/day
     - Pediatrics: 2 to 3 g/kg/day
   - Excessive carbohydrate/glucose administration can result in excessive water and carbon monoxide generation, leading to increasing edema and difficulty in weaning ventilator support.
   - Enteral feeding is preferred to parenteral nutrition.
4. Topical antimicrobial agents
   - Silver nitrate
     - Advantages: Can provide antimicrobial coverage and some hemostasis
     - Disadvantages: Must be frequently reapplied, stains tissue black, can cause electrolyte disturbances and methemoglobinemia
   - Silver sulfadiazine (Silvadene)
     - Advantages: Broad-spectrum antimicrobial coverage
     - Disadvantages: Forms a yellowish-gray pseudoeschar that must be removed before reapplication, can cause

leucopenia, cross-reactive with sulfa allergies, cannot penetrate eschar or cartilage
   - Mafenide acetate (Sulfamylon)
     - Advantages: Broad-spectrum antimicrobial coverage, penetrates eschar and cartilage, useful in setting of burn wound infection and suppurative chondritis
     - Disadvantages: Painful when applied, can cause metabolic acidosis, secondary to inhibition of carbonic anhydrase
5. Surgical management/burn reconstruction
   - Operative excision and grafting are recommended for burn wounds that are not likely to reepithelialize and heal within 3 weeks.
     - The practice of early burn wound excision and grafting has reduced mortality from burn wound sepsis.
   - Debride partial-thickness wounds with tangential excision until pinpoint bleeding is obtained, then perform skin graft.
   - Skin substitutes may be used in patients who may not have enough donor site availability for burn wound coverage.
     - Cultured epidermal autografts: Ex vivo expansion of donor keratinocytes
       - Advantages: Can obtain ~10,000-fold expansion; available in spray form
       - Disadvantages: Lack dermal component, rendering these grafts fragile and highly susceptible to sheer forces; grown with murine fibroblasts and fetal calf serum, which can contribute to rejection, infection
   - Escharotomy
     - Indications: Full-thickness circumferential skin burns that can cause ischemia to a distal extremity or part from development of compartment syndrome
     - Symptoms
       - Dry, pale/whitish skin, nonblanching, insensate
       - "5 Ps": pain, pallor, poikilothermia, paresthesia, pulselessness
     - Perform at bedside as soon as the patient stabilized
     - Make incisions in the following orientation and with a depth into the subcutaneous fat:
       - Arm/forearm: Longitudinal medial and lateral
       - Hand: Thenar/hypothenar, dorsal incisions 3× between metacarpals, digital midlateral lines
       - Chest wall: Midline, + /− transverse
       - Thigh/leg: Longitudinal medial and lateral
       - Foot: Dorsal, medial, lateral
   - Reconstruction of burn wounds can be performed through skin grafts, pedicled flaps, and/or free flaps.
     - Delay free flaps for at least 6 weeks after debridement in burn patients secondary to a hypercoagulable state; leads to an increased risk of microvascular thrombosis.

Burn Complications

1. Postburn contracture
   - Reduced motion secondary to scar contracture
     - Especially common around joints

- Can occur through extrinsic and intrinsic means
  - Extrinsic contractures: Tissue loss in distant sites leads to distortion and limitations through tension.
  - Intrinsic contractures: Distortion and limitations secondary to tissue loss within the affected area
- Can prevent functional deficits from contractures through splinting
  - Appropriate positions for postburn splinting
    - Neck: Slight extension
    - Shoulder: Fully abducted to 90 degrees
    - Elbow: Fully extended at 180 degrees
    - Wrist: Neutral or slightly extended
    - Hand: Intrinsic plus ("safe") position
- Most common locations for postburn contracture release (in order of frequency)
  - Neck
  - Axilla
  - Elbow
  - Trunk
  - Knee
  - Hand
2. Scar alopecia
   - Occurs commonly from scalp burns
   - Tissue expansion is the preferred method of treatment for large areas.
     - Can reconstruct up to 50% of the scalp through tissue expansion
3. Ectropion
   - Most common complication following burns to the eyelid
   - If ectropion is related to skin deficiency only, preferred treatment is contracture incision and placement of full-thickness skin graft.

Electrical Injury

1. Occurs often to electricians and linemen or can occur through lightning injury
2. Electrical injury is the primary cause of compartment syndrome in the burn patient.
   - Greatest risk for compartment syndrome with exposure to >1000 V (reported incidence of ~30%)
3. Deep periosseus tissues are at highest risk for injury because of the high heat capacity of bone.
4. If compartment syndrome is a concern, perform fasciotomy in standard fashion.
   - Missed compartment syndrome from electrical injury can lead to a high rate of amputation.

Frostbite

1. Frostbite injury occurs through severe vasoconstriction and intravascular ice crystal formation, leading to ischemia and tissue necrosis.

2. Initial management
   - Rapid rewarming will decrease further tissue damage by reversing vasoconstriction and preventing ice crystal formation.
     - Preferred method is hot water bath at 40° C (104° F to 107° F) for 15 to 30 minutes.
     - Do not use a radiant heat source.
   - Anti-inflammatory medications: NSAIDs or COX-2 inhibitors are beneficial for vasodilatory effects and antiplatelet aggregation.
   - Debride clear blisters that contain inflammatory mediators.
     - Do not debride hemorrhagic blisters because this can promote dessication and necrosis.
   - Allow time for tissue demarcation.
     - Early debridement and amputation only if there is evidence of infection
     - Bone scans can assist with predicting the level of amputation.
   - In severe frostbite with absent pulses: Emergent angiography and tissue plasminogen activator (tPA) infusion.
     - Decreases rate of amputation if given within 24 hours of injury

Stevens-Johnson Syndrome/Toxic Epidermal Necrolysis

1. May begin 1 to 3 weeks after starting a specific medication (e.g., phenobarbital, Dilantin, sulfa, allopurinol, various antibiotics, NSAIDs).
2. Characterized by
   - Epidermal sloughing in conjunction with mucosal inflammation and ulceration
   - Several days of nonspecific symptoms rapidly progressing to exfoliating rash
3. Slough >10% TBSA is best treated in a burn center.
4. Treatment is supportive.
   - Fluid resuscitation
   - Burn wound care including early debridement and coverage
     - Often requires use of synthetic skin substitutes
       - For example, allograft, xenograft, Biobrane

Suggested Readings

Borghese, L., Masellis, A., Masellis, M., 2013. Chapter 19: Extremity burn reconstruction. In: Neligan, P.C. (Ed.), Plastic Surgery, 3rd ed. Elsevier, pp. 435–455.

Burns, J.L., Phillips, L.G., 2006. Chapter: Burns. In: McCarthy, J.G., Galiano, R.D., Boutros, S.G. (Eds.), Current Therapy in Plastic Surgery. Saunders, pp. 71–76.

French, L.E., Prins, C., 2012. Chapter 20: Erythema multiforme, Stevens-Johnson syndrome and toxic epidermal necrolysis. In: Bolognnia, J.L., Jorizzo, J.L., Schaffer, J.V. (Eds.), Dermatology, 3rd ed. Elsevier, pp. 319–333.

Herndon, D.N. (Ed.), 2012. Total Burn Care, 4th ed. Elsevier.

Klein, M.B., 2013. Chapter 22: Reconstructive burn surgery. In: Neligan, P.C. (Ed.), Plastic Surgery, 3rd ed. Elsevier, pp. 500–510.

Spence, R.J., 2013. Chapter 21: Management of facial burns. In: Neligan, P.C. (Ed.), Plastic Surgery, 3rd ed. Elsevier, pp. 468–499.

Steinstraesser, L., Al-Benna, S., 2013. Chapter 18: Acute management of burn/electrical injuries. In: Neligan, P.C. (Ed.), Plastic Surgery, 3rd ed. Elsevier, pp. 393–434.

Benign Skin Conditions and Skin Disorders

23

Common Benign Skin Lesions

1. Keratocanthoma (see Figure 23.1)
   - Benign tumor that behaves like a squamous cell carcinoma (SCC) and is difficult to differentiate histologically
   - Characterized by rapid growth with a central crater/keratin plug
   - Can spontaneously regress
   - Treatment recommendation: Excision

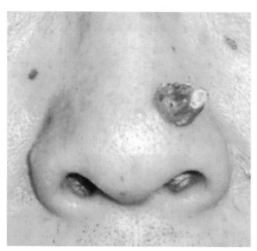

Figure 23.1. Keratoacanthoma on the nose. *(Reprinted from Neligan, P.C. [Ed.], 2013. Plastic Surgery, vol. 1, 3rd ed. Elsevier, 707–742.)*

2. Actinic keratosis (AK; also known as solar keratosis, senile keratosis; see Figure 23.2)
   - Extremely common skin lesions reportedly affecting up to 12% of the population
   - Benign, premalignant lesion that can progress to SCC
     - Estimated rate of conversion to SCC is 13% to 20% over 10 years for lesions that are untreated.
   - More than 80% occur on sun-exposed/sun-damaged areas such as the head, neck, and upper extremities (e.g., dorsal hand/forearm).
   - Risk factors: Chronic sun exposure, increasing age, male gender, fair skin
   - Characterized by a rough, erythematous papule with a white to yellowish scale or plaque
   - Treatment: Cryosurgery, photodynamic therapy, medical treatment (e.g., topical or intralesional 5-fluorouracil [5FU], topical imiquimod)

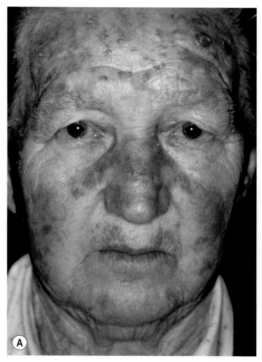

Figure 23.2. Actinic keratoses (AKs). **A,** Multiple AKs on the face of an elderly woman with fair complexion, blue eyes, and moderate-to-severe photodamage; the AKs vary in size from a few millimeters to >1 cm. On the left forehead, the red nodule with slight scale-crust represents a well-differentiated SCC.

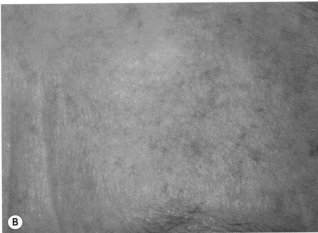

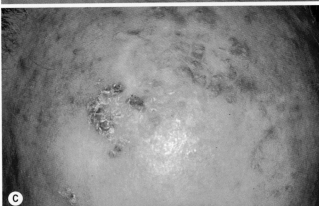

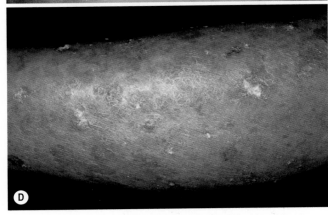

Figure 23.2, cont'd. B, Pink-colored, atrophic AK with minimal scale on the forehead. **C,** Numerous hypertrophic AKs on the bald scalp with hypopigmentation at sites of previous treatment. **D,** Multiple large, hypertrophic AKs on the shin of an elderly woman; note the thick scale. *(Reprinted from Bolognia, J.L., Jorizzo, J.L., Schaffer, J.V. [Eds.], 2012. Dermatology, 3rd ed. Elsevier, 1773–1793.* **B,** *Courtesy Iris Zalaudek, M.D.;* **D,** *Courtesy Jean L. Bolognia, M.D.)*

3. Seborrheic keratosis (SK; also known as a senile wart) (see Figure 23.3)
   - Benign skin growth originating from the basal and squamous cells of the epidermis
   - Characterized by well-circumscribed, waxy lesions that are occasionally pigmented and have a "stuck-on" appearance
   - Must be differentiated from AK, basal cell carcinoma (BCC), and melanoma
   - Sudden appearance of multiple SKs can be a marker of internal malignancy.
   - Treatment: Laser therapy, cryotherapy, electrosurgery, and excision

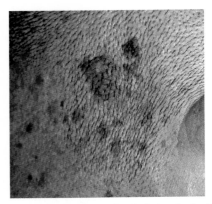

Figure 23.3. Example of a large seborrheic keratosis. Notice the waxy, stuck-on appearance. *(Reprinted from Neligan, P.C. [Ed.], 2013. Plastic Surgery, vol. 1, 3rd ed. Elsevier, 707–742. Courtesy Lorenzo Cerroni, M.D.)*

4. Nevus sebaceous ("nevus sebaceous of Jadassohn") (see Figure 23.4)
   - A benign hamartoma confined to the head and neck regions
   - Can have malignant degeneration into BCC
   - Characterized by a waxy, smooth or papillated, hairless, salmon-colored patch or thickening on the scalp that typically presents at birth
   - Treatment: Excision

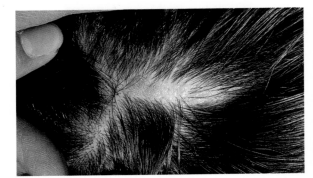

Figure 23.4. Nevus sebaceous. A typical lesion on the scalp of a prepubertal male. *(Reprinted from Habif, T.P. [Ed.], 2010. Clinical Dermatology: A Color Guide to Diagnosis and Therapy, 5th ed. Elsevier, 776–800.)*

5. Juvenile melanoma ("Spitz nevus"; see Figure 23.5)
   - Benign pigmented skin lesion typically found in children or young adults
   - Difficult to distinguish from melanoma clinically and histologically
   - Characterized by a red, pink, or brown papule or nodule with rapid growth
   - Treatment: Complete excision with negative margins; if any concern for melanoma, obtain appropriate margins based on depth.

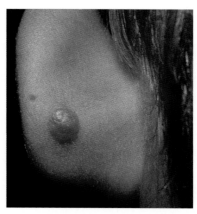

Figure 23.5. Spitz nevus. Red, dome-shaped papule on the ear of a child. *(Reprinted from Bolognia, J.L., Jorizzo, J.L., Schaffer, J.V. [Eds.], 2012. Dermatology, 3rd ed. Elsevier, 1851–1883. Courtesy Ronald P. Rapini, M.D.)*

6. Nevus of Ota (see Figure 23.6)
   - Benign blue nevus that is present within the dermatome of the first and second branches of the trigeminal nerve
   - Most commonly affects Asian females
   - Bimodal distribution: Early infancy and early adolescence
   - Caused by dermal proliferation of melanocytes
   - Treatment: Laser (e.g., Q-switched ruby, alexandrite); dermabrasion, peels, or cryotherapy have also been used.

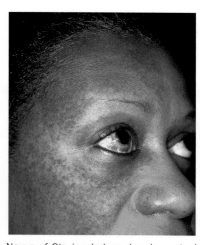

Figure 23.6. Nevus of Ota (oculodermal melanocytosis). Unilateral, bluish-gray discoloration of the face, which is either mottled or confluent. There is also involvement of the sclera. *(Reprinted from Bolognia, J.L., Jorizzo, J.L., Schaffer, J.V. [Eds.], 2012. Dermatology, 3rd ed. Elsevier, 1851–1883.)*

7. Nevus of Ito
   - Often considered a subtype of nevus of Ota
   - Occurs in the acromiodeltoid region.
   - Treatment: Similar to nevus of Ota
8. Mongolian spot (also known as congenital dermal melanocytosis; see Figure 23.7)
   - A common benign proliferative disorder that affects the majority of Native American, Asian, and Hispanic infants
   - Caused by entrapment of melanocytes within the dermis during development
   - Characterized by multiple bluish-gray spots or a large patch covering the lumbosacral region
   - Lesions typically disappear by 10 years of age.
   - Treatment: Observation because most disappear without treatment; lasers for severe cases.

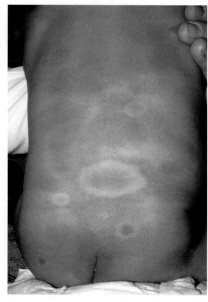

Figure 23.7. Dermal melanocytosis (Mongolian spots) in a child with type-1 neurofibromatosis. Surrounding each café-au-lait macule is an absence of the characteristic blue discoloration. *(Reprinted from Bolognia, J.L., Jorizzo, J.L., Schaffer, J.V. [Eds.], 2012. Dermatology, 3rd ed. Elsevier, 1851–1883.)*

9. Blue nevus
   - Also caused by dermal melanocytosis
   - Characterized by a well-circumscribed, firm, blue-pigmented nodule/papule
   - Three subtypes: Common, cellular (can invade the subcutaneous tissue), and combined (combined with a pigmented nevus or a Spitz nevus)
   - Treatment: Biopsy for suspicious lesions; simple excision (see Figure 23.8)
10. Rosacea ("acne rosacea"; see Figure 23.9)
    - Common, benign facial condition with both vascular (flushing/blushing) and inflammatory (papules/pustules) aspects
    - Characterized by erythema, telangiectasia, flushing/blushing, and papules and pustules on the face, especially the forehead, cheeks, nose, and periorbita

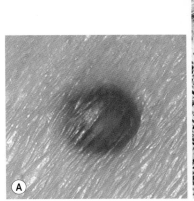
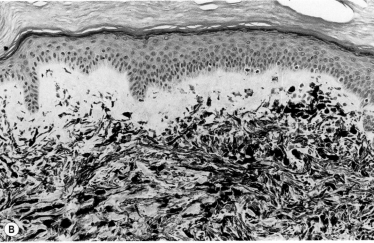

Figure 23.8. Common blue nevus. **A,** A well-circumscribed, blue, dome-shaped papule. **B,** Histologically, heavily pigmented, spindle-shaped melanocytes as well as melanophages are within the dermis; the melanocytes are denser than in dermal melanocytosis or nevus of Ota. *(Reprinted from Bolognia, J.L., Jorizzo, J.L., Schaffer, J.V. [Eds.], 2012. Dermatology, 3rd ed. Elsevier, 1851–1883.)*

- Exacerbated by hot foods and drinks, alcohol, heat, sunlight, and topical skin creams
- Treatment: Avoidance of exacerbating factors, sunscreen, topical treatment of papules/pustules (e.g., Isotretinoin), long-term oral antibiotics
- Chronic rosacea can lead to granuloma formation, deep inflammation, and scarring with subsequent irreversible hypertrophy ("granulomatous rosacea" or "rhinophyma" when it involves the nose).
  - Treatment of rhinophyma generally consists of tangential excision of involved skin, electrosurgery, and/or carbon dioxide laser resurfacing.

11. Chondrodermatitis nodularis helicis (see Figure 23.10)
    - Uncommon lesion that frequently occurs on the lateral surface of the helix and occasionally the antihelix in men over the age of 40
    - Characterized by a small, painful, dull red to white nodule with a central scale and underlying erosion or ulceration on the ear
    - Treatment: Simple excision of the nodule with removal of involved underlying cartilage to reduce recurrence

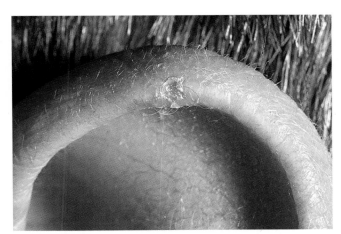

Figure 23.10. Chondrodermatitis nodularis. Shown is an early lesion with a central crust on the most common site, the apex of the helix. *(Reprinted from Habif, T.P. [Ed.], 2010. Clinical Dermatology: A Color Guide to Diagnosis and Therapy, 5th ed. Elsevier, 776–800.)*

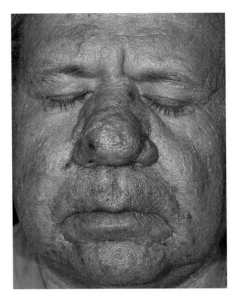

Figure 23.9. Rosacea and rhinophyma. Chronic rosacea of the nose has caused irreversible hypertrophy (rhinophyma). *(Reprinted from Habif, T.P. [Ed.], 2010. Clinical Dermatology: A Color Guide to Diagnosis and Therapy, 5th ed. Elsevier, 217–263.)*

Common Benign Skin and Soft-Tissue Masses

1. Lipoma
   - Most common benign soft-tissue tumor
   - Many subtypes and often classified based on their location (e.g., intramuscular)
   - Patients can have multiple lipomas affecting the extremities, head, neck, and trunk ("lipomatosis").
   - Has the potential for malignant degeneration to liposarcoma
     - Rapid growth is a potential sign of liposarcoma.
   - Characterized by a soft, spongy, mobile, well-circumscribed, soft-tissue mass
   - Computed tomography (CT) or magnetic resonance imaging (MRI) may be helpful in diagnosis and surgical planning.
   - Treatment: Complete surgical excision with the capsule to reduce recurrence
2. Epidermoid cyst (also known as epidermal cyst)
   - Characterized by a smooth, dome-shaped, mobile, subcutaneous, cystic mass, often with a central punctum
   - Frequently rupture spontaneously or with external pressure
   - May become inflamed and/or infected
   - Treatment: Simple excision, with care to remove the entire cyst to minimize the risk for recurrence
3. Dermoid cyst
   - Congenital subcutaneous cyst that develops along embryonic fusion lines
   - Most commonly occurs on the head and neck (e.g., lateral brow, glabella, scalp).
   - Characterized by a firm, solitary, soft-tissue mass
   - Midline dermoid cysts may have intracranial extension; investigate with CT or MRI before excision.
     - CT findings can include splaying of the nasal bones as well as defects in the foramen cecum and crista galli.
   - Treatment: Simple excision of the entire cyst; if intracranial involvement is detected, neurosurgical consultation and craniotomy is required.
4. Acrochordon ("skin tag")
   - Common benign fibroma found in an estimated 25% of adults
   - Most frequently found in the axilla, neck, and inguinal region of obese patients
   - Characterized by small, pedunculated, brownish-red, or normal skin color superficial skin lesions with a broad-to-narrow stalk
   - Treatment: Scissor excision, simple excision, cryotherapy, electrodessication
5. Pilomatricoma (also known as a pilomatrixoma or calcifying epithelioma of Malherbe; see Figure 23.11)
   - Benign, firm, cystic nodule that typically occurs in the head and neck of children
   - Calcification can be detected on radiographic studies (e.g., ultrasound, X ray, CT, and MRI).
   - Treatment: Complete excision to prevent recurrence

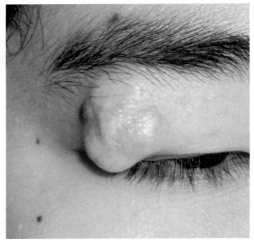

Figure 23.11. Pilomatricoma on the upper eyelid. *(Reprinted from Neligan, P.C. [Ed.], 2013. Plastic Surgery, vol. 1, 3rd ed. Elsevier, 707–742.)*

6. Trichilemmal cyst
   - Arises from the outer root sheath of the hair follicle
   - Up to 70% of patients have multiple cysts.
   - Characterized by a subcutaneous cyst within the hair-bearing portion of the scalp
   - Treatment: Complete excision
7. Dermatofibroma (also known as fibrous histiocytoma; see Figure 23.12)
   - Caused by the proliferation of fibroblasts, histiocytes, and vascular endothelial cells within the dermis
   - They may not be true tumors but, instead, a reaction to trauma, viral infection, or insect bites.
   - Typically asymptomatic but may present with pruritis and/or pain
   - Characterized by a small, firm, pink-brown nodule on the extremities, particularly the lower extremity, that retracts beneath the skin surface with attempts to compress or elevate it with the thumb and index finger ("retraction sign" or "Fitzpatrick sign")
   - Treatment: May be observed; however, simple excision is often performed for symptoms, diagnostic uncertainty, or cosmetic purposes

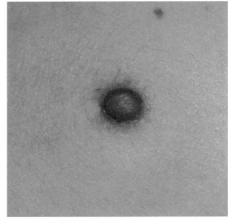

Figure 23.12. Dermatofibroma. *(Reprinted from Neligan, P.C. [Ed.], 2013. Plastic Surgery, vol. 1, 3rd ed. Elsevier, 707–742.)*

8. Neurofibroma
   - Benign tumor of the peripheral nerve sheath that arises from Schwann cells
   - Typically found in patients with neurofibromatosis (types 1 and 2)
   - Characterized by multiple small, pink or skin colored, raised nodules
   - Can undergo malignant degeneration
   - Treatment: Excision, CO_2 laser treatment, adjuvant chemotherapy, and radiation in malignant cases

9. Schwannoma (also known as "neurilemmoma")
   - Benign tumor of the peripheral nerve sheath that arises from Schwann cells
   - Most commonly occurs in the deep soft tissues, along the main nerve trunks of the extremities, especially the flexor surface of the arms, wrists, and knees
   - Characterized by a solitary, pale pink, or yellowish deep nodule that may be firm or soft and occasionally painful
     - Often, the mass is mobile in the transverse plane and not the longitudinal plane
   - MRI is useful in diagnosis; displays a well-encapsulated "egg-shaped" tumor within the nerve sheath that does not disrupt the nerve fascicles.
   - Treatment: Surgical excision

10. Desmoid tumor
    - Characterized by large, well-circumscribed, deep masses that arise from the muscular aponeurosis
    - Most commonly occur on the abdominal wall
    - Rarely metastasize, although they can be locally aggressive with a high recurrence rate
    - Diagnosis is often made by clinical exam and CT or MRI.
    - Treatment: Wide local excision with margin clearance, radiation, and hormonal therapy (e.g., Tamoxifen)

Other Skin Disorders

1. Genetic skin disorders (also known as "genodermatoses") (see Table 23.1)
2. Xeroderma pigmentosum (XP)
   - Rare, autosomal, recessive skin disorder
   - Caused by defective DNA repair mechanisms within the nucleotide excision repair (NER) pathway associated with ultraviolet (UV)- light-induced damage
   - Characterized by severe photosensitivity to UV radiation including severe burns and blistering
   - Significant risk of skin cancer, often developing within the first decade of life

Table 23.1 Key Features of Genodermatoses

SYNDROME	INHERITANCE	GENETIC MUTATION	NONCUTANEOUS FEATURES	CUTANEOUS FEATURES
Gardner syndrome (familial adenomatous polyposis)	AD	*APC*	GI polyps and adenocarcinoma, osteomas, supernumerary or unerupted teeth	Epidermoid cysts, lipomas, Gardner fibroma, desmoid tumor
Gorlin syndrome (nevoid BCC syndrome)	AD	*PTCH*	Odontogenic keratocysts, medulloblastoma, calcification of the falx, bifid ribs, ovarian fibromas, macrocephaly, frontal bossing, pectus deformity	Palmar pits, BCCs
Multiple endocrine neoplasia, type 1 (Wermer syndrome)	AD	*MEN1*	Endocrine tumors including parathyroid, pituitary, adrenocortical, gastrinoma	Multiple angiofibromas, collagenomas, lipomas
Muir-Torre syndrome	AD	*MSH2* and *MLH1*	Colorectal, breast, genitourinary cancers	Keratoacanthomas, sebaceous adenoma, sebaceous epithelioma, sebaceous carcinoma
Neurofibromatosis (von Recklinghausen disease)	AD	*Neurofibromin*	Lisch nodules of the iris, optic nerve glioma, sphenoid dysplasia	Café-au-lait macules, axillary freckling, numerous neurofibromas (often including plexiform neurofibroma)
Porphyria cutanea tarda	AD	*Uroporphyrinogen decarboxylase*	Liver function abnormalities	Blisters, erosions, milia on the dorsal hands and photoexposed sites, hypertrichosis, hyperpigmentation, sclerodermoid plaques
Tuberous sclerosis	AD	*Tuberin (TSC2)* and *hamartin (TSC1)*	Retinal nodular hamartoma, cortical tuber, subependymal nodule, subependymal giant cell astrocytoma, epilepsy, mental retardation, cardiac rhabdomyoma, lymphangiomyomatosis, renal angiomyolipoma	Adenoma sebaceum (angiofibromas), periungual fibromas, shagreen patch, hypopigmented ash leaf macules

Reprinted from Elston, D.M., Ferringer, T., Ko, C.J., et al. (Eds.), 2014. Dermatopathology, 2nd ed. Elsevier, 208–212.
AD, *Autosomal dominant*; APC, *adenomatous polyposis coli*; AR, *autosomal recessive*; BCC, *basal cell carcinoma*; GI, *gastrointestinal*; MEN1, *multiple endocrine neoplasia 1*; MLH1, *mutL homolog 1*; MSH2, *human mutS homolog 2*; PTCH, *patched*.

- Diagnosis: Largely clinical, although DNA testing is available; suspect XP in children <2 years old who present with freckling on sun-exposed skin and severe sunburn after minimal sun exposure.
- Treatment: UV protection (e.g., sunscreen, skin cover with clothing/hats, sunglasses, UV protection over windows), regular skin exams, early excision of skin cancers

3. Calcifying skin disorders (also known as "calcinosis cutis")
   - Characterized by deposition of insoluble calcium salts within the skin and subcutaneous tissues
   - Generally divided into four broad categories
     - Dystrophic: Occurs in the setting of localized tissue damage with normal metabolic calcium regulation
     - Metastatic: Occurs in the setting of dysfunction in calcium regulation (e.g., renal failure)
     - Iatrogenic: Calcification related to medial therapy or testing
     - Idiopathic: Calcification of unknown etiology
   - CREST syndrome (calcification, Raynaud's phenomenon, esophageal dysmotility, sclerodactyly, telangiectasia)
     - A form of dystrophic calcinosis cutis related to the autoimmune disease scleroderma
     - Patients typically present with small calcium deposits over bony prominences and tendons and/or on the elbows, knees, buttocks, shoulders, and hands.
     - These calcium deposits are painful and can extrude a white chalky material and ulcerate.
     - Treatment: Low-calcium and -phosphate diet, aluminum hydroxide, and bisphosphonates; surgical excision of deposits is reserved for localized painful masses that limit function.
   - Calciphylaxis
     - A form of metastatic calcinosis cutis related to renal failure that occurs secondary to progressive vascular calcification with ischemic necrosis of the skin and soft tissues
     - Patients typically present with multiple, extremely painful skin lesions that can be violaceous, ulcerated, or necrotic.

- High mortality and poor prognosis, with death often secondary to gangrene and sepsis
- Risk factors: Female gender, obesity, poor nutritional status, diabetes
- Treatment: Low-calcium and -phosphate diet, low-calcium dialysis, phosphate binders, parathyroidectomy, and aggressive local wound care; surgical excision/ debridement is generally not recommended.

Suggested Readings

Bolognia, J.L., Schaffer, J.V., Duncan, K.O., et al. (Eds.), 2014. Chapter 95: Common soft tissue tumors/proliferations. In: Dermatology Essentials. Elsevier, pp. 934–941.

Fairley, J.A., 2012. Chapter 50: Calcifying and ossifying disorders of the skin. In: Bolognia, J.L., Jorizzo, J.L., Schaffer, J.V. (Eds.), Dermatology, 3rd ed. Elsevier, pp. 729–736.

Ferringer, T., 2014. Chapter 12: Genodermatoses. In: Elston, D.M., Ferringer, T., Ko, C.J., et al. (Eds.), Dermatopathology, 2nd ed. Elsevier, pp. 208–212.

Habif, T.P., 2010. Chapter 20: Benign skin tumors. In: Habif, T.P. (Ed.), Clinical Dermatology: A Color Guide to Diagnosis and Therapy, 5th ed. Mosby Elsevier, pp. 776–800.

Habif, T.P. (Ed.), 2010. Chapter 7: Acne, rosacea, and related disorders. In: Clinical Dermatology: A Color Guide to Diagnosis and Therapy. 5th ed. Elsevier, pp. 217–263.

Habif, T.P., Campbell, J.L., Chapman, M.S., et al. (Eds.), 2011. Chapter 16: Benign skin tumors. In: Skin Disease. 3rd ed. Elsevier, pp. 424–463.

James, W.D., Berger, T.H., Elston, D.M. (Eds.), 2011. Chapter 28: Dermal and subcutaneous tumors. In: Andrews' Disease of the Skin: Clinical Dermatology. 11th ed. Elsevier, pp. 574–619.

McMasters, K.M., Uris, M.M., 2012. Chapter 32: Melanoma and cutaneous malignancies. In: Townsend, C.M., Beauchamp, R.D., Evers, B.M., et al. (Eds.), Sabiston Textbook of Surgery, 19th ed. Elsevier, pp. 742–767.

Ogawa, R., 2013. Chapter 30: Benign and malignant nonmelanocytic tumors of the skin and soft tissue. In: Neligan, P.C. (Ed.), Plastic Surgery, vol. 1, 3rd ed. Elsevier, pp. 707–742.

Rabinovitz, H.S., Barnhill, R.L., 2012. Chapter 112: Benign melanocytic neoplasms. In: Bolognia, J.L., Jorizzo, J.L., Schaffer, J.V. (Eds.), Dermatology, 3rd ed. Elsevier, pp. 1851–1883.

Soyer, H.P., Rigel, D.S., Wurm, E.M.T., 2012. Chapter 108: Actinic keratosis, basal cell carcinoma and squamous cell carcinoma. In: Bolognia, J.L., Jorizzo, J.L., Schaffer, J.V. (Eds.), Dermatology, 3rd ed. Elsevier, pp. 1773–1793.

Tamura, D., Kraemer, K.H., DiGiovanna, J.J., 2014. Chapter 249: Xeroderma pigmentosum. In: Lebwohl, M.G., Heymann, W.R., Berth-Jones, J., et al. (Eds.), Treatment of Skin Disease: Comprehensive Therapeutic Strategies, 4th ed. Elsevier, pp. 808–811.

Malignant Skin Conditions

Chapter

24

Melanoma

1. Incidence of melanoma is increasing faster than any other cancer in the United States.
2. Melanoma is most commonly located in the skin but can occur in the oral mucosa, nasopharynx, esophagus, vagina, and rectum.
3. Risk factors for melanoma
   - Fair skin (e.g., Fitzpatrick I/II), blue eyes, blond/red hair
   - Chronic exposure to ultraviolet (UV) radiation (e.g., UVA, UVB, tanning salons)
   - History of sunburns, freckles
   - Family history of melanoma (e.g., familial, atypical, multiple mole-melanoma syndromes; B-K mole syndrome)
   - Immunosuppression
   - Presence of multiple, giant congenital, or dysplastic nevi
   - Xeroderma pigmentosa, *BRCA2* mutations

4. The most important factor related to outcome is the depth of the primary lesion.
   - Regional lymph node metastasis is also associated with poorer prognosis.
5. Diagnosis of melanoma is based on histologic examination; however, clinical suspicion of lesions that follow the "ABCDE" guidelines of the American Cancer Society (ACS) should guide biopsy decisions (see Figure 24.1).
   - Asymmetry of the lesion
   - Border irregularity
   - Color changes or variation
   - Diameter >6 mm
   - Evolution of the lesion (e.g., change in size, shape, symptoms, surface characteristics, and/or color)

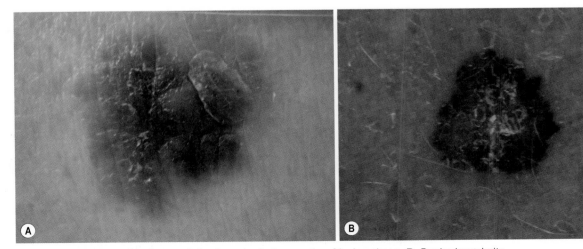

Figure 24.1. Melanoma with characteristic changes. **A,** Asymmetry of lesion shape. **B,** Border irregularity.

Continued

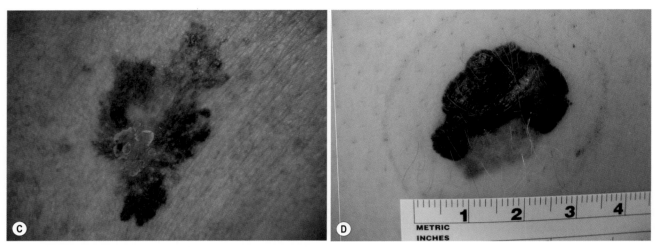

Figure 24.1, cont'd. C, Color variegation. **D,** Diameter >6 mm. *(Reprinted from Neligan, P.C. [Ed.], 2013. Plastic Surgery, vol. 1, 3rd ed. Elsevier, 743–785.)*

- "Ugly duckling sign": Unique appearance of the nevus relative to the patient's other nevi
6. Melanoma staging relies on the tumor (T), node (N), and metastases (M) system established by the ACS.

Table 24.1 Melanoma TNM Classification

TUMOR (T) CLASSIFICATION	TUMOR THICKNESS (BRESLOW DEPTH)		MITOTIC RATE/ULCERATION STATUS
Tis	In situ		None
T1	≤1.0 mm or less		a: Mitosis <1/mm^2, no ulceration b: Mitosis ≥1/mm^2, or ulceration
T2	1.01 to 2.0 mm		a: No ulceration b: Ulceration
T3	2.01 to 4.0 mm		a: No ulceration b: Ulceration
T4	>4.0 mm		a: No ulceration b: Ulceration
NODAL (N) CLASSIFICATION	**NUMBER OF METASTATIC NODES**		**NODAL METASTATIC MASS**
N1	1		a: Micrometastasis b: Macrometastasis
N2	2 to 3		a: Micrometastasis b: Macrometastasis c: In-transit metastases/satellite lesions without metastatic nodes
N3	≥4		Matted nodes, in-transit metastases/satellite lesions with metastatic nodes
METASTASES (M) CLASSIFICATION	**SITE OF METASTASES**		**SERUM LDH LEVEL**
M0	None		Normal
M1a	Skin, subcutaneous, distant lymph nodes		Normal
M1b	Lung		Normal
M1c	All other visceral sites, distant metastasis		Normal, elevated

Adapted from How Is Melanoma Skin Cancer Staged? © 2015 American Cancer Society, Inc. All rights reserved. http://www.cancer.org.
LDH, Lactase dehydrogenase.

Table 24.2 Melanoma Staging

STAGE	T	N	M
0	Tis	N0	M0
IA	T1a	N0	M0
IB	T1b or T2a	N0	M0
IIA	T2b or T3a	N0	M0
IIB	T3b or T4a	N0	M0
IIC	T4b	N0	M0
IIIA	T1a-T4a	N1a or N2a	M0
IIIB	T1b-T4b	N1a or N2a	M0
	T1a-T4a	N1b or N2b	M0
	T1a-T4a	N2c	M0
IIIC	T1b-T4b	N1b or N2b	M0
	T1b-T4b	N2c	M0
	Any T	N3	M0
IV	Any T	Any N	M1 (a, b, or c)

Adapted from How Is Melanoma Skin Cancer Staged?
© 2015 American Cancer Society, Inc. All rights reserved.
http://www.cancer.org.

7. Histologic subtypes/growth patterns
   - Superficial spreading
     - Most common pattern (50% to 80%)
     - Radial growth followed by vertical growth phase
   - Lentigo maligna melanoma
     - Typically located on sun-exposed areas and grows in a horizontal pattern
     - Develops within a preexisting lentigo maligna ("Hutchinson freckle"—flat, brown macule with variable shades of pigmentation located on sun-exposed areas in older adults; considered to be melanoma in situ)
   - Nodular
     - Second most common pattern (20% to 30%)
     - Early vertical growth phase
   - Acral lentiginous
     - Develops on the palms, soles, and subungual region
     - More common in dark-skinned individuals
     - Has the lowest 5-year survival of all melanoma (10% to 20%) and highest recurrence
   - Amelanotic and desmoplastic
     - Rare histologic forms
     - Desmoplastic melanomas are locally aggressive but rarely metastasize.
8. Biopsy recommendations
   - In small cutaneous lesions, excisional biopsy with 1- to 2-mm margins is recommended to establish the Breslow depth of the lesion
   - In larger lesions, or lesions with functional or cosmetic concerns prohibiting complete excision, an incisional biopsy (e.g., punch biopsy) can be performed.
   - Shave biopsy is generally not recommended unless it is performed for a suspicious lesion on the nail bed that is concerning for a subungual melanoma.

9. Sentinel lymph node biopsy indications
   - Breslow depth >0.76 mm without clinically palpable nodes
   - Melanoma of any depth with the presence of ulceration or high mitotic rate (e.g., >1 mitosis per high-powered field)
   - Elective or complete lymph node dissection is generally performed for patients with palpable lymphadenopathy on clinical exam or positive sentinel nodes, respectively.
10. Additional workup (see Box 24.1)

BOX 24.1 STAGING EVALUATION: TESTS RECOMMENDED FOR DETERMINATION OF PRESENCE AND EXTENT OF TUMOR SPREAD

Primary tumor (no clinical evidence of other involvement)
Physical examination
Chest radiography
Liver function tests
Lymphoscintigraphy to detect sites of sentinel nodes (if primary tumor ≥1-mm thick)

Local and regional disease (in-transit lesions or nodal involvement)
Physical examination
Liver function tests
Computed tomography (CT) scans
   Chest and abdomen (to examine lungs and liver)
   Pelvis if tumor involves lower extremities
   Neck if tumor involves the head and neck
Lymphoscintigraphy to detect sites of sentinel nodes
Additional scans as indicated by clinical signs or symptoms

Distant organ metastases
Physical examination
Liver function tests and serum lactate dehydrogenase level
CT scans, as indicated above
Magnetic resonance imaging scans if required to detect extent of soft-tissue invasion
Positron emission tomography scans to detect extent of tumor involvement of vital organs (lung, liver, brain)

Reprinted from Ariyan, S., Berger, A., 2013. Chapter 31: Melanoma. In: Neligan, P.C. (Ed.), Plastic Surgery, vol. 1, 3rd ed. Elsevier, 743–785.

11. Wide local excision: The mainstay of initial treatment to decrease the rate of local recurrence (reported to occur in 3% to 20%)
    - General recommendations for wide local excision margins
      - Melanoma in situ: 0.5-mm margins
      - Melanoma <1 mm: 1 cm
      - Melanoma 1 to 2 mm: 1 to 2 cm
      - Melanoma 2 to 4 mm: 2 cm
      - Melanoma >4 mm: 2 to 3 cm
    - If primary closure of the defect cannot be achieved, delay reconstruction until permanent pathology preparations confirming negative margins are finalized.
12. Additional treatment recommendations
    - Lentigo maligna: Treat as melanoma in situ
    - Subungual melanoma

- Can observe lesion for a short period to see if it will resolve
- If no resolution, biopsy is recommended.
- Melanoma in situ of the nail bed can be treated via excision with margin clearance and full-thickness grafting to the nail bed.
- Melanoma of the nail bed requires amputation through the closest joint (e.g., distal interphalangeal joint of the fingers or interphalangeal joint of the thumb).
- Congenital melanocytic nevi (CMN): Reported to carry an increased risk of malignant degeneration to melanoma (see Figure 24.2)
  - CMN develop from neural crest origin and can be present in the deep dermis and subcutaneous tissues and/or have neurologic involvement.
    - Neurologic involvement is suggested by large or multiple satellite posterior midline lesions and carries a poor prognosis.
  - Risk factors for malignant degeneration include truncal lesions and giant CMN (nevus expected to be >20 cm in size by adulthood).
  - Malignant degeneration of CMN carries the greatest risk in early childhood; thus, complete excision of high-risk lesions is generally recommended by 6 to 7 years of age.
  - Surgical options include serial excision (if it can be completely removed in 3 or fewer stages), tissue expansion, and skin grafting.

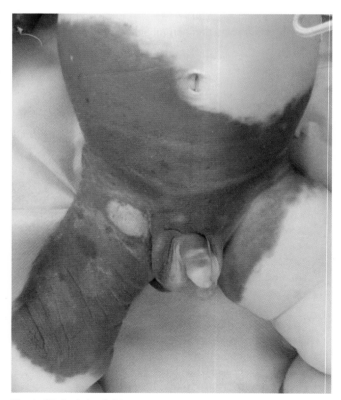

Figure 24.2. Animal-skin nevus. *(Reprinted from Neligan, P.C., [Ed.], 2013. Plastic Surgery, vol. 1, 3rd ed. Elsevier, 707–742.)*

- Adjuvant therapy
  - Interferon-α2b
    - Only approved adjuvant therapy
    - Typically reserved for stage-III disease
  - Chemotherapy (e.g., dacarbazine, interleukin-2, paclitaxel, ipilimumab)
    - Typically reserved for unresectable stage-IV (metastastic) disease
  - Isolated limb perfusion
    - Generally used for multicentric in-transit disease or recurrence in an effort to salvage the extremity

Basal Cell Carcinoma (BCC)

1. The most commonly encountered skin malignancy and the second most common malignancy of the hand.
2. Most (~86%) occur in the head and neck, particularly the upper lip, nose, scalp, and eyelid.
3. Typically confined to the skin, although they can become locally destructive; BCC rarely metastasizes.
4. Risk factors
   - Chronic sun exposure
   - Fair skin, blond/red hair
   - Personal or family history of skin cancer
   - Xeroderma pigmentosum, Gorlin syndrome (see below)
   - Nevus sebaceous
5. Multiple histologic subtypes including
   - Nodular
     - Most common
     - Characterized by a nodular/domal shape, "pearly" appearance, telangiectasia, and occasional ulceration (see Figure 24.3)
   - Adenoid and adenoid cystic
   - Superficial
     - Second most common form
     - Often involves the trunk/extremities
     - Characterized by flat, pink, scaly patches with ulcerations and crusting
   - Morpheaform (sclerosing)
     - Most aggressive subtype
     - Characterized by firm, depressed plaque surrounded by scar
     - High rate of margin involvement and recurrence
6. Diagnosis of BCC is based on histologic examination; biopsy suspicious lesions.
   - Biopsy recommendations: Excisional, incisional, and shave biopsies
7. Treatment options
   - Mainstay is excision and staged reconstruction in defects that cannot be closed primarily.
     - Wide local excision with recommended 3- to 5-mm margins for lesions <2 cm and up to 1 cm in lesions >2 cm with aggressive histology (e.g., morpheaform)
     - Mohs micrographic surgery (see below)
   - Cryotherapy and/or electrodesiccation and curettage
     - Typically reserved for multiple, superficial, low-risk, small BCC

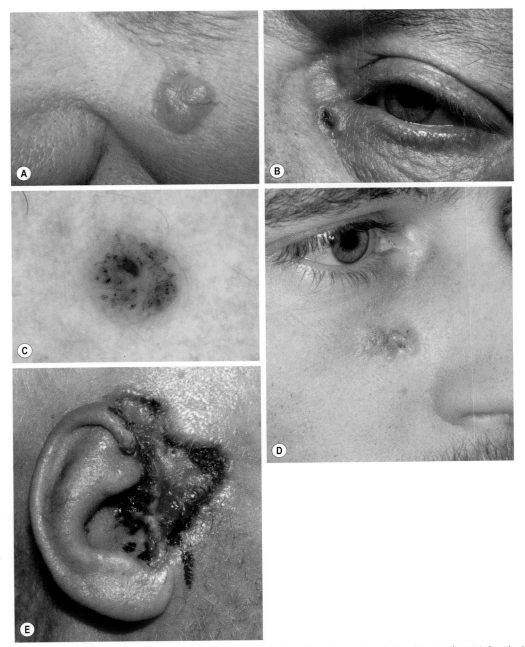

Figure 24.3. Clinical spectrum of nodular basal cell carcinoma (BCC). **A,** Translucent papulonodule with prominent telangiectasia on the infraorbital cheek. **B,** Classic presentation with a pearly, rolled border and central, hemorrhagic crust. **C,** Dermoscopy of a pigmented BCC demonstrating arborizing telangiectasia and multiple, bluish-gray, ovoid globules, pointing to the diagnosis of a small, nodular BCC; the one large, bluish-brown structure resembles, but does not fulfill all the criteria for a large, bluish-gray, ovoid nest. **D,** Larger plaque with rolled borders and multiple telangiectasia. **E,** Nodulo-ulcerative tumor of the preauricular region with translucent, rolled borders, most obvious at the 12:00 location. *(Reprinted from Bolognia, J.L., Jorizzo, J.L., Schaffer, J.V. [Eds.], 2012. Dermatology, 3rd ed. Elsevier, 1773–1793.* **A,** *Courtesy Stanley J Miller, M.D.;* **C,** *courtesy Giuseppe Argenziano, M.D.)*

- Topical therapy
  - Imiquimod (Aldara): Approved for treatment of superficial BCC, although typically reserved for lesions that are not amenable to resection
- Radiation
  - Typically reserved for patients who cannot undergo excision (e.g., elderly, significant comorbidities)

8. Gorlin syndrome (nevoid BCC syndrome)
   - Rare, autosomal dominant disorder
   - *PTCH* gene mutation
   - Characterized by
     - Multiple or early-onset BCC
     - Odontogenic keratocysts
     - Palmar and plantar pits

- Calcifications of the falx cerebri
- Skeletal abnormalities
- Patients may also develop medulloblastomas, meningiomas, and fibromas.
- BCCs typically appear after puberty but may occur in childhood.
    - Exquisitely sensitive to radiation
- Diagnosis: Requires two major or one major and two minor criteria (see Box 24.2)

BOX 24.2 DIAGNOSTIC CRITERIA FOR NEVOID BASAL CELL CARCINOMA* SYNDROME

Major criteria
1. More than two BCCs or one BCC before the age of 20 years
2. Odontogenic keratocysts of the jaw (proven by histology)
3. Three or more palmar or plantar pits
4. Bilamellar calcification of the falx cerebri
5. Bifid, fused, or markedly splayed ribs
6. First-degree relative with NBCC syndrome

Minor criteria
1. Macrocephaly (determined after adjustment for height)
2. Congenital malformations: Cleft lip or palate, frontal bossing, "coarse face," moderate or severe hypertelorism
3. Other skeletal abnormalities: Sprengel deformity,** marked pectus deformity, marked syndactyly of the digits
4. Radiographic abnormalities: Bridging of the sella turcica, vertebral anomalies such as hemivertebrae and fusion or elongation of the vertebral bodies, modeling defects of the hands and feet, flame-shaped lucencies of the hands or feet
5. Bilateral ovarian fibroma
6. Medulloblastoma

*The diagnosis of NBCC syndrome requires two major or one major and two minor criteria.
**Unilateral elevation of smaller-sized scapula.
Adapted from Kimonis, V.E., Goldstein, A.M., Pastakia, B., et al., 1997. Clinical manifestations in 105 persons with nevoid basal cell carcinoma syndrome. Am. J. Med. Genet. 69, 299–308.
BCC, Basal cell carcinoma; NBCC, Nevoid basal cell carcinoma.

- Treatment: Topical therapy, surgical excision, close observation for development of neoplasms

Squamous Cell Carcinoma (SCC)

1. Second most common skin malignancy overall; most common skin malignancy on the hand
2. Typically occurs on the face, hands, and forearms (sun-exposed areas)
    - ~60% of external ear tumors are SCC
    - Frequently involves the lower lip
    - Can also occur on the penis
3. SCC has an in situ variant and can develop from a precursor lesion (actinic keratosis [AK]) and in association with human papilloma virus (HPV) infection; also has the ability to metastasize to lymph nodes and/or hematogenously

4. Risk factors for SCC the same as for BCC but also include HPV infection, arsenic exposure, and chronic inflammatory states (e.g., chronic wounds, burn scars)
5. Risk of recurrence, metastasis, and poor prognosis are increased with poor differentiation, perineural invasion, tumors >2 cm, rapid growth, and recurrence
6. Often characterized by raised, pink, plaque-like or scaly papule, with occasional ulceration and ill-defined borders
7. Diagnosis: Similar to that of BCC
8. Histologic subtypes
    - SCC in situ: Confined to the epidermis
    - Bowen disease: "Erythroplasia of Queyrat" (SCC in situ) of the penis
    - Invasive SCC associated with AK
        - Located on sun-damaged/-exposed skin
        - Favorable prognosis with low risk of metastasis
    - De novo invasive SCC ("Marjolin's ulcer")
        - High-risk variant with high rate of metastasis and poor prognosis
        - Often occurs in immunocompromised patients and in areas with chronic inflammation (e.g., burn scars, chronic wounds, organ transplant patients; see Figure 24.4)

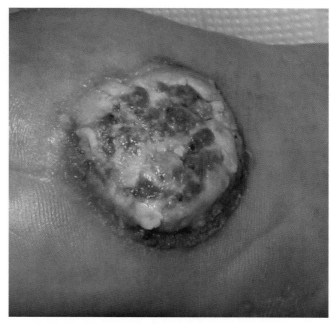

Figure 24.4. Nodulo-ulcerative tumor. SCC on the sole that has arisen from traumatic scars. *(Reprinted from Neligan, P.C. [Ed.], 2013. Plastic Surgery, vol. 1, 3rd ed. Elsevier, 707–742.)*

- Keratoacanthoma (see Figure 24.5)
    - Benign tumor that behaves like an SCC but is difficult to differentiate histologically
    - Characterized by rapid growth with a central crater/keratin plug
    - Can spontaneously regress
    - Treatment recommendation: Excision

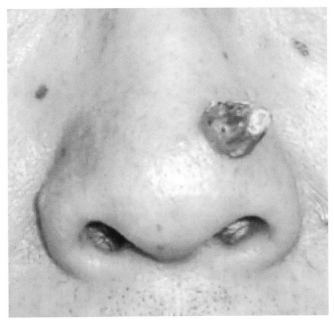

Figure 24.5. Keratoacanthoma on the nose. *(Reprinted from Neligan, P.C. [Ed.], 2013. Plastic Surgery, vol. 1, 3rd ed. Elsevier, 707–742.)*

- Adenoid SCC
  - Rare, ulcerated, nodular lesion on the face of elderly men
  - High rate of metastasis
9. Treatment options
  - Mainstay is excision and staged reconstruction in defects that cannot be closed primarily
    - Wide local excision with recommended 4-mm (low-risk) or 6-mm (high-risk) margins for lesions <2 cm and up to 1 cm in lesions >2 cm in diameter, on the hands, or with aggressive histology (e.g., perineural invasion, morpheaform subtype, Marjolin's ulcer)
    - Mohs micrographic surgery (see below)
    - Amputation at the joint proximal to the lesion is recommended for SCC that involves bone or the nail bed.
  - Sentinel lymph node (SNL) biopsy in SCC: Currently controversial, although many advocate for SLN biopsy in aggressive subtypes >2 cm in diameter.
  - Cryotherapy and/or electrodesiccation and curettage
    - Typically reserved for multiple, low-risk, small, superficial lesions
  - Topical therapy
    - Imiquimod (Aldara): May be effective in treatment of Bowen disease and invasive SCC, although typically reserved for lesions that are not amenable to resection
    - Topical 5-fluorouracil (5FU): Effective in the treatment of diffuse AK of the face
  - Radiation
    - Typically reserved for patients who cannot undergo excision (e.g., elderly, significant comorbidities), have incompletely excised large lesions, and/or high-risk tumors (e.g., deep SCC with perineural invasion)

Other Skin and Soft-Tissue Malignances

1. Merkel cell carcinoma
   - Rare, highly aggressive cancer that develops just beneath the skin and in hair follicles
   - Frequently metastasizes to lymph nodes and other organs (e.g., liver, bone, brain, lung, skin)
   - Etiology: Merkel cell polyomavirus
   - Characterized by a smooth, painless, nodular lesion on the face, head, and neck
   - Treatment: Wide local excision with 1- to 3-cm margins and SLN biopsy in clinically negative nodes; adjuvant radiation therapy is often recommended, along with chemotherapy for distant metastases.
2. Angiosarcoma
   - Malignant tumors of endothelial cells
   - Aggressive tumors with a high rate of recurrence, frequent metastases to distant sites, and poor prognosis
   - Characterized by red, violaceous, nodular, or plaque-like lesions on the face, trunk, or extremities
     - Stewart-Treves syndrome is a rare variant of lymphangiosarcoma of the upper extremity that occurs in postmastectomy patients.
     - Cutaneous angiosarcoma is commonly located on the face and scalp of older men.
   - Treatment: Surgical resection, radiation therapy, chemotherapy, and immunotherapy with interleukin-2
3. Sebaceous carcinoma
   - Arises from sebaceous glands and includes meibomian gland carcinoma (eyelid), Zeis gland carcinoma, and Montgomery gland carcinoma.
   - Characterized by nodular/raised mass that can ulcerate
   - High rate of lymph node metastases; thus, lymph node biopsy/dissection is often recommended for large lesions.
   - Treatment: Wide local excision with at least 5-mm margins; adjuvant radiation and/or chemotherapy may be useful.
4. Dermatofibrosarcoma protuberans (DFSP)
   - Also known as giant cell fibroblastoma
   - More than 90% associated with a chromosomal translocation (17:22) affecting the collagen gene (COL1A1) and the platelet-derived growth factor gene (PDGF).
   - Characterized by multiple or solitary tumors that are red, elevated, and often with a keloid appearance (see Figure 24.6)
   - Rarely metastasize but locally aggressive with high rate of local recurrence
   - Excision can be difficult because of tumor cell invasion of local tissues with "tentacle-like" projections that appear normal.
   - Treatment: Wide resection with 5-cm margins; Mohs micrographic surgery is useful for peripheral margin mapping/clearance and reduces local recurrence rates; adjuvant chemotherapy and radiation therapy may be useful.

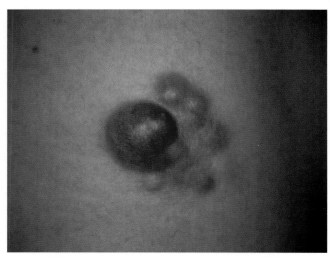

Figure 24.6. Dermatofibrosarcoma protuberans on the abdomen. *(Reprinted from Neligan, P.C. [Ed.], 2013. Plastic Surgery, vol. 1, 3rd ed. Elsevier, 707–742.)*

5. Kaposi's sarcoma
   - Caused by human herpes virus 8 and associated with human-immunodeficiency virus (HIV) and acquired immune deficiency syndrome (AIDS)
   - Characterized by red, purple, brown, or black nodules or palpable blotches found on the skin
   - Growth can be slow or rapid and can be associated with significant mortality and morbidity.
   - Treatment: Highly active antiretroviral therapy (HAART), radiation therapy, cryotherapy, and chemotherapy; surgical excision is not recommended and largely supportive

Mohs Micrographic Surgery

1. Mohs surgery can be performed for both BCC and SCC and is more frequently being used for DFSP peripheral margin mapping/clearance

2. Advantages of Mohs
   - Lower recurrence rates
   - Higher cure rates
   - Preservation of uninvolved skin in cosmetically sensitive areas
   - Same-day determination of margin clearance
3. General indications
   - Tumors >2 cm
   - Recurrent tumors or tumors in high-risk areas (e.g., eyelid, nose, ear, lips, perineum, hands)
   - Tumors with indistinct clinical margins (e.g., morpheaform) or aggressive features (e.g., perineural invasion, poorly differentiated)
   - Tumors in cosmetically sensitive areas

Suggested Readings

Ariyan, S., Berger, A., 2013. Chapter 31: Melanoma. In: Neligan, P.C. (Ed.), Plastic Surgery, vol. 1, 3rd ed. Elsevier, pp. 743–785.

Arneja, J.S., Gosain, A.K., 2007. Giant congenital melanocytis nevi. Plast. Reconstr. Surg. 120 (2), 26e–40e.

Buck, D.W., Kim, J.Y., Alam, M., et al., 2012. Multidisciplinary approach to the management of dermatofibromasarcoma protuberans. J. Am. Acad. Dermatol. 67 (5), 861–866.

Dzwierzynski, W.W., 2013. Managing malignant melanoma. Plast. Reconstr. Surg. 132 (3), p. 446e–460e.

Garbe, C., Bauer, J., 2012. Chapter 113: Melanoma. In: Bolognia, J.L., Jorizzo, J.L., Schaffer, J.V. (Eds.), Dermatology, 3rd ed. Elsevier, pp. 1885–1914.

Heitmann, C., Ingianni, G., 1999. Stewart-Treves syndrome: lymphangiosarcoma following mastectomy. Ann. Plast. Surg. 44 (1), 72–75.

McMasters, K.M., Uris, M.M., 2012. Chapter 32: Melanoma and cutaneous malignancies. In: Townsend, C.M., Beauchamp, R.D., Evers, B.M., et al. (Eds.), Sabiston Textbook of Surgery, 19th ed. Elsevier, pp. 742–767.

Netscher, D.T., Leong, M. Orengo, I., et al., 2011. Cutaneous malignancies: melanoma and nonmelanoma types. Plast. Reconstr. Surg. 127 (3), 37e–56e.

Ogawa, R., 2013. Chapter 30: Benign and malignant nonmelanocytic tumors of the skin and soft tissue. In: Neligan, P.C. (Ed.), Plastic Surgery, vol. 1, 3rd ed. Elsevier, pp. 707–742.

Soyer, H.P., Rigel, D.S., Wurm, E.M.T., 2012. Chapter 108: Actinic keratosis, basal cell carcinoma and squamous cell carcinoma. In: Bolognia, J.L., Jorizzo, J.L., Schaffer, J.V. (Eds.), Dermatology, 3rd ed. Elsevier, pp. 1773–1793.

Flaps and Microsurgery

Chapter 25

Flap Definitions

1. Axial flap: Tissue that is based on the vascular territories of named vascular pedicles with an axial alignment
2. Random flap: Tissue that is based off of an unnamed vascular supply, whereby the primary vascularity is provided through the subdermal plexus
3. Delayed flap: A flap that is incised and minimally or partially elevated and then immediately placed back in its in situ position to enhance flap circulation through the dilation of choke vessels
4. Perforator flap: A flap that is designed and elevated based on a perforating vessel within a known vascular territory, whereby the perforator is dissected down to a known source pedicle of sufficient length and diameter
5. Freestyle flap: A type of perforator flap that is designed randomly off of an identified perforating vessel within a specific region, whereby the perforator is dissected down to a pedicle of sufficient length and diameter
6. Prelaminated flap: An axial flap that is modified with grafts (e.g., mucosa, cartilage, or bone) to create composite tissue structure at the donor site before flap transfer
7. Prefabricated flap (see Figure 25.1): A flap that is created by introducing a vascular pedicle to a desired donor site that on its own does not possess an axial blood supply. This induces vascularization of the donor site from the pedicle before transfer.

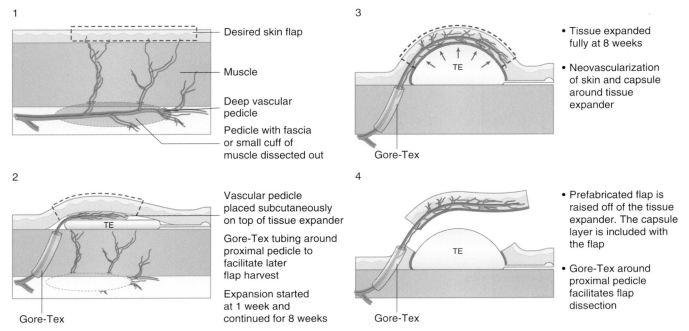

1
- Desired skin flap
- Muscle
- Deep vascular pedicle
- Pedicle with fascia or small cuff of muscle dissected out

2
TE
Gore-Tex
- Vascular pedicle placed subcutaneously on top of tissue expander
- Gore-Tex tubing around proximal pedicle to facilitate later flap harvest
- Expansion started at 1 week and continued for 8 weeks

3
TE
Gore-Tex
- Tissue expanded fully at 8 weeks
- Neovascularization of skin and capsule around tissue expander

4
TE
Gore-Tex
- Prefabricated flap is raised off of the tissue expander. The capsule layer is included with the flap
- Gore-Tex around proximal pedicle facilitates flap dissection

Figure 25.1. 1-4, Flap prefabrication technique. *TE,* Tissue expansion. *(Reprinted from Wei, F.C., Mardini, S. [Eds.], 2009. Flaps and Reconstructive Surgery. Elsevier, 103–116.)*

8. Tubed flap: A flap that is rolled on itself to serve as a conduit
9. Reverse flow flap: A flap that is supplied through retrograde flow
   • Venous flow is possible through communicating vein branches along the comitantes that allow reverse shunting of flow to bypass valves.
10. Venous flap (see Figure 25.2): A flap of skin, subcutaneous, tissue, and a venous plexus, whereby the inflow and outflow of the flap is through veins.
    • Considered for small dorsal or palmar defects, fingers, or hand requiring simultaneous reconstruction of venous outflow or arterial inflow
    • Arterialized venous flaps: An arteriovenous fistula is created by anastomosing the inflow vein to a recipient artery and the outflow vein to a vein
    • Arterialized venous "flow-through" flap: The proximal and distal veins are anastomosed to a proximal and distal artery to create a flow-through flap.

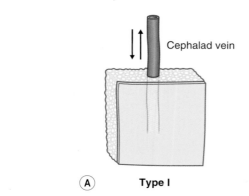

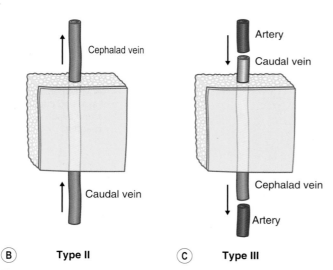

Figure 25.2. Classification of venous flaps. **A,** Type I. **B,** Type II. **C,** Type III. *(Reprinted from Neligan, P.C., Gurtner, G.C. [Eds.], 2013. Principles in Plastic Surgery, vol. 1, 3rd ed. Elsevier, 512–572.)*

Flap Classification

1. Mathes-Nahai classification
   • Type 1: Flap vascular supply via one major pedicle
   • Type 2: Via one major and one minor pedicle
   • Type 3: Via two major pedicles
   • Type 4: Via segmental pedicles
   • Type 5: Via one major and segmental pedicles (see Figure 25.3 and Box 25.1-25.5)

BOX 25.1 TYPE-I VASCULAR PATTERN MUSCLES

Abductor digiti minimi (hand)
Abductor pollicis brevis
Anconeus
Colon
Deep circumflex iliac artery
First dorsal interosseous
Gastrocnemius, medial and lateral
Genioglossus
Hyoglossus
Jejunum
Longitudinalis linguae
Styloglossus
Tensor fascia lata
Transversus and verticalis linguae
Vastus lateralis

Reprinted from Neligan, P.C., Gurtner, G.C., (Eds.), 2013. Principles in Plastic Surgery, vol. 1, 3rd ed. Elsevier, 512–572.

BOX 25.2 TYPE-II VASCULAR PATTERN MUSCLES

Abductor digiti minimi (foot)
Abductor hallucis
Brachioradialis
Coracobrachialis
Flexor carpi ulnaris
Flexor digitorum brevis
Gracilis
Hamstring (biceps femoris)
Peroneus brevis
Peroneus longus
Platysma
Rectus femoris
Soleus
Sternocleidomastoid
Trapezius
Triceps
Vastus medialis

Reprinted from Neligan, P.C., Gurtner, G.C. (Eds.), 2013. Principles in Plastic Surgery, vol. 1, 3rd ed. Elsevier, 512–572.

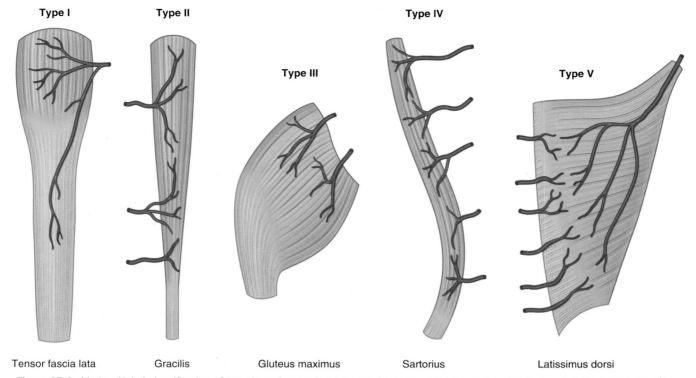

Type I	Type II	Type III	Type IV	Type V
Tensor fascia lata	Gracilis	Gluteus maximus	Sartorius	Latissimus dorsi

Figure 25.3. Mathes-Nahai classification of muscle and musculocutaneous flaps. *(Reprinted from Neligan, P.C., Gurtner, G.C. [Eds.], 2013. Principles in Plastic Surgery, vol. 1, 3rd ed. Elsevier, 512–572.)*

BOX 25.3 TYPE-III VASCULAR PATTERN MUSCLES

Gluteus maximus
Intercostal
Omentum
Orbicularis oris
Pectoralis minor
Rectus abdominis
Serratus anterior
Temporalis

Reprinted from Neligan, P.C., Gurtner, G.C. (Eds.), 2013. Principles in Plastic Surgery, vol. 1, 3rd ed. Elsevier, 512–572.

BOX 25.4 TYPE-IV VASCULAR PATTERN MUSCLES

Extensor digitorum longus
Extensor hallucis longus
External oblique
Flexor digitorum longus
Flexor hallucis longus
Sartorius
Tibialis anterior

Reprinted from Neligan, P.C., Gurtner, G.C. (Eds.), 2013. Principles in Plastic Surgery, vol. 1, 3rd ed. Elsevier, 512–572.

BOX 25.5 TYPE-V VASCULAR PATTERN MUSCLES

Fibula
Internal oblique
Latissimus dorsi
Pectoralis major

Reprinted from Neligan, P.C., Gurtner, G.C. (Eds.), 2013. Principles in Plastic Surgery, vol. 1, 3rd ed. Elsevier, 512–572.

Common Local Flaps

1. Z plasty: Useful for increasing length along a central limb
   - Degree of angles dictates the amount gained in length
     - 30 degree angle leads to a 25% gain
     - 45 degree: angle leads to a 50% gain
     - 60 degree angle leads to a 75% gain
     - 75 degree angle leads to a 100% gain
     - 90 degree angle leads to a 120% gain (see Figure 25.4)
2. W plasty: Useful for scars that cross the relaxed skin tension lines
   - Requires undermining and removal of "healthy" surrounding tissue for closure (see Figure 25.5)
3. Rhomboid flaps: A rotation flap based on a rhomboid skin design that allows closure of the donor site primarily (see Figure 25.6)

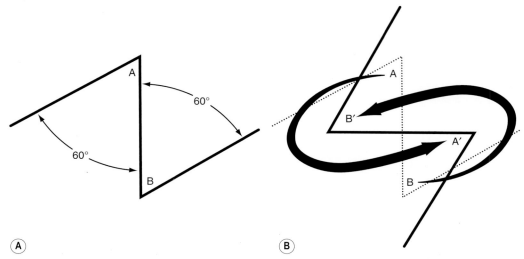

Figure 25.4. Z-plasty technique. **A,** Central limb designed along the scar. Both limbs are equal in length, and angles A and B are 60 degrees. **B,** The flaps are transposed and sutured. Note that the original central limb has been lengthened and the scar is reoriented. *(Reprinted from McCarthy, J.G., Galiano, R.D., Boutros, S.G. [Eds.], 2006. Current Therapy in Plastic Surgery. Elsevier, 3–10.)*

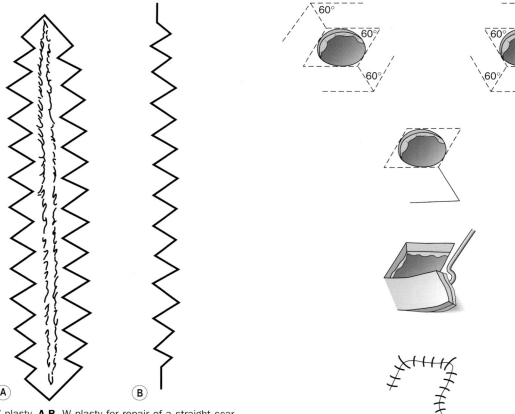

Figure 25.5. W plasty. **A,B,** W plasty for repair of a straight scar. Triangles become smaller at the end of the scar. A W plasty, however, results in excision of nonscarred skin. *(Reprinted from McCarthy, J.G., Galiano, R.D., Boutros, S.G. [Eds.], 2006. Current Therapy in Plastic Surgery. Elsevier, 3–10.)*

Figure 25.6. Rhomboid flap. *(Reprinted from McCarthy, J.G., Galiano, R.D., Boutros, S.G. [Eds.], 2006. Current Therapy in Plastic Surgery. Elsevier, 11–21.)*

4. Bilobed flaps (see Figure 25.7): A double transposition flap that allows for movement of skin over a longer distance than possible with a single transposition flap
   - Useful for reconstruction of defects within the face and nose

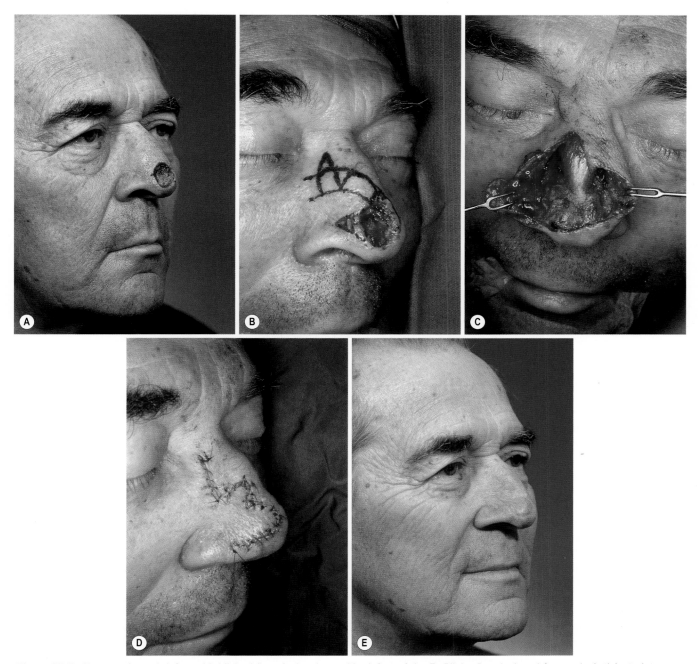

Figure 25.7. Closure of nasal defect with bilobed flap. **A,** 1 × 1 cm skin defect of tip. **B,** Bilobe flap designed for repair. Anticipated standing cutaneous deformity marked for excision in alar groove. Linear axis of each lobe designed 45° from each other, with primary lobe axis positioned 45° from axis of defect. **C,** Transfer of flap requires complete undermining of entire nasal skin. **D,** Flap in place. **E,** 1 year postoperative. No revision surgery performed. *(Reprinted from Baker, S.R., 2007. Local Flaps in Facial Reconstruction, 2nd ed. Mosby.)*

Common Flaps of the Head and Neck

1. Scalp flaps: Highly redundant blood supply allows for multiflap variations based off of a vascular pedicle.
   - Vascular supply (see Figure 25.8): Supratrochlear a. and supraorbital a. (anterior scalp); superficial temporal a. (temporal scalp); posterior auricular a. (parietal scalp); occipital a. (occipital scalp)

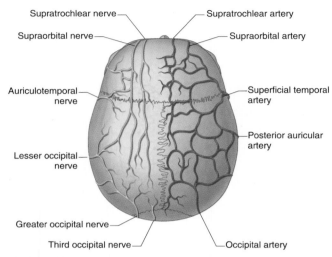

Figure 25.8. Arterial and nervous supply of the scalp. *(Reprinted from Neligan, P.C., Rodriguez, E.D. [Eds.], 2013. Plastic Surgery, vol. 3, 3rd ed. Elsevier, 105–133.)*

   - Primary closure often possible for defects <3 cm in diameter
     - May require galeal scoring to enhance tissue stretch
   - Scalp rotation flaps (e.g., orticochea) are useful for defects with a maximum diameter of 6 cm or <50% total surface area (TSA)
     - Tissue expansion can increase available soft tissue for rotation and can be used for defects up to 50% of the TSA without altering hair growth.
     - Dog ears created from rotation will most likely resolve and should not be excised at the time of rotation.
     - In some instances, the donor site from the rotation can be skin grafting as long as the pericranium is not violated during flap elevation (see Figures 25.9 and 25.10).
2. Forehead flap
   - Vascular supply: Supratrochlear a.
   - Advantages: Excellent for resurfacing of nasal defects, including the nasal tip; reliable vascular supply; excellent donor site healing
   - Disadvantages: Requires multiple stages; if flap extends into hair-bearing region, can get persistent hair growth after transfer (see Figures 25.11 and 25.12)
3. Temporoparietal fascia (TPF) flap
   - Vascular supply: Superficial temporal a.
   - Advantages: Thin flap, pliable

- Useful for coverage of tendons, exposed joints, or in areas where a thin fascial flap is desired
4. Facial artery musculomucosal (FAMM) flap
   - Vascular supply: Sacial a.
   - Dissection includes buccinators muscle
   - Can be used for oronasal defects of the palate, alveolus, and nasal septum (see Figure 25.13)
5. Submental myocutaneous flap
   - Vascular supply: Submental branch of the facial a.
   - Flap should include the platysma muscle
   - Advantages: Good contour, color, and texture for facial defects
   - Disadvantages: Donor site scar; pedicle reach often limits use of this flap to the central and lower third of the face (see Figure 25.14).

Common Flaps of the Trunk

1. Pectoralis major flap
   - Vascular supply: Thoracoacromial a. (major); internal mammary perforators (minor segmental)
   - Advantages: Excellent flap for head and neck (central to lower third), upper trunk, sternal defects; salvage flap for free-flap failures.
   - Disadvantages: Donor site morbidity; cannot use as a turnover flap for sternal coverage if the internal mammary a. has been used for a bypass procedure
2. Trapezius flap
   - Vascular supply: Occipital a. (superior third); superficial cervical a. (middle third); dorsal scapular a. (lower third).
     - 80% of flaps have a common trunk (the transverse cervical a.), which then branches into the superficial cervical and dorsal scapular arteries.
     - The transverse cervical a. is often divided during a radical neck dissection.
   - Advantages: Reliable musculocutaneous flap for posterior head and neck defects; often a salvage flap for free-flap failures.
   - Disadvantages: Donor site, skin paddle can be thick and difficult to shape, limited skin paddle availability (see Figure 25.15)
3. Latissimus dorsi flap
   - Vascular supply: Thoracodorsal a. (major); lumbar intercostal perforators (minor segmental)
   - Advantages: Reliable flap for provision of wide, pliable muscle, skin, and occasionally bone (can be harvested with portion of scapula in chimeric flap); workhorse muscle flap for free tissue transfer to the extremities, scalp, and trunk; workhorse pedicled flap option for breast reconstruction
   - Disadvantages: Donor site, limited skin paddle availability, relatively short pedicle (can be extended with interposition grafts)
4. Serratus anterior flap
   - Vascular supply: Thoracodorsal a. (inferior muscle slips); lateral thoracic a. (superior muscle slips)

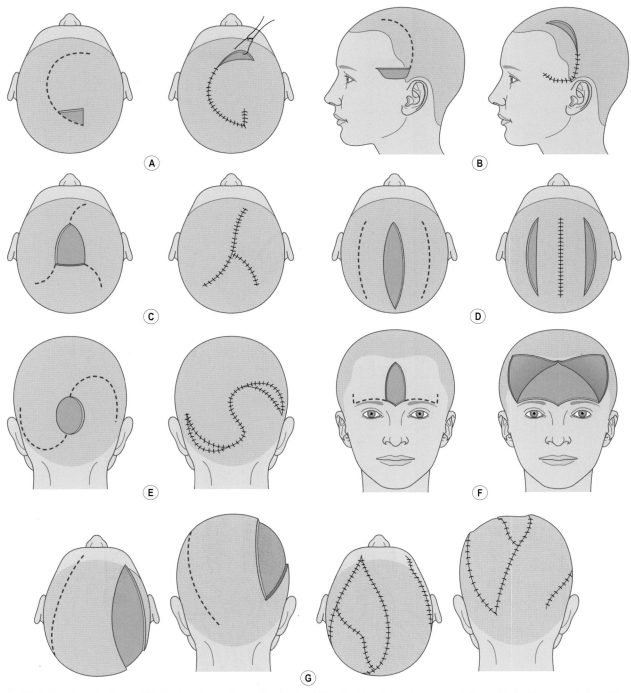

Figure 25.9. Local scalp flaps. **A,B,** Scalp rotation flaps; **C,** pinwheel flap; **D,** bipedicle advancement flaps; **E,** double opposing rotation flaps; **F,** Y to T flap; **G,** bipedicled fronto-occipital flaps. *(Reprinted from Marchac, D., 1990. Deformities of the forehead, scalp, and cranial vault. In: McCarthy, J.G. [Ed.], Plastic surgery. WB Saunders, Philadelphia, 1538.)*

- Advantages: Extremely versatile flap that can include bone (scapula), relatively long pedicle with large diameter; can be used as a functional muscle flap (long thoracic n.)
- Disadvantages: Donor site, winged scapula (must preserve superior 4 to 5 muscle slips).

5. Scapular/parascapular flap
   - Vascular supply: Circumflex scapular a. (provides a horizontal and vertical branch upon which flaps can be designed)
   - Advantages: Can provide multiple skin paddles with a high degree of independent motion through use of the

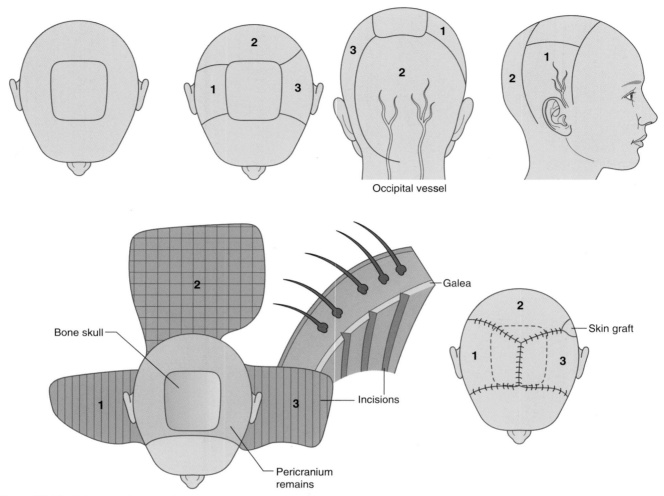

Figure 25.10. Orticochea three-flap technique. Two flaps based on the superficial temporal artery are used to reconstruct the defect. A posterior-based flap based on the occipital vessels is used to fill the donor defect. *(Reprinted from Arnold, P.G., Rangarathnam, C.S., 1982. Multiple flap scalp reconstruction: orticochea revisited. Plast. Reconstr. Surg. 69, 607.)*

Figure 25.11. Arterial supply to the paramedian forehead flap. *(Reprinted from Menick, F. [Ed.], 2009. Nasal Reconstruction: Art and Practice. Elsevier, 109–154.)*

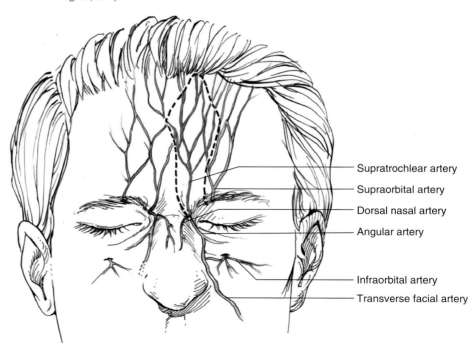

Supratrochlear artery

Supraorbital artery

Dorsal nasal artery

Angular artery

Infraorbital artery

Transverse facial artery

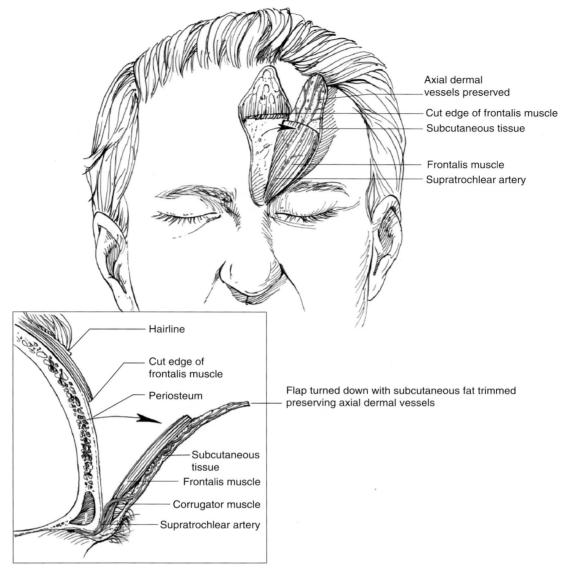

Figure 25.12. Recommended dissection plane for the paramedian forehead flap. The paramedian forehead flap can be elevated in the subcutaneous plane distally, with a transition proximally to the subperiosteal plane to include the supratrochlear artery. *(Reprinted from Menick, F. [Ed.], 2009. Nasal Reconstruction: Art and Practice. Elsevier, 109–155.)*

transverse and descending cutaneous branches, vascularized bone (lateral scapula border) for composite flaps, and be used as a perforator flap for skin-only reconstructions; useful for facial reconstruction (e.g., hemifacial microsomia, Romberg disease)
- Disadvantages: Donor site, relatively short pedicle
- Landmarks: "Quadrangular space" borders—triceps m. (lateral border), teres minor (superior border), teres major (inferior border), scapula (medial border) (see Figure 25.16)

6. External oblique turnover flap
- Vascular supply: Intercostal a. (upper half); deep circumflex iliac a. (DCIA) or iliolumbar a. (lower half; DCIA most common)
- Advantages: Useful for large, midline, back defects without other local options

7. Rectus abdominis flap
- Vascular supply: Deep inferior epigastric a. (off of external iliac a.); superior epigastric a. (off of internal mammary a.)
- Advantages: Provides reliable muscle flap with good length; workhorse as a musculocutaneous flap for breast, perineal, and chest-wall reconstruction
- Disadvantages: Less reliable as a pedicled flap in instances where ipsilateral internal mammary a. has been harvested
  - Flap based off of 8th intercostal a. in this instance
- Delay pedicled rectus myocutaneous flaps in patients with the following risk factors: Obesity, active smoking, history of radiation therapy, large volume requirements

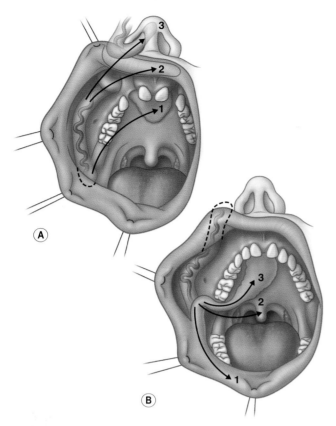

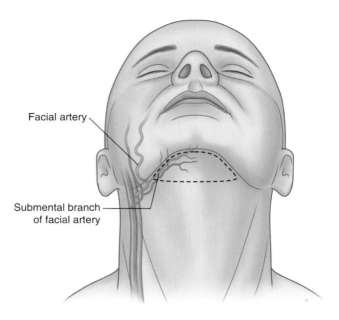

Figure 25.14. Prominent mandible angle: Mandible angle ostectomy and external corticotomy with microfat graft in older ages. *(Reprinted from Neligan, P.C., Rodriguez, E.D. [Eds.], 2013. Plastic Surgery, vol. 3, 3rd ed. Elsevier, 254–277.)*

Figure 25.13. A, Superiorly based facial artery musculomucosal (FAMM) flap may be used for defects of the anterior palate, alveolus, maxillary antrum, nose, upper lip, and orbit. **B,** Inferiorly based FAMM flap may be used for defects of the posterior palate, tonsillar fossa, alveolus, floor of mouth, and lower lip. *(Reprinted from Neligan, P.C., Rodriguez, E.D. [Eds.], 2013. Plastic Surgery, vol. 3, 3rd ed. Elsevier, 461–472.)*

- Most common complication after rectus flap reconstruction for vaginal defects is vaginal stenosis

Common Flaps of the Upper Extremity

1. Brachioradialis flap
   - Vascular supply: Radial recurrent a.
   - Advantages: Useful for coverage of anterior elbow and antecubital fossa defects, minimal donor site morbidity due to redundancy of flexors
2. Lateral arm flap
   - Vascular supply: Posterior radial collateral a. (PRCA)
   - Advantages: Provides a thin, pliable fasciocutaneous flap for coverage of the hand and other sensitive areas where thin skin flaps are desired (e.g., floor of mouth, coverage of joints); can be harvested with the posterior third of the humerus as a composite flap
   - Reverse lateral arm flap can be used for coverage of elbow defects (vascular supply off of radial recurrent a.)
     - Disadvantages: Venous congestion with rotation ≥180 degrees (see Figure 25.17)

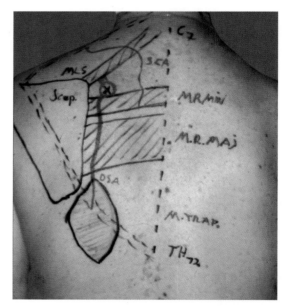

Figure 25.15. Anatomic landmarks and flap markings. Typical preoperative markings preparatory to a myocutaneous flap based on the dorsal scapular artery (DSA). *(Reprinted from Wei, F.C., Mardini, S. [Eds.], 2009. Flaps and Reconstructive Surgery. Elsevier, 249–269.)*

3. Medial arm flap
   - Vascular supply: Superior ulnar collateral a.
   - Disadvantages: Less reliable, variable anatomy
4. Posterior interosseous a. flap
   - Vascular supply: Posterior interosseus a.
   - Advantages: Provides thin, pliable skin; useful for hand reconstruction

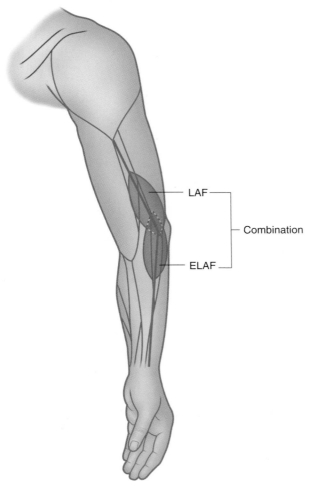

Figure 25.16. Anatomic landmarks and markings. *ELAF,* Extended lateral arm flap; *LAF,* lateral arm flap. *(Reprinted from Standring, S. [Ed.], 2005. Gray's Anatomy: The Anatomic Basis of Clinical Practice, 39th ed. Churchill Livingstone.)*

- Disadvantages: Limited reach for distal hand/finger defects, high incidence of partial flap loss
- Landmarks
  - Pivot point is located 2 cm proximal to ulnar styloid
  - Flap should be centered on a line drawn from the lateral epicondyle to the distal radioulnar joint.
5. Radial forearm flap
   - Vascular supply: Septocutaneous perforators from the radial a.
   - Advantages: Thin fasciocutaneous flap; useful for defects where thin, pliable tissue is desired (hemiglossectomy defects, floor of mouth, cheek, hand, etc.); can be harvested with bone as a composite flap
     - Radius should be harvested from radial aspect and be no greater than 40% of the cross-sectional area to reduce the risk of distal radius fracture.
     - Vascular supply to radius is via fascioperiosteal perforators within the intermuscular septum.

- Disadvantages: Donor site defect, neuroma (superficial branch of the radial nerve), venous congestion (often harvest skin paddle with cephalic vein for outflow to reduce risk for venous congestion)
- Landmarks
  - Proximal radial a. found deep to brachioradialis
  - Distal radial a. found within the intermuscular septum between the brachioradialis and flexor carpi radialis (see Figure 25.18)

Common Flaps of the Lower Extremity

1. Iliac crest osteocutaneous flap
   - Vascular supply: Deep circumflex iliac a.
   - Advantages: Can be harvested with a skin paddle up to 12 × 6 cm and an iliac crest bone segment of up to 8 cm; good contour for mandible reconstruction
   - Disadvantages: Thick and bulky cutaneous portion that is insensate and difficult to inset; risk of hernia formation at donor site
2. Groin flap
   - Vascular supply: Superficial circumflex iliac a.
   - Advantages: Provides thin soft-tissue coverage of the hand, wrist, and distal forearm; can be used as a free flap
   - Landmark
     - Arises from the common femoral a. or superficial femoral a.; travels parallel to, 1 cm deep, and 2 to 3 cm inferior to the inguinal ligament (see Figure 25.19)
3. Shaw flap
   - Vascular supply: Superficial inferior epigastric a.
   - Advantages: Useful for coverage of hand and forearm defects with better elbow position than traditional groin flap (located higher, so elbow can remain flexed)
   - Landmark
     - Pedicle found at the intersection of the inguinal ligament and femoral a. and courses to the anterior axillary line
4. Gluteal a. flap
   - Vascular supply: Superior gluteal a. (SGA) and inferior gluteal a. (IGA) off of internal iliac a.
   - Advantages: Useful for coverage of sacral wounds, defects of lumbar spine; can be harvested off of perforators as fasciocutaneous flaps for breast reconstruction
   - Disadvantages: Tedious dissection when used as free flaps; requires position change if using as free flap for anterior defects/reconstruction
   - Landmarks
     - The SGA exits lateral and deep to the sacrum above the piriformis, whereas the IGA exits below the piriformis.
       - The piriformis can be outlined by a line drawn from the greater trochanter to the midpoint between the posterior superior iliac spine (PSIS) and the coccyx.
       - The SGA will often emerge at the junction of the medial and middle thirds of a line drawn from the PSIS to the greater trochanter.

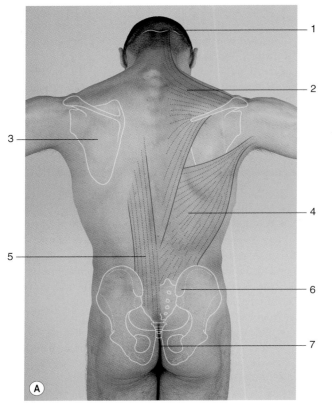

1. External occipital protuberance
2. Trapezius
3. Inferior angle of scapula
4. Latissimus dorsi
5. Erector spinae
6. Posterior superior iliac spine underlying sacral dimple
7. Rectal cleft

1. Median furrow
2. Lateral border of erector spinae
3. Gluteus maximus
4. Gluteal fold

Black: scapular flap
Blue: ascending vertical flap
Red: parascapular
Green: imecc flap

Figure 25.17. A,B, Mathes-Nahai classification of fascia/fasciocutaneous flaps. *(Reprinted from Wei, F.C., Mardini, S. [Eds.], 2009. Flaps and Reconstructive Surgery. Elsevier, 305–319.)*

5. Gracilis
   - Vascular supply: Medial circumflex femoral a. (profunda femoris a.)
   - Advantages: Reliable myofascial flap; provides thin, pliable muscle coverage; useful for groin/medial thigh defects; can be used as a functional m. for fascial reanimation (obturator n.)
   - Disadvantages: Vertical skin paddle unreliable (especially over distal third)
   - Landmarks
     - Pedicle enters the muscle 8 to10 cm below the pubic tubercle.
     - The gracilis m. is the most superficial m. in the medial thigh (between the adductor longus and brevis m.), is triangular shaped, and coalesces into a tendon distally.
   - TUG flap: Transverse upper gracilis myocutaneous flap for use in autologous breast reconstruction (see Figure 25.20)

6. Sartorius flap
   - Vascular supply: Segmental perforators from the superficial femoral a.
   - Advantages: Useful for coverage of groin defects and femoral vessels
   - Disadvantages: Relatively unreliable because of segmental blood supply
   - Landmarks
     - Most proximal pedicle located ~8 cm from anterior superior iliac spine
7. Rectus femoris flap
   - Vascular supply: Lateral circumflex femoral a.
   - Advantages: Reliable myofascial flap; useful for coverage of abdominal, groin, and hip defects
   - Disadvantages: Harvest results in 15-degree extensor lag of knee.
   - Expanded rectus femoris flap can be used to cover massive abdominal wall defects and reach the xyphoid.

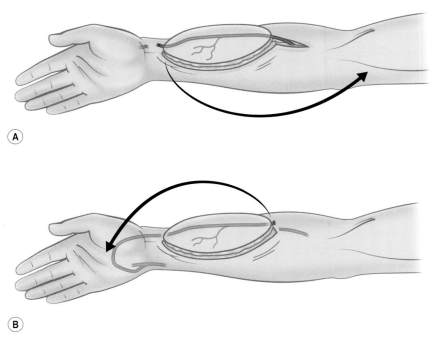

Figure 25.18. Radial forearm flap. **A,** Standard arc to antecubital fossa. **B,** Reverse arc to palmar surface of hand. *(Reprinted from Neligan, P.C., Gurtner, G.C. [Eds.], 2013. Principles in Plastic Surgery, vol. 1. Elsevier, 512–572.)*

8. Anterolateral thigh flap
   - Vascular supply: Perforators from the descending branch of the lateral circumflex femoral a.
   - Advantages: Reliable fasciocutaneous flap that has become a workhorse free flap for reconstruction of the extremities, head and neck, glossectomy defects, and trunk; can be harvested with vastus lateralis m. for bulk
   - Disadvantages: Tedious dissection for intramuscular perforators; subcutaneous tissue can be thick, resulting in a bulky flap.
   - Landmarks
     - Main pedicle lies within the septum between the rectus femoris m. and the vastus lateralis m.
     - Perforators to skin can typically be found within a 3-cm radius at the midpoint of a line from the ASIS to the superolateral patella (see Figure 25.21).

9. Medial femoral condyle flap
   - Vascular supply: Descending geniculate a.
   - Advantages: Provides reliable, small-segment vascularized bone graft

10. Gastrocnemius flap
    - Vascular supply: Medial and lateral sural a. (off of the popliteal a.)
    - Advantages: Workhorse local flap for coverage of complex knee wounds and proximal-third lower leg wounds; can be harvested with skin
    - Disadvantages: Limited reach
    - Medial head is larger and more preferred than lateral head.

11. Soleus flap
    - Vascular supply: Proximal supply via posterior tibial, popliteal, and peroneal a.; distal supply via posterior tibial a. (medial) and peroneal a. (lateral)
    - Advantages: Useful coverage for middle-third lower leg defects.
    - Reversed hemisoleus flap can occasionally be used for proximal lower-third leg defects (based medially off of perforators from posterior tibial a.)

12. Peroneal a. perforator flap
    - Vascular supply: Perforators from the peroneal a.
    - Can be used as a propeller fasciocutaneous flap for lower leg defects

13. Reverse sural a. flap
    - Vascular supply: Septocutaneous perforators from the peroneal a.
    - Can be used for distal-third leg defects
    - Improved flap survival when the saphenous vein and median cutaneous sural n. are included in the flap
    - Disadvantages: Venous congestion, partial flap loss (see Figure 25.22)

14. Free fibula flap
    - Vascular supply: Peroneal a.
    - Advantages: Reliable vascularized bone flap; useful for mandible reconstruction; can provide up to 25 cm of bone; be harvested with skin based off of peroneal perforators in the posterior intermuscular septum; include soleus m. and/or flexor hallucis longus m. to provide bulk

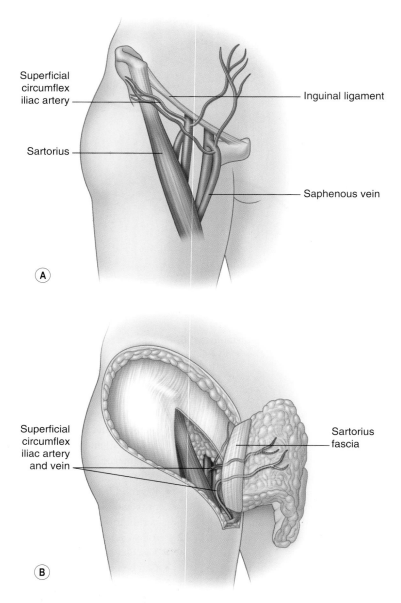

Figure 25.19. Groin flap elevation. **A,** The dominant pedicle is the superficial circumflex iliac artery; **B,** venae comitantes and superficial circumflex iliac vein. *(Reprinted from Neligan, P.C., 2013. Plastic Surgery, 3rd ed. Elsevier, 127–150.)*

- Disadvantages: Donor site morbidity, claw toes, ankle/knee instability, nerve injury
  - Must leave 6 cm of proximal fibula and distal fibula for stability of the knee and ankle joints, proximal and distal 6 cm of bone for stability
15. Medial plantar a. flap
  - Vascular supply: Medial plantar a. (off of posterior tibial a.)
  - Advantages: Useful for coverage of heel or distal foot defects
  - Disadvantages: Limited arc or rotation and reach, usually requires skin graft of donor site

16. Lateral calcaneal flap
  - Vascular supply: Lateral calcaneal a. (off of peroneal a.)
  - Advantages: Useful for coverage of lateral ankle defects; very reliable
  - Disadvantages: Limited arc of rotation and reach; typically requires skin graft of donor site
17. Great toe flap
  - Vascular supply: 1st dorsal metatarsal a. (off of dorsalis pedis in 2/3rds and deep plantar a. or plantar arch in 1/3rd)
  - Advantages: Useful for thumb reconstruction

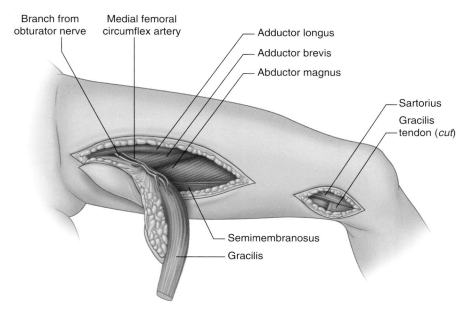

Figure 25.20. Gracilis muscle flap elevation. It is a type-II circulation pattern (the dominant pedicle is the terminal branch of the medial circumflex femoral artery, and one or two minor pedicles arise as branches of the superficial femoral artery) and can reach to cover the abdomen, ischium, groin, and perineum as a muscle or musculocutaneous flap. *(Reprinted from Neligan, P.C., 2013. Plastic Surgery, 3rd ed. Elsevier, 127–150.)*

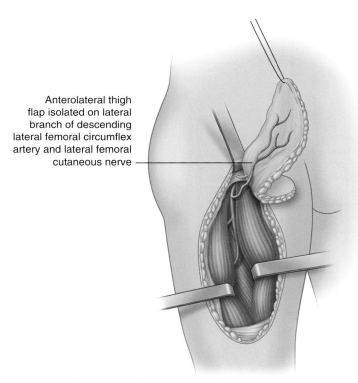

Figure 25.21. The anterolateral thigh flap. Numerous perforators are found along the region of intermuscular septum between the vastus lateralis and rectus femoris. These perforators usually drain into the descending branch of the lateral femoral circumflex artery, proceed proximally to the lateral circumflex artery, and then on to the profunda femoris artery. *(Reprinted from Neligan, P.C., 2013. Plastic Surgery, 3rd ed. Elsevier, 127–150.)*

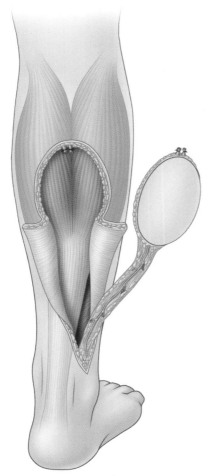

Figure 25.22. The reverse sural artery flap is a fasciocutaneous flap based on the median superficial sural artery and its communication with the perforating branch of the peroneal artery situated in the region of the lateral malleolar gutter. Reverse flow is established after elevation of the flap and with division of the sural artery and the nerve proximally. *(Reprinted from Neligan, P.C., 2013. Plastic Surgery, 3rd ed. Elsevier, 127–150.)*

Common Visceral Flaps

1. Omental flap
   - Vascular supply: Right and left gastroepiploic a.
   - Advantages: Reliable, thin, pliable flap; useful for defects of the sternum/trunk, perineum, abdomen, groin, and intrathoracic region
   - Disadvantages: Donor site morbidity, hernia formation; requires skin graft
2. Jejunal flap
   - Vascular supply: Jejunal a. (from the superior mesenteric a.)
   - Advantages: Useful for esophageal/pharyngeal reconstruction
   - Disadvantages: Donor site morbidity

General Microsurgery Considerations

1. Factors that can affect anastomosis patency include surgical precision, vessel size, vessel size mismatch, blood flow, tension, kinking, and the use of anticoagulants/antithrombotics.
   - Most influential factor on anastomotic patency is surgical precision.
   - No evidence for benefit of anticoagulation, type of anastomosis, or suture technique
   - Adequate fluid resuscitation is paramount.
     - Euvolemia is preferred because hypovolemia and volume overload can have detrimental effects on flap perfusion.
   - Although anastomotic couplers have been used for arterial anastomoses, their use is contraindicated in the setting of vessel calcification.
2. Anastomotic thrombosis
   - Most occur within the first 24 hours (~90%)
     - In head and neck cases, it is most likely to occur within 12 hours of the anastomosis
   - Venous thrombosis is more common than arterial thrombosis.
     - Signs of venous thrombosis: Flap congestion, brisk capillary refill, brisk dark bleeding from skin paddle when scratched
     - Signs of arterial thrombosis: Pale, cool flap; delayed capillary refill; no return of bright red bleeding when skin paddle is scratched; loss of Doppler signal
     - Any concern for thrombosis warrants an immediate return to the operating room with exploration of the anastomosis.
       - Rapid return to the operating room yields higher salvage rates.
   - Management of thrombosis
     - Thrombectomy and revision of the anastomosis +/− intraflap thrombolytics
     - Thrombolytics
       - Tissue plasminogen activator (tPA)
         - Mechanism of action: Activated in the presence of fibrin and catalyzes the conversion of plasminogen to plasmin
         - Preferred thrombolytic; more specific than urokinase or streptokinase
         - Disadvantages: Bleeding
       - Dextran
         - Formerly used as a thrombolytic; no longer used in the United States
         - Mechanism of action: Decreases factor VIII and von Willebrand (vWF) factor, which results in decreased platelet function and aggregation and increased susceptibility of fibrin to degrade
         - Disadvantages: Risk of anaphylaxis, flash pulmonary edema, acute respirator distress syndrome (ARDS), acute renal failure (toxic to glomeruli)

3. Flap monitoring
   - Clinical exam
     - Temperature
     - Color
     - Turgor
     - Capillary refill
     - Scratch test
       - Skin paddle scratched with an 18-gauge needle or scalpel to evaluate for bleeding
   - Doppler
     - Pencil doppler: Useful for monitoring flaps with arterial perforator signals found within the transferred skin paddle
     - Implantable venous doppler: Doppler probe is wrapped around the pedicle vessel just distal to the anastomosis.
       - Effective for monitoring, especially for flaps without a skin paddle or buried flaps in which clinical exam is difficult
       - Newer implantable dopplers are integrated within the anastomotic coupler device
   - Tissue oxygenation
     - Use of spectroscopy to detect tissue oxygenation with the flap skin paddle
     - Trends of tissue oxygenation, and subsequent changes in those trends, can be used to detect flap compromise.
     - Absolute tissue oxygenation <30% suggests flap ischemia.

Special Flap Considerations

1. Venous congestion
   - Delayed or persistent venous congestion of flaps, not related to a venous thrombus, can be treated with leeches.
     - Advantages: Leech application will provide decongestion of flap through action of hirudin.
     - Disadvantages: Risk of infection that can progress from cellulitis to sepsis, caused by *Aeromonas hydrophila*
       - Prevention via prophylactic treatment with a fluoroquinolone (e.g., ciprofloxacin) and/or aminoglycoside
       - Continue treatment until the wound is fully healed because of possibility of a delayed infection.
2. Heparin-induced thrombocytopenia (HIT)
   - An immune-mediated thrombocytopenia that can occur in patients exposed to heparin, especially those who have had prior exposure within 3 months, which can result in thrombotic events, limb ischemia, and death
   - Mechanism: Antibody binding to heparin and platelet factor 4, resulting in platelet activation, aggregation, and increase in thrombin generation
   - Diagnosis
     - A 30% decrease in baseline platelet count combined with any thrombotic event
     - Platelet aggregation test or enzyme-linked immunosorbent assay (ELISA)
   - Treatment: Stop heparin and switch to an alternative anticoagulant (e.g., argatroban, lepirudin, danaparoid) until platelet levels return to baseline.
     - Remember to discontinue heparin flushes of all intravenous lines.

Suggested Readings

Chuang, D.C.C., 2009. Chapter 29: Gracilis flap. In: Wei, F.C., Mardini, S. (Eds.), Flaps and Reconstructive Surgery. Elsevier, pp. 397–410.

Colohan, S., Saint-Cyr, M., 2013. Chapter 2: Management of lower extremity trauma. In: Neligan, P.C. (Ed.), Plastic Surgery, 3rd ed. Elsevier, pp. 63–91.

Dumanian, G.A., Heckler, F.R., Bernard, S.L., 2003. The external oblique turnover muscle flap. Plast. Reconstr. Surg. 111 (7), 2344–2348.

Guo, L., Pribaz, J.J., 2009. Chapter 11: Prefabrication and prelamination. In: Wei, F.C., Mardini, S. (Eds.), Flaps and Reconstructive Surgery. Elsevier, pp. 103–116.

Guo, L., Pribaz, J.J., 2009. Clinical flap prefabrication. Plast. Reconstr. Surg. 124 (Suppl. 6), e340–e350.

Hallock, G.G., 2009. Chapter 2: Classification of flaps. In: Wei, F.C., Mardini, S. (Eds.), Flaps and Reconstructive Surgery. Elsevier, pp. 7–15.

Hansen, S.L., Young, D.M., Lang, P., et al., 2013. Chapter 24: Flap classification and applications. In: Neligan, P.C., Gurtner, G.C. (Eds.), Principles in Plastic Surgery, vol. 1. Elsevier, pp. 512–572.

Hong, J.P., 2013. Chapter 5: Reconstructive surgery: lower extremity coverage. In: Neligan, P.C. (Ed.), Plastic Surgery, 3rd ed. Elsevier, pp. 127–150.

Jackson, I.T. (Ed.), 2007, Local Flaps in Head and Neck Reconstruction, 2nd ed. QMP, pp. 1–611.

Jackson, I.T., 2013. Chapter 18: Local flaps for facial coverage. In: Neligan, P.C., Rodriguez, E.D. (Eds.), Plastic Surgery, vol. 2, 3rd ed. Elsevier, pp. 440–460.

Jones, N.F., Lister, G.D., 2011. Chapter 51: Free skin and composite flaps. In: Wolfe, S.W., Hotchkiss, R.N., Pederson, W.C., et al. (Eds.), Green's Operative Hand Surgery, 6th ed. Elsevier, pp. 1721–1756.

Kim, S., Chung, K.C., 2009. Chapter 95: Free tissue transfer. In: Guyuron, B., Eriksson, E., Persing, J.A. (Eds.), Plastic Surgery Indications and Practice. Elsevier, pp. 1225–1237.

McCarthy, J.G., Galiano, R.D., Boutros, S.G., 2006. Chapter 1: Plastic surgery strategies. In: McCarthy, J.G., Galiano, R.D., Boutros, S.G. (Eds.), Current Therapy in Plastic Surgery. Elsevier, pp. 3–10.

Menick, F., 2009. Chapter 6: A modern approach to nasal reconstruction with a forehead flap. In: Menick, F. (Ed.), Nasal Reconstruction: Art and Practice. Elsevier, pp. 109–0154.

Morris, S.F., Maciel-Miranda, A., Hallock, G.G., 2013. Chapter 1: History of perforator flap surgery. In: Blondeel, P.N., Morris, S.F., Hallock, G.G., et al. (Eds.), Perforator Flaps, 2nd ed. QMP, pp. 3–24.

Morris, S.F., Taylor, G.I., 2013. Chapter 23: Vascular territories. In: Neligan, P.C., Gurtner, G.C., (Eds.), Principles in Plastic Surgery, vol. 1. Elsevier, pp. 479–511.

Neligan, P.C., 2013. Chapter 10: Cheek and lip reconstruction. In: Neligan, P.C., Rodriguez, E.D. (Eds.), Plastic Surgery, vol. 2, 3rd ed. Elsevier, pp. 254–277.

Pang, C.Y., Neligan, P.C., 2013. Chapter 25: Flap pathophysiology and pharmacology. In: Neligan, P.C., Gurtner, G.C. (Eds.), Principles in Plastic Surgery, vol. 1, 3rd ed. Elsevier, pp. 573–586.

Pederson, W.C., 2011. Chapter 50: Nonmicrosurgical coverage of the upper extremity. In: Wolfe, S.W., Hotchkiss, R.N., Pederson, W.C., et al. (Eds.), Green's Operative Hand Surgery, 6th ed. Elsevier, pp. 1645–1720.

Pribaz, J.J., Chan, R.K., 2013. Chapter 19: Secondary facial reconstruction. In: Neligan, P.C., Rodriguez, E.D. (Eds.), Plastic Surgery, vol. 2, 3rd ed. Elsevier, pp. 461–472.

Spector, J.A., Levine, J.P., 2006. Chapter 2: Cutaneous defects: flaps, grafts, and expansion. In: McCarthy, J.G., Galiano, R.D., Boutros, S.G. (Eds.), Current Therapy in Plastic Surgery. Elsevier, pp. 11–21.

Wei, F.C., Mardini, S. (Eds.), 2009. Flaps and Reconstructive Surgery. Elsevier.

Wei, F.C., Tay, S.K.L., 2013. Chapter 26: Principles and techniques of microvascular surgery. In: Neligan, P.C., Gurtner, G.C. (Eds.), Principles in Plastic Surgery, vol. 1, 3rd ed. Elsevier, pp. 587–621.

Wells, M.D., Skytta, C., 2013. Chapter 5: Scalp and forehead reconstruction. In: Neligan, P.C., Rodriguez, E.D. (Eds.), Plastic Surgery, vol. 2, 3rd ed. Elsevier, pp. 105–133.

Chapter

Eyelid Anatomy, Reconstruction, and Blepharoplasty

26

General Anatomy (see Figure 26.1)

1. Upper eyelid layers (superficial to deep)
   - Skin → orbicularis oculi muscle → retro-orbicularis oculi fat (ROOF) → orbital septum → orbital fat (central and medial) → levator palpebrae superioris m. → Müller's muscle → conjunctiva
2. Lower eyelid layers (superficial to deep)
   - Skin → orbicularis oculi muscle → suborbicularis oculi fat (SOOF) → orbital septum → orbital fat (lateral, central, and medial) → levator palpebrae superioris m. → Müller's muscle → conjunctiva

3. Orbital fat

- Upper eyelid
  - Two compartments: Medial and central
  - Medial fat is pale in color.
  - No lateral compartment, because the lacrimal gland occupies the lateral portion
- Lower eyelid
  - Three compartments: Medial, central, and lateral
  - Medial fat is pale in color.
  - Medial and central compartments separated by the inferior oblique m.
4. Vascular supply of the eyelids (see Figure 26.2)
   - Branches of the ophthalmic a. (medially) and lacrimal a. (laterally) via the internal carotid artery
     - Form the medial and lateral palpebral a., which anastomose to create the arterial arcades of the lid
     - The upper eyelid has two arterial arcades.
       ○ Marginal arcade runs along the surface of the tarsal plate, 2 to 3 mm above the eyelid margin
       ○ Peripheral arcade runs parallel to the marginal arcade, superior to the tarsal plate, and in between the levator m. and Müller's m.
     - The lower eyelid has only one well-developed marginal arcade.
   - Also receive arterial supply from branches of the facial a., superficial temporal a., and infraorbital a. via the external carotid a.

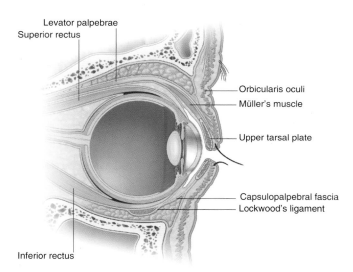

Figure 26.1. Eyelid anatomy. Each eyelid consists of an anterior lamella of skin and orbicularis muscle and a posterior lamella of tarsus and conjunctiva. The orbital septum forms the anterior border of the orbital fat. *(Reprinted from Neligan, P.C., Buck, D.W. [Eds.], 2013. Core Procedures in Plastic Surgery. Elsevier, 1–22.)*

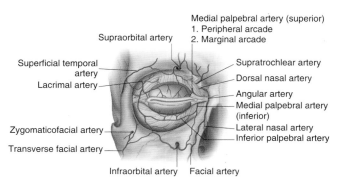

Figure 26.2. Arterial supply to the periorbital region. *(Reprinted from Neligan, P.C., Buck, D.W. [Eds.], 2013. Core Procedures in Plastic Surgery. Elsevier, 1–22.)*

5. Sensory innervation of the eyelids (see Figure 26.3): Via the ophthalmic (V1) and maxillary (V2) divisions of the trigeminal n.
   - Supraorbital n.: Upper eyelid and forehead skin
     - Exits the orbit through the supraorbital notch or supraorbital foramen
   - Supratrochlear n.: Central forehead skin and medial upper eyelid
     - Courses superiorly through the corrugator m. and is vulnerable to injury during transpalpebral resection of medial brow depressors
   - Infratrochlear n.: Medial upper and lower eyelid and medial canthal tendon
   - Lacrimal n.: Lacrimal gland, conjunctiva, and lateral portion of the upper eyelid
   - Zygomaticofacial n.: Lateral fat pad of the lower eyelid and lateral skin of the lower eyelid
   - Infraorbital n.: Lower eyelid, cheek, and upper lip

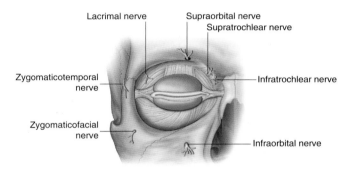

Figure 26.3. Sensory nerves of the eyelids. *(Reprinted from Neligan, P.C., Buck, D.W. [Eds.], 2013. Core Procedures in Plastic Surgery. Elsevier, 1–22.)*

6. Orbicularis oculi m. (see Figure 26.4)
   - Superficial muscle of facial expression, innervated by the facial n. (frontal and zygomatic branches)
   - Divided into three anatomical portions: Orbital, preseptal, and pretarsal
     - The orbital orbicularis m. is used in forced eyelid closure.
     - The preseptal and pretarsal orbicularis fibers are critical for blinking and voluntary winking and originate medially from a superficial and deep head associated with the medial canthal tendon.
     - The pretarsal orbicularis fibers run horizontally, anterior to the tarsus, and insert into the lateral orbital tubercle (Whitnall's tubercle) via the lateral canthal tendon.
     - Avoid injury to the pretarsal orbicularis.

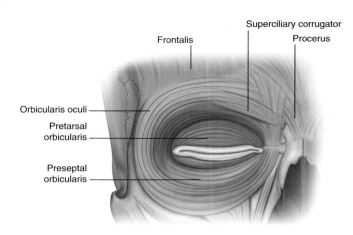

Figure 26.4. Fascial muscles of the orbital region. Note that the preseptal and pretarsal orbicularis muscles fuse with the medial and lateral canthal tendons. *(Reprinted from Neligan, P.C., Buck, D.W. [Eds.], 2013. Core Procedures in Plastic Surgery. Elsevier, 1–22.)*

7. Orbital septum
   - A connective tissue structure that functions to contain the orbital contents
   - Attaches peripherally at the orbital rim via the arcus marginalis (the periosteal extension of the septum) and fuses centrally with the lid retractors at tarsal plates at the lid margins
     - A transconjunctival approach to the lid/orbit can be performed in a pre- or postseptal plane.
8. Eyelid retractors
   - Levator complex
     - Originates at the orbital apex from the lesser wing of the sphenoid and travels horizontally until it reaches the Whitnall ligament, where it then changes to a more vertical direction before inserting onto the upper eyelid tarsal plate, orbital septum, and dermis via an aponeurosis
       - Above the level of the tarsus, the orbital septum lies anterior to the levator, and preaponeurotic fat lies posterior to the orbital septum.
       - Müller's muscle lies directly posterior to the levator m., superior to the tarsus.
     - Motor innervation via the oculomotor n. (cranial n. [CN] III).
   - Müller's muscle
     - Sympathetic smooth muscle of the upper eyelid
     - Arises from the levator complex and inserts directly on the tarsus

- Positioned posterior to the levator m., directly superior to the tarsus
- Resection of Müller's m. can provide 2 mm of eyelid elevation.
  - Capsulopalpebral fascia
    - Makes up the anteriosuperior portion of the lower eyelid retractors distal to the Lockwood ligament
    - Inserts on the inferior border of the tarsus and functions akin to the levator m. in the upper eyelid
    - Divided during the transconjunctival incision
9. Inferior oblique muscle
   - Located between the medial and central fat compartments of the lower eyelid, deep to the periosteum
   - Vulnerable to injury when performing fat excision or fat compartment manipulation during lower blepharoplasty or via inadvertent resection, cauterization, scarring, hemorrhage, edema, or suture injury while repairing the septum
     - Depending on the extent of injury, symptoms, including diplopia, can be transient or permanent.
10. Orbitomalar ligament/orbicularis retaining ligament (see Figure 26.5)
    - Attaches the orbicularis oculi muscle of the eye to the orbital rim, separating the lower eyelid from the midface
    - Contributes to the lateral canthal ligament
    - Release is required to obtain access to the midface when approaching it from the lower eyelid.

11. Whitnall ligament
    - Fascial thickening of the upper eyelid that surrounds the levator m. and tarsus to provide structural support to the lid and aids the levator m. in elevating the lid superiorly by changing the functional orientation of the m. fibers
    - Attaches laterally to the orbit at Whitnall's tubercle (lateral orbital tubercle)
12. Lockwood ligament
    - A fascial thickening of the lower eyelid that surrounds the inferior rectus and inferior oblique muscles and fuses with the capsulopalpebral fascia to support the globe
    - Analogous to the Whitnall ligament in the upper eyelid
13. Canthal tendons (see Figures 26.6 and 26.7)
    - Medial canthal tendon (or medial palpebral ligament)
      - Fibrous band that is continuous with the tarsal plates and attaches the lid to the orbital rim
      - Three limbs: Anterior, posterior, and superior
        - Posterior, or deep limb, attaches to the posterior lacrimal crest
      - Intimately related to the pretarsal and preseptal orbicular oculi m. and lacrimal system
    - Lateral canthal tendon (or lateral palpebral ligament)
      - Attaches the upper and lower tarsal plates to Whitnall's tubercle inside the lateral orbital rim and deep to the septum

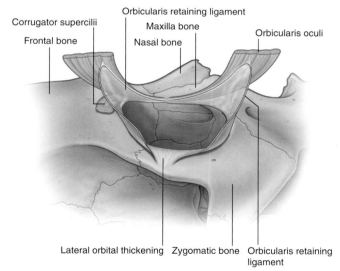

Corrugator supercilii
Frontal bone
Orbicularis retaining ligament
Maxilla bone
Nasal bone
Orbicularis oculi
Lateral orbital thickening   Zygomatic bone   Orbicularis retaining ligament

Figure 26.5. The orbicularis muscle fascia attaches to the skeleton along the orbital rim by the lateral orbital thickening (LOT) in continuity with the orbicularis retaining ligament (ORL). *(Adapted from Ghavami, A., Pessa, J.E., Janis, J., et al., 2008. The orbicularis retaining ligament of the medial orbit: closing the circle. Plast. Reconstr. Surg. 121 [3], 994–1001.)*

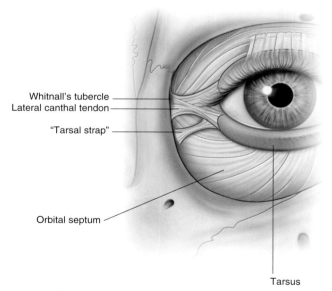

Whitnall's tubercle
Lateral canthal tendon
"Tarsal strap"
Orbital septum
Tarsus

Figure 26.6. The lateral canthal tendon inserts securely into the thickened periosteum overlying Whitnall's tubercle. The tarsal strap is a distinct anatomic structure that suspends the tarsus medial and inferior to the lateral canthal tendon to the lateral orbital wall, approximately 4 to 5 mm from the orbital rim. *(Reprinted from Neligan, P.C., Buck, D.W. [Eds.], 2013. Core Procedures in Plastic Surgery. Elsevier, 1–22.)*

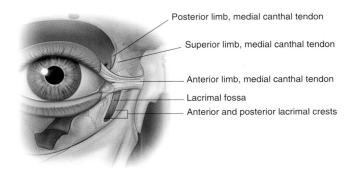

Figure 26.7. The medial canthal tendon envelops the lacrimal sac. It is tripartite, with anterior, posterior, and superior limbs. Like the lateral canthal tendon, its limbs are continuous with tarsal plates. The components of this tendon along with its lateral counterpart are enveloped by deep and superficial aspects of the orbicularis muscle. *(Adapted from Spinelli, H.M., 2004. Atlas of Aesthetic Eyelid and Periocular Surgery. Saunders, Philadelphia, 13.)*

Lacrimal/Eyelid Physiology

1. The lacrimal drainage system (see Figure 26.8)
   - Consists of the lacrima gland, punctum, ampulla, canaliculi, lacrimal sac, and nasolacrimal duct

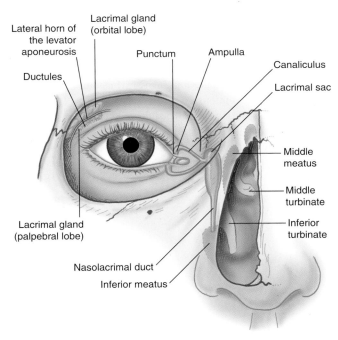

Figure 26.8. Cross section of the lower eyelid. *(Reprinted from Nerad, J.A., 2009. Techniques in Ophthalmic Plastic Surgery: A Personal Tutorial, 1st ed. Elsevier Health Sciences, Philadelphia, 43.)*

2. Eyelids open
   - The lacrimal puncta are open and in contact with the lacrimal lake at the medial aspect of the lower eyelid
   - The lacrimal sac is collapsed and empty, and the canaliculi are patent.

3. Eyelids closed
   - The lacrimal puncta are closed.
4. Normal tear flow
   - Opening the eyelids
     - The canaliculi open to allow collection of tears.
     - The lacrimal diaphragm returns to its resting position because the sphincter action of the oribularis is released.
     - Relaxation of the lacrimal diaphragm creates sufficient pressure to propel the tears from the lacrimal sac into the nasolacrimal duct.
   - Closing the eyelids
     - Tears are milked lateral to medial
     - The deep heads of the preseptal muscles contract, which
       - Shortens the canaliculi and closes their ampullae.
       - Pulls the lacrimal diaphragm laterally, creating negative pressure that opens the lacrimal sac, causing it to fill with tears
5. Lacrimal pump failure can be caused by anatomic obstruction and/or functional failure.
   - Functional failure may be due to a displaced punctum, eyelid laxity, weak orbicular muscle of the eye, or CN-VII palsy.
   - Anatomical obstruction may occur at any point along the lacrimal drainage pathway and may be congenital or acquired.
     - Primary acquired lacrimal duct obstruction: Occurs in elderly patients secondary to fibrosis
     - Secondary acquired obstruction may be caused by tumors, trauma, or mechanical obstruction.
6. Testing lacrimal function
   - Jones tests: Two tests used to evaluate for and discern among functional and obstructive etiologies of poor tear flow
     - Jones-I test: Fluorescein dye is injected into the punctum, and the examiner looks for presence of fluorescein dye drainage from the nose.
       - A positive test means that there is drainage.
       - A negative test means that there is no drainage and suggests an obstruction; requires a Jones-II test.
     - Jones-II test: Performed after a negative Jones-I test and involves cannulation of the punctum and irrigation with 1 mL of saline
       - If fluorescein-dye-stained fluid is now visualized at the inferior turbinate, there is partial obstruction of the lower canicular system (most likely at the level of the nasolacrimal duct).
       - If fluorescein-dye-stained fluid is found flowing retrograde within the tear sac, this suggests total obstruction of the nasolacrimal duct.
7. Treatment options for lacrimal pump failure
   - Can perform nasolacrimal duct dilation or stent placement in cases of distal functional pump failure.
     - Contraindicated in cases of complete obstruction
   - Conjunctivodacryocystorhinostomy (CDCR): Performed in cases of flaccid canaliculi, paralysis of the lacrimal pump,

and when the site of obstruction is proximal (punctum, canaliculi, lacrimal sac)

■ CDCR is not required when these structures are intact.

- Dacryocystorhinostomy (DCR): Performed in cases of distal obstruction (nasolacrimal duct)

Eyelid Evaluation

1. Visual acuity
   - Superior or lateral visual field loss suggests functional ptosis or pseudoptosis.
   - If superior visual field loss is present, test with the lid taped and untaped and document any improvement.
2. External examination
   - Should include examination of extra-ocular movements, pupil evaluation, signs of asymmetry, skin lesions, dry eye, conjunctivitis, and brow ptosis
      ■ Compensated brow ptosis: Constant frontalis m. contraction to elevate the ptotic brow
         ○ Important to consider because blepharoplasty alone in these patients could worsen the brow ptosis.
         ○ Diagnosed by evaluating the change in brow position with the patient in downward and frontal gaze
3. Eyelid ptosis: Defined by how much the upper limbus is covered by the lid margin at rest and forward gaze
   - Normal: 1 to 2 mm
   - Mild ptosis: 2 mm
   - Moderate: 3 mm
   - Severe: ≥4 mm
4. Eyelid laxity: Defined by relative relaxation of lid support structures and resting tone of the lid
   - Laxity determined by distance lid can be distracted away from the globe.
      ■ Mild: 1 to 2 mm
      ■ Moderate: 2 to 6 mm
      ■ Severe: >6 mm
   - Lid tone determined and graded according to the snap-back test
      ■ Snap-back test: Lid is distracted away from globe, held for a few seconds, and released. Measure the amount of time from release to the lid assuming its resting position, correlated with the degree of laxity and loss of muscle tone.
         ○ Grade 0 (normal): Lid returns to position immediately upon release
         ○ Grade I: Lid returns to position after ~2 to 3 seconds
         ○ Grade II: Lid returns to position after ~4 to 5 seconds
         ○ Grade III: >5 seconds for lid to return to position, or only occurs after blinking
         ○ Grade IV (severe): Lid never returns to position
5. Globe position: Determined by the position of anterior border of the globe relative to the most anterior point of the lateral orbital rim
   - Can be objectively measured using a Hertel exophthalmometer
      ■ Enophthalmos: <14 mm

■ Normal: 15 to 18 mm

■ Exophthalmos/proptosis: >18 mm

6. Levator function: Defined as the distance that the upper lid retracts when the globe moves from inferior gaze to upward gaze
   - Normal/excellent: 12 to 15 mm
   - Good: 8 to 12 mm
   - Fair: 5 to 7 mm
   - Poor: 2 to 4 mm
   - None: 0 mm
7. Tear production: Can elicit risk for postoperative dry eye
   - Schirmer test: After applying topical anesthetic, place filter paper strips in the lateral third of the lower eyelid, and the level of filter paper moisture is measured over time.
      ■ After 5 minutes, normal tear production should be >15 mm.
      ■ 5 to 10 mm indicates borderline tear production.
      ■ <5 mm indicates hyposecretion.

Blepharoptosis

1. Many etiologies
   - Congenital ptosis (see Figure 26.9)
      ■ Occurs in young patients
      ■ Defined by
         ○ Moderate-to-severe ptosis
         ○ Absent eyelid crease
         ○ Poor levator function
      ■ A child with progressive or acute symptoms suggests a possible tumor etiology (e.g., rhabdomyosarcoma); thus, magnetic resonance imaging (MRI) is indicated.
      ■ Treatment options
         ○ Observation can be tried for mild cases.
         ○ Frontalis sling performed for moderate-to-severe cases and in mild cases with persistent symptoms, to prevent amblyopia or other visual disturbances

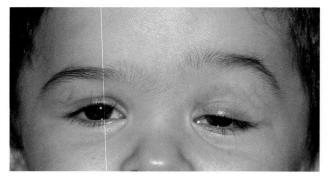

Figure 26.9. Unilateral congenital ptosis. *(Reprinted from Philandrianos, C., Galinier, P., Salazard, B., et al., 2009. J. Plast. Reconstr. Aesthet. Surg. 63 [5], 782–786.)*

- Senile/involutional ptosis
  - Occurs in elderly patients
  - Most commonly related to dehiscence or attenuation of the levator aponeurosis from the tarsal plate
  - Defined by
    - Upper eyelid ptosis
    - Superior migration of the upper eyelid crease
    - Abnormal levator function depending on severity of attenuation/dehiscence
      - The degree of levator function determines corrective options.
        - Levator plication (shortening)
        - Poor levator function: Frontalis suspension
        - Moderate function: Requires levator resection versus plication
        - Normal/excellent levator function: Levator aponeurosis reinsertion or plication, Fasanella-Servat procedure, or Müller's muscle resection (if only mild ptosis)
          - Fasanella does not address excess external skin.
- Horner syndrome
  - Occurs with disruption of sympathetic nerve action within the superior cervical ganglion
  - Defined by
    - Ptosis
    - Miosis
    - Anhidrosis
    - Normal eyelid crease position
- Myasthenia gravis
  - Occurs in young women or elderly men
  - Autoimmune disease caused by antibodies to the acetylcholine receptor at the postsynaptic neuromuscular junction
  - Defined by
    - Unilateral or bilateral ptosis that is exaggerated with fatigue
    - Diplopia with extraocular muscle involvement
  - Diagnosed by muscle fatigability on examination or pharmacologic testing (edrophonium test)
  - Treatment options
    - Acetylcholinesterase inhibitors (e.g., Neostigmine)
    - Immunosuppressants (e.g., prednisone, cyclosporine)
    - Thymectomy (high incidence of thymoma)
- Inadvertent chemodenervation of upper eyelid retractors
  - Can occur after Botox injection for glabellar rhytids secondary to medication diffusion
    - Treatment options
      - Observation
      - α-Adrenergic agonists (e.g., apraclonidine)
        - Stimulates Müller's muscle
- Compensated eyelid ptosis
  - Occurs when the frontalis muscles are used to elevate the eyebrows, resulting in functional improvement in visual fields and ptosis
    - Diagnosed by frontalis contraction and eyebrow elevation when the patient opens her eyes from the closed position

Upper Eyelid Procedures

1. Skin-only upper blepharoplasty: Excision of excess eyelid skin, with or without resection of orbicularis muscle, and/or manipulation of orbital fat
   - Generally indicated for patients with excess skin (dermatochalasis), normal ptosis, and normal levator function
   - Can be combined with levator techniques below in setting of ptosis
2. Blepharoptosis repair: Technique often determined by degree of ptosis and levator function
   - Fasanella-Servat: Full-thickness excision of conjunctiva, superior 3 mm of tarsus, and Müller's muscle
     - Indicated in patients with mild ptosis and good-to-excellent levator function
       - Disadvantage: Does not address excess external skin
   - Müller's muscle resection: Full-thickness excision of the conjunctiva and Müller's muscle, with sparing of the tarsus
     - Indicated in patients with mild ptosis and fair-to-good levator function
     - Leads to approximately 2 mm of lid elevation
     - Do not perform deep excision because levator muscle lies deep to Müller's muscle in this location.
       - Disadvantage: Does not address excess external skin
   - Levator aponeurosis reinsertion/advancement: Levator aponeurosis is advanced/resuspended to the tarsus
     - Indicated in patients with moderate ptosis and fair levator function
   - Frontalis suspension: The upper lid is connected to the brow using different sling materials (including fascia or synthetic materials) to allow frontalis m. contraction to aid in elevating the upper lid.
     - Indicated in patients with severe ptosis and poor levator function

Lower Eyelid Blepharoplasty

1. Can be approached through subciliary incision or transconjunctival incision
   - Subciliary incision allows removal of excess external skin.
   - Transconjunctival approach can be pre- or postseptal.
     - Often used for repositioning or manipulation of orbital fat compartments and release of arcus marginalis
2. Preoperative lower lid tone and laxity is important for determining additional necessary procedures.
   - Moderate-to-severe laxity (>6 mm distraction) and poor tone on snap-back test: Options include lateral canthoplasty and tarsal strip canthoplasty.
   - Mild-moderate laxity (>2 mm distraction) and poor-moderate tone: Options include horizontal wedge excision and orbicularis m. repositioning.

- If very minimal laxity, can consider temporary tarsorrhaphy for corneal protection
3. Complications
   - Lower eyelid malposition: Most common complication
     - Etiologies
       - Excessive scarring
       - Over-resection of skin
       - Over-resection of orbital fat
       - Imbrication of orbital septum
       - Orbicularis m. palsy
       - Edema
       - Hematoma
     - Risk factors
       - Malar hypoplasia
       - Proptosis
       - High myopia
       - Lower lid laxity
       - Thyroid ophthalmopathy
     - Treatment options
       - Early postoperative period: Downward massage, aggressive lubrication to protect the cornea
       - Persistent malposition may require secondary surgical intervention, depending on the cause.
   - Ectropion
     - Often secondary to lower lid laxity or lamellar scarring
     - In early postoperative period, can be managed with scar massage
     - If it persists after 6 to 9 months, consider surgical intervention depending on the likely cause.
       - For lower lid laxity: Consider canthoplasty
       - For cicatricial ectropion: Consider a scar release and skin graft
       - For midlamellar scarring: Consider lysis of adhesions and an interposition graft
       - For paralytic ectropion: Consider a tarsoligamentous sling that supports the medial and lateral canthus

Miscellaneous Eyelid Conditions

1. Epiblepharon (see Figure 26.10)
   - Most commonly occurs in the lower eyelids; may be congenital
   - More common in patients of Asian descent
   - Defined by
     - Excess pretarsal skin and orbicular muscle at the lower eyelid margin
     - Cilia inversion with contact against the globe
     - Accentuated in downward gaze
   - Treatment options
     - Observation in congenital cases because most resolve with facial growth
     - Surgical intervention indicated when the inverted eyelashes cause corneal injury and irritation
       - Surgery consists of resection of excess skin and orbicularis m., with placement of sutures between the tarsal plate and subcutaneous tissue to create adhesions.

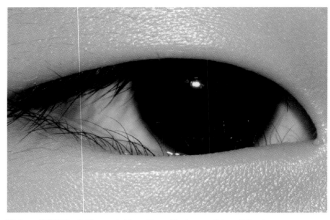

Figure 26.10. A 3-year-old male with lower lid epiblepharon. Note how the lower lid eyelashes are touching the cornea and conjunctiva. *(Reprinted from Kim, C., Shin, Y.J., Kim, N.J., et al., 2007. Conjunctival epithelial changes induced by Cilia in patients with epiblepharon or entropion. Am. J. Ophthalmol. 144 [4], 564–569.)*

2. Thyroid ophthalmopathy
   - Most common cause of proptosis and diplopia in adults
   - Symptoms include eyelid edema, conjunctival injection, lid lag, and proptosis.
   - Treatment is focused on management of underlying thyroid disorder.
3. Blepharospasm: Uncontrolled muscle contraction of the eyelid
   - Many causes, although etiology of many cases is unknown (idiopathic)
   - Botulinum toxin injection is the preferred treatment method for most patients.
4. Dry eye syndrome (dysfunctional tear syndrome)
   - Occurs as a result of deficient tear production leading to corneal irritation and can progress to corneal scarring
   - Can develop after eyelid surgery
     - Risk factors
       - Preoperative dry eye
       - Injury to orbicular oculi m.
       - Combined upper and lower blepharoplasty procedures
       - Hormone replacement therapy
       - Laser vision correction (Lasik) within 6 months of blepharoplasty
         - Affects tear production and corneal sensation
     - Consider eye lubrication pre- and postoperatively
5. Asian eyelids
   - No supratarsal crease secondary to a general lack of levator aponeurosis insertion into the dermis
   - Narrow pretarsal segment of the supratarsal lid fold when present secondary to a more caudal fusion of the orbital septum to the levator aponeurosis
   - More ROOF and SOOF fat when compared to the Caucasian eyelid
   - More likely to have epicanthal folds

6. Involutional entropion versus involutional ectropion
   - Difficult to discern in the static state because of the associated lower eyelid laxity in both cases
   - Diagnosis can be made on animation of the orbicularis m., because the lower eyelid inverts on attempted eyelid closure in cases of involutional entropion.
7. Hyphema is a traumatic hemorrhage of the anterior chamber of the eye.
8. Blepharochalasis: Inflammation of the eyelid characterized by recurrent episodic painless eyelid swelling
   - Over time, can progress to thin, atrophic eyelid skin, levator aponeurosis attenuation, and ptosis

Reconstruction

1. Reconstructive options are generally selected based on the lamellar components missing and the overall size of the defect.
   - Anterior lamellar defects (skin and orbicularis oculi m.)
     - Depending on size, options include
       - Secondary intent
       - Primary closure
       - Full-thickness skin grafts
       - Local flaps (e.g., cheek advancement, transposition flaps)
   - Posterior lamella defects
     - Conjunctival replacement
       - Mucosa graft (buccal mucosa, hard palate mucosa)
       - Conjunctival graft
     - Tarsal defects
       - Auricular or nasal septal cartilage grafts
   - Composite defects/eyelid margin defects
     - <25% (33% for upper lid): Direct layered closure
     - 25% to 50%: Lateral cantholysis with direct closure versus Hughes tarsoconjunctival flap
     - 50% to 75%: Tenzel flap, Hughes tarsoconjunctival flap
     - >75%: Cheek advancement flap with septal/auricular cartilage graft and lining graft.
2. Hughes tarsoconjunctival flap (see Figure 26.11)
   - A pedicled tarsoconjunctival flap from the upper eyelid is elevated and advanced to the lower lid defect to replace the posterior lamella and tarsus.
     - Take care to leave 3 to 4 mm of the upper tarsus intact to prevent loss of upper lid support.
     - Can reconstruct the anterior lamella by a cheek advancement flap or other local skin/muscle flap.
     - The flap pedicled is divided at 6 weeks.

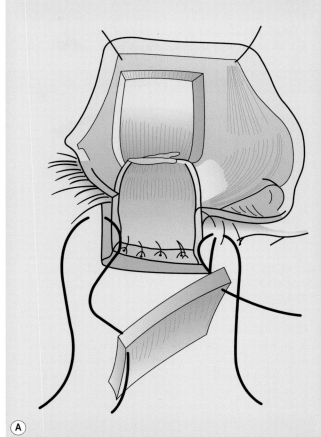

(A)

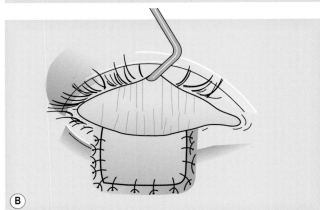

(B)

Figure 26.11. A, Tarsoconjunctival advancement flap for lower lid reconstruction (Hughes): This superiorly based advancement flap provides a conjunctival lining and tarsal support (posterior lamella) for the lower lid defect. **B,** The anterior lamella is reconstructed with a skin graft or flap. *(Reprinted from Herford, A.S., Cicciu, M., Clark, A., 2009. Traumatic eyelid defects: a review of reconstructive options. J. Oral Maxillofac. Surg. 67 [1], 3–9.)*

3. Tenzel semicircular flap (see Figure 26.12)
   - A semicircular rotation advancement musculocutaneous flap beginning at the level of the lateral canthus
   - Uses lateral orbit skin redundancy to advance into defect

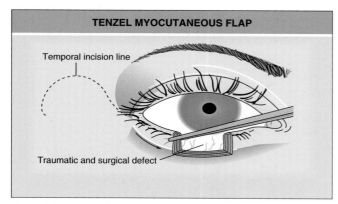

TENZEL MYOCUTANEOUS FLAP

Temporal incision line

Traumatic and surgical defect

Figure 26.12. Repair of a lower eyelid defect with the Tenzel myocutaneous flap. *(Reprinted from Yanoff, M., Duker, J.S. [Eds.], 2014. Ophthalmology, 4th ed. Elsevier, 1312–1317.)*

4. Cutler-Beard flap
   - Indicated for large central defects of the upper eyelid
   - Uses a full-thickness segment of the lower eyelid that is pedicled and passed under an intact lower lid margin bridge and inset into the defect
   - The flap pedicle is divided at 6 to 8 weeks.

Suggested Readings

Alghoul, M., Pacella, S.J., McClellan, T.W., et al., 2013. Eyelid reconstruction. Plast. Reconstr. Surg. 132 (2), 288e–302e.

Azurin, D.J., Versaci, A.D., 2010. Chapter 58: Eyelid reconstruction. In: Weinzweig, J. (Ed.), Plastic Surgery Secrets Plus, 2nd ed. Mosby, pp. 388–394.

Bashour, M., Vistnes, L.M. Upper eyelid reconstruction procedures, treatment, & Management. Found at: http://emedicine.medscape.com/article/1282054-treatment. Accessed on 8/14/14.

Bashour, M., Vistnes, L.M., Lower Lid Ectropion Blepharoplasty Workup. Found at: http://emedicine.medscape.com/article/1281565-workup. Accessed on 8/14/14.

Dudas, J.R., Hurst, E.A., 2014. Chapter 8: Eyelid (cancer and reconstruction). In: Woo, A.S., Shahzad, F., Synder-Warwick, A.K. (Eds.), Plastic Surgery Case Review: Oral Board Study Guide. Thieme, pp. 33–36.

Few, J., Ellis, M.E., 2013. Chapter 8: Blepharoplasty. In: Neligan, P.C. (Ed.), Plastic Surgery, 3rd ed. Elsevier, pp. 108–137.

Flowers, R.S., Smith, E.M., 2010. Chapter 75: Blepharoplasty. In: Weinzweig, J. (Ed.), Plastic Surgery Secrets Plus, 2nd ed. Mosby, pp. 487–497.

Gangopadhyay, N., Woo, A.S., 2014. Chapter 18: Lower lid ectropion (senile or paralytic). In: Woo, A.S., Shahzad, F., Synder-Warwick, A.K. (Eds.), Plastic Surgery Case Review: Oral Board Study Guide. Thieme, pp. 77–80.

Ge, N.N., McGuire, F., Dyson, S., et al., 2009. Nonmelanoma skin cancer of the head and neck II: surgical treatment and reconstruction. Am. J. Otolaryngol. 30 (3), 181–192.

Green, J.P., Charonis, G.C., Goldberg, R.A., 2013. Chapter 12: 11: Eyelid trauma and reconstruction techniques. In: Yanoff, M., Duker, J.S. (Eds.), Ophthalmology, 4th ed. Saunders, pp. 1312–1317.

Herford, A.S., Cicciu, M., Clark, A., 2009. Traumatic eyelid defects: a review of reconstructive options. J. Oral Maxillofac. Surg. 67 (1), 3–9.

Koh, K.S., Choi, J.W., Ishii, C.H., 2013. Chapter 10: Asian facial cosmetic surgery. In: Neligan, P.C. (Ed.), Plastic Surgery, 3rd ed. Elsevier, pp. 163–183.

Leedy, J.E., 2007. Chapter 78: Blepharoplasty. In: Janis, J.E. (Ed.), Essentials of Plastic Surgery, 1st ed. Quality Medical Publishing, pp. 795–807.

Lin, L.K., 2013. Chapter 2: Eyelid Anatomy and Function. In: Holland, E.J., Mannis, M.J., Lee, W.B. (Eds.). Ocular Surface Disease: Cornea, Conjunctiva, and Tear Film. Saunders, pp. 11–115.

Lisman, R.D., Lelli, G.J., 2009. Chapter 34: Treatment of blepharoplasty complications. In: Aston, S.J., Steinbrech, D.S., Walden, J.L. (Eds.), Aesthetic Plastic Surgery. Elsevier, pp. 393–408.

Neligan, P.C., Buck, D.W. (Eds.), 2013. Chapter 1: Blepharoplasty. In: Core Procedures in Plastic Surgery. Elsevier, pp. 1–22.

Nicoson, M.C., Myckatyn, T.M., 2014. Chapter 17: Lower lid ectropion (cicatricial). In: Woo, A.S., Shahzad, F., Synder-Warwick, A.K. (Eds.), Plastic Surgery Case Review: Oral Board Study Guide. Thieme, pp. 73–76.

Philandrianos, C., Galinier, P., Salazard, B., et al., 2009. Congenital ptosis: long-term outcome of frontalis suspension using autogenous temporal fascia or fascia lata in children. J. Plast. Reconstr. Aesthet. Surg. 63 (5), 782–786.

Potter, J.K., 2007. Chapter 30: Eyelid reconstruction. In: Janis, J.E. (Ed.), Essentials of Plastic Surgery, 1st ed. Quality Medical Publishing, pp. 287–294.

Sachanandani, N.S., Tenenbaum, M., 2014. Chapter 16: Aging upper face (brows and lids). In: Woo, A.S., Shahzad, F., Synder-Warwick, A.K. (Eds.), Plastic Surgery Case Review: Oral Board Study Guide. Thieme, pp. 69–72.

Trussler, A.P., Rohrich, R.J., 2008. Blepharoplasty. Plast. Reconstr. Surg. 121 (S1), 1–10.

Anatomy of the Nose

1. The nose is a system of two closely related layers.
   - Outer layer: Soft, elastic sleeve that slides over the semirigid inner framework
     - Skin/soft tissue: Thinner and more loosely attached over the cartilaginous and bony framework and thicker and more adherent over the nasal tip
     - Lower lateral cartilages (LLCs): Paired "alar cartilages" that contain medial, middle, and lateral crura that support the nasal tip and play a significant role in determining tip shape, size, and projection
   - Inner layer: Semirigid framework
     - Nasal bones make up the upper bony vault of the nasal dorsum and articulate with the upper lateral cartilages (ULCs) inferiorly and the nasal septum to form the "keystone area."
     - ULCs make up the cartilaginous midvault, articulate with the cephalic margin of the LLCs at the "scroll area," and contribute to the internal nasal valve (INV) (see below).
     - Septum: Formed by the perpendicular plate of the ethmoid bone; vomer, maxillary crest, crest of the palatine bone; and the septal or "quadrangular" cartilage; provides structural support to the nose and divides the airway
     - Nasal lining: Mucosal inner layer (see Figure 27.1)
2. Muscles of the nose: Crucial to dynamic function of the nasal valve and airway
   - Facial paralysis (cranial nerve [CN] VII) can cause nasal airway obstruction on side of lesion
   - Levator labii superioris: Dilates the nares; paralysis of this muscle shows collapse of the external valve.
   - Depressor septi nasi: Depresses nasal tip (see Figure 27.2)
3. Nasal valves
   - INV (between septum and ULC): 10 to 15 degrees; if <10 = spreader grafts.
     - Cottle maneuver positive
     - Contributes the most to nasal air-flow resistance
   - External nasal valve (ENV; at genu of LLC and nares): Often from **over-resection of LLC**; treatment: Alar batten grafts (see Figure 27.3)

4. Vascular supply to the nose
   - Nasal tip: Columellar artery (superior labial a. → facial a. → external carotid a.), lateral nasal a. (angular a. → facial a. → external carotid a.)
     - Limited dissection above the alar groove will spare injury to the lateral branch of the angular a., which could contribute to tissue loss if injured.
   - Nasal sidewall, dorsum: Angular a. and lateral nasal a.
     - The lateral nasal a. also perfuses the nasal tip during open rhinoplasty.
   - Posterior nasal septum: Sphenopalatine a.
   - Upper/central nasal septum: Posterior ethmoid a. (see Figure 27.4).
5. Sensory innervation of the nose
   - External branch of the anterior ethmoidal nerve: Nasal tip; vulnerable to damage during endonasal rhinoplasty procedures
     - Emanates from between the nasal bone and the lateral nasal cartilage, supplying sensation to the skin at the distal nasal dorsum and tip
   - Infraorbital nerve: Lower lateral half of the nose and columellar skin
   - Infratrochlear nerve: Cephalic portion of the nasal sidewalls and the skin overlying the radix
   - Supraorbital nerve also innervates the skin of the radix.
   - Supratrochlear nerve supplies sensation to the forehead skin.
   - Nasopalatine nerve branches from the pterygopalatine ganglion to innervate the inferior septum and travels through the incisive foramen to join the greater palatine nerve from the palate.
6. Nasal subunits
   - The nose is made up of 9 esthetic subunits.
     - Nasal sidewall (2)
     - Nasal dorsum
     - Nasal ala (2)
     - Soft triangle (2)
     - Columella
     - Nasal tip (see Figure 27.5)

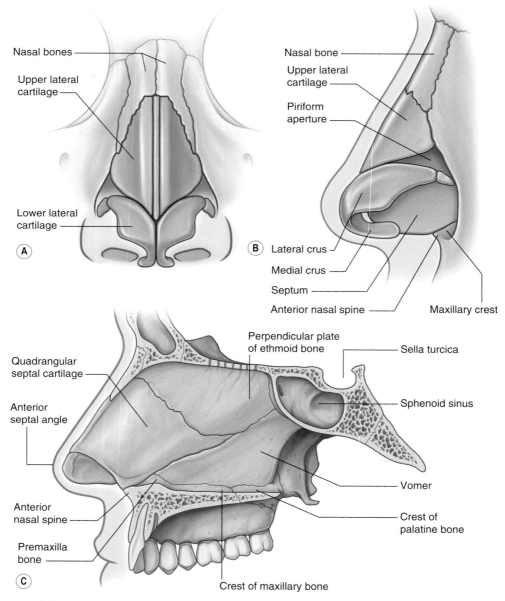

Figure 27.1. Diagrams of the cartilaginous and bony nose and septum. *(Reprinted from Aston, S.J., Steinbrech, D.S., Walden, J.L. [Eds.], 2009. Aesthetic Plastic Surgery. Saunders, 437–472.)*

Nasal Physiology

1. Nasal functions
   - Conduit for oxygenated air to enter the lungs
   - Reservoir for warming and humidifying inspired air
   - Provides sense of smell
   - Filters air and provides first-line immune defense against pathogens
2. Nasal airway obstruction
   - The middle meatus marks the path of primary air flow within the nasal cavity.
   - Causes of obstruction include any abnormality that results in increased nasal resistance and decreased air flow (e.g.,

septal deviation, trauma, nasal valve collapse, turbinate hypertrophy, intranasal masses)
   - INV incompetence and/or collapse thought to be the most common cause
   - In cases of rhinitis and turbinate hypertrophy, preoperative medical treatment is recommended.
     - Viral rhinitis: Oral/topical decongestants
     - Allergic rhinitis: Decongestants, 2nd-generation antihistamines, cromolyn sodium nasal spray (mast cell stabilizer), nasal topical corticosteroids, ipratropium bromide nasal spray (anticholinergic), and corticosteroid injection of the inferior turbinate

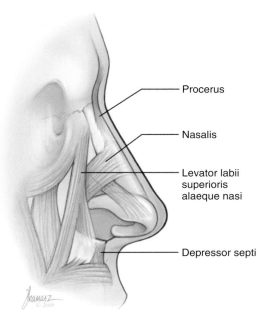

Figure 27.2. Profile view illustration depicting the nasal musculature. *(Reprinted from Guyuron, B. [Ed.], 2012. Rhinoplasty. Elsevier, 1–26.)*

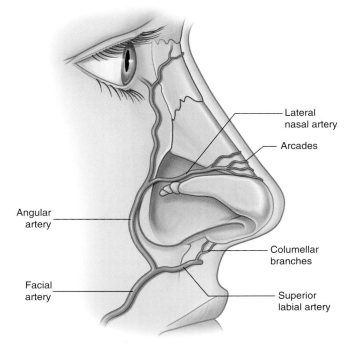

Figure 27.4. Nasal arterial anatomy. *(Reprinted from Aston, S.J., Steinbrech, D.S., Walden, J.L. [Eds.], 2009. Aesthetic Plastic Surgery. Saunders, 507–521.)*

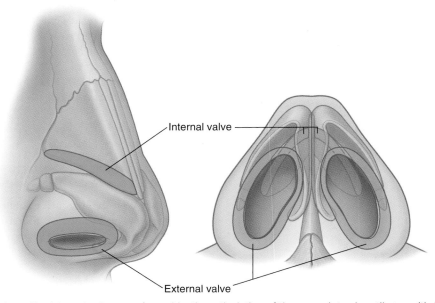

Figure 27.3. The nasal valves. The internal valves are formed by the articulation of the upper lateral cartilages with the anterior (dorsal) septal edge; the external valves are formed by the alar cartilage lateral crura and their associated, investing, soft-tissue cover. *(Reprinted from Neligan, P.C., Buck, D.W. [Eds.], 2013. Core Procedures in Plastic Surgery. Elsevier, 46–70.)*

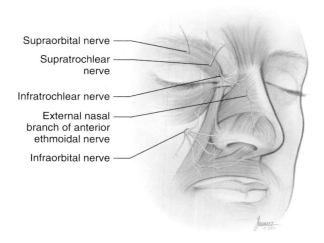

Figure 27.5. Illustration of the sensory innervation of the nose from cranial nerve (CN) V. *(Reprinted from Guyuron, B. [Ed.], 2012. Rhinoplasty. Elsevier, 1–26.)*

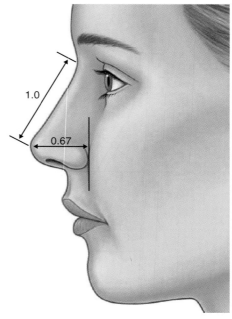

Figure 27.7. Byrd method of determining tip projection based on ideal nasal length. Using this method, the patient's nasal projection should be ⅔ their nasal length. *(Reprinted from Aston, S.J., Steinbrech, D.S., Walden, J.L. [Eds.], 2009. Aesthetic Plastic Surgery. Saunders, 507–521.)*

Ideal Nasal Analysis (see Figure 27.6)

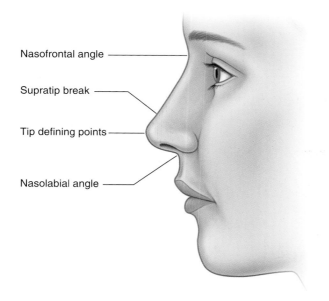

Figure 27.6. Important nasal landmarks in profile view. *(Reprinted from Aston, S.J., Steinbrech, D.S., Walden, J.L. [Eds.], 2009. Aesthetic Plastic Surgery. Saunders, 437–472.)*

1. Nasofrontal angle: Males, 120 to 130 degrees; females, 115 to 125 degrees
2. Nasolabial angle: Males, 90 to 95 degrees; females, 100 to 105 degrees
3. Tip projection: Equal to base width; 2/3 length of nose (see Figure 27.7)

4. Base width: Equal to intercanthal distance
5. Angle of divergence refers to middle crura of LLC; the angle between R and L middle crus while looking at the nose from anterioposterior (AP) view.
   - Ideal angle: 30 to 60 degrees; >60 = boxy tip, <30 = narrow tip (see Figure 27.8)
6. The nostrils should have a teardrop configuration, with the diameter of the base slightly larger than the diameter of the apex.
   - The long axis of each nostril points in a slight medial direction (see Table 27.1).

Preoperative Considerations

1. Perform a full and thorough nasal history, examination, and analysis and address areas of concern accordingly.
2. The aging nose is characterized by a drooping, elongated tip complex and is primarily related to loss of intrinsic LLC support.
3. The Asian nose is characterized by alar flare, a bulbous nasal tip, a short retracted columella (i.e., no columellar show), thick subcutaneous tissue, and a wide, flat nasal dorsum.
   - Basilar view shows a flat columella-alar triangle with hanging ala and a poorly projecting nasal tip.
   - Asian rhinoplasty generally focuses on augmentation of the nasal dorsum with an alloplastic implant.
     - Silicone implants are especially popular throughout Asia.
     - When performing nasal augmentation with an implant, consider thickness of the overlying soft tissues to reduce the risk for implant extrusion.

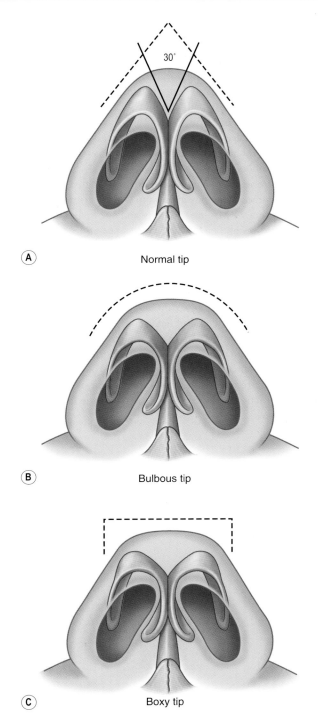

Figure 27.8. Variations in tip shape. *(Reprinted from Aston, S.J., Steinbrech, D.S., Walden, J.L. [Eds.], 2009. Aesthetic Plastic Surgery. Saunders, 507–521.)*

A — Normal tip

B — Bulbous tip

C — Boxy tip

Table 27.1 External Nasal Analysis

Frontal View	
Facial proportions	
Skin type/quality	Fitzpatrick type, thin or thick, sebaceous
Symmetry and nasal deviation	Midline, C-, reverse C-, S-, or S-shaped deviation
Bony vault	Narrow or wide, asymmetrical, short or long nasal bones
Midvault	Narrow or wide, collapse, inverted-V deformity
Dorsal esthetic lines	Straight, symmetrical or asymmetrical, well or ill defined, narrow or wide
Nasal tip	Ideal/bulbous/boxy/pinched, supratip, tip-defining points, infratip lobule
Alar rims	Gull shaped, facets, notching, retraction
Alar base	Width
Upper lip	Long or short, dynamic depressor septi muscles, upper lip crease
Lateral View	
Nasofrontal angle	Acute or obtuse, high or low radix
Nasal length	Long or short
Dorsum	Smooth, hump, scooped out
Supratip	Break, fullness, pollybeak
Tip projection	Over- or underprojected
Tip rotation	Over- or under-rotated
Alar-columellar relationship	Hanging or retracted alae, hanging or retracted columella
Periapical hypoplasia	Maxillary or soft-tissue deficiency
Lip-chin relationship	Normal, deficient
Basal View	
Nasal projection	Over- or underprojected, columellar-lobular ratio
Nostril	Symmetrical or asymmetrical, long or short
Columella	Septal tilt, flaring of medial crura
Alar base	Width
Alar flaring	Present or absent

Reprinted from Neligan, P.C., Buck, D.W. (Eds.), 2013. Core Procedures in Plastic Surgery. Elsevier, 46–70.

4. Hanging columella
   - Caused by prominence of the caudal septum or convexity of the caudal margin of the medial crura
   - Treatment options: Resection of the caudal margin of the medial crura

5. Esthetic septorhinoplasty carries a high incidence of postoperative patient dissatisfaction.
   - Patient selection is critical.
   - Most common reasons for dissatisfaction
     - Unsatisfactory results, irregularity of scar, continued nasal obstruction, asymmetry, emotional distress, and cost
     - Risk factors
       - Patients with unrealistic expectations or excessive demands
       - Patients who are indecisive, immature, secretive, motivated by others, or unstable

○ Patients with body dysmorphic disorder (BDD)
○ Patients who "doctor shop"
- Management of the dissatisfied patient: Frequent communication and follow-up
6. BDD
- Affects 7% to 15% of all plastic surgery patients
- Characterized by the degree of concern being much greater than the degree of deformity; patients are generally unaware that concerns are excessive.
  - The patient is preoccupied with appearance so much so that a significant amount of time is spent trying to camouflage or change the outward appearance with makeup.
- Most patients with BDD are single (70% never married) and up to 50% have suicidal ideation.
- Treatment recommendation: Refer to a psychiatrist to provide useful psychotherapy and pharmacotherapy.
7. Photographic documentation
- Critical for planning, demonstration of results, and patient education
- Lighting, patient positioning, and obtaining standard views are paramount for best photographic results.
  - Standard views include frontal, oblique, lateral, basilar, cephalic, and smiling lateral
  - Optimal orientation of the camera: Hold camera laterally and flash from the same side as the nose (e.g., in lateral and oblique views).

Rhinoplasty Techniques

1. Closed rhinoplasty
- Performed through infracartilaginous or intercartilaginous incisions without an "external" incision
- Advantages: Minimal scar visibility, less disruption of soft-tissue vascularity
- Disadvantages: Limited exposure and assessment of nasal structures in their "resting state"
2. Open rhinoplasty
- Performed through a columellar incision that extends into an infracartilaginous incision to "open" the nose
- Advantages: Maximal visibility and assessment of nasal structures in their "resting state," greatest degree of control over techniques
- Disadvantages: External scar burden, disrupts soft-tissue vascularity
3. Osteotomies (see Figure 27.9)
- Often performed to narrow and/or straighten the dorsum or correct an open roof deformity
- Can be performed externally or internally
  - An external osteotomy is performed at the nasofacial junction and has potential to injure the angular a.
- Infracturing of the nasal bones can result in nasal airway obstruction by inadvertently narrowing the INV (<10 to 15 degrees).

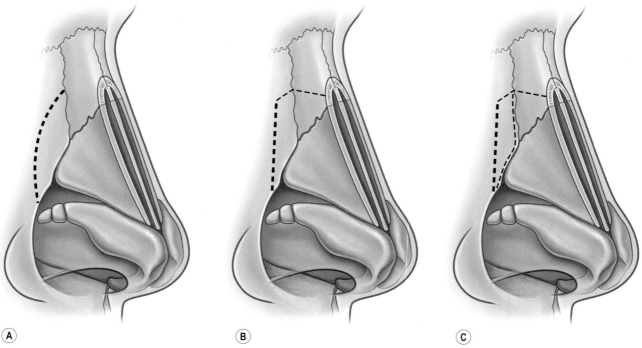

Figure 27.9. Percutaneous discontinuous lateral nasal osteotomies. **A,** Low to high; **B,** low to low; **C,** double level *(right)*. *(Reprinted from Neligan, P.C., Buck, D.W. [Eds.], 2013. Core Procedures in Plastic Surgery. Elsevier, 46–70.)*

4. Septoplasty
   - Often performed for deviated septum and nasal airway obstruction
   - Approached through an incision in the mucosa along the septal wall
     - Hemitransfixion incision: Performed on one side
     - Full-transfixion incision: Performed on both sides of the nasal wall
       - A full-transfixion incision can lead to decreased tip projection and loss of nasal tip support. In cases using a full-transfixion incision, a columellar strut graft is recommended to add tip support.
   - When removing the septum, take care to preserve a 1-cm "L strut" (1 cm of caudal septum and 1 cm of dorsal septum) to preserve strength.
     - If less than 1 cm is preserved, there is a risk of dorsal collapse and saddle nose deformity (see Figure 27.10).
5. Cephalic trim (see Figure 27.11)
   - The cephalic portion of the LLC can be trimmed to
     - De-rotate the nasal tip.
     - Reduce tip width.
     - Decrease tip fullness.
     - Increase the definition of the tip-defining points.
   - Over-resection of the LLC can lead to ENV obstruction.

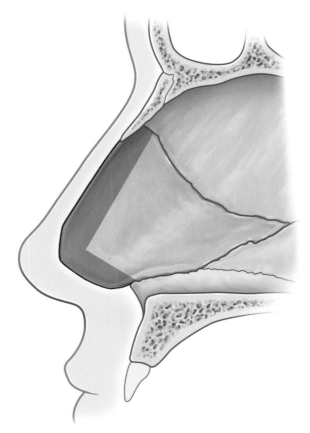

Figure 27.10. Submucoperichondrial dissection. *(Reprinted from Neligan PC, Buck DW, [Eds.], 2013. Core Procedures in Plastic Surgery. Elsevier, 46–70.)*

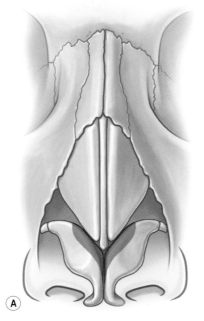 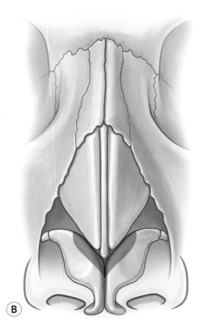

Figure 27.11. Cephalic trim. **A,** Lateral and middle crura; **B,** lateral crus *(right). (Reprinted from Neligan, P.C., Buck, D.W., [Eds.], 2013. Core Procedures in Plastic Surgery. Elsevier, 46–70.)*

6. Altering tip projection: Tip projection can be increased or decreased through varying techniques.
   - To increase tip projection
     - Cartilage tip graft
     - Medial crura sutures
     - Columellar strut graft
     - Resection of the caudal margin of the septum and cephalic alar rim can rotate the nasal tip and increase projection subtly.
   - To decrease tip projection
     - Resection of the lateral and medial crura
     - Resection of the nasal spine
     - Full-transfixion incision (through weakened tip support)

Common Grafts and Sutures Used in Rhinoplasty

1. Alar batten grafts: Cartilage placed as an only over the LLC and the "scroll area"
   - Useful to support the ENV, provide tip support, or de-rotate the tip (see Figure 27.12)
2. Alar rim grafts: Cartilage placed caudal to the LLC
   - Useful to correct alar retraction and/or asymmetry and support the ENV (see Figure 27.13)
3. Spreader grafts: Cartilage interposed between the ULC and septum
   - Useful to open the INV (increase INV angle) and straighten the dorsal esthetic line (see Figure 27.14)

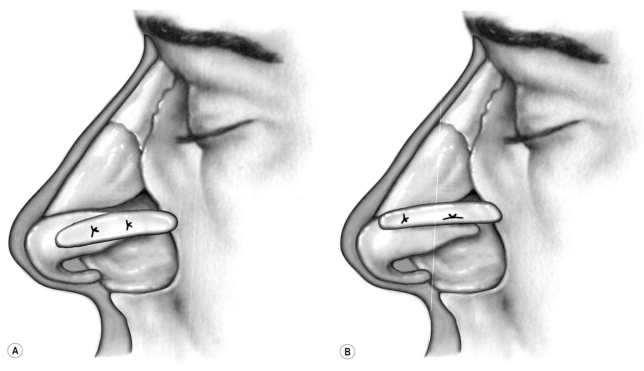

(A) (B)

Figure 27.12. A, The alar batten onlay graft provides strength to the lower lateral crus and the external nasal valve. **B,** The alar batten onlay graft can be placed superiorly over the scroll area to increase crural strength and decrease internal nasal valve collapse. *(Reprinted from Ansari, K., Asaria, J., Hilger, P., et al., 2008. Op. Tech. Otolaryn. Head Neck Surg. 19 [1], 42–58.)*

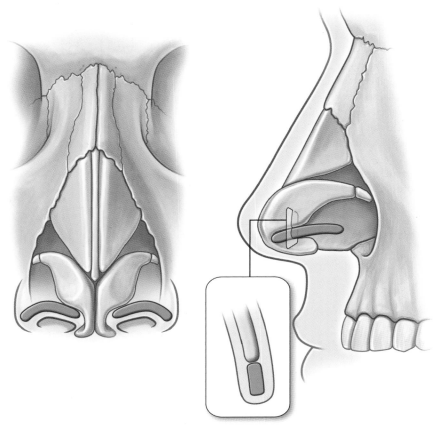

Figure 27.13. Alar contour grafts. *(Reprinted from Neligan, P.C., Buck, D.W. [Eds.], 2013. Core Procedures in Plastic Surgery. Elsevier, 46–70.)*

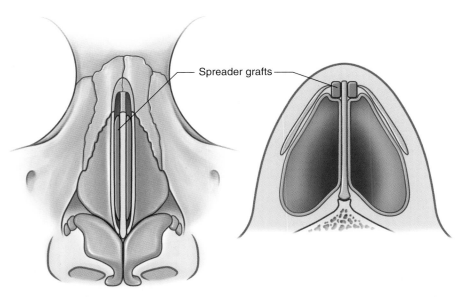

Spreader grafts

Figure 27.14. Dorsal spreader grafts. *(Reprinted from Neligan, P.C., Buck, D.W. [Eds.], 2013. Core Procedures in Plastic Surgery. Elsevier, 46–70.)*

4. Columellar strut graft: Cartilage placed between the medial crura of the LLC
    - Useful to maintain or increase tip projection, unify the nasal tip, and provide tip support (see Figure 27.15)
5. Lateral crural strut graft: Cartilage graft inserted between the vestibular lining and the lateral crus of the LLC
    - Useful to stent open a collapsed ENV (see Figure 27.16)
6. Transdomal sutures: Horizontal mattress sutures placed at the dome or in the lateral crus of the LLC
    - Useful to narrow the domes or the convexity of the lateral crura
    - May increase tip projection slightly (see Figure 27.17)
7. Interdomal sutures: Sutures between the domes
    - Useful to alter columellar projection and tip projection (see Figure 27.18)
8. Medial crural sutures: Sutures between the paired medial crura of the LLCs.
    - Useful to correct medial crura asymmetry, reduce flaring, narrow the columella, and stabilize a columellar strut (see Figure 27.19)
9. The columella-septal suture: Suture between the caudal septum and medial crura
    - Useful to rotate and strengthen the tip (see Figure 27.20)

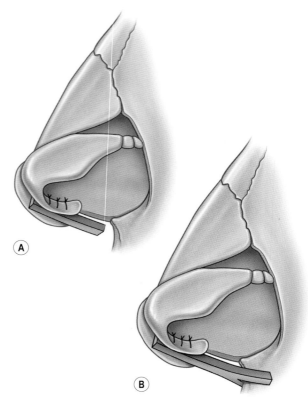

Figure 27.15. A, Floating and **B,** fixed columellar strut grafts. *(Reprinted from Neligan, P.C., Buck, D.W. [Eds.], 2013. Core Procedures in Plastic Surgery. Elsevier, 46–70.)*

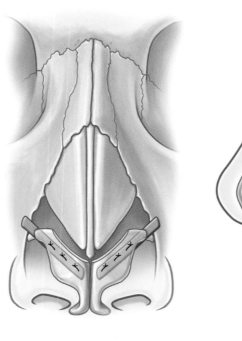
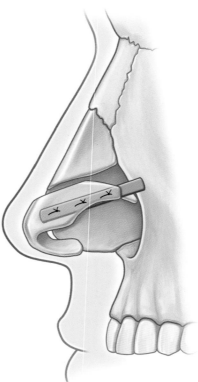

Figure 27.16. Lateral crural strut grafts. *(Reprinted from Neligan, P.C., Buck, D.W. [Eds.], 2013. Core Procedures in Plastic Surgery. Elsevier, 46–70.)*

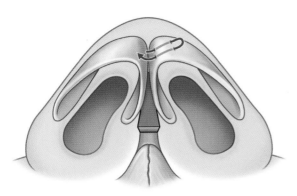

Figure 27.17. Nasal tip suturing technique (transdomal). *(Reprinted from Neligan, P.C., Buck, D.W. [Eds.], 2013. Core Procedures in Plastic Surgery. Elsevier, 46–70.)*

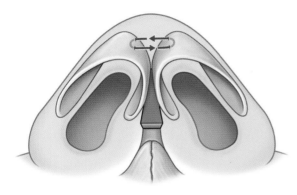

Figure 27.18. Nasal tip suturing technique (interdomal). *(Reprinted from Neligan, P.C., Buck, D.W. [Eds.], 2013. Core Procedures in Plastic Surgery. Elsevier, 46–70.)*

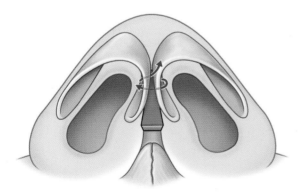

Figure 27.19. Nasal tip suturing technique (Medial crural). *(Reprinted from Neligan, P.C., Buck, D.W. [Eds.], 2013. Core Procedures in Plastic Surgery. Elsevier, 46–70.)*

Postoperative Nasal Deformities

1. Saddle nose deformity
   - Causes: Excessive resection of the nasal dorsum leading to a loss of dorsal support, septal hematoma, excessive resection of the septum, fracture of the perpendicular plate of the ethmoid, or comminution of the nasal bones during infracture

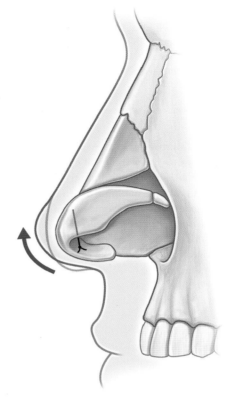

Figure 27.20. Intercrural septal suture. *(Reprinted from Neligan, P.C., Buck, D.W. [Eds.], 2013. Core Procedures in Plastic Surgery. Elsevier, 46–70.)*

   - Treatment: Often requires use of autografts (e.g., auricular cartilage, rib) or synthetic grafts
2. Open roof deformity
   - Causes: Aggressive dorsal hump reduction resulting in separation between the nasal sidewalls and the septum
   - Treatment: Nasal osteotomies with infracturing or placement of spreader grafts
3. Pollybeak deformity
   - Causes: Inadequate resection of the lower dorsal septum or excess scar formation in the supratip region
   - Characterized by fullness in the supratip area that pushes down and under; projects the nasal tip
   - Treatment
     - If <3 months since primary rhinoplasty, corticosteroid injection
     - If >3 months since primary rhinoplasty, nasal tip grafts
4. Rocker deformity
   - Causes: Medial osteotomy that goes beyond the thick radix bone, resulting in "rocking" of the fragment during manipulation
   - Characterized by contour deformity
   - Treatment: Repositioning of the cephalic fracture lower on the nasal bone
5. Inverted V deformity
   - Causes: Avulsion of the ULCs or excessive removal of the transverse portion of the ULC during dorsal septal resection
   - Treatment: Placement of spreader grafts

6. Minor contour deformities
   - If minor, and along the nasal dorsum and/or sidewalls, consider correction with soft-tissue fillers.
   - Inject filler into the subsuperficial musculoaponeurotic (sub-SMAS) plane just above the periosteum.

Other Postoperative Considerations

1. Anosmia
   - Some smell disturbance can occur after rhinoplasty.
   - This disturbance will not inhibit ability to smell irritants (e.g., ammonia), because this input travels through the trigeminal n., which is not injured during rhinoplasty.
   - If a patient complains of anosmia following rhinoplasty, including irritants, consider malingering.
2. Acute periostitis
   - Characterized by acute erythema of the nasal dorsum after dorsal hump reduction
   - Caused by retained shavings after dorsal rasping or saw osteotomy that act as a nidus for infection
   - Treatment: Oral antibiotics
     - After the erythema resolves, any residual dorsal prominence can be excised (typically wait 8 to 12 months after the initial operation).
3. Edema
   - Postoperative edema is common and can persist for several months
   - Perioperative steroid administration has been shown to decrease postoperative edema and ecchymosis.
     - Extended dosing is better than one-time dosing.

Nasal Reconstruction

1. Reconstructive options are dependent on the defect location and depth.
   - Focus analysis of the defect on location, cover, lining, and support
   - Some surgeons advocate subunit reconstruction when the defect covers ≥50% of a particular subunit.
2. Superficial, small defects (intact cartilage framework)
   - Upper 2/3rds of the nose is characterized by thin skin and is amenable to full-thickness grafts.
   - Small wounds of the sidewall or medial canthal region can be allowed to heal by secondary intent (e.g., wounds <0.5 cm in size).
   - Local flaps may also be used (especially for wounds <1.5 cm in size).
     - Dorsal nasal flap (see Figure 27.21)
       - Vascular supply: Angular a.
       - Useful option for defects of the dorsal midline (up to 2 cm in size)
       - May elevate the nasal tip and alter tip rotation

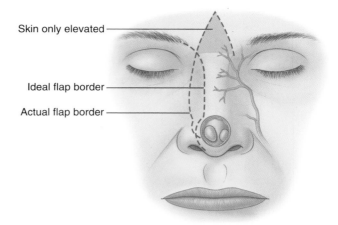

Figure 27.21. The dorsal nasal flap is based on an axial vessel and may cover defects up to 2 cm in diameter. *(Reprinted from Burget, G.C., Menick, F.J., 1994. Aesthetic Reconstruction of the Nose. Mosby, St Louis; with permission.)*

- Bilobed flap (see Figure 27.22)
  - Useful option for nasal tip and alar defects <1.5 cm in size

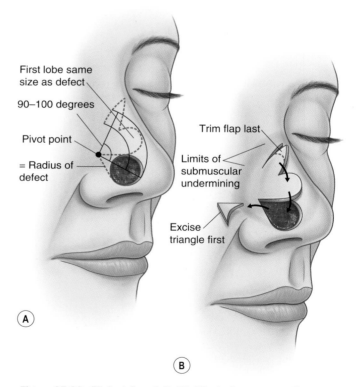

Figure 27.22. Bilobed flap. **A,B,** Zitelli's design removes the burrows triangle initially to improve the ease of flap rotation and minimize donor site contour deformities. The first lobe for rotation is set at the same size as the defect, in order to avoid distortion. The second limb is designed such that its central portion or axis represents an arc of rotation from 90 to 100 degrees. The bilobed flap is best used in defects <1.5 cm in diameter. *(**A,B,** Reprinted from Burget, G.C., Menick, F.J., 1994. Aesthetic Reconstruction of the Nose. Mosby, St Louis; Beahm, E.K., Walton, R.L., Burget, G.C., Concepts in nasal reconstruction. In: Butler, C.E., Fine, N.A. [Eds.], 2008. Principles of Cancer Reconstructive Surgery. Springer, New York; with permission.)*

- Nasolabial flap (see Figure 27.23)
  ○ Vascular supply: Perforators from the facial and angular arteries
  ○ Donor site closure occurs within the nasolabial fold.
  ○ Can be staged with pedicle division
  ○ Useful for defects of the lateral nose, ala, and total alar reconstruction

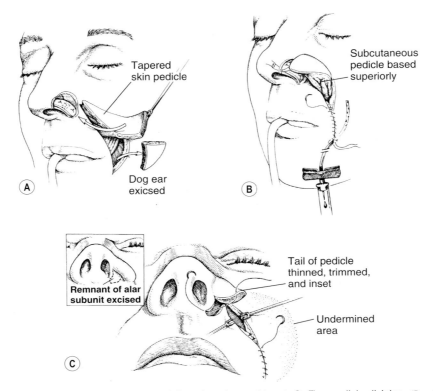

Figure 27.23. Subunit nasolabial two-stage flap. **A,B,** Initial flap elevation and inset. **C,** Flap pedicle division. *(Reprinted from Burget, G.C., Menick, F.J., 1994. Aesthetic Reconstruction of the Nose. Mosby, St Louis; with permission.)*

- Forehead flap (particularly for defects >1.5 cm in size, defects of the nasal tip, and composite defects)
  ○ Vascular supply: Supratrochlear vessels
  ○ Workhorse flap for large nasal tip defects and total nasal reconstruction
  ○ Can be extended and folded to provide nasal lining
  ○ Staged reconstruction requiring a separate pedicle division (typically 3 weeks)
  ○ For composite reconstruction, requires additional stages including flap thinning and cartilage graft placement before pedicle division (see Figure 27.24)
3. Small (<1.5 cm) full-thickness defects of the alar rim
   - Classic wound for composite graft from the helical root
4. Composite/full-thickness defects require reconstruction of the nasal lining, support, and skin.
   - Options for nasal lining reconstruction
     - Mucoperichondrial flap from the nasal septum
       ○ Vascular supply: Superior labial arteries
       ○ Can be used as a composite graft by including septal cartilage ("septal pivot flap") (see Figure 27.25)

- Folded forehead flap or skin-grafted forehead flap
- Cutaneous turnover flaps from adjacent skin
- Nasolabial flap
- Facial artery myomucosal (FAMM) flap
- Radial forearm free flap
- Options for support
  - Septal cartilage
  - Auricular cartilage (e.g., concha)
  - Rib cartilage or osteochondral rib grafts
- Options for skin
  - As above; forehead flap is the workhorse.
5. Rhinophyma
   - Localized nasal soft-tissue swelling secondary to fibrosis, sebaceous hyperplasia, and lymphedema
   - May develop spontaneously or in patients with a history of acne rosacea
   - Male predilection
   - Occasionally degenerates into a skin malignancy
   - Treatment options: Tangential surgical excision and/or laser ablation and electrosurgical excision

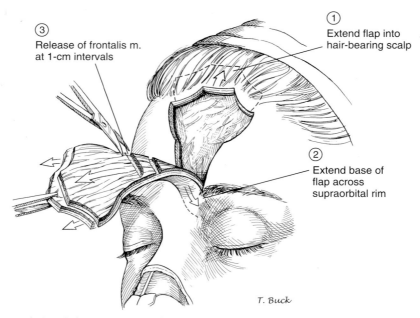

③ Release of frontalis m. at 1-cm intervals

① Extend flap into hair-bearing scalp

② Extend base of flap across supraorbital rim

T. Buck

Figure 27.24. Three ways to gain length for a paramedian forehead flap: **1,** Extend the flap into the hair-bearing scalp and depilate the flap; **2,** extend the flap 1.5 cm over the orbital rim, lifting the eyebrow with the flap, if necessary; and **3,** score only the frontalis muscle at 1-cm intervals, allowing the flap to expand up to 1.5 cm longitudinally. *(Reprinted from Mathes, S. [Ed.], 2006. Plastic Surgery, 2nd ed. WB Saunders, Philadelphia.)*

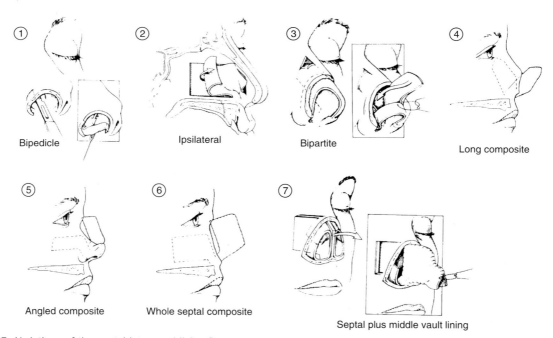

① Bipedicle   ② Ipsilateral   ③ Bipartite   ④ Long composite

⑤ Angled composite   ⑥ Whole septal composite   ⑦ Septal plus middle vault lining

Figure 27.25. Variations of the septal intranasal lining flaps. *(Reprinted from Burget, G.C., Menick, F.J., 1994. Aesthetic Reconstruction of the Nose. Mosby, St Louis; with permission.)*

Suggested Readings

Ansari, K., Asaria, J., Hilger, P., et al., 2008. Grafts and implants in rhinoplasty: techniques and long-term results. Op. Tech. Otolaryn. Head Neck Surg. 19 (1), 42–58.

Aston, S.J., Martin, J., 2009. Chapter 37: Primary closed rhinoplasty. In: Aston, S.J., Steinbrech, D.S., Walden, J.L. (Eds.), Aesthetic Plastic Surgery. Saunders, pp. 437–472.

Beahm, E., Walton, R.L., 2009. Chapter 4: Nasal reconstruction. In: Butler, C.E. (Ed.), Nasal Reconstruction. Elsevier, pp. 73–126.

Berth-Johns, J., 2014. Chapter 211: Rhinophyma. In: Lebwohl, M.G., Heymann, W.R., Berth-Jones, J., et al. (Eds.), Treatment of Skin Disease: Comprehensive Therapeutic Strategies, 4th ed. Elsevier, pp. 677–678.

Chapter 3: Rhinoplasty. In: Neligan, P.C., Buck, D.W. (Eds.), 2013. Core Procedures in Plastic Surgery. Elsevier, pp. 46–70.

Daniel, R.K., Brenner, K.A., 2009. Chapter 39: Secondary rhinoplasty. In: Aston, S.J., Steinbrech, D.S., Walden, J.L. (Eds.), Aesthetic Plastic Surgery. Saunders, pp. 481–494.

DeRosa, J., Toriumi, D., 2010. Chapter 78: Rhinoplasty. In: Weinzweig, J. (Ed.), Plastic Surgery Secrets Plus, 2nd ed. Mosby, pp. 516–525.

Fernandes, S.V., Meyers, A., medicine.com. Found at: http://emedicine .medscape.com/article/843439-overview#a17. Accessed on: September 12, 2014.

Galdino, G.M., DaSilva, D., Gunter, J.P., 2001. Digital photography for rhinoplasty. Plast. Reconstr. Surg. 109 (4), 1421–1434.

Guyuron, B., 2012. Rhinoplasty. Saunders, pp. 1–448.

Guyuron, B., Rowe, D.J., 2009. Chapter 42: Correction of the deviated septum. In: Aston, S.J., Steinbrech, D.S., Walden, J.L. (Eds.), Aesthetic Plastic Surgery. Saunders, pp. 523–530.

Hong Roy, W., Menick, F., 2010. Chapter 57: Nasal reconstruction. In: Weinzweig, J. (Ed.), Plastic Surgery Secrets Plus, 2nd ed. Mosby, pp. 381–387.

Janis, J.E., Ahmad, J., Rohrich, R.J., 2011. Chapter 55: Primary rhinoplasty. In: Nahai, F. (Ed.), The Art of Aesthetic Surgery, 2nd ed. Quality Medical Publishing, pp. 1895–1974.

Marin, V.P., Cochran, C.S., Gunter, J.P., 2009. Chapter 41: Anatomic approach for tip problems. In: Aston, S.J., Steinbrech, D.S., Walden, J.L. (Eds.), Aesthetic Plastic Surgery. Saunders, pp. 507–521.

Rohrich, R.J., Adams, W.P., Pessa, J.E., et al., 2011. Chapter 53: Applied anatomy of the nose. In: Nahai, F. (Ed.), The Art of Aesthetic Surgery: Principles and Techniques, 2nd ed. QMP, pp. 1859–1873.

Sandel, H.D., Meyers, A.R., Polly Beak Deformity in Rhinoplasy. Emedicine. com. Found at: http://emedicine.medscape.com/article/841075-overview. Accessed on: September 12, 2014.

Tabbal, N., Bogdan, M., 2009. Chapter 38: Primary open rhinoplasty. In: Aston, S.J., Steinbrech, D.S., Walden, J.L. (Eds.), Aesthetic Plastic Surgery. Saunders, pp. 473–479.

Tebbets, J.B., 2006. Open and closed rhinoplasty (minus the "versus"): analyzing processes. Aesthet. Surg. J. 26 (4), 456–459.

Toriumi, D.M., Checcone, M., 2009. Chapter 44: The Asian rhinoplasty. In: Aston, S.J., Steinbrech, D.S., Walden, J.L. (Eds.), Aesthetic Plastic Surgery. Saunders, pp. 555–571.

Rhytidectomy and Neck Rejuvenation

Essential Facial Anatomy

1. Continuous facial layers (see Figure 28.1)
2. Nerves
   - Motor nerve innervation of the muscles of facial expression (see Table 28.1 and Figure 28.2)
   - Sensory innervation of the face and neck (see Figure 28.3)
3. Anatomy of the aging face (see Figure 28.4)

Rhytidectomy

1. Techniques (see Table 28.2 and Figures 28.5-28.10)
2. Preoperative considerations
   - Blood pressure control
   - Stop all antiplatelet and anticoagulant medications at least 7 to 10 days preoperatively.
   - Smoking cessation at least 3 to 4 weeks before surgery and after surgery to reduce the risk of facial skin flap necrosis
3. Complications
   - Hematoma
     - The most common facelift complication (reported to occur in 2% to 3% of women and up to 8% of men)
     - Symptoms: Unrelenting, asymmetric ear and facial pain
     - Risk factors
       - Hypertension
       - Male gender
     - Treatment
       - Early: Operative evacuation
       - Late (days after surgery with no skin compromise): Attempt aspiration.
   - Skin loss
     - Risk factors: Excess tension, thin flaps, hematoma, tight dressings, smoking
     - Frequently occurs in the retroauricular location
     - Treatment: In general, treat skin loss conservatively (e.g., antibiotic ointment, silver sulfadiazine), with possible scar revision at a later date. If infection is present, debridement may be necessary and large areas may require skin grafting.

- Alopecia
  - Etiology: Excess tension at the incision, direct injury to follicles
    - Beveling during incision placement within the hair will reduce the risk of alopecia by promoting hair growth within the scar.
  - Secondary facelifts have a high risk for causing greater distortion of the hairline; thus, use a new incision for these procedures.
  - Large areas of alopecia may require hair transplantation, scalp rotation flaps, or even scalp expansion at a later date.
- Nerve injury
  - In general, nerve palsy following facelift procedures is managed with initial observation unless known direct nerve injury has occurred.
  - If direct injury occurs during surgery, primary repair of the nerve and/or primary grafting is recommended.
- Infection
  - Treat infections with antibiotics to reduce the risk of subsequent skin loss and scarring.
  - Rarely, pseudomonas infection can occur, particularly in patients who are colonized with pseudomonas species within the ear canal (e.g., swimmers).
    - For these patients, add ciprofloxacin for coverage.
- Malar hollowing secondary to malar fat pad resorption
  - Secondary to interruption of the angular a. during dissection

Necklift

1. Preoperative considerations
   - Degree of skin laxity
   - Cervicomental angle
   - Platysmal banding
   - Presence of excess submental fat
   - Chin position
   - Submandibular glands
   - Hyoid bone, thyroid cartilage (see Figures 28.11-28.13)

Text continued on page 292

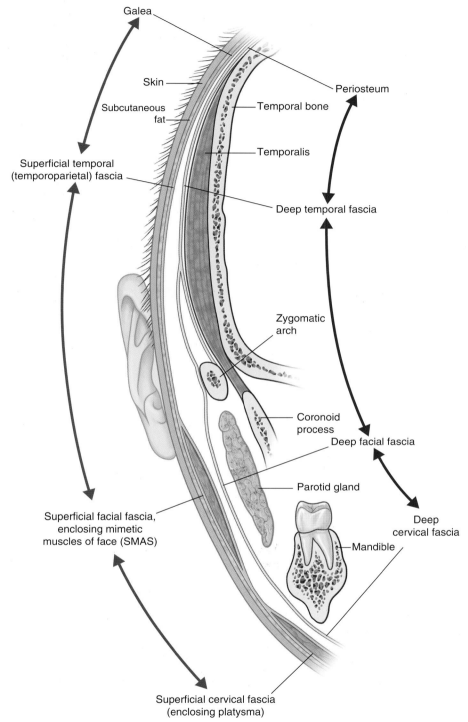

Figure 28.1. The facial layers of the scalp, face, and neck. *SMAS,* Superficial muscular aponeurotic system. *(Reprinted from Neligan, P.C., Rodriguez, E.D. [Eds.], 2013. Plastic Surgery, vol. 3, 3rd ed. Elsevier, 1–22.)*

Table 28.1 Extratemporal Facial Nerve Branches

NERVE BRANCH	LOCATION	INNERVATED MUSCLES	BRANCH INJURY	NOTES
Temporal/frontal	Pitanguy's line (0.5 cm below tragus to 1 cm above and lateral to brow); often travels with "sentinel vein"; deep to SMAS at level of the zygoma and deep to temporoparietal fascia above zygoma	Frontalis muscle, orbicularis oculi	Inability to elevate the brow, weak eyelid closure	Often neurapraxia injury from stretch; susceptible to injury at level of the zygoma with sub-SMAS techniques; neuropraxia
Zygomatic	Pierce the deep parotidomasseteric fascia 4 cm anterior to the tragus and travel toward lower lid and midcheek	Lower orbicularis oculi (primarily); also some innervation of zygomaticus major, buccinator, orbicularis oris, levator labii	Often asymptomatic because of arborization with buccal branch	
Buccal	Pierce deep parotidomasseteric fascia at anterior border of masseter	Orbicularis oculi, zygomaticus major and minor, levator labii superioris, buccinator, orbicularis oris	Often asymptomatic because of arborization with buccal branch; occasional inability to compress cheeks	Most common motor nerve injury with facelift
Marginal mandibular	Deep to platysma, can travel up to 3 to 4 cm below the mandibular border	Lower lip depressors, mentalis, orbicularis	Inability to depress lower lip (injured side higher during smile) or to purse lips	Treatment: Observation unless known direct injury; Botox to uninjured side can improve symmetry
Cervical	Deep to platysma, below mandibular border	Platysma	Inability to depress lower lip (pseudoparalysis of marginal mandibular n.)	Treatment: Observation

SMAS, *Superficial muscular aponeurotic system.*

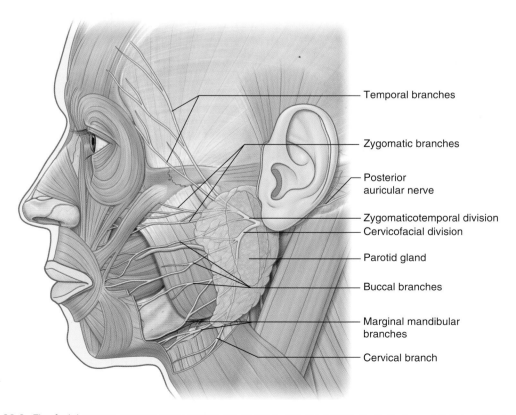

Figure 28.2. The facial nerves. *(Reprinted from Neligan, P.C., Rodriguez, E.D. [Eds.], 2013. Plastic Surgery, vol. 3, 3rd ed. Elsevier, 1–22.)*

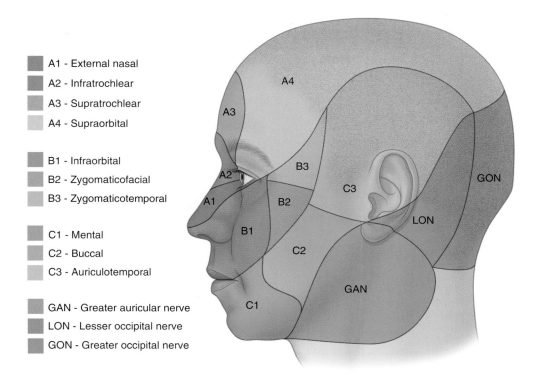

Figure 28.3. The sensory supply of the face. *(Reprinted from Neligan, P.C., Rodriguez, E.D. [Eds.], 2013. Plastic Surgery, vol. 3, 3rd ed. Elsevier, 1–22.)*

Legend:

A1 - External nasal
A2 - Infratrochlear
A3 - Supratrochlear
A4 - Supraorbital

B1 - Infraorbital
B2 - Zygomaticofacial
B3 - Zygomaticotemporal

C1 - Mental
C2 - Buccal
C3 - Auriculotemporal

GAN - Greater auricular nerve
LON - Lesser occipital nerve
GON - Greater occipital nerve

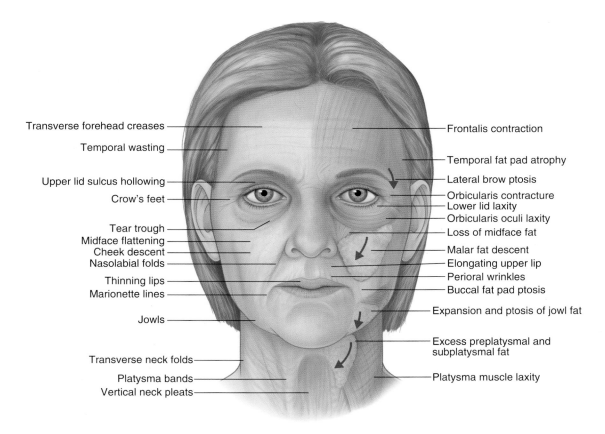

Labels:
- Transverse forehead creases
- Temporal wasting
- Upper lid sulcus hollowing
- Crow's feet
- Tear trough
- Midface flattening
- Cheek descent
- Nasolabial folds
- Thinning lips
- Marionette lines
- Jowls
- Transverse neck folds
- Platysma bands
- Vertical neck pleats
- Frontalis contraction
- Temporal fat pad atrophy
- Lateral brow ptosis
- Orbicularis contracture
- Lower lid laxity
- Orbicularis oculi laxity
- Loss of midface fat
- Malar fat descent
- Elongating upper lip
- Perioral wrinkles
- Buccal fat pad ptosis
- Expansion and ptosis of jowl fat
- Excess preplatysmal and subplatysmal fat
- Platysma muscle laxity

Figure 28.4. The aging face exhibits changes in the skin, superficial wrinkles, deeper folds, soft-tissue ptosis, loss of volume in the upper third and middle third, and increased volume in the lower third. *(Reprinted from Neligan, P.C., Warren, R.J. [Eds.], 2013. Plastic Surgery, vol. 2, 3rd ed. Elsevier, 184–207.)*

Table 28.2 Facelift Techniques

TECHNIQUE	DESCRIPTION	ADVANTAGES/DISADVANTAGES
Subcutaneous facelift	Dissection and tightening of excess skin only	Advantages: Safe, rapid recovery Disadvantages: Recurrence of ptosis because tightening relies on skin tension alone
SMAS plication	Dissection in subcutaneous plane with suture plication of the SMAS over the parotid gland	Advantages: Relatively safe, long-lasting results without need for sub-SMAS dissection Disadvantages: Potential loss of effect from suture failure
MACS lift	Limited preauricular/pretemporal hairline incision with skin elevation and purse-string suture of lower SMAS to deep temporal fascia (extended MACS lift places a 3rd suture in the SMAS to suspend the malar fat pad)	Advantages: Similar to SMAS plication, but firmer point of fixation to deep temporal fascia Disadvantages: Similar to SMAS plication
Subcutaneous facelift with SMASectomy	Similar dissection as SMAS plication, but limited strip of SMAS is removed obliquely across the cheek, and the defect is closed primarily with sutures	Advantages: Allows for skin and SMAS to be moved in different vectors, more secure than plication, more rapid than sub-SMAS lifts Disadvantages: Possible nerve injury
Deep plane facelift	Skin, fat, and SMAS are elevated in a single layer	Advantages: Long-lasting results, retaining ligaments are thoroughly released Disadvantages: Potential for nerve injury, more complex than supra-SMAS techniques above
Subperiosteal facelift	Dissection of the midface in a subperiosteal plane; occasionally adds a lower lid or intraoral incision	Advantages: Deep to all critical structures, relatively short incision, no tension on skin, can combine rejuvenation of lower lid and brow Disadvantages: Relatively complex procedure, limited effect on lower face/neck, and excess skin

MACS, *Minimal access cranial suspension;* SMAS, *superficial muscular aponeurotic system.*

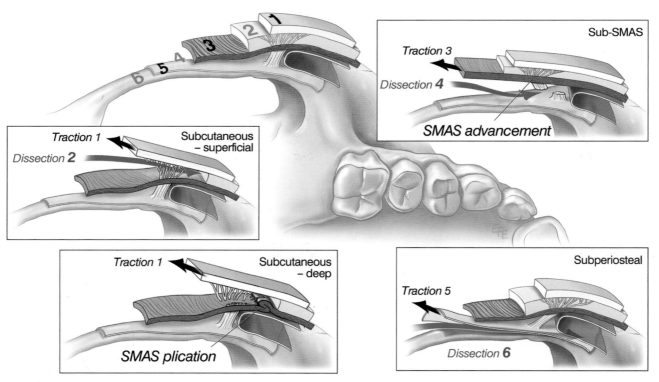

Figure 28.5. The alternative levels for dissection and redraping in facelifts. Dissection can be performed through any one of three alternate layers, namely, subcutaneous *(layer 2)*, sub-SMAS *(layer 4)*, and subperiosteal *(layer 6)* (for the upper two-thirds of the face). Redraping is performed on the mobilized layer according to the dissection plane. These are skin *(layer 1)*, SMAS *(layer 3)*, and periosteum *(layer 5)*. A subcutaneous dissection *(2)* allows not only redraping of the mobilized layer *1* but also tightening of the surface of the revealed deeper layer SMAS, where it overlies a space. *SMAS, Superficial muscular aponeurotic system. (Reprinted from Aston, S.J., Steinbrech, D.S., Walden, J.L. [Eds.], 2009. Aesthetic Plastic Surgery. Saunders, 53–71.)*

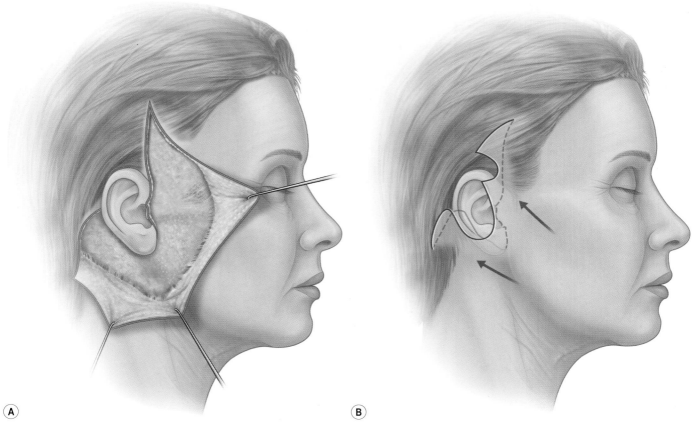

Figure 28.6. Subcutaneous facelift. *(Reprinted from Neligan, P.C., Warren, R.J. [Eds.], 2013. Plastic Surgery, vol. 2, 3rd ed. Elsevier, 208–215.)*

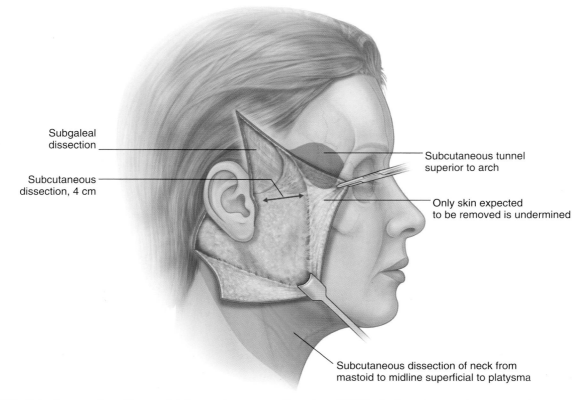

Subgaleal dissection

Subcutaneous dissection, 4 cm

Subcutaneous tunnel superior to arch

Only skin expected to be removed is undermined

Subcutaneous dissection of neck from mastoid to midline superficial to platysma

Figure 28.7. Subcutaneous flap with superficial muscular aponeurotic system (SMAS) plication. *(Reprinted from Neligan, P.C., Warren, R.J. [Eds.], 2013. Plastic Surgery, vol. 2, 3rd ed. Elsevier, 208–215.)*

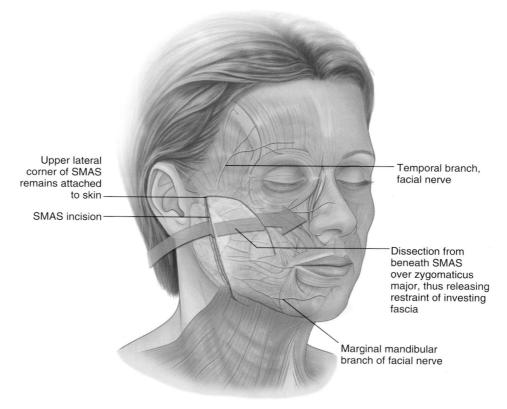

Upper lateral
corner of SMAS
remains attached
to skin

SMAS incision

Temporal branch,
facial nerve

Dissection from
beneath SMAS
over zygomaticus
major, thus releasing
restraint of investing
fascia

Marginal mandibular
branch of facial nerve

Figure 28.8. Subcutaneous flap with loop sutures for minimal access cranial suspension (MACS) lift. *SMAS,* Superficial muscular aponeurotic system. *(Reprinted from Neligan, P.C., Warren, R.J. [Eds.], 2013. Plastic Surgery, vol. 2, 3rd ed. Elsevier, 208–215.)*

Figure 28.9. Subcutaneous flap with superficial muscular aponeurotic system (SMAS) excision (SMASectomy). *(Reprinted from Neligan, P.C., Warren, R.J. [Eds.], 2013. Plastic Surgery, vol. 2, 3rd ed. Elsevier, 208–215.)*

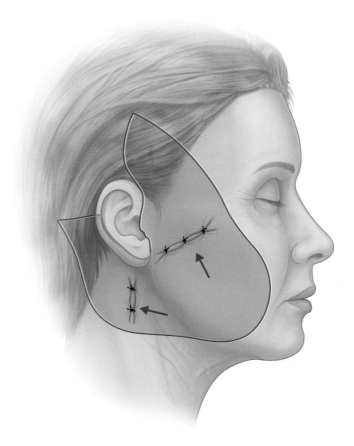

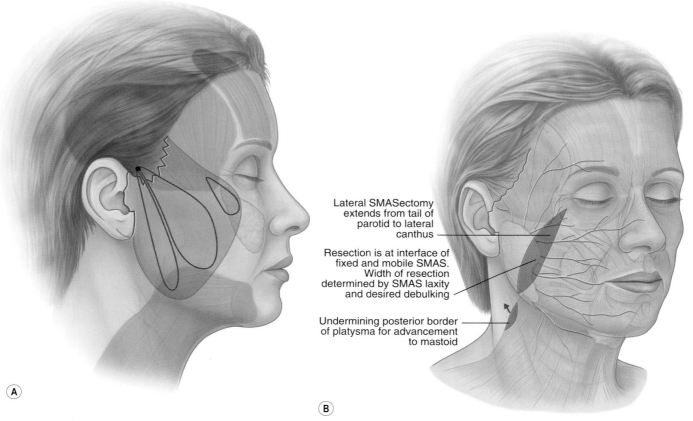

Lateral SMASectomy
extends from tail of
parotid to lateral
canthus

Resection is at interface of
fixed and mobile SMAS.
Width of resection
determined by SMAS laxity
and desired debulking

Undermining posterior border
of platysma for advancement
to mastoid

Figure 28.10. Superficial muscular aponeurotic system (SMAS) flap with skin attached (deep plane facelift). *(Reprinted from Neligan, P.C., Warren, R.J. [Eds.], 2013. Plastic Surgery, vol. 2, 3rd ed. Elsevier, 208–215.)*

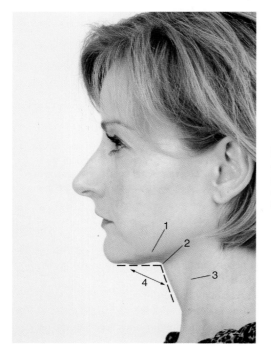

Figure 28.11. Profile view demonstrates the attributes of a youthful neck including *(1)* a cervicomental angle of ~105 degrees; *(2)* a distinct inferior mandibular border; *(3)* a slightly visible thyroid cartilage; and *(4)* a visible anterior border of the sternocleidomastoid muscle. *(Reprinted from Neligan, P.C., Warren, R.J. [Eds.], 2013. Plastic Surgery, vol. 2, 3rd ed. Elsevier, 313–326.)*

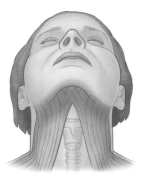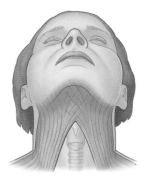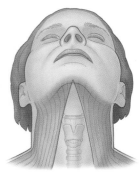

Type I
Occurs in 75% of cases (most common).
Demonstrates a limited decussation of
platysma muscles, extending 1 to 2 cm
below the mandibular symphysis.

Type II
Occurs in 15% of cases.
Demonstrates decussation of the
platysma from the mandibular
symphysis to the thyroid cartilage.

Type III
Occurs in 10% of cases.
Demonstrates no decussation
or interdigitations.

Figure 28.12. Variations in platysma anatomy in the submental region. *Type I,* Interdigitation of the platysma muscle 1 to 2 cm posterior to the mandibular symphysis. *Type II,* Interdigitation of the platysma muscles from mandibular symphysis to the thyroid cartilage. *Type III,* No interdigitation of the platysma muscles. *(Reprinted from Neligan, P.C., Warren, R.J. [Eds.], 2013. Plastic Surgery, vol. 2, 3rd ed. Elsevier, 313–327.)*

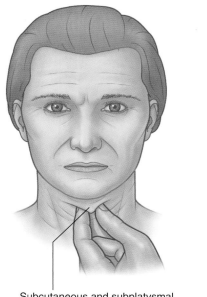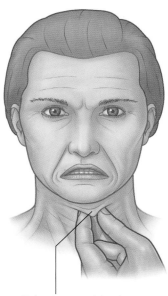

Subcutaneous and subplatysmal
fat pinched

Subcutaneous fat only

Figure 28.13. Physical exam. The figure demonstrates pinching the soft tissue at rest and with muscle contraction to distinguish the cervical bulk caused by preplatysmal fat from bulk caused by subplastysmal structures. Bulk due to subplastysmal structures "escapes" from the pinch with contraction. *(Reprinted from Aston, S.J., Steinbrech, D.S., Walden, J.L. [Eds.], 2009. Aesthetic Plastic Surgery. Saunders, 231–242.)*

2. Techniques
    - Liposuction
        - Preplatysmal fat removal with skin contraction
        - Ideal for young patients with good skin elasticity and localized submental and submandibular fat
        - Avoid overcorrection.
        - Wear elastic compression garments postoperatively.
    - Suspension sutures
        - Create a permanent artificial ligament to correct the neck deformities.
        - Long-term stability is questioned.
    - Anterior/submental open neck lift
        - Uses a submental incision for open access to the neck (see Figure 27.14)

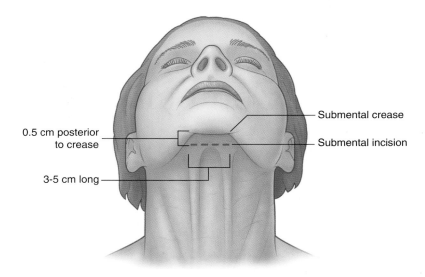

Figure 28.14. Location of submental incision 2 mm posterior to the submental crease. *(Reprinted from Aston, S.J., Steinbrech, D.S., Walden, J.L. [Eds.], 2009. Aesthetic Plastic Surgery. Saunders, 231–242.)*

- ■ Lipectomy performed by direct excision or combination of liposuction and direct excision
- ■ Platysmal banding treated with platysmaplasty
  - ○ Midline plication,
  - ○ Lateral plication, or
  - ○ Transection
- • Patients with severe skin laxity will require standard lower facelift/necklift incisions, wide undermining, and skin redraping or, in severe cases, direct excision in the midline incorporating a Z plasty.
3. Complications
  - • Similar to those found following facelift
  - • Facial nerve injury for necklift most often involves the marginal mandibular nerve.

Suggested Readings

Afifi, A.M., Djohan, R., 2013. Chapter 1: Anatomy of the head and neck. In: Neligan, P.C., Rodriguez, E.D. (Eds.), Plastic Surgery, vol. 3, 3rd ed. Elsevier, pp. 1–22.

Marten, T.J., Elyassnia, D., 2013. Chapter 12: Secondary deformities and the secondary facelift. In: Neligan, P.C., Warren, R.J. (Eds.), Plastic Surgery, vol. 2, 3rd ed. Elsevier, pp. 277–312.

Mendelson, B., 2009. Chapter 6: Facelift anatomy, SMAS, retaining ligaments, and facial spaces. In: Aston, S.J., Steinbrech, D.S., Walden, J.L. (Eds.), Aesthetic Plastic Surgery. Saunders, pp. 53–71.

Nahai, F., 2011. Chapter 50: Avoiding complications in facial aesthetic surgery. In: Nahai, F. (Ed.), The Art of Aesthetic Surgery: Principles and Techniques, 2nd ed. Quality Medical Publishing, pp. 1762–1792.

Thorne, C.H., 2007. Chapter 49: Facelift. In: Thorne, C.H. (Ed.), Grabb and Smith's Plastic Surgery, 6th ed. Elsevier, pp. 498–508.

Warren, R.J., 2013. Chapter 11.1: Facelift: principles. In: Neligan, P.C., Warren, R.J. (Eds.), Plastic Surgery, vol. 2, 3rd ed. Elsevier, pp. 184–207.

Warren, R.J., 2013. Chapter 11.2: Facelift: introduction to deep tissue techniques. In: Neligan, P.C., Warren, R.J. (Eds.), Plastic Surgery, vol. 2, 3rd ed. Elsevier, pp. 208–215.

Weinfeld, A.B., Nahai, F., 2009. Chapter 20: Deep plane procedures in the neck. In: Aston, S.J., Steinbrech, D.S., Walden, J.L. (Eds.), Aesthetic Plastic Surgery. Saunders, pp. 231–242.

Zins, J.E., Morrison, C.M., Langevin, C.J., 2013. Chapter 13: Neck rejuvenation. In: Neligan, P.C., Warren, R.J. (Eds.), Plastic Surgery, vol. 2, 3rd ed. Elsevier, pp. 313–326.

Body Contouring and Suction-Assisted Lipectomy

1. Body contouring
   - Trunk: Removal of excess skin and subcutaneous tissue, often after massive weight loss
     - Degree of skin excess, fatty excess, and muscular diastasis assists with selection of appropriate procedure.
       - Suction-assisted lipectomy: Minimal skin excess, moderate subcutaneous adiposity, no diastasis
       - Abdominoplasty: Excess anterior abdominal skin and subcutaneous tissue, with appreciable diastasis. Lower incision placed at least 5 to 7 cm superior to vulvar commissure
         - Miniabdominoplasty: Short scar, often no transposition of umbilicus, minimal diastasis
         - Full abdominoplasty: Full transverse incision; requires umbilical transposition, and possible diastasis repair
         - Fleur-de-lis: Excess skin in both transverse and vertical dimensions. By adding vertical excision, can improve vertical excess
           → In general, perform the vertical excision first.
         - Lipoabdominoplasty: Combination of full abdominoplasty and liposuction
       - Circumferential body lift/lower body lift: Excess skin and subcutaneous tissue circumferentially with ptosis of gluteal soft tissues
         - Can perform gluteal lift/autoaugmentation with gluteal artery flaps
       - Panniculectomy: Removal of abdominal pannus only to achieve improvements in hygiene, skin irritation, moisture
     - Complications: Reportedly occur in 15% to 25% of patients (50% for active smokers)
       - Pulmonary embolism: Abdominoplasty is the procedure most frequently associated with postoperative mortality.
       - Skin necrosis: Most commonly occurs in supraumbilical region
       - Seroma: Most common complication after lipoabdominoplasty and with patients following massive weight loss
       - Skin dehiscence: Most common complication when combining skin resection procedures
         - Often occurs late in massive-weight-loss patients secondary to seroma; treatment is nutrition improvement.
       - Bulge: Most commonly occurs superior to umbilicus because of failure to plicate supraumbilical rectus fascia during diastasis repair
         - Men are more likely to have a wide upper rectus muscle diastasis, whereas women are more likely to have a lower rectus muscle diastasis.
       - Encephalopathy: Most commonly associated with thiamine deficiency (Wernicke-Korsakoff encephalopathy) in the massive-weight-loss patient
         - Treatment: Intravenous thiamine supplementation, 100 mg daily; increase to 100 mg every 8 hours as needed until resolution of symptoms.
       - Pain/numbness (see Figure 29.1)
         - Lateral femoral cutaneous n.: Numbness/pain along anterolateral thigh (see Figure 29.2)
           → Danger zone: Passes through inguinal ligament to the thigh 1 cm medial to anteriosuperior iliac spine
         - Iliohypogastric n.: Numbness/pain along the inguinal crease and lateral gluteal region
           → Danger zone: Lateral lower abdominal transverse incisions near inguinal ligament
         - Ilioinguinal n.: Numbness along the medial thigh and scrotum/labia
           → Danger zone: Lateral lower abdominal transverse incisions near inguinal ligament
         - Intercostal n.: Numbness along abdominal/flank dermatomes T5 to L1
           → Danger zone: Anterior intercostal nerves pass between the internal oblique and the transversus abdominis muscle, enter the rectus abdominis m., and travel to the overlying fascia and skin. Lateral branches penetrate the intercostal muscles at the midaxillary line and travel within the subcutaneous tissue.

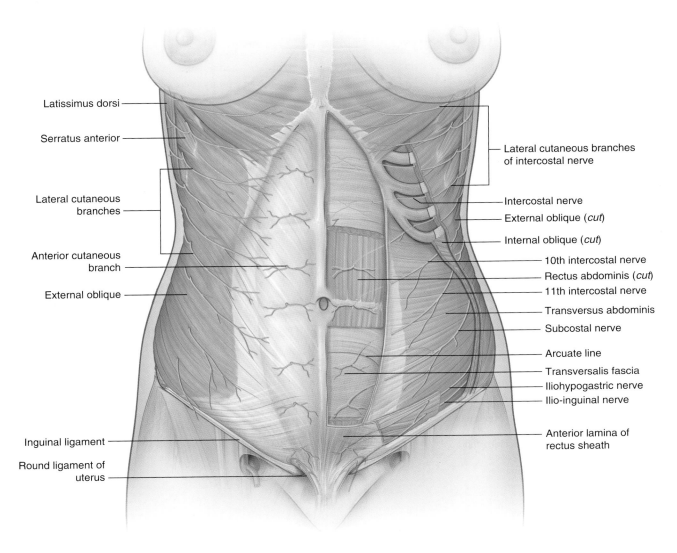

Figure 29.1. Abdominal nerves. *(Reprinted from Neligan, P.C., Buck, D.W. [Eds.], 2013. Core Procedures in Plastic Surgery, 1st ed. Elsevier, 79–90.)*

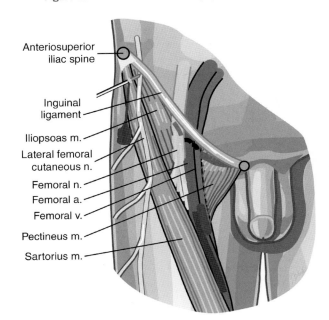

Figure 29.2. Lateral femoral cutaneous nerve. *(Reprinted from Waldman, S.D., 2004. Lateral femoral cutaneous nerve block. In: Atlas of Interventional Pain Management, 2nd ed. Saunders, Philadelphia, 457.)*

- Upper extremity/brachioplasty: Removal of excess skin and adipose tissue of the upper arm (see Figure 29.3)
  - Critical anatomy
    - Ptosis of upper arm skin is secondary to relaxation of the longitudinal fascial sling, which extends from clavipectoral and axillary fascia.
  - Key technical point
    - Re-anchoring the posteromedial upper arm soft tissue to axillary fascia with nonabsorbable suture
  - Complications: Reportedly occur in 25% to 50% of patients
    - Hypertrophic scarring (occurs in up to 40%): Most frequent complication of brachioplasty; often caused by tension, tissue mismatch, poor nutrition
      - Treatment: Conservative including compression, silicone sheeting, steroid injection
    - Wound healing complications: Seroma, wound dehiscence
    - Under-resection
    - Standing cone deformities
    - Lymphedema
  - Recurrence
    - Can be exacerbated by further weight loss
      - Best to perform brachioplasty even if still above ideal body weight rather than encourage additional weight loss
  - Nerve injury (occurs in up to 5%)
    - Medial antebrachial cutaneous n.
      - Arises from medial cord
      - Runs in close proximity to the intramuscular septum and penetrates fascia at 14 cm proximal to the medial epicondyle; especially at risk of injury here
        - Therefore, always identify nerve at this level and leave fat on deep fascia in this area.
      - Leads to paresthesia of upper arm and anterior proximal forearm
      - Treat with hand therapy and local massage, gabapentin; improves with time
    - Medial brachial cutaneous n.
      - Arises from medial cord
      - Runs with basilic vein, sends out branches at 7 cm and 15 cm proximal to the medial epicondyle

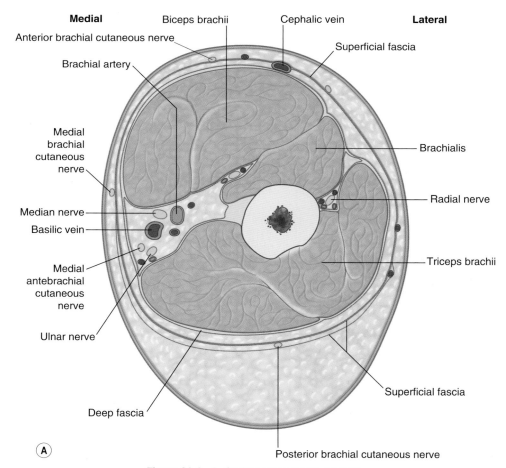

Figure 29.3. A, Sagittal view of arm anatomy.

Medial   **Lateral**

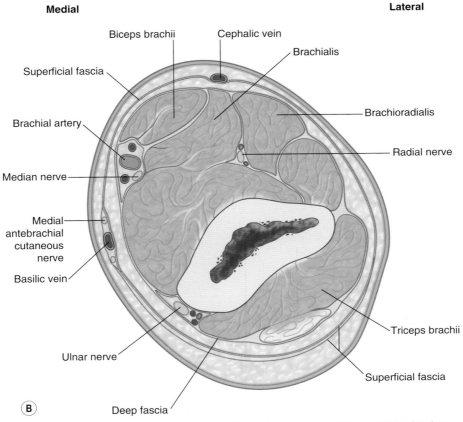

Figure 29.3., cont'd **B,** Distal portion of arm, highlighting nerves, arteries, veins, and fascial planes at this level. *(Reprinted from Capella, J.F., 2013. In: Neligan, P.C. [Ed.], 2013. Plastic Surgery, 3rd ed. Elsevier, 617–633.)*

→ Injury leads to numbness and paresthesias of the medial upper arm.

- Lower extremity/medial thighlift
  - Critical anatomy
    - Femoral triangle contains a high concentration of lymphatics draining the leg as well as the femoral neurovascular bundle (see Figure 29.4).
      - Injury can lead to bleeding, bruising, lymphedema, leg weakness, pain.
      - Borders: Inguinal ligament, adductor longus m., sartorius m.
    - Colles' fascia: Deep layer of the superficial perineal fascia that is thin, aponeurotic, and has considerable strength. It is continuous with the Scarpa's fascia of the abdomen anteriorly.
      - Helps define the perineal/thigh crease and lies deep to the subcutaneous adipose tissue of the perineum
        → Posteriorly fuses with urogenital diaphragm
      - High in elastin content, which gives it a yellow hue, thereby distinguishing it from the muscular fascia, which is white
  - Key technical points
    - Re-anchoring the medial thigh soft tissue to the Colles' fascia with nonabsorbable suture (analogous to anchoring medial arm tissues to axillary fascia in brachioplasty)

- Near femoral triangle, make depth of incision only to the subcutaneous layer to avoid injury to its contents.
  - With severe soft-tissue redundancy, can add a vertical or longitudinal component to the excision.
  - Complications: Similar to brachioplasty
    - Seroma (occurs in 4% to 20%)
    - Hypertrophic scarring
    - Recurrence
    - Labial spreading

2. Suction-assisted lipectomy
- Indications: Removal of excess adipose tissue, often with minimal excess skin
  - Mesotherapy: Subcutaneous injection of medications as an alternative to liposuction; not approved by the FDA
  - Can perform reduction mammaplasty in select female patients with liposuction alone (50% of the female breast is adipose tissue)
- Wetting solutions: Combination of saline, lidocaine, and epinephrine used to assist with anesthesia, hemostasis, and emulsification of adipocytes. Differ based on ratio of infiltrate volume to aspirate volume. In general, the combination of infiltrate volume and intravenous volume should be twice the aspirate volume.
  - Dry: No wetting solution
    - Greatest blood loss in aspirate

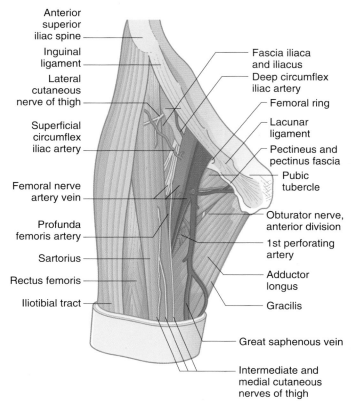

Figure 29.4. Femoral triangle with femoral artery, vein, and nerve with course of saphenous vein. *(Reprinted from Serletti, J.M., 2009. In: Wei, F.C., Mardini, S. [Eds.], Flaps and Reconstructive Surgery. Elsevier, 39–49.)*

- Wet: 100 to 300 mL of infiltrate per area, regardless of amount of aspirate
  - 25% blood loss in aspirate
- Superwet: 1:1 ratio of infiltrate volume to aspirate volume
  - 1% to 4% blood loss in aspirate
  - Approximately 70% of infiltrate remains in the body after superwet liposuction.
- Tumescent: 2 to 3:1 ratio of infiltrate volume to aspirate volume
  - Lowest blood loss in aspirate (1%)
  - Maximum safe dose of lidocaine: 35 mg/kg (doses up to 55 mg/kg have been reported)
- Complications
  - Neuropraxia: Motor weakness after liposuction
    - Treatment: Reassurance with observation; most neurapraxic injuries should resolve within 3 to 4 months.
  - Pulmonary embolism: Most common cause of death following liposuction
    - Risk factors: Increased tumescent infiltrate volume, multiple combined procedures, large-volume aspirate (defined as >5 L by American Society of Plastic Surgeons Committee on Patient Safety)

- Surface irregularities/dimpling: Commonly occur through aggressive superficial suctioning, use of large cannulas, and use of a single port site without cross-tunneling
  - Common with liposuction to buttocks due to fibrous septae
- Seroma: Most common complication of lipoabdominoplasty; more common with ultrasound-assisted liposuction than traditional suction lipectomy
- Thermal burns: More common with ultrasound-assisted liposuction
- Fat embolism: Develop petechial rash and respiratory failure. Treatment: Supportive
- Supraventricular tachycardia develops after accidental intravascular injection of wetting solution. Treatment: Discontinue infiltration, check composition of the infiltrate

Suggested Readings

Buck, D.W., II, Mustoe, T.A., 2010. An evidence-based approach to abdominoplasty. Plast. Reconstr. Surg. 126 (6), 2189–2195.

Capella, J.F., Trovato, J.M., Woehrle, S., 2013. Chapter 29: Upper limb contouring. In: Neligan, P.C. (Ed.), Plastic Surgery, 3rd ed. Elsevier, pp. 617–633.

Cruz-Korchin, N., Korchin, L., Gonzalez-Keelan, C., et al., 2002. Macromastia: how much of it is fat? Plast. Reconstr. Surg. 109, 64–68.

Friedland, J.A., Maffi, T.R., 2008. MOC-PS(SM) CME article: abdominoplasty. Plast. Reconstr. Surg. 121 (Suppl. 4), 1–11.

Gingrass, M.K., 2007. Chapter 52: Liposuction. In: Thorne, C.H., Beasley, R.W., Aston, S.J., et al. (Eds.), Grabb and Smith's Plastic Surgery, 6th ed. Lippincott Williams & Wilkins, Philadelphia, pp. 533–541.

Haeck, P.C., Swanson, J.A., Gutowski, K.A., et al., 2009. Evidence-based patient safety advisory: liposuction. Plast. Reconstr. Surg. 124 (Suppl. 4), 28S–44S.

Iverson, R.E., Pao, V.S., 2008. MOC-PS(SM) CME article: liposuction. Plast. Reconstr. Surg. 121 (Suppl. 4), 1–11.

Klein, J.A., 1990. Tumescent technique for regional anesthesia permits lidocaine doses of 35 mg/kg for liposuction. J. Dermatol. Surg. Oncol. 16, 248–263.

Knoetgen, J., III, Moran, S.L., 2006. Long-term outcomes and complications associated with brachioplasty: a retrospective review and cadaveric study. Plast. Reconstr. Surg. 117 (7), 2219–2223.

Landfair, A.S., Rubin, J.P., 2011. Chapter 75: Applied anatomy in body contouring. In: Nahai, F. (Ed.), The Art of Aesthetic Surgery: Principles and Techniques, vol. 3. Quality Medical Publishing, St. Louis, pp. 2679–2708.

Matarasso, A., 2000. Suction mammaplasty: the use of suction lipectomy to reduce large breasts. Plast. Reconstr. Surg. 105, 2604–2607.

Michaels, J., 5th, Coon, D., Rubin, J.P., 2011. Complications in postbariatric body contouring: postoperative management and treatment. Plast. Reconstr. Surg. 127 (4), 1693–1700.

Neligan, P.C., Buck, D.W. (Eds.), 2013. Chapter 4: Abdominoplasty. In: Core Procedures in Plastic Surgery, 1st ed. Elsevier, pp. 79–90.

Ostad, A., Kageyama, N., Moy, R.L., 1996. Tumescent anesthesia with a lidocaine dose of 55 mg/kg is safe. Dermatol. Surg. 22, 921–927.

Rubin, J.P. (Ed.), 2013. Body Countouring and Liposuction. Elsevier, pp. 1–603.

Schuenke, M., Schulte, E., Schumacher, U., et al., 2006. Atlas of Anatomy: General Anatomy and Musculoskeletal System. Thieme, New York.

Serletti, J.M., 2009. Chapter 5: Chest, abdomen, groin, and back. In: Wei, F.C., Mardini, S. (Eds.), Flaps and Reconstructive Surgery. Elsevier, pp. 39–49.

Seruya, M., Baker, S.B., 2008. MOC-PS(SM) CME Article: venous thromboembolism prophylaxis in plastic surgery patients. Plast. Reconstr. Surg. 122 (Suppl. 3), 1–9.

Shermak, M.A. (Ed.), 2011. Body Contouring. McGraw-Hill Professional, New York, pp. 1–304.

Shermak, M.A., 2012. Body contouring. Plast. Reconstr. Surg. 129 (6), 963e–978e.

Waldman, S.D. (Ed.), 2009. Chapter 67: The lateral femoral cutaneous nerve. In: Pain Review. Saunders, p. 123.

Wells, J.H., Hurvitz, K.A., 2011. An evidence-based approach to liposuction. Plast. Reconstr. Surg. 127 (2), 949–954.

Injectables, Skin Resurfacing, Lasers, and Hair Restoration

30

Injectables

1. Substances that are injected into the dermis or subcutaneous tissue to alter facial shape, appearance, and/or aesthetics
   - There is no ideal injectable and each carries its own individual risk/benefit profile.
   - Do not inject any injectables obtained by a patient from any other location than your office.
2. General complications of injectables
   - Inadvertent arterial injection: Immediately stop the injection and attempt to aspirate the substance. Can reduce risk by injecting slowly, using a small needle
   - Inadvertent venous injection: Treatment is conservative and includes massage, warm compresses, and nitroglycerine patch.
   - Inadvertent placement of injectable: If the patient develops problems, can try to debulk the filler (i.e., hyaluronidase)
3. Types of injectables (see Table 30.1)
   - Hyaluronic acid
     - Synthetic compound used to "fill" soft tissues (i.e., deep rhytids, etc.)
       - Nasolabial fold, perioral rhytids: Inject into subdermal space
       - Tear-trough deformity: Inject subperiosteally
     - Example products
       - Juvederm
       - Restylane
       - Perlane
     - Reversible with hyaluronidase
   - Botulinum toxin A (botulinum toxin type-A cosmetic, Dysport)
     - Chemodenervation
       - Mechanism of action: Inhibition of acetylcholine release at the neuromuscular junction
       - Useful for dynamic rhytids
     - FDA approved for glabella rhytids and crow's feet
       - May be used off-label for other sites legally but cannot be advertised for these off-label uses
     - Onset of action: 24 to 72 hours, but may take up to 2 weeks for maximum effect
     - Duration of action: 3 to 4 months
     - Example products
       - Botox cosmetic
       - Dysport
         - Cannot be used in patients with milk allergy
     - Potentiating medications
       - Penicillamine, quinine, calcium-channel blockers, and aminoglycosides
     - Common uses
       - Glabellar rhytids: Chemodenervation of the corrugators
       - Crow's feet: Chemodenervation of the lateral orbicularis oculi
         - Can lead to lateral brow elevation due to unopposed action of the frontalis m.
       - Bunny lines: Chemodenervation of the levator labii superioris alaeque nasi and nasalis
       - Forehead rhytids: Chemodenervation of frontalis m.
         - Hyperactive frontalis m. can mask eyelid ptosis; thus, chemodenervation of the frontalis can lead to upper eyelid ptosis.
           - → Treatment includes α-adrenergic eyedrops (e.g., Iopidine), which causes stimulation of Mueller's m. and elevation of the upper eyelid by 2 mm.
       - Horizontal nasal lines: Chemodenervation of the procerus m.
     - Complications
       - Unexpected brow position changes (elevation or ptosis)
         - Depends on which muscles are denervated
         - Elevators of the medial brow: Orbicularis oculi, corrugator supercilii, depressor supercilii and procerus
         - Elevators of the lateral brow: Frontalis
       - Upper eyelid ptosis
         - Diffusion of drug through the orbital septum to the levator m. (most common), which usually occurs with primary treatment to the glabellar region
         - Chemodenervation of hyperactive frontalis m.
   - Botulinum toxin type B
     - FDA approval for treatment of cervical dystonia and hemifacial spasm

Table 30.1 Common Facial Fillers Currently Available for Use in Soft-Tissue Augmentation

FILLER TYPE	NAME (MANUFACTURER)	INDICATION	DURABILITY	ADVANTAGES	DISADVANTAGES	MARKET STATUS
Autologous products	Viable fat	Deep defects	Variable; months to years	Abundant supply, safe, inexpensive	Donor site morbidity, variable reproducibility, requires processing	No FDA/EEA approval required
Autologous collagen/autolagen	Collagenesis, Beverly, MA; Isolagen, Exton, PA	Moderate to deep defects	Months to years; processed from excised skin	Can be stored up to 6 months, safe	Donor morbidity, painful, costly	FDA approved/CE mark
Bovine collagens	Zyderm 1 (3.5% dermal collagen) (INAMED, Santa Barbara, CA)	Superficial defects, fine lines, acne scars	2 to 4 months	Safe, reliable, contains lidocaine, ease of administration	Allergic reaction in 1% to 3%, short-term results, requires skin testing before use, reactivation of herpes is possible with lip injections	FDA approved/CE mark
	Zyderm 2 (6.5% collagen) (INAMED, Santa Barbara, CA)	Moderate defects, deeper acne scars, lip augmentation	2 to 6 months	Same as Zyderm 1	Same as Zyderm 1	FDA approved/CE mark
	Zyplast (3.5% cross-linked collagen) (INAMED, Santa Barbara, CA)	Deep defects, lip augmentation	2 to 6 months	Same as Zyderm 1, more viscous and resistant to degradation	Can cause skin necrosis if used in glabella, allergies in 3%, requires skin testing	FDA approved/CE mark
Cadaveric collagens	AlloDerm (acellular human dermis; comes in sheets of varying sizes) (LifeCell, Branchburg, NJ)	Deep wrinkles or scars, lip augmentation	6 to 12 months	Safe, no allergy testing required	Expensive, surgically implanted, often causes temporary swelling, occasionally palpable, shrinkage with time	FDA approved/CE mark
	Cymetra (micronized, injectable form of AlloDerm) (LifeCell, Branchburg, NJ)	Deep wrinkles or scars, lip augmentation	3 to 6 months	Safe, no allergy testing required, contains lidocaine	Can cause skin necrosis if used in glabella, costly, often clumps within needle	FDA approved/CE mark
Cell-cultured collagen	Cosmoderm (35 mg/mL collagen) (INAMED, Santa Barbara, CA)	Superficial defects, shallow wrinkles and acne scars	3 to 4 months	Safe, no allergy testing required, contains lidocaine	Short-term results, most common side effects include cold symptoms (4%), flu symptoms (2%)	FDA approved/CE mark
	Cosmoplast (35 mg/mL cross-linked collagen) (INAMED, Santa Barbara, CA)	Deeper defects and wrinkles, lip augmentation	3 to 4 months	Same as Cosmoderm	Same as Cosmoderm	FDA approved/CE mark
Avian-derived hyaluronic acids	Hylaform gel (INAMED, Santa Barbara, CA)	Moderate defects, lip augmentation	3 to 4 months	Safe, reliable, no allergy testing required	Short-term results, immunologic reactions in patient allergic to avian products (eggs)	FDA approved/CE mark
	Hylaform Plus (INAMED, Santa Barbara, CA)	Moderate to deeper defects, facial wrinkles, and folds.	3 to 4 months	Same as hylaform gel	Same as hylaform gel, superficial injection may lead to skin discoloration	FDA approved/CE mark
Bacterial-cultured hyaluronic acids	Restylane/Restylane Fine (Medicis, Scottsdale, AZ)	Superficial (Restylane Fine)-to-moderate defects, deeper wrinkle reduction, nasolabial folds, glabellar creases, lip augmentation	6 to 12 months	Safe, reliable, predictable results, no allergy testing required, longer lasting than bovine collagens	Rare immunologic reactions, higher incidence of bruising, pain, and postprocedure swelling vs. bovine collagens, higher cost	FDA approved/CE mark
	Perlane (Medicis, Montreal, Canada)	Deeper defects, shaping facial contours, lip augmentation	6 to 12 months	Same as Restylane	Same as Restylane	FDA approved/CE mark
	Captique (INAMED, Santa Barbara, CA)	Superficial defects, fine lines and wrinkles	3 to 6 months	Safe, no allergy testing required, similar to Restylane	Relatively new product, short-term results	FDA approved/CE mark
	Juvederm 18, 24, 30 (L.E.A. Derm, Paris)	Superficial (18), moderate (24), and deep (30) defects	3 to 6 months	Safe, predictable results, no allergy testing needed	Short-term results, rare immunologic reactions, relatively new product	FDA approved

Continued

Table 30.1 Common Facial Fillers Currently Available for Use in Soft-Tissue Augmentation—cont'd

FILLER TYPE	NAME (MANUFACTURER)	INDICATION	DURABILITY	ADVANTAGES	DISADVANTAGES	MARKET STATUS
Synthetics	Sculptra (poly-L-lactic acid microparticles) (Dermik Laboratories, Berwyn, PA)	Deep defects	1 to 2 years	Long-term results, safe	Rare, foreign body reaction, limited U.S. results/studies	Approved for lipoatrophy; off-label for cosmetic purposes/CE mark
	Radiesse (calcium hyodroxyapatite microspheres) (Bioform Medical, Franksville, WI)	Deep defects, nasolabial folds, vertical lip lines, acne scars, marionette lines, volume restoration around cheeks	1 to 2 years	Long-term results, no allergy testing required, no concern for antigenic or inflammatory reactions	Can rarely develop nodules if injected superficially	FDA approved/CE mark
	Artecoll/ArteFill (polymethylmethacrylate microspheres in 3.5% bovine collagen and 0.3% lidocaine) (Artes Medical, San Diego, CA)	Deep defects, glabella, nasolabial folds	Permanent after nearly 50% resorption	Unrivaled longevity, probably safe, but reports of persistent erythema at injection site	Palpable if placed superficially or excessively; thus, avoid injecting into the lips and areas with thin overlying skin; requires allergy testing	Preliminary FDA approval for cosmetic purposes/CE mark
	Reviderm Intra (dextran beads in a hylan gel) (Rofil Medical International, Breda, The Netherlands)	Deep defects, lip augmentation	Months to years	Long-term results, safe	Postprocedural swelling, relatively new product to U.S.	Not FDA approved/CE mark
	Silicone/Silikon-1000 (liquid silicone) (Alcon Laboratories, Fort Worth, TX)	Deep defects, lip augmentation	Permanent	Permanent, safe, long clinical experience	Migration, foreign body reactions, poor reputation	Off-label for cosmetic purposes
	Endoplast 50 (elastin and collagen) (Laboratories Filorgra, Paris)	Deep defects, lip augmentation	12 months	Long-term results	Allergy tests required, limited experience	Not FDA approved/CE mark
	Bio-Alcamid (96% water, 4% polyalkylimide) (Pur Medical Corp, Toronto, Canada)	Deep defects	Permanent	Long-term results, removable, no allergy testing required, biocompatible	Limited experience, inflammatory reactions, infectious complications, migration	FDA approved/CE mark for HIV lipoatrophy
	Aquamid (polyacrylamide hydrogel) (Contura International)	Deep defects, lip augmentation	Permanent	Long-term results, compound plasticity	High rate of granuloma formation, infectious complications	Not FDA approved/CE mark

Adapted from Johl, S.S., 2006. Curr. Opin. Ophthalmol. 17 (5), 471–479; Murray, C.A., Zloty, D., Warshawski, L., 2005. Dermatol. Clin. 23, 343–363; Broder, K.W., Cohen, S.R., 2006. Plast. Reconstr. Surg. 118 (Suppl. 3), 7S–14S; Eppley, B.L., Dadvand, B., 2006. Plast. Reconstr. Surg. 118 (4), 98e–106e; Sengelmann, R.D., Tull, S. Dermal Fillers. Available at: http://www.emedicine.com/derm/topic515.htm.
CE, Certification; EEA, European Economic Area; FDA, Food and Drug Administration; HIV, human-immunodeficiency virus.

- Comparison with toxin A
  - Acidic (more painful on injection), stable as a liquid, longer shelf life, shorter duration of action, faster onset, greater radius of diffusion
- Can be used if patient develops antibodies to Botox cosmetic
- Example products
  - Myobloc
- Bovine collagen
  - Example products
    - Zyderm I and II, Zyplast
  - Approximately 3% of patients will exhibit hypersensitivity reactions.
    - Must test skin 4 weeks before injecting
- Poly-L-lactic acid
  - FDA approved for human-immunodeficiency virus (HIV) lipoatrophy
  - Injected subcutaneously in the cheek, submuscularly in the orbital region, and subperiosteally in the temples region
  - Example products
    - Sculptra
  - Patients require multiple injections every 4 to 6 weeks for several months.
  - Advantages: Results may last for more than 2 years.
  - Disadvantages: Can result in nodule formation in dynamic muscles of the face (especially the lip and eye)
- Fat grafting
  - "Autologous filler"
  - Advantages: No risk of hypersensitivity
  - Disadvantages: Requires a donor site (harvest of adipocytes), with processing, before injection; resorption; unpredictable graft survival; longer recovery time
  - Method
    - Aspiration
    - Sedimentation
      - Balanced centrifugation
      - Gravity (optimal but lengthy)
    - Injection into the deep dermis
      - Small amount of fat per pass
  - Optimizing survival
    - Avoid: Large canula aspiration, filtration, rinsing, straining, or drying

Chemical and Mechanical Skin Resurfacing

1. Use of chemical or mechanical methods to damage superficial skin (epidermis and superficial dermis) to create inflammation that leads to predictable healing, resulting in skin tightening and improved skin-surface appearance
2. Pretreatment considerations
   - Personal history of perioral herpetic lesions
     - Recommended to pretreat with Acyclovir (valacyclovir or famciclovir) to reduce risk of posttreatment outbreak
       - Estimated 50% likelihood of outbreak without pretreatment

- Recommended to begin treatment starting 1 to 2 days before resurfacing and continue until reepithelialization completed
- Acyclovir can be used after resurfacing as treatment for lesions to reduce the duration of the outbreak.

3. Peels: Use of a chemical substance to damage skin and result in resurfacing; can result in hypo- or hyperpigmentation (see Table 30.2)
   - Glycolic acid peel
     - Light peel
   - Tricyclic acid (TCA) peel
     - Neutralized within the superficial dermis
     - Depth of penetration can vary (light, medium, or deep; see Figure 30.1), depending on mixture.
   - Jessner's solution
     - Light peel
     - Often used as a preparation for a TCA peel
     - Ingredients: Resorcinol USP, salicylic acid USP, and lactic acid USP; 14% each in ethanol USP
   - Phenol peel
     - Deep peel
       - Penetrates into the reticular dermis (deeper than TCA peels)
       - Liquid soap can be used to decrease depth of peel
     - Disadvantages: Longer recovery time because of depth, requires cardiac monitoring because of rare risk of arrhythmia at application

Table 30.2 Classification of Ablative Procedures by Depth

CLASSIFICATION	RESURFACING PROCEDURES	DEPTH OF ABLATION
Superficial	α- or β-hydroxy acid chemical peels (salicylic acid, 10% to 70% glycolic acid, 10% to 25% trichloracetic acid [10% to 35%]), microdermabrasion	<60 μm (stratum granulosum to immediately above superficial papillary dermis)
Jessner's solution (lactic acid, 14 mL; salicylic acid, 14 g; resorcinol, 14 g)		
Medium	Jessner's solution+35% TCA or 70% glycolic acid	60 to 450 μm (papillary dermis to upper reticular dermis)
Phenol 88% (full strength)		
Dermabrasion		
Laser and plasma resurfacing, depending on fluence and number of passes		
Deep	Baker-Gordon phenol peel	450 to 800 μm (up to midreticular dermis)
Dermabrasion		
CO_2 laser resurfacing, depending on fluence and number of passes		

Adapted from Matarasso, S.L., Glogau, R.G., 1991. Chemical face peels. Dermatol. Clin. 9, 131–150.
TCA, tricyclic acid.

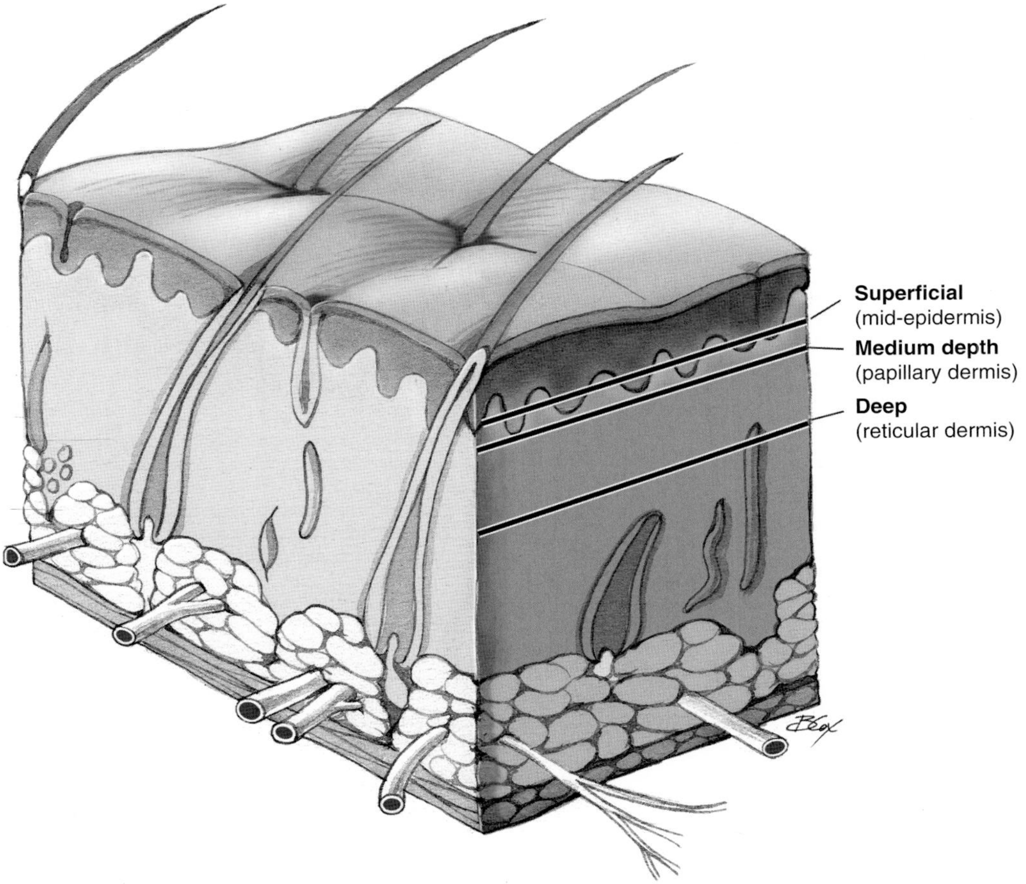

Figure 30.1. Illustration of depth of superficial, medium, and deep resurfacing procedures. *(Reprinted from Meduri, N.B., 2007. Op. Tech. Otolaryn. Head Neck Surg. 18 [3], 172–180.)*

4. Dermabrasion
   - Mechanical removal of epithelium for skin resurfacing
   - Depth determined by clinical endpoints encountered during the treatment process
     - Epithelium removed first
     - Dermal-epidermal junction characterized by smooth texture and no bleeding
     - Superficial papillary dermis characterized by sparse, punctate bleeding
     - Papillary dermis characterized by coarse texture with greater bleeding
     - Superficial reticular dermis is characterized by brisk, confluent bleeding on a coarse-tissue background.
       - This is the preferred endpoint.
       - Further dermabrasion beyond this level can lead to permanent scarring.
   - Although reepithelialization typically occurs within 7 to 10 days following dermabrasion, erythema may persist for as long as 6 weeks after treatment.
   - Disadvantages: Longer recovery, potential for permanent scarring

5. Lasers
   - **L**ight **a**mplification by **s**timulated **e**mission of **r**adiation
   - Use of light to generate heat-induced injury of the skin, leading to inflammation and repair, resulting in skin rejuvenation/tightening, depigmentation, and/or hair removal
     - Ablative: Causes epidermal vaporization to create intended effect of collagen remodeling within the dermis
     - Nonablative: Selectively injures the dermis without injuring the epidermis
   - Posttreatment erythema following laser resurfacing can be treated with ascorbic acid application.
     - Erythema is more severe when a CO_2 laser is used, compared to a fractionated CO_2 laser or the erbium:yttrium-aluminum-garnet (Er:YAG) laser.
   - Hyperpigmentation is the most common side effect of laser resurfacing and is more common in patients with darker skin.
     - Treat with hydroquinone and Tretinoin.
   - Type of laser wavelength selected is based on depth and target chromophore properties (see Table 30.3).

Table 30.3 Lasers in Plastic Surgery

LASER	WAVELENGTH (NM)	TARGET/MECHANISM	USES/BENEFITS	DRAWBACKS
Pulsed dye	595	Oxyhemoglobin Red, yellow, orange pigments/ selective fragmentation and phagocytosis	Port-wine stains, vascular lesions, scars	Can be painful, posttreatment bruising, multiple treatments necessary for effect
Q-switched ruby	694	Melanin: Rupture of cells Black, blue, violet pigments/ selective fragmentation and phagocytosis	Very effective on dark pigments, nevus of Ota, road rash, hair reduction Minimal collateral thermal injury	Not effective on red or yellow pigments, may cause breaks in the skin
Q-switched Nd:YAG (neodymium:yttrium-aluminum-garnet)	532+1064	Red, brown, orange pigments/ selective fragmentation and phagocytosis	Wider spectrum of uses, pigmented lesions, hair reduction Superior red pigment removal (532)	Uneffective on darker pigments
Alexandrite	755	Melanin Green and black pigments	Tattoos, hair reduction	Uneffective on red pigments
Intense pulsed light (IPL)	510 to 1200		Sun damage (pigmented lesions), telangiectasia, rosacea, hair reduction Simple and easy to use, no sedation necessary, nonablative, minimal complications	Nonselective, multiple treatments necessary for effect
Erbium	2940	Water	Skin resurfacing One pass yields 10 to 30 μm of ablation, affinity for H_2O is 10× that of CO_2 laser, minimal collateral damage	No visual endpoint to ablation, no limit to ablative depth, less collagen remodeling, ablative
Carbon dioxide (CO_2)	10,600	Water	Skin resurfacing One pass yields 150 to 200 μm of ablation, immediate collagen tightening, increased neocollagen formation, visual color change highlights endpoint Dermis devoid of H_2O prevents further ablation	Increased collateral tissue damage, pigmentary alterations, postoperative erythema; ablative, sedation required

Reprinted from Weinzweig, J. (ed.), 2010. Plastic Surgery Secrets Plus, 2nd ed. Elsevier, 554–560.

6. Tretinoin
   - Retinoic acid receptor activation with epidermal hyperproliferation, leading to
     - Normalization of epidermal disarray, which results in thickening of the epidermis
     - Stimulation of collagen and glycosaminoglycan deposition, which increases skin turgor and elasticity
     - Reduction in collagen degradation
     - Increased transit of keratinocytes through the epidermis.
   - Improves photoaged skin by decreasing pigmentation and fine and coarse wrinkles
   - Histologic effects
     - Epidermis: Thinning of the stratum corneum, reversal of cellular atypia, and thickening of the epidermis
     - Dermis: Increased collagen and more organized melanin granule deposition
   - Example products: Retin-A

Hair Restoration

1. Hair anatomy
   - Each hair is produced through the proliferation of matrix cells at the base of the hair follicles within reticular dermis.
     - The progeny of these cells become displaced from below and mature and then produce keratin.
   - Outermost layer: Hair cuticle, composed of hard keratin and responsible for anchoring the hair in its follicle
   - Infundibulum: Upper portion of the hair follicle above the sebaceous duct, lined by surface epithelium
   - Outer root sheath covers the inner root sheath and extends upward from the matrix cells to the entrance of the sebaceous gland duct
     - Basal layer contains inactive, pigmented, amelanotic melanocytes that can produce melanin after injury, such as chemical peels or dermabrasion, and migrate toward the epidermis.
   - Sebaceous glands produce sebum and open into the hair follicle.
   - In the scalp, hair follicles are found in the subcutaneous layer (see Figure 30.2)
2. Hair growth
   - A normal cycle of growth and rest characterized by three stages
     - Anagen: Active phase, lasts 1000 days in men and 2 to 5 years longer in women (85% to 90% hairs in this phase)

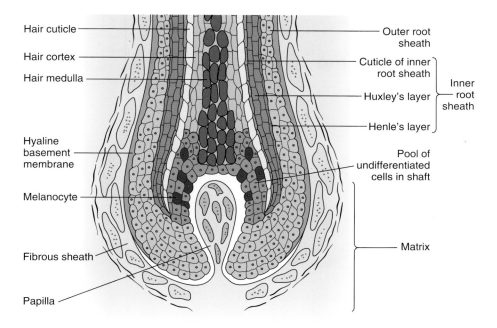

Figure 30.2. Anatomy of a hair follicle. *(Reprinted from Habif, T., 2004. Clinical Dermatology: A Color Guide to Diagnosis and Therapy, 4th ed. Mosby, St Louis.)*

- Catagen: Degradation phase, follows anagen, lasts weeks; follicular bulb atrophies and degrades.
- Telogen: Resting phase, begins after catagen and lasts 2 to 4 months (10% hairs in this phase)
  - On average, 50 to 100 telogen hairs fall out every day and are replaced with new growing hairs.
  - Male-pattern alopecia occurs when the anagen (active) phase is shortened and the telogen (resting) phase is prolonged.
  - Telogen effluvium is a temporary increase in telogen phase cycles caused by pregnancy, stress, eating disorders, chemotherapy, etc.
- Female hair loss
  - Differs from male alopecia because of the numerous hormonal and medical causes for hair loss in women
  - Generalized hair thinning with discrete areas of alopecia is the most common pattern of hair loss in women and is responsive to surgical restoration.
  - Traumatic or surgical scar alopecia may also respond to surgical restoration.
  - Women with frontal temporal alopecia may be treated in a similar manner as patients with male-pattern hair loss.
  - Etiologies
    - Hormonal/medical causes including chronic telogen effluvium (persistent, increased telogen hair shedding); usually unresponsive to surgical hair restoration
    - Psoriasis/tinea capitis: Hair loss associated with scalp changes including crusting/scaling
    - Trichotillomania: Traction alopecia from compulsive hairpulling (not diffuse, patchy)
    - Alopecia totalis: Total hair loss over entire scalp

- Female-pattern hair loss (FPHL): Androgenetic alopecia with sparing of frontal hairline
  - 10% to 40% found to be hyperandrogenic
- Polycystic ovary syndrome (PCOS): Look for menstrual irregularity, acne, hirsutism
- Alopecia areata (AA): Recurrent, nonscarring type of hair loss that can affect any hair-bearing area
  - Presents with many different patterns; medically benign but causes severe emotional and psychosocial stress
  - Etiology unknown (although possibly a T-cell-mediated autoimmune condition in genetically predisposed patients)
    - Corticosteroids have been used successfully to treat alopecia areata.
    - Intralesional steroids are the first-line treatment in localized conditions.
      - Intradermal injection every 4 to 6 weeks
    - Hair growth may persist for 6 to 9 months after a single injection.
  - For patients with extensive AA (>40% hair loss), little data exist on the natural evolution; 24% experienced spontaneous, complete or nearly complete regrowth at some stage during the observation period of 3 to 3.5 years.
  - Surgery does not have a role in this condition.
- Male-pattern alopecia
  - Genetically triggered condition in susceptible men (X-linked dominant gene)
  - Observed increase in the activity of 5-α-reductase in the susceptible follicles; plasma testosterone levels are normal in these patients.
    - Minoxidil (increases hair growth; not useful in extensive loss situations) or Propecia (Finasteride:

5-α-reductase inhibitor) recommended in treating male-pattern alopecia
- ◆ Halts the hair loss, increases number of hairs and diameter of existing hairs; only effective in patients with mild to moderate baldness

- ■ Occurs in 60% to 80% of Caucasian men; can begin as early as 20 years of age
- ■ Hamilton-Norwood classification system (see Figure 30.3): Classifies male-pattern alopecia based on the appearance of the anterior hairline and hair loss at the vertex

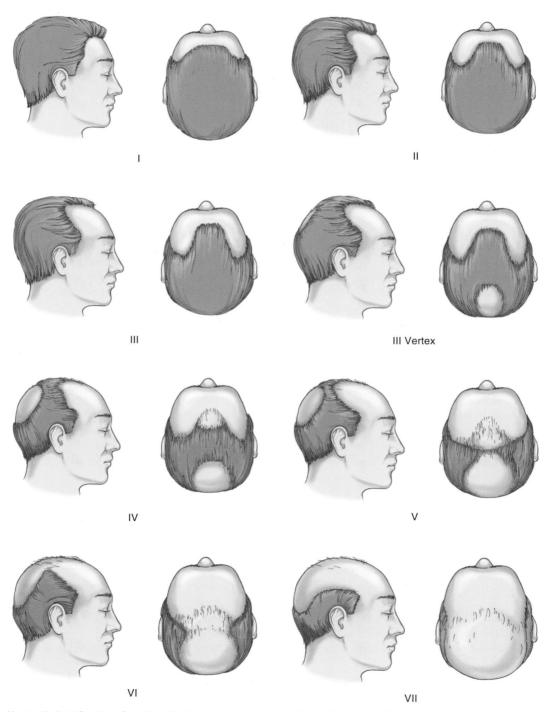

Figure 30.3. Norwood classification of androgenic alopecia. *(Reprinted from Unger, M.G., Cotterill, P.C., 2000. Hair transplantation. In: Achauer, B.M., Eriksson, E., Guyuron, B., et al. [Eds.], Plastic Surgery: Indications, Operations, and Outcomes, vol. 5: Esthetic Surgery. Mosby, St Louis, 2487; redrawn from Norwood, O.T., 1975. Male pattern baldness: classification and incidence. South Med. J. 68, 1359–1365.)*

3. Treatment
   - Scalp reduction: The most appropriate surgical management of male-pattern alopecia
     - Removal of the hairless scalp will diminish the total area that requires grafting and will assist with conservation of donor sites.
     - Sagittal excision patterns are preferred because they will remove the greatest amount of bald skin due to the excess of scalp laxity seen in the sagittal plane.
   - Micrografting hair growth cycle: Hair growth for 1 month (false growth), followed by hair loss (telogen phase), and then normal growth after 3 months at a rate of 1 cm/month
     - Typically, 6 months required for onset of permanent hair growth in grafted area
     - Hair in healthy scalp grows in 1 to 4 hairs, each with their own associated neurovascular bundles, sebaceous glands, sweat glands, and piloerectile muscles surrounded by collagen.
       - When used as micrografts, these units ("hair follicles with dermal elements") have been shown to provide excellent results in hair transplantation.
       - The macroscopic hair transplantation technique of hair plugs with multiple hair follicles, intervening skin, subcutaneous tissue, and epicranial and subepicranial tissue can successfully transplant hair but results in an unnatural appearance.
     - Donor dominance concept: Each hair follicle possesses its own individual, genetically defined life span. Therefore, hair follicles located in those areas that tend to have a longer life span will continue to possess the same life span even after they have been transplanted.
       - Occipital scalp hairs have the longest genetically defined life span in most patients (also an esthetically acceptable donor site).
       - Sideburns often have a life span that is genetically similar to the occipital area, but the donor site is quite small and usually unacceptable.

Special Considerations

1. Laser hair removal
   - Melanin is the target chromophore for laser and intense pulsed-light (IPL) hair reduction (wavelength 250 to 1200 nm).
     - Thermal injury to the melanin-containing cells of the bulb and matrix results in destruction of the hair follicle.
     - Patients with greater melanin content have darker hair and are more likely to have effective laser or IPL hair reduction.
     - In very fair-haired individuals, the limited melanin content makes hair reduction less effective.
2. Eyebrow reconstruction
   - Absence of the eyebrow resulting from trauma: Composite grafting from the scalp is the most appropriate reconstructive option.
   - Microplug hair transplantation is unreliable over scar tissue, especially traumatized soft tissue and radiated scars

Suggested Readings

Avram, M.R., Keene, S.A., Stough, D.B., et al., 2012. Chapter 157: Hair restoration. In: Bolognia, J.L., Jorizzo, J.L., Schaffer, J.V. (Eds.), Dermatology, 3rd ed. Elsevier, pp. 2535–2545.

Born, T.M., Airan, L.E., 2013. Chapter 4: Soft-tissue fillers. In: Neligan, P.C. (Ed.), Plastic Surgery, 3rd ed. Elsevier, pp. 44–59.

Buck, D.W., Alam, M., Kim, J.Y.S., 2009. Injectable fillers for facial rejuvenation: a review. J. Plast. Reconstr. Aesthet. Surg. 62, 11–18.

Carruthers, A., Carruthers, J., 2012. Chapter 159: Botulinum toxin. In: Bolognia, J.L., Jorizzo, J.L., Schaffer, J.V. (Eds.), Dermatology, 3rd ed. Elsevier, pp. 2561–2572.

Kane, M.A.C., 2013. Chapter 3: Botulinum toxin (BoNT-A). In: Neligan, P.C. (Ed.), Plastic Surgery, 3rd ed. Elsevier, pp. 30–43.

Lemperle, G., 2009. Chapter11: Avoidance and treatment of complications after dermal filler injections. In: Cohen, S.R., Born, T.M. (Eds.), Techniques in Aesthetic Plastic Surgery Series: Facial Rejuvenation with Filler. Elsevier, pp. 135–154.

Monheit, G.D., Chastain, M.A., 2012. Chapter 154: Chemical and mechanical skin resurfacing. In: Bolognia, J.L., Jorizzo, J.L., Schaffer, J.V. (Eds.), Dermatology, 3rd ed. Elsevier, pp. 2493–2508.

Saedi, N., Rotunda, A.M., Jones, D.H., et al., 2012. Chapter 158: Soft tissue augmentation. In: Bolognia, J.L., Jorizzo, J.L., Schaffer, J.V. (Eds.), Dermatology, 3rd ed. Elsevier, pp. 2547–2560.

Appendix Q&A

Chapter 1

1. A 55-year-male undergoes a liposuction procedure with a tumescent technique. Approximately 6600 cc were aspirated from multiple areas. Which of the following would represent an early sign of lidocaine toxicity?
   a. Chest pains
   b. Shortness of breath
   c. Headache with sensory changes on tongue
   d. Seizure
   e. Monocular blindness

2. A 36-year-old female previously healthy with no prior surgical history is scheduled to undergo a breast augmentation and liposuction of her abdomen and waist. She undergoes general endotracheal anesthesia without complication. Twenty minutes after the infiltration of local anesthetic along her breast augmentation incisions during the dissection of the implant pocket, what would be the initial suggestion that the patient may be experiencing malignant hyperthermia?
   a. Rapid increase in core temperature
   b. Muscle rigidity
   c. Increased end-tidal CO_2
   d. Acidosis
   e. Profuse bleeding

3. You manage a busy solo private practice and are recruiting a new practice manager. Which of the following topics can you legally inquire about?
   a. Race
   b. Child-care responsibilities
   c. Marital status
   d. Customer service experience
   e. Religion

4. You excise a 1-cm benign nevus. To close the acquired defect, you undermine local tissue and rotate local skin to facilitate reconstruction. Which of the following accurately codes the procedure for billing Medicare?
   a. Excision of benign mass 1 cm with intermediate repair 1 cm
   b. Excision of benign mass 1 cm with complex repair 1 cm
   c. Excision of benign mass 1 cm with adjacent tissue transfer closure 4 cm^2
   d. Fasciocutaneous flap closure
   e. Adjacent tissue transfer closure (4 cm^2)

5. You performed an abdominal component separation reconstruction of a recurrent ventral hernia with your general surgeon colleague, who separately performed the required lysis of bowel adhesions. Which modifier should surgeons use?
   a. 22 modifier
   b. 52 modifier
   c. 51 modifier
   d. 59 modifier
   e. 62 modifier

6. A-64-year-old woman is scheduled to undergo an abdominal panniculectomy after losing 75 lb. Her body mass index (BMI) is 31, and her past history is significant for hypertension (which resolved after weight loss) and insulin-dependent diabetes. She has a normal hemoglobin A1C level. Her American Society of Anesthesiologists (ASA) classification is
   a. ASA 1
   b. ASA 2
   c. ASA 3
   d. ASA 4

7. Malignant hyperthermia can be triggered by which of the following?
   a. Propofol
   b. Halothane
   c. Bupivacaine
   d. Rocuronium

8. A 67-year-old man undergoes an incisional hernia repair with components separation performed by you. Which of the following may be billed to Medicare in addition to the components separation?
   a. Meeting with the patient in the preoperative holding area to obtain hospital consent and mark the abdomen
   b. Office visit to remove drains on postoperative day POD 12
   c. Half-hour meeting on POD 4 with patient, family, and social worker to discuss rehab placement
   d. Office visit 6 months postop to evaluate result of repair

9. You are interviewing a candidate for your plastic surgery residency program. The candidate's personal statement indicates that her interest in plastic surgery stemmed from needing plastic surgery after a car accident. The personal statement also indicates that her favorite activity in her spare time is playing with her children. Which of the following is an acceptable question to ask during the interview?
   a. What type of child care would you use during your residency?
   b. Do you speak any foreign languages?
   c. What kind of injuries did you sustain in your accident?
   d. Is your spouse able to help you with home responsibilities?

10. A 16-year-old male is scheduled to undergo a rectus abdominis free flap to the distal right leg using a pfannensteil-type incision for harvest, with split-thickness skin graft to the flap. Which of the following maneuvers can be billed in addition to the free flap?
    a. Elevation of the lower abdominal skin to expose the rectus
    b. Exposure of the posterior tibial vessels for anastomosis to the flap through a separate incision and creation of a tunnel to the defect
    c. Split thickness skin graft
    d. Complex closure of the abdomen

Chapter 2

1. What anatomic landmark can be used to identify the approximate location of the mental nerve as it travels through the mental foramen to provide sensory innervation to the lower lip and chin?
    a. Third molar
    b. Canine
    c. Central incisor
    d. Second premolar

2. Your 55-year-old female presents to your office 3 days after undergoing a facelift procedure. She is complaining of numbness to her right earlobe. What nerve was most likely injured during the procedure to account for this finding?
    a. Auriculotemporal
    b. Greater occipital
    c. Great auricular
    d. Lesser occipital

3. A 34-year-old female presents to your office 1 day after suffering a deep laceration to the right cheek and neck, which was repaired in the emergency room. She now has an asymmetric smile concerning for concomitant nerve injury. The function of what muscle can help distinguish between a marginal mandibular nerve injury and a cervical branch injury?
    a. Mentalis
    b. Orbicularis oris
    c. Risorius
    d. Buccinator

4. What structure passes through the foramen rotundum?
    a. Internal carotid artery
    b. Maxillary division of the trigeminal nerve
    c. Facial nerve
    d. Mandibular division of the trigeminal nerve

5. Which of the following structures does NOT pass through the superior orbital fissure?
    a. Oculomotor nerve
    b. Abducens nerve
    c. Optic nerve
    d. Trochlear nerve

6. A 29-year-old male presented to the emergency room 3 hours ago with a deep, vertical laceration over the left posterior zygomatic arch. On exam, the patient is unable to elevate the left eyebrow. How long after the injury is it possible to electrically stimulate the transected distal nerve end and evaluate muscle contraction?
    a. 12 hours
    b. 24 hours
    c. 48 hours
    d. 72 hours

7. The facial nerve courses in which fascial layer within the temporal region?
    a. Superficial temporal fascia
    b. Superficial layer of deep temporal fascia
    c. Temporal fat pad
    d. Deep layer of deep temporal fascia

8. Your 39-year-old patient presents to the emergency room with pronounced ipsilateral cheek edema 2 days status post direct end-to-end repair of a transected buccal branch of the facial nerve. The patient noted the increased edema after resuming eating. What injury was most likely missed at the time of presentation?
    a. Facial artery transection
    b. Parotid duct transection
    c. Submandibular parenchymal injury
    d. Intraoral laceration

9. A 45-year-old female presents to your office 6 months after resolution of Bell's palsy with concerns regarding difficulty opening her eyes when moving her mouth. These symptoms began only in the last 2 to 3 weeks. She does not have difficulty opening her eyes at any other time. What is the most likely diagnosis?
    a. Hypertonicity
    b. Atrophy
    c. Ectropion
    d. Synkinesis

10. A 3-year-old male is brought to your clinic with his parents for evaluation of a mass on the central neck. The mass has been draining fluid for 2 weeks. On exam, the mass does not appear acutely infected, and you note that it moves when the patient swallows and protrudes his tongue. In addition to the mass, what structure will most likely require excision?
    a. Central portion of the hyoid bone
    b. Anterior edge of sternocleidomastoid muscle
    c. Thyroid cartilage
    d. Lymph node

Chapter 3

1. Related to salivary gland tumors, all of the following statements are correct, except
   a. Hemangioma is the most common parotid tumor in children.
   b. Mucoepidermoid carcinoma is the most common salivary gland malignancy.
   c. Adenoid cystic carcinoma usually presents as a painless, nonfixed mass without facial nerve dysfunction. Superficial parotidectomy with nerve preservation is the treatment of choice.
   d. Pleomorphic adenoma is treated by superficial parotidectomy and facial nerve preservation.

2. A 25-year-old male presents with a mandibular swelling. On imaging, a large well-demarcated radiolucency in the posterior mandible is identified. An incisional biopsy confirms an odontogenic keratocyst (keratocystic odontogenic tumor). All of the following with respect to management of this tumor are correct except
   a. For smaller cysts, enucleation with removal of the entire cyst lining is appropriate.
   b. For larger, multilocular lesions, enucleation alone is associated with higher recurrence rates.
   c. If multiple cysts are present, nevoid basal cell carcinoma syndrome (Gorlin syndrome) must be ruled out.
   d. Close follow-up of the patient is unnecessary.

3. In tongue reconstruction, identify the incorrect treatment plan for a given defect or tumor.
   a. Small defect: can often be closed primarily or with skin graft
   b. Larger tumor involving 1/3 to 1/2 of the tongue and requiring adjuvant radiotherapy: A flap that provides adequate lining and prevents tethering of the remaining tongue is required, such as radial forearm free flap.
   c. Subtotal glossectomy: A flap that provides bulk for restoration of speech and facility with oral diet is necessary, such as the anterolateral thigh (ALT) flap.
   d. Total glossectomy: skin graft

4. Risk factors for developing bisphosphonate-related osteonecrosis (medication-related osteonecrosis of the jaw [MRONJ]) include
   a. Oral bisphosphonates
   b. Intravenous bisphosphonates
   c. Dental infection, periodontal disease, or tooth extraction
   d. Chemotherapy
   e. All of the above

5. With regard to vascular malformations and hemangiomas, choose the correct pairs:
   a. Vascular malformations are present at birth; hemangiomas usually appear within the first 4 weeks of life.
   b. Vascular malformations demonstrate proportionate growth with age; hemangiomas have a rapid growth phase followed by involution.
   c. Low-flow venous malformation can be treated by sclerotherapy followed by surgical excision; asymptomatic hemangiomas may be observed.
   d. Vascular malformations of an extremity are present in Klippel-Trenaunay syndrome and retinal hemangiomas are present in von Hippel-Lindau syndrome.
   e. All of the above

6. An otherwise healthy 68-year-old man is evaluated for bilateral 1.5-cm parotid masses. Physical examination does not demonstrate facial muscle weakness. Fine-needle aspiration of one of the lesions reveals mucoid fluid, lymphoid tissue nodules, and papillary cysts. What is the most likely diagnosis?
   a. Squamous cell carcinoma (SCC)
   b. Pleomorphic adenoma
   c. Mucoepidermoid carcinoma
   d. Warthin's tumor

7. A 58-year-old woman underwent left superficial parotidectomy for a pleomorphic adenoma 2 years ago. She presents with complaints of occasional perspiration and redness of the left cheek and ear after eating. Which of the following nerves is the most likely source of these complaints?
   a. Great auricular
   b. Frontal branch of the facial nerve
   c. Auriculotemporal
   d. Lingual

8. Which of the following is the most appropriate initial treatment for a 4-year-old boy with a painful venous malformation of the cheek and neck with obvious facial asymmetry?
   a. Resection
   b. Embolization
   c. Sclerotherapy
   d. Systemic corticosteroid therapy

9. Which of the following is the most appropriate treatment for a T4aN0M0 floor-of-mouth SCC with mandibular cortical invasion?
   a. Wide local excision, neck dissection, and segmental mandibulectomy
   b. Wide local excision alone
   c. Wide local excision and segmental mandibulectomy
   d. Wide local excision and neck dissection

10. A 69-year-old woman who underwent previous resection, radiation, and chemotherapy for oropharyngeal cancer presents with halitosis and left-sided jaw pain. Intraoral examination reveals a 1-cm area of exposed yellow mandibular bone. A subsequent computed tomography (CT) scan does not reveal any evidence of fracture. What is the most appropriate initial management?
   a. Hyperbaric oxygen (HBO) therapy
   b. Antimicrobial mouthwash, antibiotics, and observation
   c. Resection of the exposed mandible and reconstruction with a fibular free flap
   d. Debridement of the exposed bone

Chapter 4

1. A 45-year-old male presents to the emergency room after a motor vehicle collision. He is unconscious and intubated. On examination, he has right periorbital ecchymosis and swelling. When a light is shined on his left eye, both pupils constrict, and when the light is shined on his right eye, the right pupil dilates. Which of the following is the most likely etiology of this finding?
   a. Entrapment of the inferior rectus muscle
   b. Injury to the optic nerve
   c. Hyphema
   d. Enophthalmos

2. A 29-year-old male was involved in a bicycle accident and presents to the emergency room with a palpable step-off of the left hemimandible and malocclusion. A CT scan reveals a displaced fracture of the left mandibular body near the 3rd molar. Which of the following is an indication for extraction of the 3rd molar during fixation of this fracture?
   a. The 3rd molar is near the fracture line.
   b. The 3rd molar enamel is chipped and would require dental treatment.
   c. The 3rd molar is impacted.
   d. The 3rd molar contains dental caries.

3. An 8-year-old boy presents to the emergency room after being struck in the face with a baseball. On examination, he has left periorbital ecchymosis and swelling with restricted upward gaze. He is vomiting and bradycardic. A CT scan reveals a minimally displaced orbital floor fracture. Which of the following is the most appropriate treatment?
   a. Reassurance and observation
   b. Ophthalmology follow-up
   c. Emergent operative reduction and orbital floor reconstruction
   d. Elective operative reduction and orbital floor reconstruction within 7 days

4. A 2-year-old girl presents to your office with orbital dystopia and a growing skull fracture. Nine months ago, she fell and fractured her right superior orbital rim and orbital roof and was treated nonoperatively. Which of the following is the most likely etiology of her presentation?
   a. Unrecognized craniofacial cleft
   b. New craniofacial trauma
   c. Unrecognized dural tear at the time of her initial injury
   d. Metabolic disorder

5. A 34-year-old female presents to the emergency room after a motor vehicle accident. On examination, she has bilateral periorbital ecchymosis, telecanthus, and upturning of the nasal tip. A CT scan reveals a type-III naso-orbital ethmoid fracture. Which of the following is the appropriate position for placement of the medial canthal tendon at the time of repair?
   a. Posterior and superior to the lacrimal fossa
   b. Anterior and superior to the lacrimal fossa
   c. Posterior and inferior to the lacrimal fossa
   d. Anterior and inferior to the lacrimal fossa

6. A 45-year-old male presents to the emergency department after a head-on motor vehicle collision. Examination shows a stellate laceration and a palpable deformity in the frontal region. A CT scan shows a displaced and comminuted fracture of the anterior wall of the frontal sinus and a nondisplaced fracture of the posterior wall. The frontonasal duct is not patent. Which of the following is the most appropriate treatment?
   a. Open reduction and internal fixation (ORIF) of the anterior wall of the frontal sinus
   b. Obliteration of the sinus and nasofrontal duct
   c. Cranialization of the sinus and obliteration of the nasofrontal duct
   d. ORIF of the anterior wall of the frontal sinus and stenting of the nasofrontal duct

7. A 27-year-old male was struck in the face during an altercation. Examination demonstrates right periorbital ecchymosis and edema. A CT scan shows a right orbital floor and comminuted medial orbital wall fracture. Which incision is preferred?
   a. Bicoronal
   b. Subciliary
   c. Transconjunctival
   d. Subtarsal

8. Which of the following is the optimal treatment of noncomminuted mandibular body fracture?
   a. A Champy plate
   b. Maxillomandibular fixation (MMF)
   c. Inferior border compression plate and superior miniplate
   d. Inferior border locking plate and arch bar

9. A 25-year-old female presents with a displaced zygomaticomaxillary complex fracture and a palpable step-off along the inferior orbital rim. Proper alignment of which of the following structures is most important to confirm adequate reduction?
   a. Zygomaticofrontal suture
   b. Zygomaticomaxillary buttress
   c. Zygomaticotemporal suture
   d. Zygomaticosphenoid suture
   e. Inferior orbital rim

10. A 30-year-old male presents to the emergency department 2 weeks after ORIF of a parasymphyseal and angle fracture of the mandible. On exam, he has significant facial swelling and purulent drainage from his intraoral incision. A CT scan shows fluid collection, but the hardware is still in place without evidence of osteomyelitis. He still has his arch bars on but is not in MMF. The most appropriate management would be
   a. intravenous (IV) antibiotics
   b. Incision and drainage (I&D)
   c. I&D with plate and arch bar removal
   d. I&D with plate removal and use of the arch bars to put him in MMF

Chapter 5

1. Robin sequence is a clinical diagnosis characterized by
   a. Micrognathia
   b. Glossoptosis
   c. Upper airway obstruction
   d. All of the above

2. A 7-month-old boy presents to your clinic with the chief complaint of abnormal head shape since birth. Physical exam shows flattening of the right forehead and supraorbital rim with elevation of the eyebrow. Which of the following is your recommended treatment?
   a. Total vault reconstruction
   b. Endoscope-assisted strip craniectomy and helmet therapy
   c. Fronto-orbital advancement
   d. Cranial distraction

3. A 2-month-old presents with eyelid ptosis, telecanthus, bilateral frontal retrusion, increased head height, and low frontal hairline. A CT scan shows bilateral coronal synostosis. The most likely genetic mutation involves
   a. FGFR2
   b. FGFR3
   c. TWIST1
   d. TCOF1

4. Which of the following sutures is the first to close?
   a. Sagittal
   b. Metopic
   c. Coronal
   d. Lambdoid

5. A 3-year-old presents to your office with bilateral malar deficiency, lower eyelid coloboma, and retrognathia. Which of the following is the most likely diagnosis?
   a. Treacher Collins syndrome
   b. Robin sequence
   c. Apert syndrome
   d. Craniofacial microsomia

6. A facial bipartition is planned for a 7-year-old female with an anterior interorbital distance of 40 mm (normal mean = 21.5 mm). Which of the following diagnoses best accounts for these findings?
   a. Craniofrontonasal dysplasia with hypertelorbitism
   b. Craniofrontonasal dysplasia with telecanthus
   c. Goldenhar syndrome with epibulbar dermoids
   d. Crouzon syndrome with exorbitism

7. A Pi procedure is planned for an infant with sagittal craniosynostosis. Which of the following best characterizes the objectives of this procedure?
   a. AP lengthening, biparietal widening
   b. AP shortening, biparietal narrowing
   c. AP lengthening, biparietal narrowing
   d. AP shortening, biparietal widening

8. Which of the following features is consistent with a right unilateral lambdoid craniosynostosis as opposed to right posterior deformational plagiocephaly?
   a. Anterior displacement of the right ear
   b. Right occipitomastoid flattening
   c. Right frontal bulging
   d. Parallelogram-like head shape from the posterior view

9. A newborn is evaluated in the NICU for respiratory distress. The examination is notable for down-slanting palpebral fissures, eyelid colobomata, malar hypoplasia, severe mandibular retrognathia, and bilateral hypoplastic thumbs. A CT scan shows abnormal temporomandibular joints. The patient's features are most consistent with which craniofacial syndrome?
   a. Pfeiffer
   b. Nager
   c. Treacher Collins
   d. Apert

10. A 17-year-old female with Binder syndrome is scheduled to undergo orthognathic surgery to address deficiency at the level of the nasion and maxillary occlusal plane. This is best achieved with
    a. Fronto-orbital advancement
    b. LeFort I osteotomy
    c. LeFort II osteotomy
    d. Surgically assisted rapid palatal expansion (SARPE)

Chapter 6

1. A 3-month-old child presents with Goldenhar syndrome characterized by microtia, macrostomia, VIIth nerve palsy, epibulbar dermoid, hypoplastic mandibular ramus without a defined right mandibular condyl/glenoid fossa, and a hypoplastic maxilla. Which branchial arches are involved with this condition?
   a. 2nd and 3rd branchial arches
   b. 1st and 2nd branchial arches
   c. 1st, 2nd, and 3rd branchial arches
   d. 2nd and 4th branchial arches

2. NICU consults plastic surgery to see a 2-day-old infant with the following findings: small recessed lower jaw, a high-arched U-shaped cleft palate, and chest retractions. Which of the following syndromes can be associated with these findings?
   a. Stickler syndrome, velocardiofacial syndrome (VCFS)
   b. Crouzon syndrome, Apert syndrome
   c. Parry Romberg syndrome, cherubism
   d. van der Woude, ectrodactyly–ectodermal dysplasia–cleft syndrome (EEC)

3. A child presents with a typical cleft lip that starts at what would have been the left philtral column but courses more laterally, disrupting the left alar base cheek junction as it continues superiorly to the medial lower eyelid canthal region. The child presents with which Tessier cleft number?
   a. Tessier 4 cleft
   b. Tessier 2 cleft
   c. Tessier 3 cleft
   d. Tessier 5 cleft

4. Parents bring a 16-year-old girl to your office because she is unhappy with the appearance of her nose and chin. She has a history of a left cleft lip and palate. She presents with a significantly asymmetrical nasal tip and alar base. Additional physical findings that would be consistent include
   a. Caudal septal deviation to the right
   b. The dome of the left lower lateral cartilage is higher than the dome on the right side.
   c. Caudal septal deviation to the left
   d. Proximal septal deviation to the right

5. Further examination of the 16-year-old girl interested in cleft nasal rhinoplasty revealed that she has an acute nasal labial angle, short vertical lip, and no show of her front teeth (−2 mm). When asked to smile, she does not show any gingiva, and she has a significant anterior cross bite (−9 mm) missing the left lateral incisor, and left posterior crossbite. Lateral cephalometric radiographs show that she a sella-nasion-subspinale (SNA) angle of 76° (82°) and an SNB of 85° (80°). The appropriate surgical sequence would be
   a. Cleft rhinoplasty followed by LeFort I with setback genioplasty
   b. Bilateral sagittal split osteotomy (BSSO) setback followed by cleft rhinoplasty
   c. Cleft rhinoplasty with genioplasty setback
   d. LeFort I advancement and BSSO setback followed by cleft rhinoplasty

6. A pregnant mother suffers an insult while she is in the 9th week of gestation. She is concerned about the potential of a cleft deformity. During a prenatal consult with this family, what type of cleft(s) should you discuss as a likely possibility?
   a. Cleft lip only
   b. Cleft palate only
   c. Cleft lip and palate
   d. Cleft lip and primary palate

7. A child with a previously repaired cleft palate presents with a new diagnosis of velopharyngeal insufficiency. As videonasoendoscopy is being performed, the otolaryngologist notes clear evidence of pulsatility in the posterior pharynx. What is the likely diagnosis on this patient?
   a. van der Woude syndrome
   b. Treacher Collins syndrome
   c. Stickler syndrome
   d. 22q11.2 deletion syndrome (DS)

8. Which of the muscles of the velopharynx is NOT innervated by the pharyngeal plexus (IX, X, and XI)?
   a. Levator veli palatini
   b. Tensor veli palatini
   c. Palatoglossus
   d. Superior pharyngeal constrictor

9. A 10-year-old girl presents with velopharyngeal dysfunction and severe sleep apnea. Videonasoendoscopy and videofluoroscopy are performed, demonstrating little to no velar or lateral wall movement of the palate during speech examination. Her speech is pervasively hypernasal. Which management strategy is most reasonable for this patient?
   a. Furlow double-opposing Z plasty
   b. Pharyngeal flap
   c. Sphincter pharyngoplasty
   d. Palatal prosthesis

10. An 18-year-old female enters for orthognathic evaluation. On examination, she has class-III occlusion with a negative overjet of 9 mm. Cephalograms demonstrate an SNA angle of 75 degrees and an SNB angle of 80 degrees. What procedure should be offered to this patient?
   a. LeFort I advancement and bilateral sagittal split osteotomies (BSSOs) of the mandible
   b. LeFort I advancement alone
   c. BSSOs of the mandible alone
   d. LeFort I osteotomy with distraction

Chapter 7

1. A 65-year-old man presents to you with a large SCC of the superior helix. What nodal basin primarily drains this region?
   a. Level-I cervical nodes
   b. Level-II cervical nodes
   c. Level-III cervical nodes
   d. Parotid nodes

2. Which of the following is the primary blood supply to the ear?
   a. Superficial temporal artery
   b. Occipital artery
   c. Posterior auricular artery
   d. Transverse facial artery

3. Which of the following is not a common cause of prominent ear?
   a. Conchoscaphal angle >90 degrees
   b. Deepened conchal bowl
   c. Prominent lobule
   d. Auriculocephalic angle <25 degrees

4. A 7-year-old boy is brought to your office by his parents regarding their concern for the appearance of his right ear. On examination, the superior helix of the right ear is abnormally adherent to the temporal skin. Gentle retraction on the helix allows it to be pulled out to a normal position. What is the most likely diagnosis?
   a. Lop ear
   b. Stahl's ear
   c. Cup ear
   d. Cryptotia

5. A 45-year-old female was involved in an accident and suffered an injury to her left ear. On examination, she has a defect of the superior helical rim that is ~1.5 cm in length. Which of the following is the best method for reconstruction of this defect?
   a. Primary closure
   b. Posterior auricular transposition flap
   c. Antia-Buch chondrocutaneous flap
   d. Orticochea chondrocutaneous flap

6. Which of the following statements is not true for autogenous total auricular reconstruction?
   a. The Tanzer method uses full-thickness lobule rotation.
   b. The Nagata method uses split-lobule rotation.
   c. When creating a skin pocket for cartilage framework implantation, 5 mm is the ideal thickness of the skin flap for optimal definition.
   d. There is often insufficient costal cartilage for an adequate autogenous reconstruction if the chest circumference is less than 60 cm.

7. Which of the following statements is not true regarding microtia associated with craniofacial deformities?
   a. Microtia in hemifacial microsomia is associated with low-set, anteriorly located vestige skin and low hairline.
   b. Microtia in hemifacial microsomia is associated with an atypical course of superficial temporal vessels.
   c. For bilateral microtia with craniofacial deformities, it is imperative to refer the child for hearing assistance; bone-anchored hearing aids (BAHA) or external hearing aids need to be placed at an earlier age to help the development of the child.
   d. Autogenous auricular reconstruction is contraindicated in microtia with severe craniofacial deformities.

8. What is the embryologic origin of the superior helix?
   a. First branchial arch
   b. First branchial cleft
   c. Second branchial arch
   d. Second branchial cleft

9. Which of the following statements is false regarding the proper anatomy, dimensions, and proportion of the auricle?
   a. The auricle is located 6.5 to 7.5 cm posterior to the lateral orbital rim.
   b. The axis of the auricle is inclined 10 to 20 degrees posteriorly.
   c. A well-proportioned auricle width is 50% to 55% of the length.
   d. The top of the auricle is on line with the lateral canthus.

10. What is the optimal timing for nonsurgical correction of external ear deformity using external splinting?
    a. Immediately after birth
    b. Three months after birth
    c. Before the age of 1 year
    d. At any age

Chapter 8

1. Describe the dominant arterial blood supply to the breast.
   a. Intercostal artery perforators
   b. Lateral thoracic artery perforators
   c. Second and third internal mammary artery (IMA) perforators
   d. Thoracoacromial artery perforators

2. In the youthful, nonptotic breast, what is the normal distance between the nipple and the inframammary fold (IMF)?
   a. Nine to 10 cm
   b. Ten to 11 cm
   c. Five to 6 cm
   d. Seven to 8 cm

3. What is the normal diameter of the nipple-areolar complex (NAC)?
   a. Twenty to 30 mm
   b. Twenty-five to 35 mm
   c. Thirty five to 45 mm
   d. Forty to 50 mm

4. The pectoralis major muscle originates on the medial sternal half of the clavicle and lateral aspect of the sternum/costochondral region and is the major component of the anterior axillary fold. Which nerve provides motor innervation to the lateral and inferior portion of the pectoralis major muscle?
   a. Lateral pectoral nerve
   b. Medial pectoral nerve
   c. Third and fourth medial intercostal nerves
   d. Long thoracic nerve

5. A 35-year-old female undergoes bilateral breast reduction with an inferior pedicle design. What is the dominant arterial supply to the inferior pedicle of the breast?
   a. Intercostal artery perforators
   b. Lateral thoracic artery perforators
   c. Second and third IMA perforators
   d. Thoracoacromial artery perforators

6. An 11-year-old female presents to her primary care physician for a routine physical exam. On exam, she has a palpable breast bud and the areola is slightly elevated. She meets criteria for which Tanner stage of breast development?
   a. Stage I
   b. Stage II
   c. Stage III
   d. Stage IV

7. Incomplete involution of the mammary ridge during gestation results in accessory breast tissue (polymastia) and supernumerary nipples (polythelia). What is the most common location of accessory breast tissue and supernumerary nipples, respectively?
   a. Inframammary area and axilla
   b. Supramammary area and pelvis
   c. Axilla and inframammary area
   d. Axilla and supramammary area

8. During dissection along the lateral border of the pectoralis major muscle, a nerve is injured resulting in reduced sensation to the NAC. Which nerve was likely injured?
   a. Supraclavicular branches of the cervical plexus
   b. Cutaneous branch of 4th intercostal nerve
   c. Cutaneous branch of 3rd intercostal nerve
   d. Cutaneous branch of 6th intercostal nerve

9. The internal mammary/parasternal lymph nodes receive efferent lymph drainage from what portion of the breast parenchyma?
   a. Upper inner quadrant
   b. Lower inner quadrant
   c. Upper inner and lower inner quadrants
   d. All breast quadrants

10. A 14-year-old female presents with bilateral diffuse breast enlargement. She complains of shoulder pain, tender breasts, and a chronic rash along the IMFs bilaterally. Which of the following is true regarding juvenile breast hypertrophy?
    a. The breast enlargement is always bilateral.
    b. Estrogen levels are typically elevated in these patients.
    c. Hormone receptors are overexpressed in the breast parenchyma of these patients.
    d. First-line therapy is reduction mammoplasty.

11. A 17-year-old female presents with right unilateral Poland syndrome with severe breast hypoplasia, including a superiorly malpositioned NAC. What is the likely etiology of her disrupted pectoralis major development?
    a. Abnormal migration of mesenchymal tissue during the eighth and ninth weeks of gestation
    b. Hypoplasia of the branches of the brachial artery
    c. An extrinsic disturbance in morphogenesis such as amniotic bands
    d. Hypoplasia of the internal thoracic artery

12. A 16-year-old female presents with a rapidly enlarging mass in her left breast. The growth has caused considerable asymmetric enlargement of the breast. You suspect a giant fibroadenoma. What is the most appropriate next step in the management of this patient?
    a. Reassurance and follow-up in 6 months
    b. Core needle biopsy
    c. Surgical excision
    d. Mammography

13. A 42-year-old male presents with complaints of bilateral breast enlargement. On exam, he has moderate breast enlargement with excess skin overlying the breast tissue. What Simon grade correctly correlates with his physical exam findings?
    a. Grade I
    b. Grade IIA
    c. Grade IIB
    d. Grade III

14. A 15-year-old male presents with a chief complaint of bilateral breast enlargement. Laboratory studies reveal elevated human chorionic gonadotropin (HCG) and estrogen/androgen ratio. Luteinizing hormone (LH), follicle-stimulating hormone (FSH), and thyroid function tests are within normal limits. Which of the following should be ordered as a follow-up to the elevated HCG and estrogen/androgen ratio?
    a. Adrenal CT scan
    b. Liver function tests
    c. Chest X ray
    d. Ultrasound of the testes

15. Which of the following medications is known to cause gynecomastia as a side effect?
    a. Ketoconazole
    b. Amoxicillin
    c. Losartan
    d. Cephalexin

16. A 61-year-old woman post-3-vessel coronary artery bypass graft using the IMA presents with symptomatic mammary hypertrophy. Her cardiac function is excellent and she has clearance from her cardiologist to have a reduction mammaplasty. Based on optimizing the vascularity to the NAC, which pedicle would place the nipple at highest risk?
    a. Inferior
    b. Medial
    c. Superior
    d. Central mound

17. A 15-year old girl presents to the clinic because of abnormal right breast development. Physical findings include a normal left breast, presence of the pectoralis major muscle, and absence of glandular tissue with a nipple present. What is the most likely diagnosis?
    a. Poland syndrome
    b. Atheia
    c. Jeune syndrome
    d. Amastia

18. A 20-year-old woman presents with irregular breast development and an unusual shape. She is diagnosed with a tuberous breast deformity. All of the following are characteristic of a tuberous breast except
    a. Constricted IMF
    b. Herniation of the NAC
    c. Lowered IMF
    d. Narrowed breast base

19. A 25-year-old woman presents for bilateral breast augmentation. Physical examination demonstrates a "pigeon's chest" appearance. The most likely diagnosis is
    a. Thoracic hyperplasia
    b. Thoracic hypoplasia
    c. Pectus excavatum
    d. Pectus carinatum

20. A 35-year-old woman presents for correction of a Poland deformity. The classic findings include all of the following except
    a. Absence of the clavicular head of the pectoralis major
    b. Hypoplasia or aplasia of the breast or nipple
    c. Deficiency of subcutaneous fat and axillary hair
    d. Abnormalities of the rib cage
    e. Upper extremity anomalies

Chapter 9

1. Which is the extra information you can get from an angio-CT before starting a free perforator flap breast reconstruction compared to a duplex Doppler study?
    a. Determination of the size and position of the dominant perforator
    b. Better evaluation of the recipient site
    c. Three-dimensional (3D) anatomy of the branches of the perforator in between the skin and the deep fascia
    d. Quantification and direction of flow
    e. Determination of the course of the perforator through the muscle

2. Which of the statements below is NOT true? Autologous breast reconstruction, compared to implants, provides
    a. Better sensation of the breast
    b. Easier oncologic follow-up
    c. Better control of the breast cancer
    d. Ultimately less expensive treatment
    e. More esthetically pleasing and long-lasting result

3. For a patient undergoing lumpectomy and irradiation, the following treatment is the least indicated:
    a. No reconstruction
    b. Contralateral breast reduction
    c. Reconstruction with a thoracodorsal artery perforator (TDAP) or pedicled latissimus dorsi flap
    d. Temporarily filling the lumpectomy cavity with liquids or a small prosthesis
    e. A small deep inferior epigastric artery perforator (DIEAP) flap

4. A surgeon can increase the safety of the dissection of a perforator flap by
    a. Creating and maintaining a dry surgical field
    b. Working with a wide exposure of the surgical field
    c. Starting the dissection from one side only
    d. Staying close to the perforator vessels
    e. Preserving every perforator until a bigger one is found
    f. All of the above

5. Which of the following statements on autologous breast reconstruction is incorrect?
    a. Tissue expanders do not work well for radiated chest-wall breast reconstructions.
    b. The nipple must always be resected in cases of invasive breast cancer at <2.5 cm of the areola.
    c. Primary reconstruction is usually better than secondary reconstruction.
    d. Skin-sparing mastectomy yields more local recurrences.
    e. Breast reconstruction with autologous tissue has no interference on local recurrences.

6. The lifetime risk of breast cancer for women with the *BRCA* mutation is
    a. 55%
    b. 65%
    c. 75%
    d. 85%

7. Which of the following mammographic findings are suggestive for malignancy?
    a. Popcorn-like calcifications
    b. Large rod-like calcifications
    c. Linear or branching calcifications
    d. Dystrophic/coarse calcifications

8. Which of the following conditions, although often treated as cancer, is not actually cancer?
    a. Ductile carcinoma in situ (DCIS)
    b. Invasive ductal carcinoma
    c. Invasive lobular carcinoma

9. Contraindications to breast conservation therapy include
    a. Large tumor relative to breast size
    b. History of previous radiation therapy to the breast area
    c. Multifocal breast cancer
    d. All of the above

10. The risk of breast cancer recurrence following a skin-sparing mastectomy is ___ % at 4 years?
    a. 1%
    b. 2%
    c. 6%
    d. 8%

11. Options for women for whom the need of radiation therapy is unknown include
    a. Placement of a tissue expander keeping all options open
    b. Free transverse rectus abdominis myocutaneous (TRAM) flap
    c. Delayed reconstruction
    d. All of the above

12. Reported complications from the transverse upper gracilis (TUG) myocutaneous flap include which of the following?
    a. Size limitation
    b. Visibility of donor site scar
    c. Lower extremity lymphedema
    d. All of the above
13. Management considerations in mastectomy skin flap loss associated with an expander reconstruction include
    a. The presence of muscle or vascularized tissue beneath the area of necrosis
    b. Need for postoperative chemotherapy/radiation therapy
    c. Both A and B
    d. Neither A nor B

Chapter 10

1. Relative to subglandular breast implant placement, placement of a breast implant deep to the pectoralis major muscle will result in
    a. Increased risk of visible rippling
    b. Increased risk of pseudoptosis
    c. Decreased risk of capsular contracture
    d. Increased risk of edge visibility
    e. Increased risk of implant movement with muscle contraction
2. Which of the following is NOT part of triple-antibiotic breast irrigation solution?
    a. Cefazolin
    b. Gentamycin
    c. Clindamycin
    d. Bacitracin
3. Which of the following is NOT a characteristic of the tuberous breast deformity?
    a. Herniation of breast tissue through NAC
    b. Constricted breast base
    c. High IMF
    d. Increased distance from IMF to nipple
4. A 26-year-old woman will undergo breast augmentation with a transaxillary approach for subpectoral placement of breast implants. Which of the following nerves is at greatest risk of injury during a transaxillary approach for breast augmentation?
    a. Axillary nerve
    b. Fourth intercostal nerve
    c. Thoracodorsal nerve
    d. Intercostobrachial nerve
    e. Long thoracic nerve
5. A 42-year-old woman presents with an acutely swollen breast 8 years after having breast augmentation. During surgery, a periprosthetic fluid collection is found that appears to be consistent with a late seroma. What immunohistochemical marker should be tested for when sending periprosthetic fluid for cytology?
    a. CD8
    b. CD20
    c. CD30
    d. CD38

6. A 26-year-old female presents with an enlarged areola further deformed by parenchymal herniation, a narrow base diameter, and constricted lower pole. Which of the following procedures should not be offered to this patient?
    a. Staged reconstruction with placement of a tissue expander followed thereafter by a breast implant
    b. Aggressive capsular lower pole parenchymal scoring followed by placement of a form-stable breast implant
    c. Autoaugmentation of the breast with an inferiorly based parenchymal flap through a periareolar approach
    d. Autologous fat grafting
    e. Lateral intercostal artery perforator flap (LICAP)
7. From which commonly used dermoglandular pedicle is blood supply to the nipple areola the least robust?
    a. Medial pedicle
    b. Bipedicle (superior and inferior)
    c. Inferior pedicle
    d. Superomedial pedicle
    e. Lateral pedicle
8. Form-stable breast implants confer all of the following advantages relative to smooth, round, silicone implants when placed in a submuscular or biplanar location, except
    a. Less rippling
    b. Lower rate of capsular contracture at 8 years
    c. Greater range of device volumes
    d. Lower leak rates at 8 years
    e. Greater upper pole fullness
9. Which combination of implant location and shell surface characteristic is associated with the highest rate of capsular contracture?
    a. Submuscular; textured
    b. Biplanar; smooth
    c. Biplanar; textured
    d. Subglandular; smooth
    e. Subglandular; textured
10. Which etiology is least associated with capsular contracture?
    a. Patient age
    b. Subclinical infection or biofilm formation
    c. Radiation
    d. Incision selection for implant placement
    e. Perioperative hemostasis

Chapter 11

1. For complex abdominal-wall reconstruction with synthetic mesh, it is widely accepted that increasingly contaminated wound classes are associated with progressively higher complication rates. Which Centers for Disease Control (CDC) wound classification is associated with the worst major complication profile (i.e., recurrent hernia, mesh infection, mesh explantation) for complex abdominal-wall reconstruction with **bioprosthetic** mesh?
    a. Class I (clean)
    b. Class II (clean-contaminated)
    c. Class III (contaminated)
    d. Class IV (dirty/infected)
    e. None of the above

2. For patients undergoing abdominal-wall reconstruction, which of the following medical comorbidities has **not** been shown to be associated with a fourfold increase in surgical site infection rates?
   a. Obesity
   b. Diabetes
   c. Steroid use
   d. Smoking
   e. Chronic obstructive pulmonary disease (COPD)

3. A 60-year-old diabetic male with a 15 × 20-cm² recurrent ventral hernia that was originally repaired with bridged synthetic mesh presents for a second operation to address his defect. He now presents with wound breakdown and exposure of the mesh. Which is the most appropriate technique to repair this patient's recurrent ventral hernia?
   a. Minimally invasive component separation with inlay bioprosthetic mesh
   b. Primary fascial closure without mesh
   c. Open components separation with onlay synthetic mesh
   d. Bridging technique with bioprosthetic mesh

4. An 87-year-old male with advanced Alzheimer's disease presents from an extended care facility with a left-sided pressure sore overlying his greater trochanter. The wound extends through the entire thickness of the skin down to visible tendon, but no bone is visible at the base of the wound. What is the stage of this pressure sore?
   a. Stage I
   b. Stage II
   c. Stage III
   d. Stage IV

5. A 36-year-old, otherwise healthy paraplegic woman presents with a clean, recurrent, stage-3 sacral decubitus ulcer. This sacral pressure ulcer was previously closed with bilateral V-Y gluteus maximus advancement flaps. Which of the following is the most appropriate surgical technique to surgically close her wound?
   a. Tensor fascia lata flap
   b. Gluteus maximus musculocutaneous rotation flap
   c. Readvancement of V-Y gluteus maximus flaps
   d. Transverse back flap

6. An ambulatory 45-year-old male with spina bifida presents with a 7-cm stage-4 sacral decubitus ulcer. The most appropriate management would be reconstruction using which of the following?
   a. Full-thickness skin graft
   b. Bilateral gluteal myocutaneous advancement flaps
   c. Unilateral superior gluteal perforator flaps
   d. Unilateral inferior gluteal artery myocutaneous rotational flap
   e. Posterior thigh flap

7. A 24-year-old male with a 10-year history of T10 paraplegia from a traumatic motor vehicle accident now presents with a large stage-4 right greater trochanteric decubitus ulcer. MRI shows communication with the hip joint. What is the most appropriate next step in management?
   a. IV antibiotics followed by flap coverage in 6 weeks
   b. Coverage with a posterior thigh flap
   c. Coverage with a pedicle ALT flap
   d. Coverage with a tensor fascia lata flap
   e. Resection of the femoral head

8. A 30-year-old male with history of multiple previous abdominal procedures now presents for evaluation of a large ventral hernia with a 25-cm fascial defect. Abdominal-wall reconstruction using the technique of component separation and mesh is planned. What is the plane of dissection to maintain innervated muscle flaps?
   a. Between skin and the fascia
   b. Between the fascia and the external oblique
   c. Between the external oblique and the internal oblique
   d. Between the internal oblique and the transversalis fascia
   e. Between the transversalis fascia and the peritoneum

9. A 48-year-old female with history of rectal cancer status postradiation and low anterior resection is now presenting with recurrent rectal cancer. Imaging studies are consistent with invasion into the posterior vaginal wall in addition to perineal involvement. She is scheduled to undergo abdomino-perineal resection, hysterectomy, and posterior vaginal resection. What would be the best single-stage reconstructive option for this patient?
   a. Pedicle vertical rectus abdominis muscle flap
   b. Bilateral Singapore flaps
   c. Primary closure of perineal and vaginal defects
   d. Skin grafting
   e. Vastus lateralis flap

10. A 32-year-old female is scheduled to undergo female-to-male gender reassignment surgery. A radial fasciocutaneous flap is being designed for creation of a neophallus. The procedure involved neurorrhaphy of the lateral antebrachial cutaneous nerve to the terminal branch of which of the following nerves?
    a. Pudendal nerve
    b. Lateral femoral cutaneous nerve
    c. Posterior femoral cutaneous nerve
    d. Ilioinguinal nerve
    e. Iliohypogastric nerve

Chapter 12

1. Two days ago, a 45-year-old male suffered a sharp laceration to his hand. He presented to the emergency room, where the wound was cleaned and primarily closed. At present, he notes numbness and tingling primarily at the small finger. What is the best course of action?
   a. Observation for recovery
   b. Electrodiagnostic studies
   c. Exploration and repair/graft as needed
   d. Reverse end-to-side transfer to the ulnar nerve

2. A 27-year-old computer programmer presents 3 years after he inadvertently put his arm through a plate glass window. Ever since then, he notes loss of finger and thumb extension. He was just covered by health insurance and wants surgery to restore the best function possible. What do you recommend?
   a. Distal median-to-radial nerve transfers to restore individual finger and thumb flexion
   b. Supinator-to-posterior interosseous nerve transfer
   c. Tendon transfer of FCR to finger extensors and PL to thumb extensor
   d. Direct repair and decompression of the posterior interosseous nerve

3. Which of the following is TRUE of nerve root avulsion brachial plexus injuries?
   a. Peripheral nerves do not undergo regeneration.
   b. The Schwann cell body for motor nerves is located in the descending columns.
   c. Regeneration can occur across a gap of 2 cm or less.
   d. The sensory nerve action potential (SNAP) is intact.

4. Which of the following would be present in a neurapraxia-type nerve injury?
   a. An advancing Tinel's sign as recovery occurs
   b. Normal distal and proximal conduction
   c. Wallerian degeneration within but not between fascicles
   d. None of the above

5. A patient has an extensive ulnar nerve injury at the level of the elbow. All of the following are reasonable approaches EXCEPT
   a. Exploration and direct repair with the elbow flexed to allow for tension-free repair
   b. Exploration and repair using an interposed sural nerve graft
   c. Exploration and distal tendon and/or nerve transfers to restore critical function
   d. Exploration and repair using interposed medial antebrachial nerve graft
   e. Exploration, ulnar nerve transposition, and direct tension-free repair.

6. A 19-year-old man presents to the emergency room shorty after an altercation in which he was stabbed just above the right clavicle. On exam, he demonstrates normal elbow flexion and extension but decreased strength with wrist flexion. There is also weakness of index, long-, ring-, and little-finger flexion and difficulty with palmar abduction against resistance. Finger, thumb, and wrist extension is intact. Which structure is most likely to be injured?
   a. Median nerve
   b. Lateral cord
   c. Middle trunk
   d. Ulnar nerve
   e. Medial cord

7. Diminished amplitude on a nerve conduction study (NCS) is indicative of which of the following changes to the structure of the nerve being evaluated?
   a. Decreased myelination
   b. Decreased number of intact axons
   c. Fewer nodes of Ranvier
   d. Fewer Schwann cells
   e. Increased Schwann-cell senescence

8. A 32-year-old man sustained injuries to the right upper extremity after being ejected from a motor vehicle. Four weeks later, he presents to your office with a flaccid and insensate left upper extremity, with NCSs demonstrating preservation of sensory nerve action potentials. Testing of the paravertebral muscles, biceps, triceps, and deltoids reveals fibrillations and denervation in the motor action potentials. The nerve injury is most likely located at which of the following levels of the nerve?
   a. Lateral cord
   b. Suprascapular nerve
   c. Preganglionic root
   d. Posterior division
   e. C5 and C6 trunk

9. A 60-year-old man presents with numbness and difficulty in moving his ring and little fingers for the past year. Physical examination shows inability to abduct and adduct the ring and little fingers as well as first web-space atrophy and a positive Froment's sign. Sensation to light touch is diminished. Electromyography (EMG) and NCS are consistent with severe cubital tunnel syndrome. In addition to ulnar nerve release at the elbow, which of the following is the most appropriate management to restore intrinsic muscle function?
   a. Simultaneous Guyon's tunnel release
   b. End-to-side anterior interosseous nerve (AIN)-to-ulnar nerve transfer
   c. Sural nerve grafting at the elbow
   d. Fascicular neurolysis
   e. Vascularized nerve grafting at the elbow

10. A 29-year-old football player presents 3 months following a right knee hyperextension injury that resulted in extensive ligamentous injury in addition to a peroneal nerve palsy. EMG/NCS obtained immediately prior to his office visit demonstrated a persistent peroneal mononeuropathy. What procedure has the best chance of providing the patient with active dorsiflexion?
   a. Ankle/foot orthosis
   b. Peroneal decompression at the fibular head
   c. Sural nerve grafting of the damaged peroneal nerve segment
   d. Partial tibial nerve transfer to the tibialis anterior
   e. Peroneal neurolysis in the posterior fossa

Chapter 13

1. Which of the following descriptions of the etiology of lymphedema is incorrect?
   a. Filariasis is the most common primary lymphedema in the world.
   b. Lymphedema praecox is defined as the onset of primary lymphedema between ages 2 and 35.
   c. Secondary lymphedema is attributed to the obstruction of lymphatic channels and an imbalance between the production of lymph and the excretion of lymph in the affected region.
   d. Breast-cancer-related upper limb lymphedema is the most common secondary lymphedema in developed countries.

2. Which of the following descriptions of nonsurgical procedures for treatment of lymphedema is incorrect?
   a. Risk-reduction education is important for the cancer survivor to maximize self-management and adherence to treatment.
   b. Complete decongestive therapy is the first choice. In addition, the effective combination of techniques to decongest soft-tissue swelling of lymphedematous limbs is also important.
   c. There is no requirement that lymphedema patients who undergo liposuction of the extremity continuously wear compression garments 6 months after surgery.
   d. Skin care, avoiding limb constriction, and use of compression garments are important risk-reduction practices.

3. Which of the following descriptions of surgical procedures for treatment of lymphedema is incorrect?
   a. Charles procedure and liposuction are the options for reduction of the volume and soft tissue of lymphedematous limbs.
   b. Charles procedure was first introduced for the treatment of scrotum lymphedema and is now used for advanced-stage lymphedematous limb, a lower limb lymphedema.
   c. Toe infections and cellulitis will not occur after Charles procedure because there is almost no soft tissue preserved on the affected extremity.
   d. Radical reduction of the lymphedematous limb may be combined with the preservation of perforator technique for reducing complications such as skin loss and blood loss during surgery.

4. Which of the following descriptions of surgical procedures for treatment of upper limb lymphedema is incorrect?
   a. Vascularized lymph node flap transfer is one of the most effective surgical approaches for the treatment of extremity lymphedema and is the first choice for all stages of lymphedema.
   b. Superficial groin lymph nodes are mostly located below the inguinal ligament and are medial to the sartorius. This group of lymph nodes can be transferred partially, as an entire flap, or combined with a lower abdominal flap to treat upper limb lymphedema.
   c. There are at least 3 recipient sites available for vascularized lymph node flap transfer for upper limb lymphedema, including axilla, elbow, and wrist.
   d. There is evidence showing that the wrist as a recipient site for vascularized groin lymph node flap transfer had better circumferential reduction in the elbow than using the elbow as a recipient site.

5. Which of the following descriptions of surgical procedures for treating lymphedema is incorrect?
   a. Lymphovenous anastomosis, lymphaticovenular anastomosis, lymphovenous bypass, and lymphovenous shunting are almost the same terms regarding drainage of excessive lymph into the venous system.
   b. Lymphovenous anastomosis was further modified to lymphaticovenular anastomosis by using supermicrosurgery for the subdermal venular vessels and/or for lymphatic ducts <0.8 mm.
   c. Indocyanine green with fluorescence can be preoperatively used to detect the functional lymphatic ducts for better surgical outcome of lymphovenous anastomosis.
   d. With recent indocyanine lymphography, lymphovenous anastomosis is very effective in early and advanced lower limb lymphedema.

6. Several irreversible pathological changes occur when lymphedema progresses. Which of the following is TRUE of morphological characteristics in collecting lymphatic channels?
   a. Increase in endothelial cells
   b. Constriction of valves
   c. Destruction of smooth-muscle cells
   d. None of above

7. A 52-year-old woman presents to the clinic with lymphedema in the right upper extremity. When she underwent radical mastectomy 2 years ago, edema of the right upper extremity appeared and continued for 6 months, with ineffective use of compression therapy. What is the most appropriate next step for surgical treatment?
   a. Debulking operation
   b. Liposuction
   c. Lymph node transfer
   d. Lymphovenous bypass

8. Which of the following is NOT an aggravating factor for lymphedema?
   a. Postoperative radiotherapy
   b. Sex
   c. Recurrent phlegmone
   d. Lymph node dissection

9. A 68-year-old woman presents to the clinic with skin changes on her right arm. She underwent radical mastectomy and adjuvant postoperative radiation therapy 20 years ago and had long-standing lymphedema in her right arm afterward. Clinical examination revealed numerous bluish skin nodules. Which of the following is the most likely diagnosis?
   a. Lymphangiosarcoma
   b. Melanoma
   c. Blue nevus
   d. Basal cell carcinoma

10. Which of the following correctly describes the state of lymphedema?
   a. It is immunologically vulnerable.
   b. It is characterized by an increase in lymph fluid circulation.
   c. The skin becomes soft.
   d. It is associated with a high resistance to infection.

Chapter 14

1. The standard time to release a simple, incomplete syndactyly of the 3rd webspace is
   a. Newborn period
   b. Under 6 months of age
   c. Between 1 and 2 years of age
   d. Over 2 years but before school age

2. Following surgical correction of a Wassel-type-IV radial polydactyly, long-term complications include all of the following EXCEPT
   a. Diminished size of retained thumb
   b. Angular deformity
   c. Stiffness
   d. Diminished sensation

3. The most common congenital hand malformation is
   a. Syndactyly
   b. Polydactyly
   c. Amniotic band syndrome
   d. Radial dysplasia

4. Which of the following structures is NOT typically divided during a standard pollicization?
   a. Index-finger metacarpal
   b. A1 pulley
   c. Digital artery
   d. Thumb metacarpal

5. The following clinical features may be useful in distinguishing symbrachydactyly and amniotic band syndrome EXCEPT
   a. Multiple limb involvement
   b. Fenestrations (sinus tracts) between the fingers
   c. Absent family history
   d. Absent ipsilateral pectoralis major muscle

6. A 3-month-old child presents with facial anomalies and bilateral hand complex syndactyly, consistent with Apert syndrome. What gene or mutation is involved with these anomalies?
   a. Sonic hedgehog (SSH)
   b. Fibroblast growth factor receptor type 2 (FGFR-2)
   c. Wnt7a
   d. Trisomy 13
   e. 22q11.2 deletion

7. You are asked to consult on a newborn child with absent thumbs bilaterally. On exam, you identify a prominent heart murmur. What syndrome is likely to be the diagnosis?
   a. Fanconi anemia
   b. Turner syndrome
   c. Thrombocytopenia–absent radius syndrome
   d. Holt-Oram syndrome
   e. Amniotic band syndrome

8. A 3-year-old presents with curvature of the right small finger and a radiograph showing a triangular-shaped phalanx. The diagnosis is
   a. Camptodactyly
   b. Symbrachydactyly
   c. Clinodactyly
   d. Pouce flottant
   e. Brachydactyly

9. The development of the upper limb and hand is completed by which gestational week?
   a. 4 weeks
   b. 5 weeks
   c. 6 weeks
   d. 8 weeks

10. A mother brings her 18-month-old boy with thumb hypoplasia to learn about his surgical options. On exam, the patient demonstrates instability of the carpometacarpal (CMC) joint, and on radiographs the patient demonstrates a hypoplastic CMC joint. A Blauth type-IIIB classification is made. The most appropriate surgical intervention is
   a. Amputation of the residual thumb
   b. Big-toe-to-thumb transfer
   c. Opponensplasty with ulnar collateral ligament repair
   d. Second-toe-to-thumb transfer
   e. Amputation of the residual thumb and index pollicization

Chapter 15

1. A 25-year-old right-hand-dominant accountant reports persistent pain in the proximal phalanx of his left middle finger for several months. The pain is relieved by ibuprofen. X rays of his wrist and hand suggest osteoid osteoma. What is the most likely radiographic appearance of the lesion?
   a. Poorly defined lytic lesion with stippled calcifications, cortical expansion, soft-tissue extension
   b. Small lucency surrounded by a rim of sclerotic bone
   c. Well-defined lobulated lytic lesion
   d. Moth-eaten lytic appearance with an aggressive "sunburst" periosteal reaction

2. A 36-year-old left-hand-dominant woman presents with subungual longitudinal pigmentation that has been present on her left thumb for 3 months. The lesion occupies 1/3 of the width of her nail. She states that it has not changed in appearance since it first appeared. What is your initial management?
   a. Nail-plate removal, matrix biopsy
   b. Continued observation
   c. Ray amputation
   d. Complete excisional biopsy with sentinel lymph node biopsy (SLNB)

3. Which of the following structures does not contribute to the spiral cord in Dupuytren's disease?
   a. Pretendinous band
   b. Lateral digital sheet
   c. Cleland's ligament
   d. Grayson's ligament
   e. Natatory ligament

4. A 45-year-old construction worker comes to the clinic complaining of ulnar-sided-palmar small and ring-finger pain. On exam, there is a pulsatile mass over ulnar side of the palm, and he has ulceration at the tips of his small and ring fingers. Which of the following is not part of the typical workup for this condition?
   a. X ray
   b. Ultrasound
   c. Angiogram
   d. EMG

5. A 21-year-old man sustained a distal radius fracture when his left arm was pinned under a motorcycle. Closed reduction of the distal radius was performed and a short arm splint applied. Six hours later, he returned to the emergency room with increasing pain in his forearm. His fingers are warm. What is the next most appropriate step?
   a. Administration of IV pain medication
   b. Splint removal
   c. Discharge with oral pain medication
   d. Complete blood count (CBC), erythrocyte sedimentation rate (ESR), C-reactive protein (CRP) test
   e. CT scan

6. A 68-year-old patient presents with pain at the distal interphalangeal (DIP) joint of her index finger. Palpation reveals a 6-mm fixed mass at the dorsal aspect of the DIP. A small osteophyte is seen on X ray. What is the most likely etiology of the mass?
   a. Synovial sarcoma
   b. Mucous cyst
   c. Osteoid osteoma
   d. Glomus tumor
   e. Enchondroma

7. A 44-year-old patient complains of 2-year history of episodic severe sharp pain in his middle finger. Physical exam demonstrates a slight ridge in the nail plate, the proximal aspect of which is profoundly tender to palpation. X ray shows localized scalloping on the dorsal aspect of the distal phalanx. What is the most likely diagnosis?
   a. Mucous cyst
   b. Subungual melanoma
   c. Glomus tumor
   d. Giant cell tumor
   e. Osteoid osteoma

8. A 56-year-old construction worker presents with painful ulcerations on the small and ring fingers of his dominant hand for the last 3 months. He has arterial Doppler signals in all 5 digits. There is a palpable pulse in Guyon's canal. What would most likely be seen on ultrasonography?
   a. Ulnar artery occlusion
   b. Ulnar artery aneurysm
   c. Incomplete palmar arch
   d. Normal radial and ulnar arteries
   e. Bacterial endocarditis

9. A patient with Dupuytren's disease and proximal interphalangeal (PIP) joint contracture is scheduled for open palmar fasciectomy. Which specific cord type places the neurovascular bundle at greatest risk for surgical injury?
   a. Spiral cord
   b. Central cord
   c. Natatory cord
   d. Lateral cord
   e. Retrovascular cord

10. Which of the following anatomic structures does not contribute to formation of Dupuytren's cords?
   a. Lateral digital sheet
   b. Spiral band
   c. Pretendinous band
   d. Grayson's ligament
   e. Cleland's ligament

Chapter 16

1. What allows for greater tolerance of apex dorsal angulation deformity of 5th metacarpal neck fractures?
   a. Greater flexion arc at 5th MPJ masks the angulation.
   b. The cam effect of the 5th MPJ prevents further fracture displacement.
   c. Extension at 5th CMC joint helps compensate for the apex dorsal angulation.
   d. Relative laxity of the 5th MPJ volar plate prevents a flexion deformity of the joint.

2. If a minimally displaced distal phalanx fracture presents with an associated subungual hematoma involving a third of the area of the nail plate, the most appropriate treatment is
   a. Nail trephination and closed treatment of the fracture
   b. Nail trephination and percutaneous pin fixation
   c. Nail removal and closed treatment of the fracture
   d. Nail removal and percutaneous pin fixation

3. A 35-year-old patient presents with a 3-month history of finger swelling and stiffness after an axial load injury. Plain films demonstrate a PIP joint fracture dislocation with no associated arthrosis. The comminuted volar fracture fragment involves 2/3 of the joint surface seen on the lateral plain film. The most appropriate treatment is
   a. Force-coupler dynamic pinning
   b. ORIF
   c. Closed reduction and percutaneous pinning
   d. Hemi-hamate arthroplasty

4. Of the following, the best treatment for a symptomatic gamekeeper's thumb with >30 degrees of laxity compared to the contralateral side is
   a. Cast immobilization for 6 weeks
   b. Percutaneous pin fixation
   c. Primary ligament repair
   d. Ligament reconstruction with tendon graft

5. The deforming forces of a Bennett fracture that must be overcome during the reduction maneuver originate from
   a. Abductor pollicis brevis and abductor pollicis longus (APL)
   b. Flexor pollicis longus and abductor pollicis brevis
   c. Adductor pollicis and APL
   d. Adductor pollicis and abductor pollicis brevis

6. A 35-year-old male sustains an axial load injury to his nondominant middle finger with a gross flexion deformity. Lateral plain films demonstrate a distal phalanx dorsal base avulsion fracture involving 20% of the joint surface. The best treatment is
   a. ORIF
   b. Closed reduction and percutaneous pin fixation
   c. Closed treatment with clamshell splint
   d. Excision of bony avulsion fragment and sutured anchor repair of tendon insertion

7. A 40-year-old male presents to the emergency room after a basketball injury that results in a nonreducible deformity of the 3rd metacarpal phalangeal joint. Plain films demonstrate a dorsal dislocation. After 3 attempts, the emergency room calls for further assistance. Which of the following structures is NOT typically implicated in the complex dislocation?
   a. Flexor tendon
   b. Volar plate
   c. Lumbrical
   d. Intermetacarpal ligament
   e. A1 pulley

8. A patient presents 8 years after an untreated soft-tissue mallet injury. What is the expected associated deformity?
   a. Swan-neck deformity
   b. Boutonnière deformity
   c. Camptodactyly
   d. Clinodactyly

9. The most appropriate treatment of a comminuted 1st metacarpal base (Rolando) fracture is
   a. Cast immobilization with outrigger
   b. ORIF
   c. External fixator application with axial traction across trapeziometacarpal joint
   d. Trapeziectomy, ligament reconstruction, and tendon interposition

10. A 33-year-old surgical resident presents with a fracture dislocation of the dominant middle-finger PIP joint. The lateral radiograph shows a <10% avulsion fragment involving the base of the middle phalanx. Using live fluoroscopy in the office, the joint becomes unstable at 20 degrees of PIP-joint flexion. The most appropriate treatment is
    a. Dorsal blocking splint set at 15 degrees of PIP flexion
    b. Dorsal blocking pin allowing a 40 to 110 degree flexion arc
    c. Force-coupler dynamic pinning
    d. Volar plate arthroplasty

Chapter 17

1. A 43-year-old male is brought to the emergency room immediately after sustaining a laceration of the left thumb while using a table saw at home. He has loss of skin and subcutaneous tissue on the volar aspect of the thumb from the metacarpophalangeal joint (MPJ) flexion crease to the interphalangeal joint flexion crease. The flexor tendon and digital neurovascular bundles are exposed at the wound base, but perfusion and sensation of the tip of the thumb are intact. Which of the following is the most appropriate management?
   a. Full-thickness skin grafting
   b. Reconstruction with a first dorsal metacarpal artery (FDMA) flap
   c. Reconstruction with a thenar flap
   d. Reconstruction with a volar advancement (Moberg) flap

2. Replantation is most likely to be contraindicated in which of the following patients who have sustained an amputation of a single digit at the level of the proximal interphalangeal joint?
   a. A 4-year-old girl with an amputation through the index finger
   b. A 28-year-old construction worker with an amputation through the index finger
   c. A 33-year-old piano player with an amputation through the long finger
   d. A 45-year-old carpenter with an amputation through the thumb

3. A 37-year-old male comes to the emergency room after sustaining an amputation at the fingertip of the long finger of the dominant hand while attempting to unclog a lawnmower. Physical examination shows pulp loss of 1 × 1.2 cm. Which of the following is the most appropriate method of reconstruction to maximize sensation and function?
   a. Cross-finger flap from the ring finger
   b. Full-thickness skin graft harvested from the hypothenar eminence
   c. Moist dressing changes until healing is complete
   d. V-Y advancement flap

4. A 12-year-old girl is brought to the office 2 years after she sustained a crush injury to the nail bed of her left ring finger. Her mother says that the nail grows but then lifts off the finger and catches onto her clothes. The patient complains that the nail looks ugly. On examination, the germinal matrix is intact, but 95% of the sterile matrix is scarred. Which of the following is the most appropriate treatment to improve her nail deformity?
   a. Full-thickness nail-bed grafting from the long finger
   b. Lateral paronychial-releasing incisions with central advancement flap
   c. Release of the sterile matrix scar and acellular dermal matrix grafting
   d. Split-thickness nail-bed grafting from the great toe

5. A 38-year-old male is brought to the emergency room 5 hours after sustaining an amputation of the right thumb when it was caught in a log-splitter. The amputated part was wrapped in moist saline gauze and placed on ice within 15 minutes of the injury. The amputated thumb has a long flexor tendon attached to it, with remnants of muscle attached to the proximal end of the tendon. Which of the following factors is most likely to limit the success of replantation of the thumb?
   a. Initial treatment of digit
   b. Mechanism of injury
   c. Possibility of infection
   d. Warm ischemia time

6. A 28-year-old male sustains an avulsion injury to the index finger of his nondominant left hand after it is caught in a piece of machinery while at work. He says he needs to return to his job as a manual laborer as soon as possible. The bone of the proximal phalanx is exposed. The avulsed segment of the finger includes the distal and middle phalanges and soft tissue to the level of the midproximal phalanx, along with segments of tendons, nerves, and vessels. Which of the following is the most appropriate management?
   a. Coverage with a groin flap
   b. Microvascular replantation
   c. Revision amputation
   d. Skin grafting

7. A 52-year-old male is brought to the emergency room after sustaining an injury to the right thumb and index finger from a snowblower. Physical examination demonstrates amputation of the right thumb at the CMC joint and amputation of the index finger at the head of the middle phalanx. The amputated thumb was wrapped in a moist gauze towel immediately after the injury and appears to be severely mangled. Which of the following would be the optimal management of the thumb acutely?
   a. Great-toe-to-thumb transfer
   b. Osteoplastic thumb reconstruction
   c. Replantation of the thumb
   d. Residual index-finger pollicization

8. During coverage of a defect with a reverse cross-finger flap, which of the following is the most appropriate location for application of a full-thickness skin graft?
   a. Dorsal surface of the middle phalanx of the donor finger
   b. Dorsal surface of the middle phalanx of the recipient finger
   c. Volar surface of the distal phalanx of the donor finger
   d. Volar surface of the distal phalanx of the recipient finger

9. A 31-year-old male comes to the office 12 weeks after sustaining an amputation of the tip of the long finger that healed by secondary intention and has resulted in a hook nail deformity. Physical examination shows the residual nail growing over the residual tip of the finger. Which of the following is the most likely cause of this patient's current condition?
   a. Dorsal-sided tissue loss with loss of eponychial fold
   b. Dorsal-sided tissue loss with loss of germinal matrix
   c. Volar-sided tissue loss with the nail bed folding over the residual tip
   d. Volar-sided tissue loss with nail-bed overgrowth by eponychial fold

10. A 13-year-old girl is brought to the emergency room because of persistent pain and bruising under the fingernail of her left small finger 4 hours after sustaining a crush injury. Physical examination demonstrates a subungual hematoma that is contained to a portion distal to the lunula, consisting of ~40% of the nail. The surrounding nail plate is adherent and intact, and the nail plate is not torn or lifted. Which of the following is the most appropriate management for this patient?
   a. Digital block with epinephrine
   b. Elevation
   c. Nail-plate removal and sterile matrix graft
   d. Trephination

Chapter 18

1. A 47-year-old female presents with pain, swelling, and limited range of motion of the right wrist after sustaining a fall on the outstretched hand. X-ray imaging of the wrist demonstrates a distal radius fracture. All of the following are radiographic indications for operative ORIF except
   a. Intra-articular fracture with >2 mm of articular step-off
   b. Radial shortening (positive ulnar variance) of >3 mm
   c. Loss of >10 degrees of volar angulation
   d. Nondisplaced intra-articular fracture with radial styloid involvement

2. A 26-year-old male presents with persistent wrist pain 3 weeks following a fall from a ladder at work. Initial radiographs obtained in the emergency department showed no evidence of fracture or dislocation. A repeat standard anteroposterior (AP) radiograph in the office demonstrates a 3-mm gap of the SL interval. A SL ligament injury is suspected. Which of the following additional radiographic views may be helpful in making the diagnosis?
   a. Radial deviated posteroanterior (PA) view
   b. Clenched fist AP view
   c. Pronated oblique view
   d. Roberts view

3. An 18-year-old male has persistent pain and limited range of motion at 6 months following nonvascularized bone grafting from the ipsilateral distal radius for a scaphoid proximal pole fracture nonunion. Radiographs in clinic are consistent with persistent nonunion. What is the next best step in management?
   a. Repeat nonvascularized bone graft (iliac crest, tibia, distal radius)
   b. Total wrist arthroplasty
   c. Vascularized bone graft (retrograde distal radius bone flap, medial femoral condyle flap)
   d. Total wrist arthrodesis

4. When considering partial wrist arthrodesis with a proximal row carpectomy (PRC), which articular surfaces must be free of arthritic/degenerative changes seeing as they will become the main articulation ("hinge joint") of the wrist following excision of the proximal row?
   a. Capitate and lunate fossa of the radius
   b. Hamate and lunate fossa of the radius
   c. Capitate and scaphoid fossa of the radius
   d. Hamate and lunate fossa of the radius

5. A 62-year-old female with severe rheumatoid arthritis complains of tenderness overlying the A1 pulley of the index finger with intermittent flexion "locking" throughout the day. An index trigger finger is diagnosed and corticosteroid injection is performed. If steroid injection fails and operative intervention is considered, which of the following should be performed in this patient?
   a. Release of the A1 pulley
   b. Flexor tenosynovectomy and intratendinous nodule excision
   c. Release of the A1 pulley with pulley reconstruction
   d. Release of the A1 and A2 pulleys

6. A 35-year-old male suffers a complete tear of his scapholunate (SL) interosseous ligament. Over time, if left untreated, which of the following relationships would you expect to develop?
   a. A dorsal intercalated segment instability (DISI) deformity, including a SL angle of 90 degrees and a gap of >3 mm between the scaphoid and lunate
   b. A DISI deformity, including a SL angle of 45 degrees, and a gap of >3 mm between the scaphoid and lunate
   c. A volar intercalated segment instability (VISI) deformity, including a SL angle of 90 degrees and a gap of >3 mm between the scaphoid and lunate
   d. A DISI deformity, including a SL angle of 90 degrees and a gap of <2 mm between the scaphoid and lunate
   e. A VISI deformity, including a SL angle of 45 degrees and a gap of >3 mm between the scaphoid and lunate

7. A 28-year-old man falls from a second-story window and is evaluated for pain in his right wrist. On exam, he has pain with wrist extension and palpation in the snuffbox. Radiographs reveal a radiolucency across the proximal scaphoid with 2 mm of displacement. If not treated appropriately, he is at risk for developing all of the following except
   a. Carpal arthritis
   b. Humpback deformity
   c. Proximal pole avascular necrosis
   d. SL advanced collapse (SLAC) wrist

8. A 60-year-old male with chronic wrist pain presents to the office. There is a remote history of an untreated scaphoid fracture, and radiographs obtained in the office reveal significant wrist arthritis. After unsuccessful conservative measures have been attempted, a PRC is planned. Significant arthritic changes of what articular surface would preclude moving forward with this treatment plan?
   a. Radioscaphoid
   b. Scapholunate
   c. Capitolunate
   d. Lunotriquetral
   e. Scaphotrapeziotrapezoidal

9. Four-corner fusion involves arthrodesis of all of the following carpal bones EXCEPT
   a. Scaphoid
   b. Lunate
   c. Triquetrum
   d. Capitate
   e. Hamate

10. A professional baseball player is evaluated for hand pain that affects his ability to hit a ball. A hook of hamate fracture is suspected. What type of radiograph will help identify this fracture?
   a. Roberts view
   b. PA
   c. Lateral
   d. Oblique
   e. Carpal tunnel view

11. In a complete lunate dislocation (Mayfield stage-IV perilunate dislocation), in order for the lunate to become dislocated out of the lunate fossa, which two ligaments are completely torn?
    a. SL and short radiolunate
    b. SL and lunotriquetral
    c. Lunotriquetral and radioscaphocapitate
    d. Lunotriquetral and dorsal intercarpal ligament
    e. Radioscaphocapitate and dorsal intercarpal ligament

12. Several months out from a distal radius fracture, a patient suffers a tendon rupture. On exam, what action is most likely to be impaired?
    a. Thumb extension
    b. Radial wrist extension
    c. Extension of the index finger
    d. Radial wrist flexion
    e. Thumb abduction

13. A 25-year-old male injured his right wrist after a fall from a motorcycle accident 1 year ago. Radiographs reveal no fracture, but lateral X rays of his wrist reveal his scaphoid to be in a flexed position and at a SL angle of 80 degrees. What structure is most likely injured?
    a. Lunotriquetral interosseous ligament
    b. Radioscaphocapitate ligament
    c. SL interosseous ligament
    d. Short radiolunate ligament
    e. Long radiolunate ligament

14. A 68-year-old male complains of constant hand pain. He has difficulty opening jars and his grind test is positive. X rays will likely reveal arthritic changes at the
    a. Radioscaphoid joint
    b. Thumb metacarpal phalangeal joint
    c. Trapeziometacarpal joint
    d. Index-finger proximal interphalangeal joint
    e. Thumb interphalangeal joint

Chapter 19

1. Which of the following statements regarding the contents of the carpal canal is false?
    a. The flexor digitorum superficialis (FDS) tendons to the ring and middle finger lie dorsal to the FDS tendons to the index and small.
    b. The FDP tendons lie on the dorsal floor of the carpal canal.
    c. The FPL tendon lies along the radial aspect of the carpal canal.
    d. The FDS tendons to the ring and middle finger lie volar to the FDS tendons to the index and small.

2. Which of the following can adversely affect the strength of a tendon repair?
    a. Increasing number of core strands across the repair site
    b. Epitendinous sutures
    c. Immobilization
    d. Locking sutures

3. Which of the following muscles is the prime wrist extensor?
    a. Extensor carpi ulnaris
    b. Extensor carpi radialis brevis (ECRB)
    c. Extensor carpi radialis longus
    d. Extensor digitorum communis (EDC)

4. A 45-year-old female presents to your office complaining of right-radial-sided wrist pain. On examination, she has tenderness and swelling proximal to the radial styloid. The pain is exacerbated when the wrist is forced into ulnar deviation with the thumb adducted into the palm. Which of the following tendons are involved?
    a. APL and extensor pollicis brevis
    b. Extensor pollicis longus
    c. Adductor pollicis
    d. Extensor carpi radialis longus and ECRB

5. A 35-year-old male with cerebral palsy is brought to your office by his mother for evaluation of his hand disorder. On examination, he has flexion contractures of his digits, such that it is difficult to get his fingers out of the palm for daily hygiene. Which of the following tendon transfers could be used to help correct this deformity?
    a. PL to extensor pollicis longus (EPL) transfer
    b. FCR to EDC transfer
    c. FDS to flexor digitorum profundus (FDP) transfer
    d. Extensor indicis proprius (EIP) to EPL transfer

6. A patient is brought to the operating room for a laceration in zone 7 with loss of index- and long-finger extension. A muscular mass that extends the long finger is encountered adjacent to the EDC tendon. What is this anomalous muscle's innervation?
    a. Median nerve
    b. Ulnar nerve
    c. Dorsal ulnar nerve
    d. Posterior interosseous nerve

7. A boxer presents to your clinic with an inability to extend the long finger after he makes a fist. This occurred suddenly after a match. The patient had no laceration. When asked to extend the finger, he extends at the MPJ of each digit, except for the long finger. The PIP and DIP extend normally. When passively extended, he can hold the position. There is a snap with active flexion. What structure is injured?
    a. Extensor digitorum longus
    b. Terminal tendon
    c. Sagittal band
    d. Oblique retinacular ligament

8. Following repair of a deep laceration of the volar forearm with multiple tendons involved, the patient bends her thumb when attempting to bend the index. Which of the following statements, if true, can be used to prevent this complication?
    a. The FDS of the index finger is superficial to the palmaris longus.
    b. The flexor digitorum pollicis is deep to the FDS of the index.
    c. The flexor pollicis longus is radial to the FDP.
    d. The flexor pollicis longus is ulnar to the FDP.

9. Which pulleys are the most anatomically significant and must be preserved or reconstructed in the event of injury?
   a. A1 and A4
   b. A2 and A4
   c. C2 and C4
   d. A2 and A3

10. A 60-year-old female patient presents to your office 9 months following a degloving injury of the dorsal proximal forearm, including avulsion of the radial nerve. She was reconstructed with a free flap to cover widely exposed radius and ulna. Her complaint is inability to extend the fingers, wrist, or thumb. Passive motion is adequate. The distal forearm is uninvolved. What is the most appropriate treatment strategy to improve her motion?
    a. FDS IV to ECRB, flexor carpi ulnaris (FCU) to EDC, PL to EPL tendon transfers
    b. Pronator teres (PT) to ECRB, FCU to EDC, brachioradialis (BR) to EPL tendon transfers
    c. PT to ECRB, FCU to EDC, PL to EPL tendon transfers
    d. Wrist arthrodesis

Chapter 20

1. Two days ago, a 45-year-old male suffered a deep laceration to his right lower extremity. He presented to the emergency room where the wound was cleaned and primarily closed. At present, what is the predominant cell type within the healing wound?
   a. Neutrophil
   b. Fibroblast
   c. Macrophage
   d. Platelet

2. A 27-year-old male pedestrian was struck by a motor vehicle, resulting in avulsion of 50% of his scalp. The wound was closed temporarily with a split-thickness skin graft along with the placement of scalp tissue expanders. Which of the following correctly describes the properties of newly expanded skin?
   a. The total collagen content and surface area is increased, and the tensile strength and elasticity are decreased.
   b. The total collagen content, surface area, and tensile strength is increased, and the elasticity is decreased.
   c. The surface area is increased, and collagen content, tensile strength, and elasticity are decreased.
   d. The total collagen content, surface area, tensile strength, and elasticity are increased.

3. Which of the following is TRUE of keloid scars?
   a. Keloid scars have increased myofibroblasts.
   b. Keloid scars are contained by the original boundaries of the scar.
   c. Keloid scars often produce contractures and occur over flexor surfaces.
   d. Keloid scars occur more frequently in darker pigmented patients.

4. Which of the following effects does negative pressure wound therapy (NPWT) exert on a wound?
   a. Macrodeformation of wound edges
   b. Increases matrix metalloproteinases
   c. Dessication of the wound
   d. None of the above

5. Which of the following is the most likely mechanism by which silicone affects wound healing?
   a. Alters cytokine levels within the wound
   b. Directly affects the healing cascade
   c. Increases oxygen tension within the wound
   d. Increases hydration within the wound

6. You are called on to evaluate a patient on the oncology service who has just had an infiltration of an unknown amount of intravenous chemotherapy medication into the forearm. The skin around the infiltration site is cool, painful, and quite swollen. In the hand, the fingers have good capillary refill and the hand shows no sensory deficits. What is the most reasonable option for treatment?
   a. Decompressive fasciotomies of the compartments of the forearm and hand
   b. Decompressive fasciotomies of the compartments of the forearm only
   c. Injection of saline and hyaluronidase into the area of infiltration injury
   d. Operative debridement of the skin infiltrated with the chemotherapy medication

7. What is a major benefit of enzymatic debriders in the management of chronic wounds?
   a. They are FDA approved as a means of enabling closure of all types of wounds.
   b. They are a gentle means of assisting removal of biofilm from wounds.
   c. They are a form of autolytic ointment.
   d. They can be used with any dressing.

8. What are some reasons why chronic wounds do not heal?
   a. Age
   b. Ischemia
   c. The presence of bacteria
   d. All of the above

9. A 38-year-old female of Asian ancestry undergoes an abdominoplasty. Six months after the procedure, she returns complaining of a thickened, raised, red, and pruritic scar at the midportion of the scar, which follows the borders of the original incision. Which therapy is most likely to be useful in managing this problematic scar?
   a. Excision followed by focused external beam radiation
   b. Cryotherapy
   c. Laser treatment of the hypertrophic scar
   d. Anti–transforming growth factor-β (anti-TGF-β) antisense medication

10. A 55-year-old female patient with a history of heart disease, severe rheumatoid arthritis, and right breast cancer treated 10 years prior with lumpectomy and radiation presents with a nonhealing wound of her left lower back. It resulted from a scratch and has enlarged during the last 6 weeks to a size of 2 × 3 cm. It is painful, bleeds easily, and has a mild amount of slough on it. She is referred to you because her wound-care doctor has been treating it with serial debridements and silver-containing dressings without improvement and appears to be progressively getting larger. What is a reasonable next option in your plan for treatment?
   a. Debridement followed by coverage with a skin graft
   b. Hyperbaric oxygen treatment to enhance healing of the wound
   c. Biopsy of the wound
   d. Treatment with systemic steroids

Chapter 21

1. A 20-year-old male presents to the emergency room with significant hand and forearm tenderness 2 hours after being bit in the hand by his friend's pet rattlesnake. On examination, he is mildly tachycardic with stable blood pressure. Focused examination of his upper extremity reveals mild diffuse swelling and moderate-to-severe pain with palpation of the forearm and flexion/extension of the fingers. Two small puncture wounds are noted in the first webspace. The most appropriate first treatment is
   a. Operative exploration of puncture wounds with aggressive debridement and forearm compartment release
   b. Administration of crotalidae polyvalent immune fab ovine (CroFab)
   c. Administration of piperacillin and tazobactam
   d. Upper extremity elevation
   e. Regional anesthetic block for pain control

2. An 18-year-old male presents to the emergency room with 24 hours of right-middle-finger pain and swelling over his knuckle. He was in a fight two nights ago and has multiple small wounds across the dorsum of his hand. On focused examination, he has significant swelling and pain around the middle-finger metacarpal phalangeal joint with further pain on axial loading. His white blood cell count is 16,000 cells/mL. Radiographs are negative for fracture and foreign bodies. What is the most important step in management?
   a. Irrigation of wounds in the emergency room
   b. Administration of metronidazole IV
   c. Elevation of extremity with close observation
   d. Operative exploration of the MPJ
   e. Operative exploration of flexor tendon sheath

3. A 60-year-old male with poorly controlled diabetes mellitus presents to the emergency room with tachycardia, significant hypotension, and leukocytosis. After initial stabilization, physical examination demonstrates significant erythema and crepitance of the scrotum and perineum, which his spouse reports was not present yesterday. The most appropriate next step should be
   a. Urgent, radical, surgical debridement of scrotum and perineum
   b. STAT skin biopsy to evaluate for cellulitis
   c. Scrotal ultrasound to evaluate for testicular torsion
   d. Pelvic CT scan to evaluate for subcutaneous air
   e. Intravenous metronidazole for anaerobic coverage

4. A 6-year-old girl presents with a 1-week history of a 4-cm area of slowly increasing induration and swelling of her right thigh with a 1-day history of a central opening with a small amount of pus and necrotic-appearing tissue. Her pediatrician started her on cephalexin 3 days ago. She has no allergies. After performing an adequate bedside drainage, the Gram stain shows Gram-positive cocci in clusters. What is the most appropriate antibiotic for home therapy?
   a. Vancomycin
   b. Cephalexin
   c. Linezolid
   d. Sulfamethoxazole/trimethoprim
   e. Tetracycline

5. A 40-year-old woman presents to the emergency room with a 24-hour history of worsening index-finger pain and swelling after her cat bit that finger 2 days ago. Which of the following signs would NOT be consistent with a suppurative flexor tenosynovitis?
   a. Flexion of the PIP joint at rest
   b. Fusiform swelling of the digit
   c. Pain on passive extension of IP/MCP joints
   d. Pain on palpation along flexor tendon sheath into palm
   e. Fingers held in an intrinsic plus position

6. A 63-year-old male presents to the emergency department with a complaint of fever, lethargy, and severe pain of the genitals and lower abdomen. He has a history of poorly controlled diabetes mellitus. Examination is notable for a BMI of 42 kg/m², a temperature of 101, HR of 113 bpm, and blood pressure of 87/25 mmHg. There is erythema and tenderness of the scrotum extending into the groin and lower abdomen. Following the administration of intravenous hydration and antibiotics, what is the most appropriate next step in management?
   a. Observation alone
   b. Hyperbaric oxygen
   c. CT scan of the abdomen
   d. Surgical debridement of affected tissues

7. A 27-year-old, otherwise healthy hiker is brought to the emergency room complaining of a copperhead bite to his left lower leg 2 hours earlier. The patient does not remember his immunization history. His vital signs are stable, and examination reveals a bite wound of the left lower leg with mild surrounding edema. He has no other findings of note. In addition to immobilization and administration of broad-spectrum antibiotics, what is the most appropriate next step in management?
   a. Administration of antivenin
   b. Administration of tetanus toxoid
   c. Wide debridement of the bite wound and fasciotomy
   d. Application of a tourniquet and elevation of the extremity

8. A 31-year-old female is referred to the office with a 10-year history of recurrent pain and drainage in both armpits. History includes multiple I&D procedures and courses of antibiotics. Physical examination reveals affected areas >10 cm in diameter, with multiple sinus tracts and tender nodules in each axilla. Which of the following should be the next step in management?
   a. Laser hair removal
   b. Injection of botulinum toxin
   c. I&D of abscesses
   d. Complete excision of the affected area

9. A 24-year-old male presents to the emergency room complaining of increasing pain and stiffness in the right ring finger. He states that he was involved in a fistfight three days ago. Examination shows dorsal erythema and tenderness of the MPJ of the right ring finger with an adjacent healing laceration. Radiographs show no fractures. What is the most appropriate next step in management?
   a. Splinting and elevation
   b. Discharge with oral antibiotics
   c. Surgical drainage of the joint
   d. Surgical washout of the flexor tendon sheath

10. A 52-year-old female has swelling and severe pain of the index and middle fingers of her dominant hand for the past 2 days. On physical examination, you note a sausage-like swelling of the digits and tenderness on palpation of the volar surface of the fingers. There is severe pain on passive extension. Radiographs are unremarkable. In addition to administration of broad-spectrum antibiotics, which of the following is the most appropriate management?
   a. Admission for observation
   b. Incision and irrigation of the flexor sheaths
   c. Wide debridement of the involved tissues
   d. Amputation of the involved digits

Chapter 22

1. A 50-year-old woman sustains full-thickness circumferential burns to her entire left upper extremity, partial-thickness burns to the anterior surface of her entire left lower extremity, and first-degree burns to her entire face (not scalp). What is the total body surface area (TBSA) of burn used to calculate her fluid requirements?
   a. 18%
   b. 22%
   c. 36%
   d. 40%

2. A 30-year-old sustains a 25% TBSA burn injury. According to the Parkland formula, the initial IV fluid used for resuscitation therapy should be
   a. Hypotonic saline
   b. Normal saline
   c. Ringer's lactate
   d. 5% dextrose and water

3. A 35-year-old worker spilled sodium hydroxide on his hand. What is the initial Rx?
   a. Apply calcium gluconate gel to neutralize.
   b. Apply mineral oil to neutralize.
   c. Rinse with a dilute solution of boric acid to neutralize.
   d. Rinse with water.

4. A 35-year-old female applied a petrolatum-based hair-straightening product to her hair and then lit a cigarette. She presents with 6% TBSA burns of scalp and ears. What topical treatment should be used on the ears to prevent chondritis?
   a. Silver sulfadiazine
   b. Silver nitrate
   c. Mafenide acetate
   d. Mupurocin

5. A 38-year-old homeless man presents with deep frostbite of his hands. Initial treatment should be to
   a. Warm hands in water bath at 37 °C
   b. Warm hands in water bath at 40 °C
   c. Warm hands with hot packs wrapped in a towel
   d. Obtain arteriogram

6. A 35-year-old electrician sustains contact with a 10,000-V line. He presents with fixed flexion of his right wrist with charring, a pulseless hand, and a tense forearm. After cardiopulmonary resuscitation, patient should undergo
   a. EMG
   b. Intravenous infusion of mannitol
   c. Decompressive fasciotomies
   d. Amputation at proximal wrist

7. A 4-year-old spilled hot noodles on his lap, sustaining superficial and deep partial-thickness burns to the genitalia, groin, and thigh, totaling 3% TBSA. According to American Burn Association (ABA), this burn would be classified as a
   a. Minor burn
   b. Moderate burn
   c. Intermediate burn
   d. Major burn

8. What percent TBSA scald burn will trigger a systemic inflammatory response (SIR) in most adults?
   a. >10%
   b. >15%
   c. >20%
   d. >30%

9. Electrical injury may be classified as low or high voltage. The distinction between high and low voltage is at
   a. >100 V
   b. >1000 V
   c. >10,000 V
   d. >100,000 V

10. During initial fluid resuscitation, a burned child is more susceptible than an adult to which of the following:
    a. Hypoglycemia
    b. Hyperglycemia
    c. Hypophosphatemia
    d. Hyperphosphatemia

Chapter 23

1. If left untreated, a nevus sebaceous may transform into which of the following?
   a. Atypical nevus
   b. Melanoma
   c. Basal cell carcinoma
   d. Dermatofibrosarcoma protuberans

2. What are the recommended surgical margins for an atypical pigmented nevus?
   a. 1 mm
   b. 5 mm
   c. 10 mm
   d. 20 mm

3. Which of the following is a syndrome characterized by the development of multiple, symmetric lipomas?
   a. Madelung's disease
   b. Wartenburg's disease
   c. Hirschsprung's syndrome
   d. Gorlin syndrome

4. Which of the following is an acceptable treatment for a dermatofibroma?
   a. Observation
   b. Excisional biopsy
   c. Local excision
   d. All of the above

5. Which of the following is a common childhood skin lesion that is characterized by dermal and subdermal calcifications as well as ghost cells and basaloid cells on histology?
   a. Pilomatrixoma
   b. Nevus sebaceous
   c. Pyogenic granuloma
   d. Hamartoma

6. A 40-year-old man is referred for a tender raised lesion of the helix rim of the ear, which did not respond to topical steroids. A principal diagnostic consideration is
   a. Chondrodermatitis nodularis helixis
   b. Seborrhoeic dermatitis
   c. Linear epidermal nevus of Ota
   d. Inflamed hemangioma

7. One definitive treatment for the above is
   a. Topical radiation
   b. 5-fluorouracil
   c. Wedge excision of underlying skin and cartilage
   d. Continued observation

8. An individual cutaneous neurofibroma
   a. Indicates a total body exam for cafe au lait spots
   b. Obligates a family history for von Recklinghausen's
   c. Is usually located in the head and neck
   d. Is a benign Schwann cell tumor

9. Congenital dermal melanocytosis (Mongolian spot)
   a. Characteristically involves the lumbosacral skin
   b. Persists into adult life
   c. Is treated by wide excision and skin graft
   d. Has a typical blue-black appearance

10. Which of the following statements about lipomata is untrue? Lipomata
    a. Are commonly multiple
    b. Can be bilateral and symmetrical (Madelung's disease)
    c. Have subgroups or variants (hemangio-neuro)
    d. Occur commonly after trauma

11. Epidermoid cysts are
    a. Best excised while acutely inflamed
    b. Have different cytology in different body areas
    c. Treated as malignant if rapidly growing
    d. Filled with a harmless, foul-smelling skin protein

Chapter 24

1. Which of the following lesions are not premalignant?
   a. Leukoplakia
   b. Hutchinson's freckle
   c. Keratoacanthoma
   d. Clear cell acanthoma

2. All of the following are risk factors for basal cell carcinoma, except
   a. UVA radiation
   b. UVB radiation
   c. Gamma radiation
   d. Gorlin syndrome

3. A 71-year-old male is referred to your clinic with biopsy-proven squamous cell cancer of the scalp, measuring 10 mm in diameter. What is the best course of treatment?
   a. Curettage and electrodessication
   b. Surgical excision with a 4-mm margin
   c. Surgical excision with a 6-mm margin
   d. Mohs micrographic surgery

4. Punch biopsy of a 38-year-old female with a suspicious dark lesion reveals melanoma that has invaded the papillary dermis but does not penetrate the reticular dermis. What is the Clark classification of this lesion?
   a. Level II
   b. Level III
   c. Level IV
   d. Level V

5. A 45-year-old male with a recent punch biopsy showing melanoma with a Breslow depth of 1.3 mm is referred to your clinic. He does not have palpable lymph nodes. What is the appropriate management?
   a. Surgical excision with 1-cm margin
   b. Surgical excision with 1-cm margin and SLNB
   c. Surgical excision with 2-cm margins
   d. Surgical excision with 2-cm margins and SLNB

6. A 42-year-old, fair-haired woman with Fitzpatrick skin-type I presents to the office with an irregular, darkly pigmented skin lesion on her left calf. After appropriate biopsy, it is determined to be a melanoma. Which of the following is the most common melanoma in the United States?
   a. Lentigo maligna melanoma
   b. Superficial spreading melanoma
   c. Acrolentiginous melanoma
   d. Nodular melanoma

7. Which of the following is the strongest indication for SLNB in a patient with nodular melanoma?
   a. Age younger than 35 years
   b. Tumor location on the face and scalp
   c. Tumor thickness of 2.0 mm
   d. Palpable lymphadenopathy

8. A 55-year-old man presents with a 1.5-cm-diameter, firm, painless nodule on his left forearm. Excisional biopsy shows a Merkel cell carcinoma. Which of the following statements about his disease is true?
   a. This is a neuroendocrine tumor associated with systemic immunosuppression.
   b. Expected 5-year survival is less than 50% in the absence of metastases.
   c. Metastases are hematogenous and rarely involve the lymph nodes.
   d. Radiotherapy in not effective in the treatment of Merkel cell carcinoma.

9. Which of the following features of SCC is most strongly associated with high metastatic potential?
   a. Verrucous and exophytic appearance
   b. Tumors arising from sun-induced skin changes
   c. Tumors developing on the trunk
   d. Tumors associated with Margolin's ulcer

10. Which of the following tumor types is least suitable for Mohs micrographic excision of cutaneous malignancies?
    a. Recurrent tumors in areas of previous radiation
    b. Tumors with discontiguous growth patterns
    c. Dermatofibrosarcoma protuberans
    d. Extramammary Paget's disease

Chapter 25

1. A 14-year-old male presents to your office with an oronasal fistula. He has a history of a cleft lip and palate that was repaired in China when he was an infant. The fistula measures ~2 cm in diameter. What muscle is included with a facial artery musculomucosal flap?
   a. Palatopharyngeus
   b. Palatoglossus
   c. Buccinator
   d. Levator labii superioris

2. A 74-year-old female has a sternal wound that you plan to reconstruct with a pedicled rectus abdominis myocutaneous flap. She has a history of coronary artery bypass grafting with harvest of her bilateral IMAs. What would be the primary blood supply of your flap in this instance?
   a. Superior epigastric
   b. Eighth intercostal artery
   c. Inferior epigastric
   d. Lateral epigastric

3. What is the dominant vascular pedicle to a reverse lateral arm flap?
   a. Radial recurrent artery
   b. Posterior radial collateral artery
   c. Radial artery
   d. Brachial artery

4. A 25-year-old patient has a large lower abdominal wound for which you plan to reconstruct using a pedicled rectus femoris flap. What is the expected functional morbidity from use of this flap?
   a. None
   b. Ten to 15 degrees of extensor lag
   c. Immobility
   d. No knee extension

5. Ten days ago, a 40-year-old male underwent reconstruction of his abdominal wound with a transverse fascial lata myocutaneous flap. He is noted to have persistent venous congestion and you have decided to begin leech therapy. Which of the following bacteria can be associated with infection from this treatment?
   a. *Streptococcus pneumoniae*
   b. *Staphylococcus aureus*
   c. *Pseudomonas aeruginosa*
   d. *Aeromonas hydrophila*

6. The ALT flap
   a. Is supplied by the transverse branch of the circumflex femoral artery
   b. Is supplied by perforators that can be found in a 3-cm radius in the middle of a line drawn from the greater trochanter to the superolateral border of the patella
   c. Can be harvested with vastus lateralis for bulk but requires a separate pedicle
   d. Is supplied by perforators from the descending branch of the lateral circumflex femoral artery
   e. Is unreliable as a pedicled flap because of pressure on the pedicle

7. The superior gluteal artery perforator (SGAP) flap is supplied by the SGA. This can be found lateral to the sacrum and related to the piriformis muscle because
   a. The artery is found at the junction of the middle and lateral thirds of the piriformis.
   b. The piriformis is found by drawing a line from the greater trochanter to the tip of the coccyx.
   c. The SGA is found just above the junction of the middle and medial thirds of the piriformis.
   d. The SGA lies just below the piriformis.
   e. The SGA passes through the piriformis muscle at the junction of middle and medial thirds.

8. The radial forearm flap donor site can be associated with neuroma of
   a. The posterior interosseous nerve
   b. The superficial radial nerve
   c. The median nerve
   d. The ulnar nerve
   e. All of the above

9. According to the Mathes-Nahai classification system, the sartorius muscle is
   a. Type 1
   b. Type 2
   c. Type 3
   d. Type 4
   e. Type 5

10. In harvesting the scapular system flaps based on the circumflex scapular artery, the quadrangular space is an important landmark. It is bordered by all of the following except the
    a. Latissimus dorsi
    b. Teres major
    c. Teres minor
    d. Triceps
    e. Scapular border

Chapter 26

1. Which branch of the facial nerve is responsible for normal resting lid tone?
   a. Zygomatic
   b. Buccal
   c. Temporal
   d. Marginal mandibular

2. During lower lid blepharoplasty via an external approach, the surgeon elects to redrape retroseptal fat across the orbital rim to soften contours across the lid-cheek junction. To maximize motion of the central and lateral fat pads, which structure between these two fat pads should be released from the lower orbital rim?
   a. Whitnall's ligament
   b. Arcuate expansion of Lockwood's ligament
   c. Lateral horn of the levator palpebrae superioris muscle
   d. Inferior crus of the lateral canthal tendon

3. In patients with prominent eyes, Hertel exophthalmometer measurements should be in excess of what value? Measurements describe the distance from the corneal surface to which bony landmark?
   a. Ten mm; inferior orbital rim
   b. Fourteen mm; lateral orbital rim
   c. Sixteen mm; inferior orbital rim
   d. Eighteen mm; lateral orbital rim

4. A patient underwent lower lid blepharoplasty 1 year before her current presentation. She now presents with ectropion and lower scleral show that is not correctable with the examiner's single digit pushing upward at the lateral canthus. She does not have a skin shortage. In conjunction with a lateral canthal tightening procedure, which adjuvant lower lid treatment would be most effective in returning the lower lid to its native resting position at the lower corneoscleral limbus?
   a. Middle lamellar spacer graft
   b. Skin graft from the postauricular location
   c. Skin graft from the supraclavicular location
   d. Levator recession procedure

5. A patient presents following Mohs excision of the lateral lower lid with a full-thickness defect measuring ~40% of the lower lid width. Which of the following reconstructive options would be most appropriate for closure and restoration of normal eyelid contour?
   a. Hughes tarsoconjunctival flap
   b. Cutler-Beard bridge flap
   c. Nasolabial transposition flap
   d. Tenzel rotation-advancement flap

6. A 58-year-old man presents for his first postoperative appointment 1 week after transcutaneous lower eyelid blepharoplasty with canthopexy. On examination, he demonstrates severe chemosis of the left eye, impairing his ability to close his eyelids. What is the best management plan?
   a. Administration of 2.5% phenylephrine ophthalmic drops
   b. Administration of tobramycin/dexamethasone ophthalmic drops
   c. Snip conjunctivotomy
   d. Conjunctival plication

7. One year after undergoing an ORIF of an orbital floor fracture, a 19-year-old man presents with right lower eyelid ectropion and trichiasis. The surgeon reconstructed the floor with titanium mesh through a transconjunctival approach. What is the next step in management?
   a. Eyelid massage
   b. Intralesional kenalog injection into the lower eyelid fornix
   c. Cicatricial release with posterior lamellar palatal grafting
   d. CT scan followed by hardware removal

8. Injection of 1 to 2 U of botulinum toxin into the lateral aspect of the upper eyelid creates what change on eyelid position?
   a. Minimizes complications of lagophthalmos after aggressive blepharoplasty
   b. Simulates the effects of ptosis correction
   c. Temporarily addresses the deformity of upper eyelid retraction
   d. No observable change of the eyelid esthetics

9. Orbital fat resuspension during lower eyelid blepharoplasty requires dissection and division of what structure?
   a. Orbitomalar ligament
   b. Capsulopalpebral fascia
   c. Lateral orbital retaining ligament
   d. Lockwood ligament

10. Six hours after undergoing a transconjunctival lower eyelid blepharoplasty, a 61-year-old woman returns to the emergency room complaining of severe pain. After ruling out a retrobulbar hematoma, what is the next most likely diagnosis?
   a. Blepharospasm
   b. Bacterial conjunctivitis
   c. Dry eye syndrome
   d. Corneal abrasion

Chapter 27

1. A 22-year-old woman with a crooked nose and bulbous nasal tip will undergo rhinoplasty through an open approach. Which of the following blood vessels will be disrupted?
   a. Lateral nasal artery
   b. Internal maxillary artery
   c. Columellar artery
   d. Dorsal nasal artery

2. A 38-year-old woman will undergo secondary rhinoplasty for asymmetrical dorsal esthetic lines and internal valve collapse. Which of the following maneuvers can improve internal valve function?
   a. Alar contour graft
   b. Anatomic cap graft
   c. Infratip graft
   d. Spreader graft

3. Which of the following maneuvers should be avoided during open rhinoplasty?
   a. Transposition of the lower lateral crus
   b. Alar base excisions that are inferior to the alar groove
   c. Percutaneous lateral nasal osteotomies
   d. Subdermal defatting of the nasal tip

4. A 62-year-old man will require subtotal nasal reconstruction for a defect of the nasal skin that involves the nasal tip, right and left nasal alae, and inferior half of the nasal dorsum. A right forehead flap is planned. What is the pedicle of the forehead flap?
   a. Supraorbital artery
   b. Anterior branch of the superficial temporal artery
   c. Posterior branch of the superficial temporal artery
   d. Supratrochlear artery

5. At the level of the orbital rim, where is the major blood supply of the forehead flap located?
   a. Subdermal plexus
   b. Deep to the periosteum
   c. Superficial to the periosteum
   d. Within the frontalis muscle

6. A 52-year-old man presents with a chief complaint of difficulty breathing. A Cottle maneuver is positive. Which of the following would be best suited to correct this problem?
   a. Septoplasty
   b. Tip grafts
   c. Spreader grafts
   d. Inferior turbinate reduction

7. A 33-year-old woman undergoing cosmetic rhinoplasty desires more projection of the nasal tip. Which of the following would NOT increase tip projection?
   a. Cartilage tip graft
   b. Transdomal sutures
   c. Columellar strut graft
   d. Resection of the medial crura

8. Which of the following deformities can occur from excessive reduction of the nasal dorsum?
   a. Pollybeak deformity
   b. Rocker deformity
   c. Saddle nose deformity
   d. Alar retraction

9. An 82-year-old woman undergoes Mohs micrographic surgery to remove a SCC. The defect is a 1-cm partial-thickness defect of the nasal dorsum in the middle third of the nose. Which of the following flaps would NOT be the best option to reconstruct this defect?
   a. Miter flap
   b. V-Y advancement flap
   c. Forehead flap
   d. Bilobed flap

10. A 25-year-old woman comes in seeking cosmetic rhinoplasty. Her nasolabial angle is 87 degrees. What is closest to the ideal nasolabial angle in this patient?
   a. Less than 80 degrees
   b. Ninety degrees
   c. One hundred and five degrees
   d. More than 120 degrees

Chapter 28

1. A 62-year-old female has complete numbness of the left earlobe 4 weeks after undergoing rhytidectomy. The nerve that was most likely injured can be found along the surface of which of the following muscles?
   a. Digastric
   b. Sternocleidomastoid
   c. Omohyoid
   d. Trapezius
   e. Stylohyoid

2. A 58-year-old male has increasing pain and swelling on the left side of his face 8 hours after a rhytidectomy. Which of the following perioperative interventions is most likely to have prevented this complication?
   a. Use of drains
   b. Use of fibrin glue
   c. Use of antianxiety medications postop
   d. Control of blood pressure postop
   e. Placement of a firm compressive dressing

3. A 65-year-old woman has a persistent asymmetric smile following a facelift. Physical examination shows elevation of the right oral commissure. She has a full denture smile normally but is able to purse and evert her lower lip. Which branch of the facial nerve was injured?
   a. Zygomatic
   b. Frontal
   c. Marginal mandibular
   d. Cervical
   e. Buccal

4. A 55-year-old male with a history of hypertension undergoes a routine rhytidectomy. Postoperatively, the nurse notifies the surgeon that the patient has severe ear and facial pain on one side. What is the most likely diagnosis?
   a. Anesthetic reaction
   b. Injury to Arnold's Nerve
   c. Hematoma
   d. Injury to greater auricular nerve
   e. Trigeminal neuralgia

5. What is the facelift technique called when it involves a dissection beneath the superficial muscular aponeurotic system (SMAS) layer?
   a. Minimal access cranial suspension (MACS) lift
   b. Short scar facelift
   c. Subcutaneous facelift
   d. Deep plane facelift
   e. SMAS plication

6. What is the incidence of hematoma in a female patient?
   a. 1%
   b. 3%
   c. 6%
   d. 10%
   e. 20%

7. What is the incidence of hematoma in a male patient?
   a. 1%
   b. 4%
   c. 8%
   d. 15%
   e. 30%

8. A 58-year-old female patient presents for a neck lift. She has had massive weight loss and is unhappy with her neckline. What is the normal range of the cervical mental angle?
   a. 85 to 100 degrees
   b. 105 to 120 degrees
   c. 125 to 140 degrees
   d. 145 to 160 degrees
   e. None of the above

9. On evaluation of a patient who presents for a neck lift, the surgeon notes a prominent submandibular gland. What nerve is at greatest risk with attempted resection of the gland?
   a. Zygomatic
   b. Frontal
   c. Marginal mandibular
   d. Cervical
   e. Buccal

10. The SMAS layer is continuous with which tissue layer superiorly?
    a. Temporoparietal
    b. Parotid fascia
    c. Deep temporal fascia
    d. Masseteric fascia
    e. Temporal fat pad

Chapter 29

1. A 39-year-old female presents 3 months after lipoabdominoplasty with complaints of tingling, numbness, and burning sensation along the anterior and lateral aspect of her thigh. What is the most likely diagnosis?
   a. Iliohypogastric neuralgia
   b. Lateral femoral cutaneous neuralgia
   c. Ilioinguinal neuralgia
   d. Intercostal neuralgia

2. A 45-year-old woman undergoes a brachioplasty procedure and experiences postoperative numbness of the ulnar side of the left forearm after surgery. After 6 weeks of conservative management, the numbness continues. After 3 months of further observation, the patient has developed a painful nodule in the arm under her incision. Reexploration is planned and the most likely intraoperative finding is
   a. Severed lateral antebrachial cutaneous nerve of the arm with neuroma formation.
   b. Severed medial antebrachial cutaneous nerve of the arm with neuroma formation.
   c. Entrapment of the ulnar nerve at the elbow
   d. Lymphocele

3. A 32-year-old female presents for consultation for body contouring surgery. She had gastric bypass surgery and lost 120 lbs. She now has a hanging pannus that blocks a portion of her genitals and thighs and a moderate upper role at the umbilicus with laxity of the epigastric area. The best treatment option for her is
   a. Abdominoplasty with aggressive liposuction of the upper abdomen
   b. Abdominoplasty with fleur-de-lis vertical component
   c. Miniabdominoplasty
   d. Circumferential lower body lift

4. A 40-year-old woman who has had two successful pregnancies presents for an abdominoplasty. Her BMI at the time of surgery is 28. Eight weeks postoperatively, she presents with superior abdominal fullness above the level of the umbilicus. She states that she feels like it has been there since surgery. The most likely diagnosis is
   a. Seroma
   b. Residual epigastric adiposity
   c. Failure to adequately plicate the rectus fascia above the umbilicus
   d. Redundant skin laxity

5. A 23-year-old woman presents for liposuction of her flanks to improve her waistline. In order to reduce the risk of blood loss during the procedure, the best technique to achieve this is
    a. Dry technique
    b. Wet technique
    c. Superwet technique
    d. Tumescent technique

6. A 49-year-old multiparous woman undergoes standard abdominoplasty. When insetting the umbilicus, it should be placed
    a. At the midline, 14 cm above the pubis
    b. At the midline, 14 cm below the xyphoid
    c. At the intersection of a line connecting the highest point of the iliac crest with the midline
    d. At the intersection of a line connecting the anterosuperior iliac spine with the midline
    e. At the point where the umbilicus is found lying beneath the abdominal flap

7. A 37-year-old woman has widening of the labia 3 months after undergoing a medial thigh lift. Which of the following is the most likely cause?
    a. Failure to suture the flap to Colles' fascia
    b. Excessive adjunctive suction lipectomy
    c. Abnormal scar contracture
    d. Failure of appropriate preoperative markings

8. Which of the following is the most common complication following ultrasound-assisted liposuction?
    a. Pulmonary embolism
    b. Thermal skin injury
    c. Infection
    d. Hematoma
    e. Seroma

9. During brachioplasty, permanent suturing of the medial arm skin flaps to which of the following structures will decrease unfavorable scarring and contour irregularities?
    a. Pectoralis major muscle
    b. Triceps muscle
    c. Latissimus dorsi muscle and fascia
    d. Axillary fascia
    e. Biceps brachii muscle and fascia

10. Two days after undergoing abdominoplasty, a 37-year-old woman presents to the emergency room with a firm painful cord in the medial thigh, tachycardia, hypoxia, and mental status changes. Immediate workup should include evaluation for
    a. Pulmonary embolism
    b. Incarcerated hernia
    c. Infected seroma
    d. Urinary tract infection
    e. Acute psychotic episode

Chapter 30

1. A 32-year-old female with a history of cystic acne presents for skin resurfacing. What is the recommended length of time that the patient should be off Accutane (isotretinoin) prior to her treatment?
    a. 1 month
    b. 3 months
    c. 6 months
    d. 1 year

2. A 63-year-old female presents for treatment of fine facial rhytids. Which of the following is not a component of Jessner's Peel?
    a. Salycilic acid
    b. Lactic acid
    c. Croton oil
    d. Resocinol

3. A 72-year-old female patient with deep perioral rhytids undergoes a deep chemical peel with phenol. What is the most serious medical side effect of this treatment?
    a. Hypopigmentation
    b. Chemical necrosis of the outer layer of the skin
    c. Increased collagen synthesis
    d. Cardiac arrhythmias

4. How is the depth of a phenol peel controlled?
    a. Croton oil concentration
    b. Time of application
    c. Number of applications
    d. Strength of solution

5. A 33-year-old male presents for tattoo removal. Which of the following pigments is not targeted by your Nd:YAG laser?
    a. Green
    b. Red
    c. Brown
    d. Orange

6. A 62-year-old female presents for laser resurfacing of fine periorbital rhytids. Which of the following chromophores is the target of your ablative CO_2 laser?
    a. Heme
    b. Melanin
    c. Orange pigment
    d. Water

7. A 56-year-old female with facial volume depletion associated with aging presents for treatment with injectable fillers. Which of the following is not an ingredient in a currently approved dermal filler?
    a. Silicone
    b. Hyaluronic acid
    c. Poly-L-lactic acid
    d. Calcium hydroxyapatite

8. A 45-year-old male presents with male-pattern baldness. Which of the following is not a phase of hair follicle growth?
    a. Anagen
    b. Pilogen
    c. Telogen
    d. Catagen

9. A 56-year-old male undergoes hair transplantation for treatment of male-pattern baldness. When can he expect restoration of normal hair growth?
   a. 2 weeks
   b. 1 month
   c. 3 months
   d. 1 year

10. A 59-year-old female presents for treatment of her glabellar frown lines. Which of the following is the mechanism of action of the botulinum neurotoxin?
   a. Sodium-channel binding
   b. Blockade of presynaptic acetylcholine release
   c. β-adrenergic antagonism
   d. Calcium-channel blockade

Self-Assessment Answers

Chapter 1

ANSWER 1: C.

ANSWER 2: C.

ANSWER 3: D.

ANSWER 4: E. Adjacent tissue transfer includes all tissue rearrangements but also includes excision of a lesion.

ANSWER 5: E. The 62 modifier identifies that the procedure was performed with a cosurgeon, during which each surgeon does a separately documented part of the operation.

ANSWER 6: B. This patient has well-controlled diabetes (systemic disease). Past history of hypertension that is resolved does not impact her current ASA status.

ANSWER 7: B.

ANSWER 8: D. Options a–c are included in the global period.

ANSWER 9: B. Fluency in a foreign language is a potential job skill.

ANSWER 10: C. The remainder are global to the procedure. Exposure to harvest the flap, closure of the donor site, and preparation of the recipient site are all inclusive to the flap code.

Chapter 2

ANSWER 1: D. The mental foramen can be found near the inferior mandibular cortex at the level of the second premolar and first molar.

ANSWER 2: C. The great auricular nerve provides sensory innervation to the earlobe and lower half of the ear. It can be injured during face and neck rejuvenation procedures, resulting in numbness in this region.

ANSWER 3: A. The marginal mandibular branch of the facial nerve innervates the mentalis muscle. Thus, the ability to evert the lower lip in the above setting suggests a functioning mentalis muscle and injury to the cervical branch of the facial nerve, creating "pseudoparalysis of the marginal mandibular nerve."

ANSWER 4: B. The foramen rotundum is a circular foramen within the sphenoid bone of the skull base, through which the maxillary division of the trigeminal nerve passes.

ANSWER 5: C. The superior orbital fissure is located within the greater wing of the sphenoid bone and transmits the lacrimal nerve, frontal nerve, trochlear nerve, and superior and inferior branches of the oculomotor nerve, nasociliary nerve, and abducens nerve. The optic nerve and ophthalmic artery travel through the optic canal, which is located within the lesser wing of the sphenoid.

ANSWER 6: D. Neurotransmitters remain sufficient in the distal nerve end to allow muscular contraction with electrical stimulation for 72 hours after transection.

ANSWER 7: A. The facial nerve courses in the superficial temporal fascia, or temporoparietal fascia, in this region.

ANSWER 8: B. The patient most likely has a sialocele resulting from injury to the parotid duct or parotid gland. The buccal branches are typically located adjacent to the parotid duct.

ANSWER 9: D. Synkinesis refers to unwanted facial movements that occur in addition to desired movements. Synkinesis is only a regeneration phenomenon, making the history of recovered Bell's palsy important.

ANSWER 10: A. The patient most likely has a thyroglossal duct cyst and is best managed with the Sistrunk procedure, which includes excision of the central portion of the hyoid bone to decrease risk of recurrence.

Chapter 3

ANSWER 1: C. Adenoid cystic carcinoma usually presents as a painful, firm, and fixed mass to the underlying tissues, with involvement of the facial nerve. Treatment is by total parotidectomy and sacrifice of the involved facial nerve.

ANSWER 2: D. Recurrence rates after enucleation alone have been reported to be between 2.5% and 62%. Although surgical bony resection is more curative, it carries higher morbidity. Consideration of the preferred treatment depends on the tumor and patient-related factors. Close follow-up is an essential part of the management of this pathology.

ANSWER 3: D. Total glossectomy reconstruction requires adequate bulk of vascularized tissue. These patients often require adjuvant chemotherapy and radiotherapy. A flap that provides adequate bulk and diversion of oral diet to minimized aspiration is desired. A skin graft is inappropriate for this reconstruction.

ANSWER 4: E. Bisphosphonates, steroids, chemotherapy, dental trauma, or infection are all associated with development of MRONJ. The 2014 update of a position paper from the American Association of Oral and Maxillofacial Surgeons recommended changing the name of bisphosphonate-related osteonecrosis of the jaw (BRONJ) to MRONJ due to the increased number of jaw osteonecrosis cases that have been associated with other antiresorptive (denosumab) or antiangiogenic agents.

ANSWER 5: E.

ANSWER 6: D. Warthin's tumors typically occur in men, and 10% of tumors are bilateral.

ANSWER 7: C. Aberrant regeneration of parasympathetic auriculotemporal nerve fibers after parotidectomy is thought to underlie Frey's syndrome.

ANSWER 8: C. Sclerotherapy is the most appropriate initial treatment for symptomatic venous malformations.

ANSWER 9: A. The most appropriate treatment for moderately advanced oral cavity SCCs with mandibular cortical invasion is wide local excision, segmental resection of the portion of mandible with cortical tumor invasion, and staging with neck dissection, given the high probability of occult metastases.

ANSWER 10: B. The most appropriate initial management of medication-related osteonecrosis of the mandible in the absence of pathologic fracture is antimicrobial mouthwashes, antibiotics, and observation.

Chapter 4

ANSWER 1: B. The patient has an injury to the optic nerve, which results in a "Marcus Gunn" pupil, characterized by abnormal pupillary dilation in the presence of light.

ANSWER 2: D. The indications for tooth extraction in the setting of mandible fractures include the presence of dental caries, the presence of periapical infection, injury or fracture of the tooth root, or inability to obtain proper fracture reduction because of the condition of the tooth.

ANSWER 3: C. The patient has suffered a trapdoor orbital floor fracture with entrapment of the inferior rectus muscle. He is exhibiting an oculocardiac reflex, which results in nausea and bradycardia. This patient requires emergent operative reduction and orbital floor reconstruction.

ANSWER 4: C. The patient's dystopia and growing skull fracture is most likely caused by a missed dural tear sustained at the time of her initial injury. Because of the dural injury, the fracture line is unable to heal, resulting in a growing defect as the skull enlarges with age.

ANSWER 5: A. In type-III NOE fractures, there has been extensive bony comminution of the NOE complex along with disruption of the medial canthal tendon. When performing transnasal wiring of the medial canthal tendon, it is important to position the canthus posterior and superior to the lacrimal crest with slight overcorrection.

ANSWER 6: B. Frontal sinus fractures can be assessed by whether the fracture involves the anterior and posterior wall of the sinus and by patency of the nasofrontal duct. If the nasofrontal duct is not patent, obliteration of the sinus and duct is recommended to reduce the risk of a mucocele or pyomucocele. If there is displaced or comminuted fractures of the posterior table in the presence of nasofrontal duct injury, cranialization of the sinus with duct obliteration is recommended.

ANSWER 7: C. Transconjunctival approach can be extended medially as a transcaruncular approach to access the medial orbit. A coronal incision also gives access to the medial orbit but not to the orbital floor. Subciliary and subtarsal incisions do not allow access to the medial orbit.

ANSWER 8: D. An inferior border locking plate will address the compression forces, and the arch bar acts as a superior plate to counteract the tension forces. Compression plates are not recommended. A Champy plate is for angle fractures, and MMF alone is less optimal than ORIF because of the morbidity of immobility.

ANSWER 9: D. Proper alignment and reduction of the lateral orbital wall/zygomaticosphenoid suture is most important to reduce the risk of postoperative enophthalmos and/or malar flattening.

ANSWER 10: B. Management of infection requires adequate I&D. It is important that rigid internal fixation be maintained until the bone fracture segments have ossified, because nonrigid fixation, such as external or maxillomandibular fixation, can lead to worsening of infection. Removal of the internal hardware is rarely necessary unless the hardware is actively infected and loosened because of bone involvement (osteomyelitis).

Chapter 5

ANSWER 1: D. Pierre Robin first described this clinical triad. This developmental disorder is now thought to be initiated by mandibular undergrowth or retropositioning. There is an associated syndrome in 34% to 46% of patients with Robin sequence. Cleft palate is present in up to 90% of patients with Robin sequence, although it is not required to make the diagnosis.

ANSWER 2: C. The patient has classic features of unilateral coronal synostosis. Due to age at presentation, he is not a candidate for endoscopic-assisted strip craniectomy and helmet therapy. This procedure is ideally done between the ages of 2 and 4 months, with helmet therapy recommended up to 12 months of age. Cranial distraction is not standard for unilateral coronal synostosis but has been used for posterior expansion in syndromic patients with bilateral coronal synostosis. Total or subtotal vault reconstruction has many variations and is used to treat patients with sagittal synostosis. Fronto-orbital advancement is the most appropriate treatment to correct the patient's forehead.

ANSWER 3: C. The patient likely has Saethre-Chotzen syndrome. Characteristic exam findings are eyelid ptosis and low hairline. The most common gene mutation in this syndromic craniosynostoisis is TWIST1.

ANSWER 4: B. Metopic suture undergoes physiologic closure between 2 and 9 months. The remaining sutures close in adulthood: sagittal suture (22 years of age), coronal suture (24 years), lambdoid suture (26 years), and squamosal suture (>60 years).

ANSWER 5: A. Edward Treacher Collins described this syndrome in 1900 and it is also known as mandibulofacial dysostosis. It is autosomal dominant with variable penetrance. Other abnormalities include cleft palate, microtia, anterior open bite, and macrostomia.

ANSWER 6: A. These findings are consistent with a midline craniofacial disorder characterized by increased interdacryon, or interorbital, distance. Hypertelorbitism most accurately describes this abnormality, which may be found in craniofrontonasal dysplasia. Telecanthus is distinguished from hypertelorbitism based on an increased intercanthal, rather than interorbital, distance.

ANSWER 7: D. Sagittal synostosis is characterized by increased AP length (scaphocephaly) and a relatively narrow biparietal width. Reconstruction involves shortening the AP dimension and widening the biparietal width.

ANSWER 8: D. Lambdoid synostosis is characterized by a unilateral lamboid ridge, ipsilateral occipitomastoid bulging, posteroinferior displacement of the ipsilateral ear, a parallelogram shape to the head when viewed posteriorly, and a trapezoid shape to the head when viewed from the vertex. Posterior plagiocephaly is characterized by a parallelogram shape when viewed from the vertex, anterior displacement of the ipsilateral ear, and ipsilateral frontal bulging.

ANSWER 9: B. The features are most consistent with Nager syndrome.

ANSWER 10: C. A LeFort II advancement will allow correction of the nasomaxillary hypoplasia that characterizes Binder syndrome.

Chapter 6

ANSWER 1: B.

ANSWER 2: A. The newborn presents with a Pierre Robin sequence (PRS). Although PRS can occur in isolation, it frequently occurs as a component of syndromic conditions. These include Stickler, VCFS, Treacher Collins, and Nager, and all must be ruled out.

ANSWER 3: C. Tessier clefts 1, 2, and 3 begin at the vermilion as the typical or "common" cleft lip. However, as the cleft involvement progresses superiorly to involve the nose, Tessier clefts 1, 2, and 3 diverge. Tessier 1 involves the dome, Tessier 2 the lateral crus, and Tessier 3 separates the alar base from the cheek junction. Tessier 4 begins lateral to the philtrum, spares the alar base, and courses medial to the infraorbital foramen toward the medial aspect of the lower eyelid. Tessier 5 begins medial to the oral commissure and courses lateral to the infraorbital rim to involve the lateral lower eyelid.

ANSWER 4: A. The caudal septum deviates to the noncleft side; however, the proximal component of the septum defects toward the cleft side.

ANSWER 5: D. Cleft rhinoplasty should be delayed until after the maxillary-mandibular skeletal foundation is properly established. This is because the cartilaginous septum and vomer must be separated from the maxilla to perform a LeFort I, disrupting previous cleft rhinoplasty surgery. Moreover, with maxillary advancement, the nasal tip would be expected to be elevated and the nasal labial angle more obtuse. The chin position will be altered frequently in a clockwise direction.

ANSWER 6: B. Cleft lip deformities develop during the 3rd to 7th week of gestation, whereas cleft palate deformities develop between the 5th and 12th weeks. By the 9th week, fusion of the medial nasal processes of the frontonasal prominence to the maxillary prominences has already occurred.

ANSWER 7: D. Patients with velocardiofacial syndrome (22q11.2 DS) frequently will demonstrate medialization of the carotid arteries. This anatomic finding is of critical importance because the carotids may be injured during velopharyngeal surgery, resulting in exanguination.

ANSWER 8: B. The tensor veli palatini is innervated by the mandibular branch of the trigeminal nerve (V3).

ANSWER 9: D. In this circumstance, a palatal prosthesis would be the best option, because it may help speech to some degree and can also be removed at night to prevent worsening of sleep apnea. Both pharyngeal flap and sphincter pharyngoplasty procedures have been noted to increase the risk of sleep apnea. Furlow double-opposing Z-plasty is unlikely to help when no significant levator function is identified.

ANSWER 10: A. To establish a normal dental relationship with an overjet of 2 mm, the maxilla must be advanced 11 mm relative to the mandible. This is unlikely to be able to be accomplished with LeFort I advancement alone. In standard practice, a setback of the mandible with bilateral sagittal split osteotomies is typically performed. A distraction procedure is typically unnecessary for an advancement of 11 mm.

Chapter 7

ANSWER 1: D. The structures that arise from the first branchial arch primarily drain to the parotid lymph nodes. This includes the superior helix, tragus, and helical root. The structures that arise from the second branchial arch primarily drain to the cervical lymph nodes.

ANSWER 2: C.

ANSWER 3: D. The prominent ear is often characterized by a conchoscaphal angle >90 degrees, hypertrophy of the concha cavum with a depth >1.5 cm, a prominent lobule, and an auriculocephalic angle >25 degrees.

ANSWER 4: D. Cryptotia is characterized by an abnormal adherence of the superior helix to the temporal skin, with varying degrees of severity. In some cases, the helix can be pulled out to the normal position.

ANSWER 5: C. Rim-only defects that are 1.5 cm or less in length can be reconstructed with an Antia-Buch chondrocutaneous flap.

ANSWER 6: C. To achieve definition of the auricle, it is crucial to have a well-vascularized, supple, uniform, and thin skin envelope. This can be achieved by meticulous skin pocket dissection, with the aim of creating a 2-mm-thick skin flap using blunt, straight scissors.

ANSWER 7: D. Autogenous auricular reconstruction in microtia with craniofacial deformities is challenging, because of atypical anatomy (e.g., dislocated vestige, atypical superficial temporal arteries, low hairline) and associated skeletal deformities. However, with careful planning by an experienced surgeon, auricular reconstruction in these patients is possible and therefore not contraindicated.

ANSWER 8: A. The superior helix is derived from the anterior hillocks (1 to 3) of the first branchial arch.

ANSWER 9: D. The auricle is located approximately one ear length (6.5 to 7.5 cm) behind the lateral orbital rim. The top of the auricle is on line with the eyebrow, and the bottom of the auricle is on line with the base of the columella or slightly below. The normal auricle is inclined posteriorly 10 to 20 degrees, and the width is ~50% to 55% of the length.

ANSWER 10: A. The optimal timing of ear molding is immediately after birth. After 1 month of age, ear molding becomes less effective. The duration of the treatment is ~6 to 8 weeks.

Chapter 8

ANSWER 1: C. Although all of the choices listed contribute to breast blood supply, the dominant supply is from internal IMA perforators.

ANSWER 2: D.

ANSWER 3: C.

ANSWER 4: B. The medial pectoral nerve supplies the lateral and inferior portions of the pectoralis major, whereas the lateral pectoralis major supplies the medial portion of the muscle. This is somewhat confusing because they are named according to their origin, with the medial nerve arising from the medial cord of the brachial plexus and the lateral nerve arising from the lateral cord.

ANSWER 5: A. Intercostal artery perforators are the dominant blood supply to the inferior pedicle of the breast.

ANSWER 6: B. Characteristics of Tanner stage-II breasts include darkening and widening of the areola as well as an areola that is elevated from the underlying palpable breast bud.

ANSWER 7: C.

ANSWER 8: B. Cutaneous branches of the 4th intercostal nerve supply the NAC.

ANSWER 9: D. Dye flow studies report that both the axillary and parasternal lymphatic groups receive lymph from all quadrants of the breast.

ANSWER 10: D. Reduction mammoplasty is first-line therapy after breast size has stabilized for 1 year or more. Reduction mammoplasty can be performed even if the patient is younger than 18 years.

ANSWER 11: D. Reduction in blood flow or hypoplasia of the internal thoracic artery can lead to disruption of pectoralis major development. Hypoplasia of the branches of the brachial artery during development could lead to upper extremity/hand deformities.

ANSWER 12: C. Like juvenile breast hypertrophy, giant fibroadenomas result from abnormal sensitivity of the breast tissue to normal hormonal levels. They are discrete benign tumors that enlarge rapidly. Treatment is surgical excision, with possible concurrent matching procedures to achieve symmetry.

ANSWER 13: C. Moderate breast enlargement with excess skin describes Simon grade IIB gynecomastia.

ANSWER 14: D. Ultrasound of the testes should be performed to rule out tumor. Tumors known to cause gynecomastia include Leydig cell and Sertoli cell tumors as well as choriocarcinomas.

ANSWER 15: A. Ketoconazole inhibits CYP450 enzymes, including 11β-hydroxylase, necessary for adrenal androgen production.

ANSWER 16: B. Because the internal mammary vessels were previously harvested for the bypass, reliability of a medial pedicle based on the IMA perforators may be compromised.

ANSWER 17: C. Jeune syndrome is characterized by glandular tissue that can be congenital, surgical, or radiation induced.

ANSWER 18: C. The IMF is elevated with a tuberous breast deformity.

ANSWER 19: D. Pectus carinatum is convex or anteriorly projecting sternum and ribs. It is commonly referred to as a pigeon's chest deformity.

ANSWER 20: A. Poland syndrome is characterized by an absence of the sternal head of the pectoralis major muscle.

Chapter 9

ANSWER 1: C. The main advantage of duplex Doppler is the additional information on flow quantity and direction. However, flow is very variable and dependent on cardiac output and the state of constriction of the vessel. More important is the knowledge that vessels spread in all directions into the subdermal plexus. This, together with the ability to compare relative perforator vessel sizes in one radiological document, gives us more reliability in identifying the dominant perforator in the lower abdominal wall.

ANSWER 2: C. The oncological risk for loco-regional or distant metastasis is comparable for both reconstructive techniques and is certainly not higher compared to ablative surgery without reconstruction.

ANSWER 3: E. Taking into account the increased risk of local recurrence after conservative breast surgery, the DIEAP flap should be reserved for full breast reconstruction in case that is needed in a later phase. Flaps with a smaller volume and skin surface than the DIEAP flap (TDAP, LICAP, anterior intercostal artery perforator [AICAP], and glandular flaps) should be used as a first choice.

ANSWER 4: F. These are 5 of the 8 elementary rules that form the basis for safe perforator pedicle dissection for any type of free or pedicled perforator flaps.

ANSWER 5: D. Sufficient scientific data are now available to show that skin- and areola-sparing mastectomies have no increased risk for loco-regional recurrence or distant metastasis as long as the tumor is 1 inch (2.5 cm) away from the nipple. Primary reconstructions are as safe as secondary reconstructions but provide a better esthetic outcome.

ANSWER 6: D. Both *BRCA1* and *2* carry an 85% risk for breast cancer; ovarian cancer risk is higher with *BRCA1*.

ANSWER 7: C. Linear or branching calcifications may suggest malignancy, as may pleomorphic/granular calcifications.

ANSWER 8: A. Although treated in most instances as though it were cancer, and given the unique definition of "stage 0," due to the likely progression to invasive ductal carcinoma, DCIS is NOT cancer; it is a premalignant condition.

ANSWER 9: D. Large tumor-to-breast size may cause unacceptable deformity. Previous external beam radiation therapy (XRT) complicates the need for postlumpectomy XRT, and multifocal disease is a risk for higher recurrence rate.

ANSWER 10: B.

ANSWER 11: D. Radiation therapy complicates all aspects of breast reconstruction. With an expander, XRT planning is made more difficult: Treatment of the internal mammary nodes is limited and tightness from XRT fibrosis is a problem. However, there is no information suggesting that risk of mortality is altered and that XRT skin problems may be alleviated with a flap procedure. With a free TRAM flap, XRT planning is more difficult due to the fixed volume of the TRAM flap that does not flatten in the supine position, as a natural breast would. Post-XRT, a TRAM flap may shrink unpredictably and will not increase in size with time if the woman gains weight, a typical advantage of the TRAM flap. With delayed reconstruction, XRT is not impacted, but skin is lost and will be fibrotic, making it harder to perform a successful reconstruction. This can be psychologically problematic.

ANSWER 12: D. The upper inner thigh is an area with loose skin and subcutaneous fat and can provide an autologous reconstructive option, especially for thinner women with smaller breasts, but the above limitations may complicate the procedure.

ANSWER 13: C. If the area of necrosis or dehiscence is small and overvascularized tissue AND there is no need for timely postoperative chemotherapy or radiation therapy, this area may be left to heal secondarily. If the problem is larger or other therapies are planned, excision and reclosure, either in the office or operating room, is indicated.

Chapter 10

ANSWER 1: E. Subpectoral breast implant placement may result in a dynamic deformity of the breast during contraction of the pectoralis major muscle.

ANSWER 2: C. Triple-antibiotic breast irrigation is a strategy to reduce biofilm formation and capsular contracture. It includes the use of Cefazolin, Gentamycin, and Bacitracin.

ANSWER 3: D. The tuberous breast deformity may include herniation of breast tissue through NAC, a constricted breast base, and a high IMF. The distance from the IMF to the nipple is typically decreased.

ANSWER 4: D. The intercostobrachial nerve crosses the axilla from the second rib and supplies sensation to the medial and posterior aspect of the proximal arm. During a transaxillary approach for breast augmentation, dissection should remain superficial until the border of the pectoralis major muscle is reached.

ANSWER 5: C. Anaplastic large-cell lymphoma associated with breast implants may present as a late seroma. Breast-implant-associated anaplastic large-cell lymphoma is commonly found to be CD30 positive.

ANSWER 6: E. The LICAP is predominantly used for lumpectomy defects and for autoaugmentation of the breast in postbariatric breast rejuvenation surgery or to supplement postmastectomy reconstruction. Tuberous breast deformities can be reconstructed with breast implants with (a) or without (b) antecedent tissue expansion; in inferiorly based periareolar autoaugmentation (c), or, more recently, with autologous fat grafting (d).

ANSWER 7: C. Dye injection studies (Taylor GI, Palmer JH. The vascular territories (angiosomes) of the body: experimental study and clinical applications. *British Journal of Plastic Surgery*. 1987;40:113-41) suggest that the inferior pedicle provides the least significant vascular supply to the NAC.

ANSWER 8: C. Form-stable implants have less rippling (a), lower capsular contracture rates than smooth gel devices (b), lower leak rates at 8 years (d), and tend to have greater upper pole fullness than round devices. However, they are currently available in a more limited volume range relative to round, smooth, traditional silicone implants.

ANSWER 9: D. The majority of data suggest that subglandular placement of smooth implants is most commonly associated with capsular contracture.

ANSWER 10: A. Patient age has not been consistently shown to significantly impact capsular contracture rates. In contrast, factors that impact periprosthetic inflammation, such as the biofilm theory, radiation, incision selection, and perioperative hemostasis, have all been linked to capsular contracture.

Chapter 11

ANSWER 1: E. In contrast to synthetic mesh, the degree of wound contamination does not appear to significantly affect the chance of developing major complications such as recurrent hernia, mesh infection, or mesh explantation following abdominal-wall reconstruction with bioprosthetic mesh.

ANSWER 2: B. Records from the National Surgical Quality Improvement Program (NSQIP) determined that obesity, COPD, steroid use, smoking, and low preoperative serum albumin level were all independent risk factors for a fourfold increase in wound infection rates. Diabetes was not found to be as significant a risk factor.

ANSWER 3: A. This patient has failed hernia repair with a simple bridged synthetic mesh repair and now presents with a contaminated wound healing complication; therefore, bioprosthetic mesh is indicated. It is important to provide the best possible reconstruction in this patient because the rate of reoperation increases with each subsequent hernia repair. Component separation will allow for primary fascial coaptation of the hernia defect without excessive tension over the inlay bioprosthetic, thus creating a reinforced repair with a significantly lower recurrence rate than another bridged repair. Finally, preserving the periumbilical perforating vessels from the epigastric arteries with the minimally invasive component separation technique will help preserve the perfusion of the overlying skin to avoid future wound necrosis.

ANSWER 4: D. Stage-IV pressures sores are defined as full-thickness wounds that extend beyond the subcutaneous fat into the underlying muscle, tendon, or bone, as seen in this patient.

ANSWER 5: C. This young paraplegic patient is at great risk of having future pressure sores. As such, effort should be made to maximize future flap-coverage options. The simplest option is to readvance the flaps that she already has, which simultaneously avoids burning any future reconstructive bridges. *a* is incorrect because it would be difficult to cover a sacral decubitus ulcer with a tensor fascia lata flap; *b* is incorrect because it would be more difficult to perform a gluteus maximus musculocutaneous rotation flap in the setting of a previous bilateral V-Y gluteus maximus advancement flap than to simply readvance the V-Y flaps; and *d* is similarly incorrect because readvancement of the V-Y flap would be simpler than creating a new transverse back flap and would preserve future options for reconstruction.

ANSWER 6: C. Superior gluteal artery perforator flaps provide adequate soft-tissue coverage while preserving the superior and inferior gluteal muscles. This minimizes donor site morbidity, which is important in this ambulatory patient. Gluteal myocutaneous advancement and rotational flaps would both provide the soft-tissue coverage but would involve harvest of the superior and inferior gluteal muscles, which would increase morbidity. Full-thickness skin graft does not provide stable coverage of a stage-4 sacral decubitus ulcer with exposed bone.

ANSWER 7: E. This patient has involvement of the hip joint, which is consistent with osteomyelitis. He will need adequate bony debridement, most likely involving resection of the femoral head (also known as the Girdlestone procedure), followed by vascularized tissue transfer to obliterate the dead space and cover the defect. IV antibiotics alone are not sufficient for treating the osteomyelitis. Tensor fascia lata flap, vastus lateralis flap, and ALT flaps are good options for coverage of a trochanteric decubitus ulcer, but the wound has to be adequately debrided to clear the infective process before final flap coverage.

ANSWER 8: C. The muscles of the abdominal wall are innervated by the intercostal nerves T7 to T12, and these nerves run in the plane below the internal oblique. Hence, staying in the plane between the external oblique and the internal oblique will preserve the innervation to the muscles flaps during component separation.

ANSWER 9: A. Several options exist for vaginal reconstruction but the pedicled vertical rectus abdominis myocutaneous (VRAM) flap remains the gold standard for vaginal reconstruction. It has a reliable blood supply and can be harvested with a large skin paddle that can be used to resurface both the vagina and perineum. It can be also harvested as a rectoperitoneal flap, including a cuff of peritoneum that can be used to resurface the peritoneum. Primary closure of both perineal and vaginal defects is not the best option in a radiated patient with large defects. The ALT flap has been described for perineal reconstruction but VRAM remains the preferred option for vaginal reconstruction. The McIndoe procedure involves using a split-thickness skin graft along with a mold for vaginal reconstruction especially in cases of vaginal agenesis. It usually requires serial dilations with obturators and is not the ideal option for this patient.

ANSWER 10: A. The dorsal nerve of the clitoris is analogous to the dorsal nerve of the penis and is responsible for most of the erogenous sensation associated with the clitoris. The dorsal nerve of the clitoris is the terminal branch of the pudendal nerve. Studies have shown that neurorrhaphy between the dorsal nerve of the clitoris and the donor cutaneous nerve is associated with superior sensory outcomes in phalloplasty. The posterior femoral cutaneous nerve provides sensory innervation to the posterior aspect of the thigh and perineum. The ilioinguinal nerve provides innervation to the medial thigh and the labia majora and minora. The iliohypogastric nerve provides innervation to the mons pubis. The lateral femoral cutaneous nerve arises from the lumbar plexus and innervates the lateral thigh.

Chapter 12

ANSWER 1: C. Timely exploration and surgical repair is indicated for all sharp lacerations with distal nerve deficit. Electrodiagnostic studies are not necessary. The working diagnosis should be nerve transection.

ANSWER 2: C. At 3 years postinjury, nerve repair/transfer are not options because the muscle is terminally denervated. Tendon transfers are his only available option.

ANSWER 3: D. The cell body for the sensory nerves is located in the dorsal root ganglia. This is important in cases of nerve root avulsion injuries because the electrodiagnostic study of the motor and sensory roots will show a disconnect. There will be no recordable motor action potentials at that avulsed level, but the SNAPs will actually be normal because the cell-body-to-nerve connection is intact and located distal to the site of injury.

ANSWER 4: B. A neurapraxia is by definition a conduction block. There is no Wallerian degeneration and no advancing Tinel's sign. However, if the nerve is explored and stimulated distal to the site of injury/neurapraxia, stimulation can produce distal muscle

stimulation because the conduction block is the only issue preventing function.

ANSWER 5: A. Tension-free repair means no tension through the full range of motion; joints should not be artificially flexed to attain that goal.

ANSWER 6: E. The patient has median and ulnar nerve deficits; thus, an isolated median nerve injury is unlikely. Intact elbow flexion means the lateral cord is intact. Preserved elbow flexion and extension rule out a middle trunk injury. There are median nerve deficits in addition to the ulnar nerve deficits; thus, an isolated ulnar nerve injury is unlikely. Impaired median and ulnar nerve function with preservation of lateral cord function and posterior cord function implicate the median cord as the site of injury.

ANSWER 7: B. Nerve amplitude is a proxy for the number of functional axons within the nerve being evaluated.

ANSWER 8: B. Preservation of sensory nerve action potentials in the setting of diffuse muscular palsy is pathognomonic for a preganglionic injury, because the dorsal root ganglion remains attached to the distal nerve and can thus receive nerve action potentials.

ANSWER 9: B. An end-to-side transfer from the anterior interosseous nerve to the motor branch of the ulnar nerve provides innervation necessary to preserve the intrinsic muscle motor end plates and increases the likelihood of improved intrinsic function following ulnar nerve release in the setting of severe cubital tunnel syndrome.

ANSWER 10: D. Of the options listed, a nerve transfer from the tibial nerve branch to the flexor hallucis longus (FHL) or flexor digitorum longus (FDL) to the peroneal motor branch to the tibialis anterior offers the greatest potential to restore active dorsiflexion.

Chapter 13

ANSWER 1: A. Filariasis is the most common secondary lymphedema in the world due to infection of the filarial worm, especially in Africa and India.

ANSWER 2: C. Most patients who underwent liposuction for their lymphedematous limbs require life-long compression garment usage; otherwise, the lymphedema will recur.

ANSWER 3: C. Toe infections, hyperkeratosis, residual or progressive lymphedema, and cellulitis of the lower limb are common complications developing post-Charles procedure.

ANSWER 4: A. The indications of vascularized lymph node flap transfer include total occlusion of lymphoscintigraphy, partial occlusion of lymphoscintigraphy with poor response to complete digestive therapy for 6 months, no acute infection, and no cancer recurrence/distal metastasis.

ANSWER 5: **D.** Lymphovenous anastomosis is more effective in early breast-cancer-related upper limb lymphedema.

ANSWER 6: **C.** The destruction of smooth muscle cells results in decreases of the tunica media and dilation of the lymphatic channel.

ANSWER 7: **D.** Lymphovenous bypass is most effective in patients with an earlier stage of lymphedema.

ANSWER 8: **B.** Sex difference does not contribute to aggravation of the lymphedema.

ANSWER 9: **A.** Lymphangiosarcoma is one of the lymphedema-related malignancies known as Stewart-Treves syndrome.

ANSWER 10: **A.** Chronic lymph stasis impairs local immune surveillance by disrupting trafficking of the immunocompetent cells in the lymphedematous region.

Chapter 14

ANSWER 1: **C.** Typically, a simple, incomplete syndactyly of a central webspace can be released between 1 and 2 years of age. Border digits, especially the thumb, may require earlier release.

ANSWER 2: **D.** Sensory function of the retained thumb should be within normal limits following correction of radial polydactyly.

ANSWER 3: **B.** Polydactyly is the most common congenital hand malformation, affecting ~1 in 500 live births.

ANSWER 4: **D.** The thumb metacarpal is not usually present or is hypoplastic and cannot be resected in most patients undergoing pollicization. Division of this structure is not typically performed.

ANSWER 5: **C.** Symbrachydactyly and amniotic band syndrome are both typically sporadic; thus, patients would not typically have a family history of either condition.

ANSWER 6: **B.** Apert syndrome and its anomalies are the result of a mutation of the *FGFR-2* gene.

ANSWER 7: **D.** Holt-Oram syndrome is the likely diagnosis for a child who has bilateral absent thumbs and cardiac septal defect. The most common cardiac anomaly is an atrial septal defect. This is an autosomal dominant disorder with wide variability in expression of cardiac and limb anomalies.

ANSWER 8: **C.** The patient demonstrates right small-finger clinodactyly with a delta phalanx visible on radiographs.

ANSWER 9: **D.**

ANSWER 10: **E.** A Blauth type-IIIB classification indicates an unstable CMC joint. The best option would be for amputation of the hypoplastic thumb and index pollicization.

Chapter 15

ANSWER 1: **B.** An osteoid osteoma, seen in young patients (2nd and 3rd decades of life) is typically seen as a >1-cm "lucent nidus" (occasionally with a calcified central core) surrounded by reactive sclerosis. An enchondroma is a well-defined, lobulated lytic lesion; a chondrosarcoma is usually poorly defined with stippled calcifications, extreme cortical expansion, and soft-tissue extension; an osteoscarcoma appears as a lytic lesion with an aggressive "sunburst" periosteal reaction.

ANSWER 2: **A.** The differential diagnosis of subungual pigmentation includes benign melanonychia striata, hematoma, pyogenic granuloma, and melanoma. If unchanged in appearance for >4 to 6 weeks, biopsy is recommended.

ANSWER 3: **C.** The spiral cord forms from elements of the pretendinous band, the lateral digital sheet, Grayson's ligament, the natatory ligament, and the spiral band.

ANSWER 4: **D.** A typical workup for hypothenar hammer syndrome begins with physical exam looking for a pulsatile mass. Imaging studies include MR or CT angiogram and X ray to evaluate any bony masses/hamate fractures. EMG is not part of the typical workup.

ANSWER 5: **B.** Crush injuries to the forearm are at risk for development of compartment syndrome. Any patient who develops increasing pain after a crush injury should have a thorough physical exam looking for the "5 Ps" (pain, pallor, poikilothermia, paresthesia, pulselessness), and warm fingers do not exclude the diagnosis.

ANSWER 6: **B.** Mucous cysts are ganglion cysts originating from the DIP joint. They are associated with degenerative joint disease. Although mucous cysts are not visualized on plain radiographs, they are typically associated with osteophytes of the DIP joint. Treatment consists of debridement of the mucous cyst and removal of the osteophytes and often requires a local rotation-advancement flap for coverage.

ANSWER 7: **C.** Glomus tumors present with severe episodic pain and extreme tenderness to palpation, usually localized to the mass. These tumors often appear in the subungual region. X rays may show a lytic lesion in the bone. The mass appears on MRI as a hyperintense signal. Treatment consists of simple excision and often requires removal of the nail plate.

ANSWER 8: **B.** Hypothenar hammer syndrome is described as an aneurysm of the ulnar artery resulting from repeated blunt trauma. This may lead to clot formation and distal embolization, resulting in distal ulceration. Treatment consists of excision of the aneurysm and reconstruction with arterial or venous grafts.

ANSWER 9: **A.** The spiral cord is formed by the pretendinous band, spiral band, lateral digital sheet, and Grayson's ligament. It wraps around the neurovascular bundle and contracts, displacing the bundle centrally and superficially and giving the appearance that the bundle spirals around the cord. The bundle is often found immediately deep to the skin and may be easily injured on incision or initial dissection.

ANSWER 10: E. Cleland's ligament is not involved in Dupuytren's pathoanatomy. The lateral digital sheet contributes to spiral and lateral cords. The spiral band and Grayson's ligament each contribute to spiral cords. The pretendinous band is the key element of the central cord and also contributes to spiral cords.

Chapter 16

ANSWER 1: C. The 5th CMC joint has a larger arc, often >20 degrees. The greater degree of extension allows for greater flexion deformity of the fracture fragment, compared with adjacent digits.

ANSWER 2: A. If the subungual hematoma involves <50% of the nail surface area, trephination alone is adequate. Minimally displaced fracture responds well to closed treatment.

ANSWER 3: D. Given the chronicity of the injury and the comminution, these preclude ORIF, closed reduction percutaneous pinning (CRPP), or force-coupler dynamic pinning, which are usually used in the acute setting. The hemi-hamate gives the best chance at an anatomic reconstruction and long-term function.

ANSWER 4: D. By definition, gamekeeper's thumb is a chronic injury with attenuated tissue that is irreparable. Therefore, it will not respond to treatment modalities intended for an acute injury.

ANSWER 5: C. The adductor pollicus (AP) and the APL result in adduction of the 1st metacarpal with proximal and dorsal subsidence of the metacarpal relative to the articular fracture fragment. The reduction maneuvers to overcome these forces are axial traction, abduction, and pronation of the thumb.

ANSWER 6: C. If there is minimal articular surface involvement, closed treatment alone is usually sufficient to restore the extensor function at the distal interphalangeal joint (DIPJ).

ANSWER 7: D. The volar plate can impinge in the joint space. The other structures can create a noose around that metacarpal head that can tighten with axial traction, thereby making repeated attempts at closed reduction more difficult.

ANSWER 8: A. The flexion deformity at the DIPJ will lead to long-term imbalance of the flexors and the extensors, resulting in compensatory hyperextension at the PIP joint. This is known as a swan-neck deformity.

ANSWER 9: C. Given the degree of comminution and instability, open fracture and closed treatment alone are usually unable to control the fracture fragments or provide the necessary axial distraction forces to maintain the reduction. On the other hand, the ligamentotaxis provided by an external fixator can allow for proper

reduction without disrupting the soft-tissue envelope around the bone. *d* may be offered as a salvage if there is significant secondary posttraumatic arthrosis.

ANSWER 10: B. Dorsal blocking, whether by splint or temporary pin, should maintain a flexion arc within the confines in which the joint remains concentrically reduced. Therefore, *a* is not optimal. Because the PIP joint is stable and concentrically reduced past 20 degrees of flexion, the force-coupler is unnecessary.

Chapter 17

ANSWER 1: B. The described defect is quite large, and the FDMA flap could be used to provide coverage of this area of the thumb. The other options are inappropriate for the described defect.

ANSWER 2: B. Replantation of single digits amputated within the zone-II level is relatively contraindicated due to postoperative stiffness. It is also contraindicated when the postoperative rehabilitation will significantly delay the patient's ability to return to work, as in the case of the construction worker in *b*. Replantation should be considered for any digit in healthy children and for all thumb amputations.

ANSWER 3: C. In small-fingertip injuries without a bony amputation or with minimum exposed bone (<0.5 mm), the most appropriate method of reconstruction to obtain good sensation and function is to allow the wound to heal by secondary intention with the use of moist dressings.

ANSWER 4: D. In the patient described, the majority of the sterile matrix is scarred, and the nail cannot adhere to the nail bed. Reconstruction requires removal of the scarred sterile matrix, followed by split-thickness nail-bed grafting. Of note, reconstruction of the germinal matrix, unlike the sterile matrix, requires a full-thickness nail-bed graft, typically from the toes.

ANSWER 5: B. The flexor tendons in the scenario described have been avulsed from the musculotendinous junction, which is indicative of significant injury to the digital arteries that will severely limit the success of replantation.

ANSWER 6: D. For this manual laborer who desires to return to work quickly, the most appropriate management is revision amputation, especially given the avulsive nature of his injury.

ANSWER 7: D. Pollicization can be used for amputations of the thumb between the middle of the first metacarpal and at the CMC joint, but it works best for amputation at the level of the CMC joint. In this patient, the index finger is injured and will otherwise have minimal function. Therefore, the injured index finger should be pollicized to reconstruct the thumb reconstruction and serve as a stable post.

ANSWER 8: B. A reverse cross-finger flap is used to cover soft-tissue defects on the dorsum of an adjacent digit. The skin on the donor finger is incised on the side closest to the recipient finger and elevated off of the underlying dorsal subcutaneous tissue. The dorsal subcutaneous tissue of the donor finger is raised as a flap based on the side closest to the recipient finger. The flap is sutured to the recipient finger and is used as a bed to receive a full-thickness skin graft. The native skin is then returned to the dorsum of the middle phalanx of the donor finger.

ANSWER 9: C. Hook nail deformity results from a loss of nail support following trauma to the distal fingertip, causing the nail to curve in a volar direction. The severity of hook nail deformity depends on the degree of bone loss, the amount of remaining nail bed, and the degree of scar contracture at the hyponychial-pulp interface.

ANSWER 10: D. Subungual hematomas secondary to nail-bed injuries cause pressure in the closed space between the nail plate and nail bed, resulting frequently in throbbing pain. When the hematoma is <50% of the nail, trephination can be performed for pain relief. The hole should be large enough to allow for prolonged drainage.

Chapter 18

ANSWER 1: D. Non- or minimally displaced fractures, regardless of styloid involvement or intra-articular nature, may be treated with closed reduction, splinting, and close clinical and radiographic follow-up. Indications for ORIF include intra-articular fractures with >2 mm cortical step-off or displacement, loss of radial height (positive ulnar variance) of >3 mm, loss of volar angulation of 10 degrees or more, and any fractures (intra- or extra-articular) with significant displacement or comminution.

ANSWER 2: B. SL ligament injury or disruption is suspected when the SL interval is >2 mm. The "clenched fist" draws the capitate proximally and emphasizes the SL interval. Ideally, the clenched fist view should be performed in supination and ulnar deviation. Radial deviation has the opposite effect and decreases the SL gap. If a ligamentous injury is suspected based on radiographic SL widening, comparison to the unaffected contralateral wrist is often key in establishing the diagnosis. The pronated oblique view is helpful for assessing the scapho-trapezoid-trapezial (STT) joint. The Roberts view is used to optimize visualization of the thumb CMC joint.

ANSWER 3: C. Waist and proximal pole fractures of the scaphoid are prone to nonunion and avascular necrosis, secondary to the retrograde vascular supply of the bone. Scaphoid nonunion or malunion "humpback deformity" can progress to arthritis and scaphoid nonunion advanced collapse (SNAC) wrist deformities. Management relies on either nonvascularized or vascularized bone grafting to achieve union. In a young patient in whom nonvascularized bone grafting has failed, a vascularized graft affords the best chance of successful bony union. Total wrist arthoplasty and total wrist fusion are options for recalcitrant wrist arthritis and chronic pain. Performance of either option in an active young patient would significantly limit range of motion and activity long term.

ANSWER 4: A. PRC involves excision of the proximal row of the carpus (scaphoid, lunate, triquetrum). The capitate then articulates with the lunate fossa of the radius and therefore must be free of arthritic disease. In such cases, alternative forms of partial wrist fusion (four-corner fusion) or complete wrist fusion should be pursued.

ANSWER 5: B. Trigger finger is one of the most common complaints in hand surgery. Initial management involves corticosteroid injection(s), which is curative for many patients. Surgical release of the A1 pulley is performed in patients who fail corticosteroid injection. However, the A1 pulley should never be released in patients with rheumatoid arthritis because this can result in worsening of ulnar drift of the involved digit. In such patients, tenosynovectomy and excision of intratendinous nodules is the procedure of choice.

ANSWER 6: A. After disruption of the SL interosseous ligament, there is dissociation of the scaphoid and lunate resulting in a DISI deformity. This is characterized by a SL angle >60 degrees and a gap of >3 mm (Terry Thomas sign).

ANSWER 7: D. If left untreated, displaced fractures of the proximal scaphoid are at risk for developing proximal pole avascular necrosis (AVN) and humpback deformity due to scaphoid nonunion. This nonunion is termed SNAC and can progress to pancarpal arthritis. This is different from a SLAC wrist, which develops from an untreated SL ligament tear.

ANSWER 8: C. A PRC involves removal of the scaphoid, lunate, and trapezium, allowing the capitate to act as the main contact point between the radius and carpus as it articulates with the radius in the lunate fossa. Arthritic changes of the head of the capitate are a contraindication to PRC, and other salvage procedures must be used.

ANSWER 9: A. Four-corner fusion is a salvage procedure to treat wrist arthritis. It involves removal of the scaphoid and fusion of the lunate, triquetrum, capitate, and hamate.

ANSWER 10: E. A carpal tunnel view allows the hamate to be seen in an axial view, which is useful for identifying fractures of the hook of hamate.

ANSWER 11: B. In a Mayfield stage-IV perilunate dislocation, the lunate becomes dislocated volarly out of the lunate fossa. For this to happen, its attachments to the scaphoid and triquetrum must be completely disrupted. These are the SL and lunotriquetral ligaments, respectively.

ANSWER 12: A. The EPL is most at risk for rupture following a distal radius fracture. The EPL is responsible for thumb extension, which is absent after rupture. Treatment includes tendon transfers to restore thumb extension.

ANSWER 13: C. Complete tear of the SL interoseous ligament will result in a DISI deformity over time. With complete dissociation of the scaphoid and lunate, the scaphoid assumes a flexed position and the lunate an extended position, which increases the SL angle >60 degrees.

ANSWER 14: C. The trapeziometacarpal joint, or basilar joint, is the most common site of arthritis in the hand. Patients often complain of difficulty opening jars and pain at the base of the thumb.

Chapter 19

ANSWER 1: A. The carpal canal contains 9 tendons and the median nerve. The anatomic relationships to the carpal canal are consistent: FDS tendons to the ring and middle finger lie most volar, with the FDS tendons to the index and small fingers immediately deep or dorsal to this. The FDP tendons lie on the dorsal floor of canal, and the FPL tendon lies radial, deep, and adjacent to the scaphoid and trapezium.

ANSWER 2: C. The strength of a tendon repair can be increased by an increasing number of core suture strands across the repair site, locking sutures, epitendinous sutures, and early mobilization and range of motion.

ANSWER 3: B. Because of its insertion onto the base of the third metacarpal, the ECRB is considered the prime wrist extensor.

ANSWER 4: A. The patient in this scenario has the classic signs and symptoms of de Quervain's tenosynovitis. This is characterized by entrapment of the APL and extensor pollicis brevis within the first extensor compartment.

ANSWER 5: C. The classic treatment for the "fist-in-palm" deformity is the FDS-to-FDP or superficialis-to-profundus (STP) transfer.

ANSWER 6: D. The extensor digitorum brevis manus (EDBM) muscle is an anomalous muscle identified in 2% to 3% of the population. In addition to the EDC and extensor indices proprius, this finger extensor can extend the index, long, or ring finger. Its presence should be noted to be sure the distal EIP muscle and this anomalous muscle are not mistaken for one another. Its repair is optional in the setting of intact EDC. It may also be identified in the dorsal wrist as a painful mass. The EDBM is innervated by the posterior interosseous nerve, which is the distal extension of the radial nerve.

ANSWER 7: C. Closed injury of the sagittal band can lead to subluxation of the extensor tendon off of the metacarpal head into the intermetacarpal space ulnar to the joint. In this setting, the patient can maintain active passive finger extension, and there is an associated subluxation when the finger is placed back in flexion. In these cases, active extension of the finger is often not possible. This is seen in rheumatoid patients due to attritional rupture and ulnar drift. It is also seen following blows to the MPJ, most commonly of the prominent long finger. Extension splinting or repair is indicated.

ANSWER 8: C. The flexor pollicis longus is deep and radial within the carpal tunnel. Its distal end will flex the tip of the thumb. Finding its proximal end can be difficult but very important to avoid the above complication and need for reoperation. This tendon is usually the radial-most tendon in the carpal tunnel. It takes origin distal in the forearm, leading to the lowest amount of stretch when passively extended. Unlike the FDS and FDP, it will not share a common muscle belly. It lies deep to the FDP.

ANSWER 9: B. The 2nd and 4th annular pulleys have been shown in multiple biomechanical and clinical studies to be the most important structures for preventing bowstringing of the flexor tendons and maintenance of normal joint biomechanics in the finger.

ANSWER 10: A. The classic tendon transfers to restore function for radial nerve injury are (1) PT to ECRB; (2) FCU, FCR, or FDS IV to EDC; and (3) PL to FDS to EPL. However, in this patient, the PT was likely avulsed or injured from the degloving, which also involved the adjacent radial nerve. In this setting, *a* is the only choice that avoids zone of injury and allows improved motion.

Chapter 20

ANSWER 1: C. The macrophage is the predominant cell within a healing wound at 48 to 72 hours.

ANSWER 2: A. In expanded skin, the total collagen content and total surface are increased, but tensile strength and elasticity are decreased. Likewise, the dermis is thinner, but the epidermis shows apparent increased thickness.

ANSWER 3: D.

ANSWER 4: A. The most likely mechanism by which NPWT exerts healing is through macro- and microdeformation of the wound.

ANSWER 5: D. The most widely accepted mechanism by which silicone improves wound healing is through increased hydration from occlusion.

ANSWER 6: C. A reasonable approach to extravasation/infiltration injuries consists of elevation, warmth, and occasionally, if a toxic substance is infiltrated, dilution of the offending drug assisted with hyaluronidase to limit toxic concentrations in the skin. Debridement may be necessary as the injury evolves and the area of skin necrosis declares itself. There is no evidence of compartment syndrome in this patient.

ANSWER 7: B. The only FDA-approved enzymatic debrider in the United States currently is collagenase (Santyl). It is approved as a debrider and should not be used for closure, but only when there is nonviable material such as slough in the wound. A major mechanism of action is by removing biofilm. Most film and hydrogel dressings work in part by encouraging autolytic debridement (the body's own enzymes and cells debride the wound), whereas an enzymatic debrider is a pharmacologic means of active debridement. Silver ions, in particular, and pH changes can inactivate an enzymatic ointment.

ANSWER 8: D. Chronic wounds usually have a variety of causes that contribute to their nonhealing status. Regardless of the type of wound (venous, diabetes-related, pressure sore, or arterial ulcer), most chronic wounds share the common causal factors of occurring in patients who are older, having the presence of a decrease in tissue perfusion (as a result of swelling, microvascular impairments, or vascular disease), and are all colonized with a critical level of bacteria in the form of biofilm. Successful management of these wounds requires attention to all of these parameters.

ANSWER 9: C. The patient has developed a hypertrophic scar, which is more common in patients of Asian descent and in areas of tension, such as the midportion of an abdominoplasty scar. These are best treated with conservative measures, including scar ointments and silicone gel sheeting (both of which likely work by increased hydration of the epidermis), massage, and steroid injections as first-line treatments. Excision followed by radiation treatment would likely be useful but better indicated for treatment of problematic keloids. It is not indicated for the treatment of this 6-month-old hypertrophic scar. Therapeutics targeting TGF-β in the form of antisense compounds are not approved nor available. Lasers have been shown to be quite useful for the treatment of problem scars and are rapidly becoming accepted therapies for many types of problematic scars. Pulsed-dye lasers, Nd:YAG lasers, and fractionated ablative and nonablative CO_2 lasers all have a place in treating hypertrophic and problematic scars.

ANSWER 10: C. The patient likely has an inflammatory ulcer, such as pyoderma gangrenosum, or a vasculitic ulcer. These most commonly present in patients with a systemic condition such as arthritis or inflammatory bowel disease. The back is unlikely to have ischemia that impairs healing, and most wounds here (even in patients on arthritis medications) should heal uneventfully. The progressive nature of the enlarging wound despite presumably good wound care is suggestive of either an inflammatory ulcer or a malignancy, and a diagnostic biopsy of the wound edges is essential to differentiating between these two possibilities to enable proper therapy. If an inflammatory ulcer is indicated, these usually respond dramatically to systemic steroids and proper wound care. A skin graft usually is unsuccessful in these wounds, nor is HBO. Steroids should only be used once the possibility of a malignancy has been excluded.

Chapter 21

ANSWER 1: B. Venomous rattlesnake bites are best treated primarily with antivenom (CroFab) early. Although the clinical presentation can often be similar to a compartment syndrome, compartment pressures are often normal on formal testing and if mildly elevated will often improve with the administration of antivenom.

ANSWER 2: D. The "fight bite" wound can easily lead to inoculation of the MPJ when the MPJ is flexed (as it would be when punching). The inoculation can then get trapped in the joint space as the extensor tendon slides back, resulting in a septic arthritis that is best treated with exploration and washout of the MPJ.

ANSWER 3: A. Fournier gangrene is a necrotizing fasciitis of the genitals and perineum. This life-threatening infection requires urgent surgical debridement to optimize outcomes.

ANSWER 4: D. Community-acquired methicillin-resistant *Staphylococcus aureus* (MRSA) infections are increasingly common, especially within the pediatric population. Of the options presented, sulfamethoxazole/trimethoprim (Bactrim) is the most appropriate oral antibiotic for pediatric MRSA infections.

ANSWER 5: E. Kanavel's cardinal signs for suppurative flexor tenosynovitis include all of the answers except for the fingers being held in an intrinsic plus position, which would include having the interphalangeal joints extended (and not flexed).

ANSWER 6: D. The patient described has clinical findings consistent with a necrotizing soft-tissue infection. The initial management of this group of conditions includes resuscitation, administration of broad-spectrum IV antibiotics, and extensive debridement of involved tissues.

ANSWER 7: B. The most appropriate next step is to update his tetanus status and observe for signs of envenomation.

ANSWER 8: D. The patient described has Hurley stage-III hidradenitis suppurativa. Nonsurgical management will not be effective. The patient requires excision of the affected axillary skin and subsequent reconstruction.

ANSWER 9: C. The patient described has a bite injury involving the MCP joint, with established infection. In this scenario, he should undergo immediate surgical drainage of the joint to prevent joint destruction and osteomyelitis. Administration of IV antibiotics, splinting, and elevation are important, but given alone would be insufficient.

ANSWER 10: B. The patient has signs and symptoms suggestive of flexor tenosynovitis.

Chapter 22

ANSWER 1: A. First-degree burns are not used in calculating TBSA for fluid resuscitation. Upper extremity surface area is 9% and anterior surface of lower extremity is 9%.

ANSWER 2: C. Parkland formula calls for Ringer's lactate as the initial resuscitation fluid of choice.

ANSWER 3: D. The initial treatment for most chemical burns is copious irrigation with water. The exception to that rule is in the initial treatment of elemental metal burns, for which water is contraindicated. Calcium gluconate gel is used after water irrigation of hydrofluoric acid.

ANSWER 4: C. Mafenide acetate penetrates eschar and cartilage and is the topical of choice for the treatment or prevention of *Pseudomonas* and *Staphylococcus,* the most common organisms found in chondritis.

ANSWER 5: B. Rewarming in 40-degree water has been shown to be the best way to initially treat frostbite.

ANSWER 6: C. Findings suggest compartment syndrome, which should be treated with fasciotomies.

ANSWER 7: D. Even small burns involving critical areas (hands, feet, face, and genitalia) are considered major burns according to the ABA.

ANSWER 8: D. SIRs are generally triggered after a burn involving >30% TBSA.

ANSWER 9: B. The distinction between high and low voltage is generally considered to be above 1000 V (although some make that distinction at 500 V).

ANSWER 10: A. Small children have limited glycogen stores.

Chapter 23

ANSWER 1: C. In rare circumstances, a nevus sebaceous may also transform into sebaceous carcinoma.

ANSWER 2: B. Although this is somewhat controversial, most agree that for atypical pigmented nevi, 2- to 5-mm margins of excision are recommended.

ANSWER 3: A. Madelung's disease is a rare condition characterized by the development of symmetric lipomas. The disease seems to be correlated with alcohol abuse, and symptoms are usually localized to the trunk and upper limbs.

ANSWER 4: D. Dermatofibromas are benign growths, typically on the extremities. If they are asymptomatic, they can be observed or removed, depending on preference.

ANSWER 5: A. Pilomatrixoma is a relatively common childhood dermal or subdermal lesion. It typically presents as a firm nodule that may or may not exhibit skin discoloration. Treatment is wide local excision, and with clean margins, the lesions do not usually recur.

ANSWER 6: A. Chondrodermatitis is a tender red nodule found on the helical rim. Choices *b* and *c* are not credible. An inflamed or infarcting hemangioma might be confused, but should be purplish, deeper in the skin, and, even inflamed, compressible.

ANSWER 7: B. The treatment of chondrodermatitis, which also yields a pathology specimen, is conservative wedge excision of both skin and cartilage.

ANSWER 8: D. A cutaneous neurofibroma, a benign Schwann cell tumor, can occur in any part of the body. A single lesion is not indicative of von Recklinghausen's nor is a cafe au lait spot alone.

ANSWER 9: A. A Mongolian spot is a childhood skin discoloration usually located in the lumbosacral skin. The spots are not darkly colored, usually disappear in later childhood, and seldom require formal excision.

ANSWER 10: C. Lipomata are commonly multiple, can be bilateral and symmetrical, and have histologically different subgroups that are not clinically important. They are not caused by trauma.

ANSWER 11: D. Epidermoid cysts contain the skin protein keratin, which has an odor. Rapid growth may indicate inflammation, and inflammation may necessitate I&D, with excision deferred. Most have the same histology.

Chapter 24

ANSWER 1: D. Clear cell acanthoma is a common, benign tumor of the skin, occurring primarily on the lower extremities. It appears as a shiny, red papule or plaque measuring up to 2 cm in diameter. The surface is frequently crusted. Histologically, the lesion consists of a proliferation of pale, glycogenated keratinocytes within the epidermis. The differential diagnosis of clear cell acanthoma includes SCC, nodular malignant melanoma, and pyogenic granuloma. Leukoplakia, Hutchinson's freckle (also known as lentigo maligna or melanoma in situ), and keratoacanthoma are all premalignant lesions.

ANSWER 2: C. UVA, which penetrates the skin more deeply than UVB, has long been known to play a major part in skin aging and wrinkling (photoaging); it damages keratinocytes in the basal layer of the epidermis, contributing to squamous call and basal cell carcinoma. UVB radiation damages DNA and its repair system and alters the immune system, resulting in progressive genetic alterations, contributing to basal cell carcinoma. Even small exposures to gamma radiation are well known to cause a variety of cancer such as lymphoma, multiple myeloma, breast cancer, and colon cancer, although not skin cancer.

ANSWER 3: C. Curettage and electrodessication is limited to small (<1 cm), well-defined, and well-differentiated tumors. Mohs micrographic surgery is a specialized technique used to achieve the narrowest margins necessary to avoid tumor recurrence, while maximally preserving cosmesis (not a concern in the scalp). In a prospective case series of 141 SCCs, a 4-mm margin was adequate to encompass all subclinical microscopic tumor extension in more than 95% of well-differentiated tumors up to 19 mm in diameter. Wider margins of 6 to 10 mm were needed for larger or less-differentiated tumors or tumors in high-risk locations (e.g., scalp, ears, eyelids, nose, and lips). Although the diameter of this lesion is less than 19 mm, it is located on the scalp, which is a high-risk location.

ANSWER 4: B. The Clark classification is as follows:
Level I—Lesions involving only the epidermis (in situ melanoma); not an invasive lesion.
Level II—Invasion of the papillary dermis; does not reach the papillary-reticular dermal interface
Level III—Invasion fills and expands the papillary dermis but does not penetrate the reticular dermis.
Level IV—Invasion into the reticular dermis but not into the subcutaneous tissue
Level V—Invasion through the reticular dermis into the subcutaneous tissue

ANSWER 5: B. A randomized trial compared narrow margins (1 cm) with wide margins (≥3 cm) in patients with melanomas no thicker than 2 mm; no difference was observed between the two groups in the development of metastatic disease, disease-free survival (DFS), or overall survival (OS). Evidence suggests that lesions no thicker than 2 mm may be treated conservatively with radial excision margins of 1 cm. Indications for SLNB are any lesion >.76 mm depth, without any palpable nodes; therefore, this patient may benefit from SLNB.

ANSWER 6: B. Melanomas are divided into four common types, based on growth patterns. Superficial spreading melanoma is the most common type (50% to 80%) and is generally a flat-appearing lesion with variations in color and possible nodular components. It can develop in an existing lesion or de novo. These are typically slow growing and grow horizontally before undergoing a vertical growth phase. Nodular melanoma, comprising ~20% to 30% of all melanomas, are more aggressive, with an earlier vertical growth phase and a higher incidence of ulceration and metastases. Acrolentiginous melanomas are significantly less common lesions that are found on the distal extremities, such as the palms and soles, and subungually. They occur in all ethnicities but are the more common type of melanoma in blacks and other darker-complected individuals. They grow rapidly with an early vertical growth phase. Because of their aggression and location, they are often diagnosed in advanced stages. Lentigo maligna melanomas are an unusual variant. They are classically described as melanoma in situ, but on resection, they frequently have areas of invasive disease. Lentigo maligna melanomas commonly occur on the face and hands with the appearance of a brownish-red patch. They can be quite large and have indistinct margins, which may lead to incomplete resection.

ANSWER 7: C. SLNB is a method of examining regional lymph nodes in the absence of other evidence of metastatic disease. Current recommendations for examination and staging of patients with melanoma include SLNB for patients with melanoma exceeding 0.76 to 1 mm in thickness and with no other evidence of metastatic disease. Selected patients with melanomas measuring <1 mm thick can be considered for SLNB if the primary melanoma is ulcerated, a Clark level IV, or shows extensive regression. Patients with palpable lymphadenopathy require additional screening for metastatic disease, lymph node biopsy, and possible completion lymphadenectomy.

ANSWER 8: A. Immunosuppression profoundly increases the odds of developing Merkel cell carcinoma. It is seen 30 times more frequently in patients with chronic lymphocytic leukemia, and solid organ transplant recipients have a 10-fold-increased risk compared with the general population. Patients with smaller tumors (<2 cm) that have not yet metastasized have an expected 5-year survival rate of more than 80%. Once a lesion has metastasized regionally, the rate drops to ~50%. Merkel cell carcinomas invade locally, typically metastasize early to regional lymph nodes, and also spread aggressively through the blood vessels. Adjuvant radiotherapy has been shown to be effective in reducing rates of recurrence and in increasing the survival of patients.

ANSWER 9: D. SCCs resulting from Marjolin's ulcer or xeroderma pigmentosum have a much greater tendency to metastasize than do tumors resulting from sun-induced skin changes. SCCs of the ears, nostrils, scalp, and extremities are more prone to metastasize than those of the trunk. Of the two general types of SCC, the verrucous and exophytic type is a slow-growing variety that may be locally invasive but less likely to metastasize. The second general type is more nodular and indurated and associated with rapid growth and early ulceration.

ANSWER 10: B. Mohs surgery is least useful with tumors with discontiguous growth patterns because the technique involves successive excision of tissue specimens until the margins are judged to be free of tumor. The most suitable tumors are those that are seen easily microscopically, tend to grow in a continuous pattern, are located in anatomically sensitive areas, and have ill-defined margins clinically. Mohs surgery has use in the treatment of dermatofibrosarcoma protuberans, where the tumor extends far beyond the clinical margins into the local surrounding soft tissue, and in extramammary Paget's disease, where margin-controlled surgical excision of the involved epidermis is the most effective treatment.

Chapter 25

ANSWER 1: C. The buccinator muscle is often included with the facial artery myomucosal (FAMM) flap to enhance vascularity.

ANSWER 2: B. In instances where the IMA has been harvested, a rectus abdominis flap can be based off of the 8th intercostal artery, although it provides less reliable vascularity.

ANSWER 3: A. The reverse lateral arm flap is often used for coverage of defects of the antecubital fossa and olecranon. Its dominant pedicle is off of the radial recurrent artery.

ANSWER 4: B. Harvest of the rectus femoris muscle will often result in 10 to 15 degrees of extensor lag.

ANSWER 5: D. Leech therapy can place patients at risk for infectious complications related to inoculation with *Aeromonas hydrophila*. To reduce this risk, patients undergoing leech therapy should receive prophylactic antibiotics from the fluoroquinolone and/or aminoglycoside families.

ANSWER 6: D. The ALT is supplied by perforators arising from the descending branch of the lateral femoral artery.

ANSWER 7: C. The landmark for finding the SGA is the junction of the middle and medial thirds of the piriformis, and the artery is usually above or cephalad to the piriformis at this point.

ANSWER 8: B. The superficial radial nerve can be and not infrequently is damaged if great care is not taken with harvest of the radial forearm flap.

ANSWER 9: D. The sartorius is a type 4 because it is supplied by segmental vessels.

ANSWER 10: A. The latissimus dorsi does not border the quadrangular space; it lies just distal to it.

Chapter 26

ANSWER 1: B. The extracanthal portion of the orbicularis (lateral to the medial canthus) is responsible for forceful eyelid closure, squeezing, and strong animated movements of the eyelid. The intracanthal portion is responsible for blinking, tone of the eyelid, and the lacrimal pumping mechanism. The intracanthal portion is innervated by the buccal branch of the facial nerve. This explains why subciliary incisions, which violate the zygomatic branches of the facial nerve, do not disrupt normal, resting lid tone.

ANSWER 2: B. The arcuate expansion of Lockwood's ligament is the anatomic structure that separates the central and lateral lower lid retroseptal fat pads. Its release from the orbital rim facilitates retroseptal fat repositioning across the inferior orbital rim in patients with a distinct palpebral-malar groove, otherwise known as a defined lid-cheek junction.

ANSWER 3: D. Prominent eyes measure 18 mm or greater with a Hertel exophthalmometer. The device rests upon the lateral orbital rim, and this reference point is the bony landmark from which the measurement to the corneal surface is made. Prominent eyes place lower eyelids at risk for malposition following lower eyelid surgery.

ANSWER 4: A. If the examiner cannot correct lower lid malposition with a single finger directed upward at the lateral canthus, it is unlikely that a lateral canthal tendon tightening procedure alone will be effective in correcting the deformity. Correction achieved with upward pressure of a second figure at the midpoint of the lower lid, in the absence of skin shortage, generally indicates that a middle lamellar graft, in conjunction with lateral canthal tightening, will be effective in restoring the lower lid to its native resting position at the lower corneoscleral limbus.

ANSWER 5: D. The most commonly used flap for reconstructing small-to-moderate lid defects (<50% width) is the Tenzel rotation-advancement flap. It can be used to reconstruct the anterior lamella. Conjunctiva, advanced from the fornix, can be used to line the posterior aspect of the flap. Occasionally, a periosteal flap, or alternative graft material, may be necessary for middle lamellar reinforcement.

ANSWER 6: C. In cases of impaired eyelid closure or failure of eye pressure patching, conjunctivotomy with release of fluid should be performed. This procedure can be easily performed in the office with administration of 2.5% phenylephrine and topical tetracaine drops.

ANSWER 7: C. In cases of severe cicatricial entropion, grafts to the posterior lamella can increase its height and reconstruct a smooth conjunctival surface against the globe.

ANSWER 8: B. Superficial injection of Botox into the lateral aspect of the eyelid chemodenervates the pretarsal orbicularis. As a result, the lid margin will elevate temporarily, simulating the effect of a ptosis repair.

ANSWER 9: A. The arcus marginalis formally separates the lower eyelid from the cheek. It sends fascial extensions to the skin, known as the orbitomalar ligament, that must be divided to access the cheek for a midface lift or resuspending orbital fat.

ANSWER 10: D. Corneal abrasions are a common injury when patients are under anesthesia, especially if they are undergoing a blepharoplasty. Common preventive tactics include using scleral shields and ocular lubricants.

Chapter 27

ANSWER 1: C. A transcolumellar incision divides the columellar artery during the open approach.

ANSWER 2: D. A spreader graft placed between the dorsal septum and upper lateral cartilage can improve airflow through the internal valve and the appearance of dorsal esthetic lines.

ANSWER 3: D. Subdermal defatting of the nasal tip in combination with the open approach can compromise blood supply to the nasal tip.

ANSWER 4: D.

ANSWER 5: C. At the level of the orbital rim, the supratrochlear artery is located superficial to the periosteum.

ANSWER 6: C. Spreader grafts would correct airway obstruction due to the internal valve. Septoplasty and turbinate reduction can be useful to address other causes of airway obstruction. Tip grafts would be more likely used for cosmetic refinement of the nasal tip rather than to address airway obstruction.

ANSWER 7: D. Resection of the medial crura will decrease tip projection. The other answers all contribute to increasing tip projection.

ANSWER 8: C. Saddle nose deformity can be caused by overresection of the nasal dorsum as well as excessive resection of the nasal septum, leading to loss of dorsal structural support.

ANSWER 9: C. A forehead flap would cover the defect, but would require multiple stages and incur a greater likelihood of complications in an elderly woman with a relatively small defect size. Local flaps are therefore preferable.

ANSWER 10: C. The ideal nasolabial angle in a female patient is approximately 100 to 110 degrees. In men, the nasolabial angle is closer to 90 degrees.

Chapter 28

ANSWER 1: B. The great auricular nerve, a branch of C2 and C3, travels on the superficial surface of the sternocleidomastoid muscle and enters the lower, posterior surface of the ear. Its branches supply the lobule as well as the helix, antihelix, and most of the cranial surface of the ear.

ANSWER 2: D. Hematomas are one of the most common complications after rhytidectomy, particularly in males. The treatment of a hematoma is immediate evacuation. Blood pressure control is the most important preventive measure; however, vomiting, coughing, anxiety, and pain should be controlled. Drains do not prevent hematomas but can help with postoperative swelling/bruising.

ANSWER 3: D. The cervical branch innervates the platysma, which plays a role in depression of the oral commissure in patients with full denture smile. The other possibility of a marginal mandibular branch injury is unlikely because the patient is able to evert and purse the lower lip.

ANSWER 4: C. A male patient is at increased risk for a hematoma, especially if he has a history of hypertension. The clinical presentation of unrelenting, asymmetric ear and facial pain is a hematoma until proven otherwise.

ANSWER 5: D. A deep plane facelift denotes dissection deep to the SMAS layer. The other techniques do not involve any dissection beneath the SMAS layer.

ANSWER 6: B. The incidence in females ranges from 2% to 4% in most series in the literature.

ANSWER 7: C. The incidence in males is more than twice that in females and is thought to be ~8%.

ANSWER 8: B.

ANSWER 9: C. The marginal mandibular nerve typically lies just superficial to the submandibular gland capsule, deep to the platysma, and is therefore at greatest risk for injury with attempted resection of the gland.

ANSWER 10: A. The SMAS is continuous with the temporoparietal fascia superiorly and the platysma inferiorly. The parotid fascia and masseteric fascia are both deep to the SMAS and help protect the underlying facial nerve.

Chapter 29

ANSWER 1: B. The lateral femoral cutaneous nerve is at risk for injury during abdominoplasty. The nerve emerges superficially ~2 cm medial to the anterior superior iliac spine (ASIS), and dissection in this area should be superficial to protect the nerve and reduce the risk of developing neuralgia paresthetica, a syndrome characterized by numbness, tingling, and burning pain.

ANSWER 2: B. The most likely finding is a neuroma of the medial antebrachial cutaneous nerve of the arm. This nerve extends down the ulnar side of the arm, medial to the brachial artery, pierces the deep fascia with the basilic vein (about the middle of the arm), and divides into a volar and an ulnar branch. Injury is uncommon but may occur if dissection down to the basilic vein occurs distally.

ANSWER 3: B. The best option for treating vertical and horizontal excess of the abdomen is the abdominoplasty with a fleur-de-lis or vertical component. Failure to excise skin in the vertical dimension will leave a significant amount of epigastric laxity and this will appear worse with abdominal plication.

ANSWER 4: C. The most likely cause of an upper abdominal bulge 8 weeks out from surgery is failure to adequately plicate the tissues above the level of the umbilicus. Failure to plicate all the way to the xiphoid can also produce a prominent bulge postoperatively.

ANSWER 5: D. The tumescent technique has the lowest amount of blood loss in the aspirate (1%).

ANSWER 6: C. The landmarks most commonly used for repositioning the umbilicus is the intersection of a line connecting the highest point of the iliac crest with the midline.

ANSWER 7: A. During closure of a medial thigh lift, the medial thigh flap is advanced upward, and the deep dermis is sutured to the Colles' fascia. This helps to support and pull the skin flap upward and relieves tension on the skin closure. If this is not performed, distortion of the vulva can result.

ANSWER 8: E. The most common complication directly related to ultrasound-assisted liposuction is the formation of a seroma, defined as a fluid collection at the operative site of >50 mL and/or requiring repeated aspiration for control. This complication is observed in ~10% of patients following large-volume ultrasound-assisted liposuction of the abdomen.

ANSWER 9: D. During brachioplasty, the risk for contour deformities and unfavorable scarring will be reduced if the skin flaps are permanently sutured to the axillary fascia.

ANSWER 10: A. Of all body contouring procedures, abdominoplasty is most strongly associated with deep venous thrombosis and pulmonary embolism. In any patient presenting with systemic systems after abdominoplasty, pulmonary embolism should be suspected and ruled out.

Chapter 30

ANSWER 1: D. At least 1 year should pass after stopping Accutane in order to allow adnexal healing and proper reepithelialization.

ANSWER 2: C. Croton oil is a component of the Baker-Gordon phenol peel.

ANSWER 3: D. Skin coagulation and collagen synthesis are desired effects of chemical peels. Hypopigmentation is problematic but cardiotoxicity is the most serious side effect of phenol peels.

ANSWER 4: A. Croton oil concentration has been found to be a more powerful determinant of depth of penetration of phenol than other factors.

ANSWER 5: A. The Nd:YAG laser targets red, orange, and brown pigments.

ANSWER 6: D. Water is the target chromophore for ablative CO_2 lasers.

ANSWER 7: A. The FDA currently recognizes injectable silicone only for ophthalmic use.

ANSWER 8: B. The phases of hair growth are anagen (active growth), catagen (active hair loss), and telogen (quiescence).

ANSWER 9: C. Hair transplantation is followed by one month of hair growth, then hair loss, then normal growth after three months.

ANSWER 10: B. Botox works through preventing the release of acetylcholine at the neuromuscular junction leading to flaccid paralysis and muscle atrophy.

Index